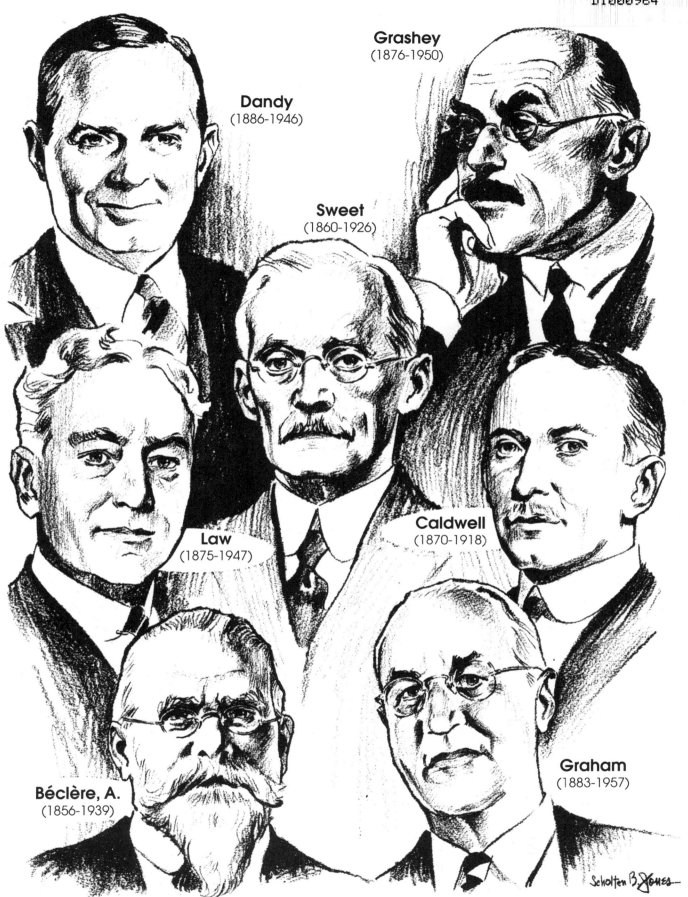

Dandy
(1886-1946)

Grashey
(1876-1950)

Sweet
(1860-1926)

Law
(1875-1947)

Caldwell
(1870-1918)

Béclère, A.
(1856-1939)

Graham
(1883-1957)

Evolve®

YOU'VE JUST PURCHASED
MORE THAN
A TEXTBOOK!

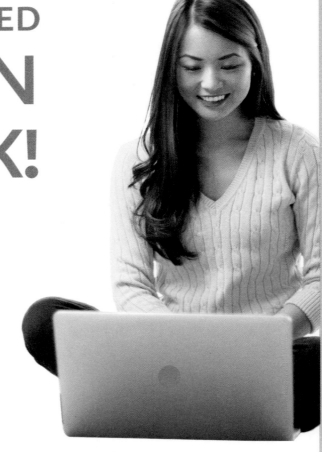

Evolve Student Resources for *Long/Rollins/Smith:*
Merrill's Atlas of Radiographic Positioning & Procedures,
fourteenth edition, **include the following:**

- Image Collection

Activate the complete learning experience that comes with each
textbook purchase by registering at

http://evolve.elsevier.com/MerrillsAtlas/

REGISTER TODAY!

2018v1.0

MERRILL'S ATLAS OF

RADIOGRAPHIC POSITIONING & PROCEDURES

FOURTEENTH EDITION | VOLUME ONE

MERRILL'S ATLAS OF
RADIOGRAPHIC POSITIONING & PROCEDURES

Bruce W. Long, MS, RT(R)(CV), FASRT, FAEIRS
Director and Associate Professor
Radiologic Imaging and Sciences Programs
Indiana University School of Medicine
Indianapolis, Indiana

Jeannean Hall Rollins, MRC, BSRT(R)(CV)
Associate Professor
Medical Imaging and Radiation Sciences Department
Arkansas State University
Jonesboro, Arkansas

Barbara J. Smith, MS, RT(R)(QM), FASRT, FAEIRS
Instructor, Radiologic Technology
Medical Imaging Department
Portland Community College
Portland, Oregon

ELSEVIER

ELSEVIER

3251 Riverport Lane
St. Louis, Missouri 63043

MERRILL'S ATLAS OF RADIOGRAPHIC POSITIONING
AND PROCEDURES, FOURTEENTH EDITION

ISBN: 978-0-323-56768-8 (vol 1)
ISBN: 978-0-323-56767-1 (vol 2)
ISBN: 978-0-323-56766-4 (vol 3)
ISBN: 978-0-323-56667-4 (set)

Notices

Practitioners and researchers must always rely on their own experience and knowledge in evaluating and using any information, methods, compounds or experiments described herein. Because of rapid advances in the medical sciences, in particular, independent verification of diagnoses and drug dosages should be made. To the fullest extent of the law, no responsibility is assumed by Elsevier, authors, editors or contributors for any injury and/or damage to persons or property as a matter of products liability, negligence or otherwise, or from any use or operation of any methods, products, instructions, or ideas contained in the material herein.

Previous editions copyrighted 2016, 2012, 2007, 2003, 1999, 1995, 1991, 1986, 1982, 1975, 1967, 1959, and 1949.

International Standard Book Number: 978-0-323-56667-4

Executive Content Strategist: Sonya Seigafuse
Director, Content Development: Laurie Gower
Content Development Specialist: Betsy McCormac
Publishing Services Manager: Julie Eddy
Book Production Specialist: Clay S. Broeker
Design Direction: Brian Salisbury

Printed in the United States of America

Last digit is the print number: 9 8 7 6 5 4 3

Working together
to grow libraries in
developing countries

www.elsevier.com • www.bookaid.org

PREVIOUS AUTHORS

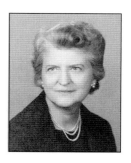

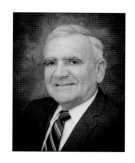

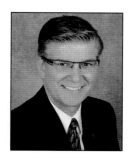

Vinita Merrill
1905-1977

Vinita Merrill was born in Oklahoma in 1905 and died in New York City in 1977. Vinita began compilation of *Merrill's* in 1936, while she worked as Technical Director and Chief Technologist in the Department of Radiology and Instructor in the School of Radiography at the New York Hospital. In 1949, while employed as Director of the Educational Department of Picker X-Ray Corporation, she wrote the first edition of the *Atlas of Roentgenographic Positions*. She completed three more editions from 1959 to 1975. Seventy-four years later, Vinita's work lives on in the fourteenth edition of *Merrill's Atlas of Radiographic Positioning & Procedures*.

Philip W. Ballinger, PhD, RT(R), FASRT, FAEIRS, became the author of *Merrill's Atlas* in its fifth edition, which published in 1982. He served as author through the tenth edition, helping to launch successful careers for thousands of students who have learned radiographic positioning from *Merrill's*. Phil currently serves as Professor Emeritus in Radiologic Sciences and Therapy, Division of the School of Health and Rehabilitation Sciences, at The Ohio State University. In 1995, he retired after a 25-year career as Radiography Program Director and, after ably guiding *Merrill's Atlas* through six editions, he retired as *Merrill's* author. Phil continues to be involved in professional activities such as speaking engagements at state, national, and international meetings.

Eugene D. Frank, MA, RT(R), FASRT, FAEIRS, began working with Phil Ballinger on the eighth edition of *Merrill's Atlas* in 1995. He became the coauthor in its ninth, 50th-anniversary edition, published in 1999. He served as lead author for the eleventh and twelfth editions and mentored three coauthors. Gene retired from the Mayo Clinic/Foundation in Rochester, Minnesota in 2001 after 31 years of employment. He was Associate Professor of Radiology in the College of Medicine and Director of the Radiography Program. He also served as Director of the Radiography Program at Riverland Community College, Austin, Minnesota, for 6 years before fully retiring in 2007. He is a Fellow of the ASRT and AEIRS. In addition to *Merrill's*, he is the coauthor of two radiography textbooks, *Quality Control in Diagnostic Imaging* and *Radiography Essentials for Limited Practice*. He now works in hospice through Christian Hospice Care and helps design and equip x-ray departments in underdeveloped countries.

THE MERRILL'S TEAM

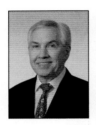 **Bruce W. Long, MS, RT(R)(CV), FASRT, FAEIRS,** is Director and Associate Professor of the Indiana University Radiologic and Imaging Sciences Programs, where he has taught for 33 years. A Life Member of the Indiana Society of Radiologic Technologists, he frequently presents at state and national professional meetings. His publication activities include 28 articles in national professional journals and two books, *Orthopaedic Radiography* and *Radiography Essentials for Limited Practice,* in addition to being coauthor of the *Atlas.* The fourteenth edition is Bruce's fourth on the Merrill's team and second as lead author.

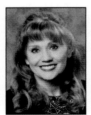 **Jeannean Hall Rollins, MRC, BSRT(R) (CV),** is an Associate Professor in the Medical Imaging and Radiation Sciences department at Arkansas State University, where she has taught for 27 years. She presents regularly at national meetings. Her publication activities include articles, book reviews, and chapter contributions. Jeannean's first contribution to *Merrill's Atlas* was on the tenth edition as coauthor of the trauma radiography chapter. The fourteenth edition is Jeannean's fourth on the Merrill's team and second as a coauthor. Her previous role was writing the workbook, *Mosby's Radiography Online,* and the Instructor Resources that accompany *Merrill's Atlas.*

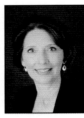 **Barbara J. Smith, MS, RT(R)(QM), FASRT, FAEIRS,** is an instructor in the Radiologic Technology program at Portland Community College, where she has taught for 34 years. The Oregon Society of Radiologic Technologists inducted her as a Life Member in 2003. She presents at state, regional, national, and international meetings, is a trustee with the American Registry of Radiologic Technologists (ARRT), and is involved in professional activities at these levels. Her publication activities include articles, book reviews, and chapter contributions. As coauthor, her primary role on the Merrill's team is working with the contributing authors and editing Volume 3. The fourteenth edition is Barb's fourth on the Merrill's team.

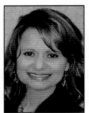 **Tammy Curtis, PhD, RT(R)(CT)(CHES),** is an associate professor at Northwestern State University, where she has taught for 18 years. She presents at the state, regional, and national levels and is involved in professional activities at the state and national levels. Her publication activities include articles, book reviews, and book contributions. Previously, Tammy served on the advisory board and submitted several projects to the *Atlas.* In particular, for the twelfth edition, Tammy submitted an updated photo of the original author, Vinita Merrill, which she discovered after a 3-year search of historical records. Her primary role on the Merrill's team is to update the workbook and work with the coauthors of the textbook to review content for all three volumes. The fourteenth edition is Tammy's second on the Merrill's team.

ADVISORY BOARD

This edition of *Merrill's Atlas* benefits from the expertise of a special advisory board. The following board members have provided professional input and advice and have helped the authors make decisions about *Atlas* content throughout the preparation of the fourteenth edition:

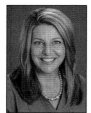

Kimberly Cross, MSRS, RT(R)(CT)
Clinical Coordinator and Assistant Program
    Director
Emory University Medical Imaging Program
Emory Department of Radiology and Imaging
    Sciences
Atlanta, Georgia

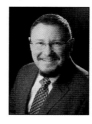

James G. Murrell, MSRS, RT(R)(M)(QM) (CT), CRT(R)(F), FAEIRS
Dean of Imaging Sciences and Radiologic
    Technology Program Director
Brightwood College
Los Angeles, California

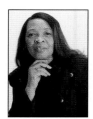

Parsha Y. Hobson, MPA, RT(R)
Professor, Program Director, and Chairperson
Radiography, Public Health, Health Sciences,
    and Health Information
Passaic County Community College
Paterson, New Jersey

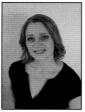

Christine Preachuk, RT(R), CAE
Clinical Educator, Health Sciences Centre,
    Winnipeg Regional Health Authority
Clinical Faculty Member, Medical Radiologic
    Technology Program, Red River College
Winnipeg, Manitoba, Canada

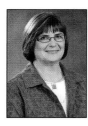

Robin J. Jones, MS, RT(R)
Associate Professor and Clinical Coordinator
Radiologic Sciences Program
Indiana University Northwest
Gary, Indiana

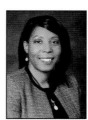

Marilyn J. Lewis Thompson, MBA, RT(R)(M)
Clinical Coordinator
Saint Luke's School of Radiologic
    Technology at Saint Luke's Hospital of
    Kansas City
Saint Luke's College of Health Sciences
Kansas City, Missouri

CHAPTER CONTENT EXPERTS

Valerie F. Andolina, RT(R)(M)
Mammography Technologist
Radiology
Lee Health
Fort Myers, Florida

Leila Bussman-Yeakel, MEd, RT(R)(T)
Program Director and Assistant Professor
Radiation Therapy Program
Mayo Clinic School of Health Sciences
Rochester, Minnesota

Derek Carver, MEd, RT(R)(MR)
Manager of Education and Training
Department of Radiology
Boston Children's Hospital
Boston, Massachusetts

Rex T. Christensen, MHA, RT(R)(MR)(CT), CIIP, MRSO
Associate Professor and MRI Program
Director
School of Radiologic Sciences
Weber State University
Ogden, Utah

Cheryl DuBose, EdD, RT(R)(MR)(CT)(QM), MRSO
Department Chair
Medical Imaging and Radiation Sciences
Arkansas State University
Jonesboro, Arkansas

Angela Franceschi, MEd, CCLS
Certified Child Life Specialist
Radiology
Boston Children's Hospital
Boston, Massachusetts

Steven G. Hayes Jr., MSRS, RT(R)
Radiology Supervisor
IU Health
Methodist Hospital
Indianapolis, Indiana

Tracy Iversen, RT(R)(M)(QM)
Rapid City, South Dakota

Nancy M. Johnson, MEd, RT(R)(CV)(CT)(QM), FASRT
Dean, Professional and
    Technical Education
Academic Affairs
GateWay Community College
Phoenix, Arizona

Raymond J. Johnson, BS, CNMT, PET
Certified Nuclear Medicine Technologist/
    Certified PET Technologist
Radiology/Nuclear Medicine
John Peter Smith Health Network
Fort Worth, Texas

Lois J. Layne, MSHA, RT(R)(CV)
Privacy Specialist
Centralized Privacy
Covenant Health
Knoxville, Tennessee

Cheryl Morgan-Duncan, MAS, RT(R)(M)
Instructor
Radiography Program
Passaic County Community College
Staff Mammographer
Mammography
St Joseph's Regional Medical Center
Paterson, New Jersey

Susanna L. Ovel, RT, RDMS, RVT
Senior Sonographer
Medical Imaging
Sutter Medical Foundation
Sacramento, California

Paula Pate-Schloder, MS, RT(R)(CV)(CT)(VI), FAEIRS
Department Chair
Medical Imaging
Misericordia University
Dallas, Pennsylvania

Lynette Petrie, MEd, RT(R)(CV)
Vascular and Interventional Radiologic
    Technologist
New Hanover Regional Medical Center
Wilmington, North Carolina

Bartram J. Pierce, BS, RT(R)(MR), MRSO
MRI Safety Officer/MR Technologist II
Radiology—MRI
The Corvallis Clinic, PC
Corvallis, Oregon
Adjunct Professor
Medical Imaging
Portland Community College
Portland, Oregon

Jessica L. Saunders, RT(R)(M)
Senior Technologist
Mammography
Elizabeth Wende Breast Care
Rochester, New York

Raymond Thies, BS, RT(R)
Radiologic Technologist II
Radiology
Boston Children's Hospital
Boston, Massachusetts

Sharon R. Wartenbee, RTR, BD, CBDT, FASRT
Senior DXA Technologist
Avera Medical Group
McGreevy Clinic
Sioux Falls, South Dakota

Gayle K. Wright, BS, RTR, CT, MR
Instructor, Radiography
Instructor, Program Coordinator—CT
    and MRI
Medical Imaging
Portland Community College
Portland, Oregon

PREFACE

Welcome to the fourteenth edition of *Merrill's Atlas of Radiographic Positioning & Procedures*. This edition continues the tradition of excellence begun in 1949, when Vinita Merrill wrote the first edition of what has become a classic text. Over the past 70 years, *Merrill's Atlas* has provided a strong foundation in anatomy and positioning for thousands of students around the world who have gone on to successful careers as imaging technologists. *Merrill's Atlas* is also a mainstay for everyday reference in imaging departments all over the world. As the coauthors of the fourteenth edition, we are honored to follow in Vinita Merrill's footsteps.

Learning and Perfecting Positioning Skills

Merrill's Atlas has an established tradition of helping students learn and perfect their positioning skills. After covering preliminary steps in radiography, radiation protection, and terminology in the introductory chapters, the first two volumes of the *Atlas* teach anatomy and positioning in separate chapters for each bone group or organ system. The student learns to position the patient properly so that the resulting radiograph provides the information the physician needs to correctly diagnose the patient's problem. The *Atlas* presents this information for commonly requested projections as well as for those less commonly requested, making it the only reference of its kind in the world.

The third volume provides basic information about a variety of special imaging modalities, such as mobile and surgical imaging, pediatrics, geriatrics, computed tomography (CT), vascular radiology, magnetic resonance imaging (MRI), sonography, nuclear medicine technology, bone densitometry, and radiation therapy.

Merrill's Atlas is not only a comprehensive resource to help students learn but also an indispensable reference as they move into the clinical environment and ultimately into practice as imaging professionals.

New to This Edition

Since the first edition of *Merrill's Atlas* in 1949, many changes have occurred. This new edition incorporates many significant changes designed not only to reflect the technologic progress and advancements in the profession but also to meet the needs of today's radiography students. The major changes in this edition are highlighted as follows.

ORGANIZATION

The fourteenth edition of the *Atlas* has been completely reorganized to emphasize all procedures listed in the Content Specifications for the ARRT Radiography Examination and in the ASRT Radiography Curriculum and to better reflect the order in which the majority of educators teach radiographic positioning and procedures. Most notably, the thoracic viscera and abdomen chapters are now the first two positioning and procedures chapters. Outdated chapters were removed, while still relevant materials were moved to appropriate chapters and updated to current practice. Selected chapter titles and anatomic terms have been updated to ensure consistency with the ARRT Content Specifications and the ASRT Curriculum Guide.

NEW PATIENT PHOTOGRAPHY

All patient positioning photographs have been replaced in Chapter 7. Additional new patient positioning photographs have been strategically added to better reflect current practice. The new photographs show positioning detail to a greater extent and in some cases from a more realistic perspective. In addition, the equipment in these photos is more modern, and computed radiography plates and occasionally direct digital detectors are used. The use of electronic central ray angle indicators enables a better understanding of where the central ray should enter the patient.

NEW IMAGES

Updated digital images were added to selected chapters, including Chapters 11, 12, 15, and 17. Many MRI images in the sectional anatomy chapter (24) were replaced by images with improved contrast.

IMAGE RECEPTORS AND COLLIMATION

Descriptions and sizes of image receptors on each projection page have been updated to include only those used in current practice. Greater emphasis has been placed on collimation size and field light coverage. This is increasingly important as many imaging departments use only a single, large IR size. A constant reminder has been added to properly place a radiographic marker in the exposure field.

REVISED IMAGE EVALUATION CRITERIA

All image evaluation criteria have been revised and reorganized to improve the student's ability to learn what constitutes a quality image. In addition, the criteria are presented in a way that improves the ability to correct positioning errors.

SIGNIFICANT VOLUME 1 CHAPTER UPDATES

Radiographic compensating filter material has been moved to Chapter 1 to place it with the rest of the general concepts material. Appropriate soft tissue neck material from the deleted anterior part of the neck chapter was moved to the thoracic viscera chapter (3) and updated to reflect current practice. Appropriate long bone measurement material from the deleted long bone measurement chapter was moved to the lower extremity chapter (7) and updated to reflect current practice. Scoliosis radiography material was updated in the vertebral column chapter (9) to reflect current practice.

SIGNIFICANT VOLUME 2 CHAPTER UPDATES

New projections have been added to the trauma chapter (12) to ensure complete coverage of procedures tested by the ARRT. In chapter 15, the modified barium swallow (swallowing dysfunction study) and other contrast media procedures of the GI tract have been updated to reflect current practice. Outdated procedures have been removed from the urinary system and venipuncture chapter (16), while sonography images of urinary anatomy have been added, as has the latest information on the relationships between radiographic contrast media administration and BUN, creatinine, and GFR. The chapter on the reproductive system (17) has been updated to include sonography of the male reproductive system.

SIGNIFICANT VOLUME 3 CHAPTER UPDATES

The vascular, cardiac, and interventional radiography chapter (27) has been significantly updated, especially with regard to ancillary equipment and interventional procedures, to reflect current practice. The nuclear medicine chapter (29) has been reorganized, and radiopharmaceuticals material has been updated.

Learning Aids for the Student

POCKET GUIDE TO RADIOGRAPHY

The new edition of *Merrill's Pocket Guide to Radiography* complements the revision of *Merrill's Atlas*. Instructions for positioning the patient and the body part for all of the essential projections are presented in a complete yet concise manner. Tabs are included to help the user locate the beginning of each section. Space is provided for the user to write in specifics of department techniques.

RADIOGRAPHIC POSITIONING AND PROCEDURES WORKBOOK

The new edition of this workbook features extensive review and self-assessment exercises that supplement the first 25 chapters in *Merrill's Atlas* in one convenient volume. To complement the textbook, similar content was merged and rearranged to better reflect the order in which the majority of students learn radiographic positioning and procedures. Chapters were removed to coincide with changes in the *Atlas*. Relevant material was updated to current practice and integrated into appropriate chapters. Terminology was updated to match the Content Specifications for the ARRT Radiography Examination, the ASRT Radiography Curriculum, and the evolution of digital imaging. The features of the previous editions, including anatomy labeling exercises, positioning exercises, and self-tests, are still available. However, this edition features more image evaluations to give students additional opportunities to evaluate radiographs for proper positioning and more positioning questions to complement the workbook's strong anatomy review. The comprehensive multiple-choice tests at the end of each chapter help students assess their comprehension of the whole chapter. New exercises in this edition focus on improved understanding of essential projections and the need for appropriate collimated field sizes for digital imaging. Additionally, review and assessment exercises in this edition have been expanded for the chapters on pediatrics, geriatrics, vascular and interventional radiography, sectional anatomy, and computed tomography in Volume 3. Exercises in these chapters help students learn the theory and concepts of these special techniques with greater ease. Answers to the workbook questions are found on the Evolve website.

Teaching Aids for the Instructor

EVOLVE INSTRUCTOR ELECTRONIC RESOURCES

This comprehensive resource provides valuable tools such as lesson plans, PowerPoint slides, and an electronic test bank for teaching an anatomy and positioning class. The test bank includes more than 1500 questions, each coded by category and level of difficulty. Four exams are already compiled in the test bank to be used "as is" at the instructor's discretion. The instructor also has the option of building new tests as often as desired by pulling questions from the ExamView pool or using a combination of questions from the test bank and questions that the instructor adds.

Evolve may be used to publish the class syllabus, outlines, and lecture notes; set up "virtual office hours" and e-mail communication; share important dates and information through the online class Calendar; and encourage student participation through Chat Rooms and Discussion Boards. Evolve allows instructors to post exams and manage their grade books online. For more information, visit *www. evolve.elsevier.com* or contact an Elsevier sales representative.

MOSBY'S RADIOGRAPHY ONLINE

Mosby's Radiography Online: Merrill's Atlas of Radiographic Positioning & Procedures is a well-developed online course companion for the textbook and workbook. This online course includes animations with narrated interactive activities and exercises, as well as multiple-choice assessments that can be tailored to meet the learning objectives of your program or course. The addition of this online course to your teaching resources offers greater learning opportunities while accommodating diverse learning styles and circumstances. This unique program promotes problem-based learning with the goal of developing critical thinking skills that will be needed in the clinical setting.

EVOLVE—ONLINE COURSE MANAGEMENT

Evolve is an interactive learning environment designed to work in coordination with *Merrill's Atlas*. Instructors may use Evolve to provide an Internet-based course component that reinforces and expands on the concepts delivered in class.

We hope you will find this edition of *Merrill's Atlas of Radiographic Positioning & Procedures* the best ever. Input from generations of readers has helped to keep the *Atlas* strong through 13 editions, and we welcome your comments and suggestions. We are constantly striving to build on Vinita Merrill's work, and we trust that she would be proud and pleased to know that the work she began 70 years ago is still so appreciated and valued by the imaging sciences community.

Bruce W. Long
Jeannean Hall Rollins
Barbara J. Smith
Tammy Curtis

ACKNOWLEDGMENTS

In preparing for the fourteenth edition, our advisory board continually provided professional expertise and aid in the decision making on the revision of this edition. The advisory board members are listed on p. vii. We are most grateful for their input and contributions to this edition of the *Atlas*.

Contributors

The group of radiography professionals listed below contributed to this edition of the *Atlas* and made many insightful suggestions. We are most appreciative of their willingness to lend their expertise.

We would like to extend special recognition and appreciation to Chris Brown, BS, RT(R); radiography student Madison Kolthoff; and the imaging professionals at Eskenazi Health in Indianapolis, Indiana, for their assistance with on-site photography for scoliosis and long bone measurement radiography. We would also like to thank Sally Powell, RT(R), imaging supervisor at Riley Hospital for Children, and student radiographer Madeline Pfister for their assistance with on-site photography for scoliosis radiography.

We would like to extend special recognition and appreciation to the imaging professionals and Gena Morris, RT(R), RDMS, PACS administrator at NEA Baptist Hospital in Jonesboro, Arkansas, for their time, effort, and expertise during this revision process. Additionally, we would also like to thank the imaging professionals and Mitzi Pierce, MSHS, RT(R) (M), radiology educator at St. Bernard's Medical Center in Jonesboro, Arkansas.

We would like to extend special recognition and appreciation to April Apple, RT(R), Senior Staff Technologist, Duke University Medical Center, for providing a new and more accurate image for the West Point method of the shoulder.

Finally, our deepest appreciation to our faith, family, and colleagues, whose support and encouragement remain an indispensable part of this work.

CONTENTS

1

PRELIMINARY STEPS
IN RADIOGRAPHY

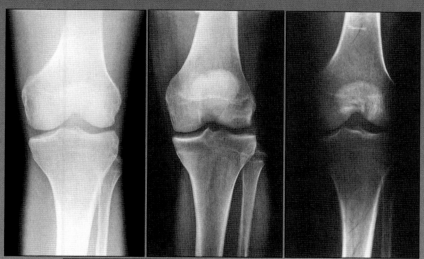

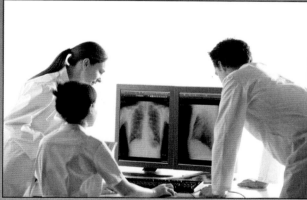

The Radiographer

Radiologic technology is a health care profession that includes all diagnostic imaging technologists and radiation therapists. A radiographer is a radiologic technologist who administers ionizing radiation to perform radiographic procedures. The radiographer produces radiographic images at the request of a licensed medical practitioner, usually a physician.

Radiographers interact with patients to produce diagnostic images, using technical skills combined with knowledge of physics, anatomy, physiology, and pathology. They must evaluate images for technical quality, accuracy, and appropriateness relative to the diagnosis or the reason for the procedure. This requires critical thinking and application of professional judgment. A fundamental responsibility of the radiographer is to ensure that each radiation exposure is "as low as reasonably achievable," or *ALARA*.

Patient care responsibilities of the radiographer include communication, assessment, monitoring, and support. The patient is questioned to ensure that the procedure ordered is consistent with the clinical history. It is the patient's right to know what is to be done and to consent to the procedure. Patient assessment before the procedure and monitoring while the patient is under the care of the radiographer are essential to ensure the patient's safety and well-being. Both physical and emotional support may be necessary during the procedure and until the patient is released from the radiographer's care.

As members of the health care team, radiographers have a shared responsibility to support and advance the mission of the health care provider for whom they work. This includes continually assessing their professional performance, as well as actively participating in quality improvement initiatives. To ensure patient safety and quality of care, each radiographer must adhere to the moral and ethical code of the profession, as well as work within the practice standards that describe the scope of practice.

Radiography Practice Standards

The Radiography Practice Standards are written and maintained by the American Society of Radiologic Technologists (ASRT). They define the practice of radiography, describe necessary education and certification, and include the Radiographer Scope of Practice. In addition, the practice standards include Clinical Performance Standards, Quality Performance Standards, and Professional Performance Standards. The full text of the most current Radiography Practice Standards can be found on the ASRT website at ASRT.org.

Ethics in Radiologic Technology

Ethics is the term applied to a health professional's moral responsibility and the science of appropriate conduct toward others. The work of the medical professional requires strict rules of conduct. The physician, who is responsible for the welfare of the patient, depends on the absolute honesty and integrity of all health care professionals to carry out orders and report mistakes.

The American Registry of Radiologic Technologists (ARRT) created and maintains the Standards of Ethics that apply to all radiologic technologists who are certified by the organization. The purpose is to describe professional values that translate into practice that is in the best interests of patients. The Standards of Ethics include a Code of Ethics and Rules of Ethics.

The ARRT Code of Ethics serves as a professional behavior guide to which radiologic technologists may aspire. It is intended to assist in maintaining a high level of ethical conduct in the profession.

1. The radiologic technologist conducts himself or herself in a professional manner, responds to patient needs, and supports colleagues and associates in providing quality patient care.
2. The radiologic technologist acts to advance the principal objective of the profession: to provide services to humanity with full respect for the dignity of humankind.
3. The radiologic technologist delivers patient care and service unrestricted by concerns of personal attributes or the nature of the disease or illness, and without discrimination, regardless of gender, race, creed, religion, or socioeconomic status.
4. The radiologic technologist practices technology founded on theoretic knowledge and concepts, uses equipment and accessories consistent with the purpose for which they have been designed, and uses procedures and techniques appropriately.
5. The radiologic technologist assesses situations; exercises care, discretion, and judgment; assumes responsibility for professional decisions; and acts in the best interest of the patient.
6. The radiologic technologist acts as an agent through observation and communication to obtain pertinent information for the physician to aid in the diagnosis and treatment management of the patient. He or she recognizes that interpretation and diagnosis are outside the scope of practice for the profession.
7. The radiologic technologist uses equipment and accessories; uses techniques and procedures; performs services in accordance with an accepted standard of practice; and demonstrates expertise in minimizing radiation exposure to the patient, self, and other members of the health care team.
8. The radiologic technologist practices ethical conduct appropriate to the profession and protects the patient's right to quality radiologic technology care.
9. The radiologic technologist respects confidence entrusted in the course of professional practice, respects the patient's right to privacy, and reveals confidential information only as required by law or to protect the welfare of the individual or the community.
10. The radiologic technologist continually strives to improve knowledge and skills by participating in educational and professional activities, sharing knowledge with colleagues, and investigating new and innovative aspects of professional practice.

The ARRT Standards of Ethics also contains 22 Rules of Ethics that are "mandatory standards of minimally acceptable professional conduct for all Certificate Holders and Candidates. The Rules of Ethics are enforceable."[1] The full list and descriptions of the Rules of Ethics can be found on the ARRT website at ARRT.org.

The Canadian Association of Medical Radiation Technologists (CAMRT) Member Code of Ethics and Professional Conduct has been developed by members to articulate the ethical behavior expected of all medical radiation technologists and to serve as a means for reflection and self-evaluation.

The code includes the following aspects of professional practice:
- Patient-centered care
- Maintaining competence
- Evidence-based and reflective practice
- Providing a safe environment
- Acting with professional integrity

The complete and current document can be found on the CAMRT website at CAMRT.ca.

Advanced Clinical Practice

In response to increased demands on the radiologist's time, a level of advanced clinical practice has developed for the radiographer. This advanced clinical role allows the radiographer to act as a "radiologist extender," similar to the physician assistant for a primary care physician. These radiographers take a leading role in patient care activities, perform selected radiologic procedures under the radiologist's supervision, and may be responsible for making initial image observations that are forwarded to the supervising radiologist for incorporation into the final report. The titles of *radiologist assistant* (RA) and *radiology practitioner assistant* (RPA) are currently used to designate radiographers who provide these advanced clinical services in the diagnostic imaging department. Requirements for practice include certification as a radiographer by the ARRT, pertinent additional education, and clinical experience under the supervision of a radiologist preceptor. The title of RA or RPA may be used only after passing an advanced level certification examination.

Care of the Radiographic Room

The radiographic procedure room should be as scrupulously clean as any other room used for medical purposes. The mechanical parts of the x-ray machine, such as the table, supporting structure, and collimator, should be wiped daily with a clean, damp (not soaked) cloth. The metal parts of the machine should be periodically cleaned with a disinfectant. The overhead system, x-ray tube, and other parts that conduct electricity should be cleaned with alcohol or a clean, dry cloth. Water is never used to clean electrical parts.

The tabletop should be cleaned after each patient procedure with a department-approved disinfectant cleaner. Accessories, such as gonad shields and nonporous positioning devices, should be cleaned daily and after any contact with a patient. Adhesive tape residue left on image receptors (IRs) should be removed, and all surfaces should be disinfected. IRs should be protected from patients who are bleeding, and disposable protective covers should be manipulated so that they do not come in contact with ulcers or other discharging lesions, if possible. Use of stained or damaged IRs is inexcusable and does not represent professional practice.

The radiographic room should be prepared for the procedure before the patient arrives. The room should look clean and organized—not disarranged from the previous procedure (Fig. 1.1). A fresh pillowcase should be put on the pillow, and accessories needed during the procedure should be placed nearby. Performing these preprocedure steps requires only a few minutes but creates a positive, lasting impression on the patient.

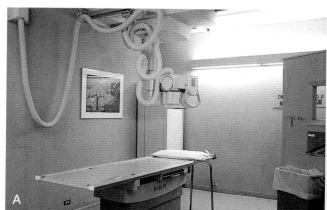 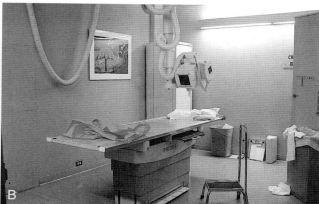

Fig. 1.1 (A) Radiographic room should always be clean and straightened before any examination begins. (B) This room is not ready to receive a patient. Note devices stored on the floor and previous patient's gowns and towels lying on the table. This room does not present a welcoming sight for a patient.

Control of Pathogen Contamination

For the protection of health care workers and patients, the US Centers for Disease Control and Prevention (CDC) provides directives for infection control. The foundation of infection control practices is included in the Standard Precautions for All Patient Care. "They're based on a risk assessment and make use of common sense practices and personal protective equipment use that protect healthcare providers from infection and prevent the spread of infection from patient to patient."[2] Standard precautions include the following aspects of professional practice:

- Perform hand hygiene (Fig. 1.2A).
- Use personal protective equipment (PPE) whenever there is an expectation of possible exposure to infectious material (Box 1.1).
- Follow respiratory hygiene/cough etiquette principles.
- Ensure appropriate patient placement.
- Properly handle and properly clean and disinfect patient care equipment and instruments/devices; clean and disinfect the environment appropriately (see Fig. 1.2B).
- Handle textiles and laundry carefully.
- Follow safe injection practices; wear a surgical mask when performing lumbar punctures.
- Ensure health care worker safety, including proper handling of needles and other sharps (Fig. 1.3).
- Transmission-based precautions are used in addition to standard precautions for patients with known or suspected infections.

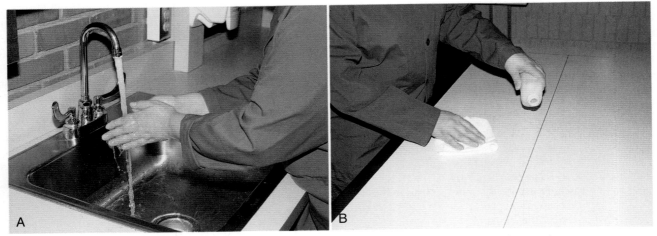

Fig. 1.2 (A) Radiographers should practice scrupulous cleanliness, which includes regular handwashing. (B) Radiographic tables and equipment should be cleaned with a disinfectant according to department policy.

BOX 1.1

Body fluids that may contain pathogenic microorganisms

Blood
Any fluid containing blood
Amniotic fluid
Pericardial fluid
Pleural fluid
Synovial fluid
Cerebrospinal fluid
Seminal fluid
Vaginal fluid
Urine
Sputum

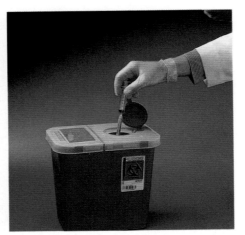

Fig. 1.3 All needles should be discarded in puncture-resistant containers.

Standard Precautions

Radiographers are engaged in caring for sick patients and should be thoroughly familiar with *standard precautions*. They should know the way to handle patients who are on isolation status without contaminating their hands, clothing, or apparatus, and radiographers must know the method of disinfecting these items when they become contaminated. Standard precautions are designed to reduce the risk for transmission of unrecognized sources of pathogens in health care institutions.

Handwashing is the easiest and most convenient method of preventing the spread of microorganisms (see Fig. 1.2A). Radiographers should wash their hands before and after working with each patient. Hands must always be washed, without exception, in the following specific situations:

• After examining patients with known communicable diseases
• After coming in contact with blood or body fluids
• Before beginning invasive procedures
• Before touching patients who are at risk for infection

As one of the first steps in aseptic technique, radiographers' hands should be kept smooth and free from roughness or chapping by the frequent use of soothing lotions. All abrasions should be protected by bandages to prevent the entrance of bacteria.

For the protection of the health of radiographers and patients, the laws of asepsis and prophylaxis must be obeyed. Radiographers should practice scrupulous cleanliness when handling all patients, whether or not the patients are known to have an infectious disease. If a radiographer is to examine the patient's head, face, or teeth, the patient should ideally see the radiographer perform handwashing. If this is not possible, the radiographer should perform handwashing and then enter the room drying the hands with a fresh towel. If the patient's face is to come in contact with the IR front or table, the patient should see the radiographer clean the device with a disinfectant or cover it with a clean drape. Under all circumstances, the radiographer must wear disposable gloves.

A sufficient supply of gowns and disposable gloves should be kept in the radiographic room to be used to care for infectious patients. After examining infectious patients, radiographers must wash their hands in warm, running water and soapsuds and rinse and dry them thoroughly. If the sink is not equipped with a knee control for the water supply, the radiographer opens the valve of the faucet with a paper towel. After proper handwashing, the radiographer closes the valve of the faucet with a paper towel.

Before bringing a patient from an isolation unit to the radiology department, the transporter should drape the stretcher or wheelchair with a clean sheet to prevent contamination of anything the patient might touch. When the patient must be transferred to the radiographic table, the table should be draped with a sheet. The edges of the sheet may be folded back over the patient so that the radiographer can position the patient through the clean side of the sheet without becoming contaminated.

When a free IR is used, it may be placed under the sheet. When possible, the gloved radiographer should position the patient using the sheet. If the radiographer must handle the patient directly, an assistant should position the tube and operate the equipment to prevent contamination. If a patient has any moisture or body fluids on the body surface that could come in contact with the IR, a nonporous cover should be placed over the IR before positioning under the patient.

When the examination is finished, the contaminated linen should be folded with the clean side out and is disposed of according to the established policy of the institution. All radiographic tables must be cleaned after patients have touched them with their bare skin and after patients with communicable diseases have been on the table (see Fig. 1.2B).

Minor Surgical Procedures in the Radiology Department

Procedures that require a rigid aseptic technique, such as cystography, intravenous urography, spinal puncture, arthrography, and angiography, are performed in the radiology department (Fig. 1.4). Although the physician needs the assistance of a nurse in certain procedures, the radiographer can make the necessary preparations and provide assistance in many procedures.

For procedures that do not require a nurse, the radiographer should know which instruments and supplies are necessary and how to prepare and sterilize them. Radiographers may make arrangements with the surgical supervisor to acquire the education necessary to perform these procedures.

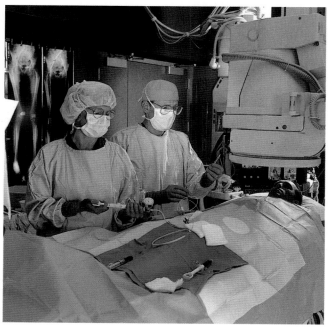

Fig. 1.4 Many radiographic procedures require strict aseptic technique, as seen in this procedure involving passing a catheter into the patient's femoral artery.

Control of Contamination Outside the Radiology Department

The radiographer is frequently required to provide imaging services to patients in hospital departments outside of radiology. These most often involve mobile radiography and C-arm fluoroscopy procedures in areas such as the emergency department (ED), intensive care units, medical-surgical units, and pain clinics.

Strict adherence to standard precautions will help to ensure the safety of the radiographer, patients, and other health care workers. In addition to standard precautions, the radiographer must practice transmission-based precautions and isolation precautions when the situation warrants. Carelessness by the radiographer can result in the spread of infection to other health care workers or between patients. In the case of immuno-compromised patients in a protective environment, failure of the radiographer to adhere to strict aseptic guidelines can result in a serious patient infection.

Providing imaging services in the operating room (OR) requires additional cleanliness considerations beyond those required in other hospital areas. The radiographer must safely enter and perform imaging procedures without contaminating the sterile surgical field. This requires experience and a high level of caution when moving imaging equipment in the surgical environment.

Chapter 21 of this atlas contains comprehensive information about the radiographer's work in the OR. A radiographer who has not had extensive patient care education must exercise extreme caution to prevent contaminating sterile objects in the OR. The radiographer should perform handwashing and wear scrub clothing, a scrub cap, and a mask and should survey the particular setup in the OR before bringing in the x-ray equipment. By taking this precaution, the radiographer can ensure that sufficient space is available to do the work without the danger of contamination. If necessary, the radiographer should ask the circulating nurse to move any sterile items. Because of the danger of contamination of the sterile field, sterile supplies, and persons scrubbed for the procedure, the radiographer should never approach the operative side of the surgical table unless directed to do so.

After checking the room setup, the radiographer should thoroughly wipe the x-ray equipment with a damp (not soaked) cloth before taking it into the OR. The radiographer moves the mobile machine, or C-arm unit, to the free side of the operating table—the side opposite the surgeon, scrub nurse, and sterile layout (Fig. 1.5). The machine should be maneuvered into a general position that makes the final adjustments easy when the surgeon is ready to proceed with the examination.

The IR is placed in a sterile covering for some procedures. The surgeon or one of the assistants holds the sterile case open while the radiographer gently drops the IR into it, being careful not to touch the sterile case. The radiographer may give directions for positioning and securing the cassette for the exposure.

The radiographer should make the necessary arrangements with the OR supervisor when performing work that requires the use of a tunnel or other special equipment. When an IR is being prepared for the patient, any tunnel or grid should be placed on the table with the tray opening to the side of the table opposite the sterile field. With the cooperation of the surgeon and OR supervisor, a system can be developed for performing radiographic examinations accurately and quickly without moving the patient or endangering the sterile field (Fig. 1.6).

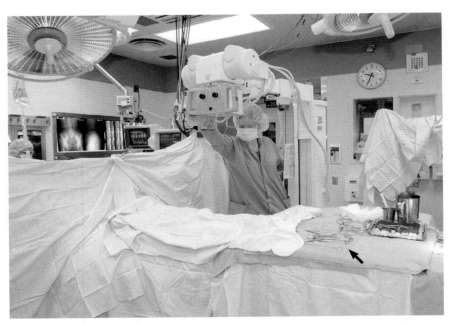

Fig. 1.5 Radiographer carefully positioning mobile x-ray tube during a surgical procedure. The sterile incision site is properly covered to maintain a sterile field. Note the sterile instruments in the foreground (*arrow*). The radiographer should never move radiographic equipment over uncovered sterile instruments or an uncovered surgical site.

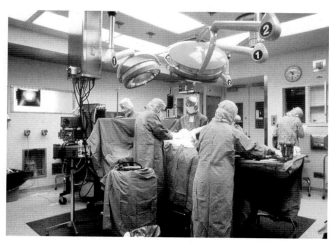

Fig. 1.6 Radiographer must exercise extreme caution to prevent contaminating sterile objects in the OR.

Interacting With Patients

Patients who are coherent and capable of understanding should be given an explanation of the procedure to be performed. Patients should understand exactly what is expected and be made comfortable. If patients are apprehensive about the examination, their fears should be alleviated. If the procedure will cause discomfort or be unpleasant, such as with cystoscopy and intravenous injections, the radiographer should calmly and truthfully explain the procedure. Patients should be told that it will cause some discomfort or be unpleasant, but because the procedure is a necessary part of the examination, full cooperation is necessary. Patients usually respond favorably if they understand that all steps are being taken to alleviate discomfort. Patients with special needs, such as autism or Alzheimer disease, may require specialized strategies to gain their cooperation during radiography procedures. See Chapters 22 and 23 for recommendations for effectively interacting with these patients.

Because the entire procedure may be a new experience, patients usually respond incorrectly when given more than one instruction at a time. For example, when instructed to get up on the table and lie on the abdomen, a patient may get onto the table in the most awkward possible manner and lie on his or her back. Instead of asking a patient to get onto the table in a specific position, the radiographer should first have the patient sit on the table and then give instructions on assuming the desired position. If the patient sits on the table first, the position can be assumed with less strain and fewer awkward movements. The radiographer should never rush a patient. If patients feel hurried, they will be nervous and less able to cooperate. When moving and adjusting a patient into position, the radiographer should manipulate the patient gently but firmly; a light touch can be as irritating as one that is too firm. Patients should be instructed and allowed to do as much of the moving as possible.

X-ray grids move under the radiographic table, and with floating or moving tabletops, patients may injure their fingers. To reduce the possibility of injury, the radiographer should inform patients to keep their fingers on top of the table at all times. Regardless of the part being examined, the patient's entire body must be adjusted with resultant motion or rotation to prevent muscle pull in the area of interest. When a patient is in an oblique (partially rolled to the side) position, the radiographer should use support devices and adjust the patient to relieve any strain. Immobilization devices should be used whenever necessary but not to the point of discomfort.

When making final adjustments to a patient's position, the radiographer should stand with the eyes in line with the position of the x-ray tube, visualize the internal structures, and adjust the part accordingly. Although there are a variety of ways to position patients, many repeat examinations can be eliminated by following these guidelines. (See Chapters 22 and 23 for specific recommendations for interacting with pediatric and geriatric patients.)

ILL OR INJURED PATIENTS

Great care must be exercised in handling trauma patients, particularly patients with skull, spinal, and long bone injuries. A physician should perform any necessary manipulation to prevent the possibility of fragment displacement. The positioning technique should be adapted to each patient and should necessitate as little movement as possible. If the tube-body part-imaging plane relationship is maintained, the resultant projection is the same regardless of the patient's position.

When a patient who is too sick to move alone must be moved, the following considerations should be kept in mind:

1. The patient should be moved as little as possible.
2. The radiographer should never try to lift a helpless patient alone.
3. To prevent straining the back muscles when lifting a heavy patient, one should flex the knees, straighten the back, and bend from the hips.
4. When a patient's shoulders are lifted, the head should be supported. While holding the head with one hand, one slides the opposite arm under the shoulders and grasps the axilla so that the head can rest on the bend of the elbow when the patient is raised.
5. When moving the patient's hips, the patient's knees are flexed first. In this position, patients may be able to raise themselves. If not, lifting the body when the patient's knees are bent is easier.
6. When a helpless patient must be transferred to the radiographic table from a stretcher or bed, he or she should be moved on a sheet or moving device by at least four and preferably six people. The stretcher is placed parallel to and touching the table. Under ideal circumstances, at least three people should be stationed on the side of the stretcher and two on the far side of the radiographic table to grasp the sheet at the shoulder and hip levels. One person should support the patient's head, and another person should support the feet. When the signal is given, all six people should *smoothly and slowly* lift and move the patient in unison (Fig. 1.7A). Often, radiographers use the three-person move for patients who are not in a critical condition (see Fig. 1.7B).

Many hospitals now have a specially equipped radiographic room adjoining the ED. These units often have special radiographic equipment and stretchers

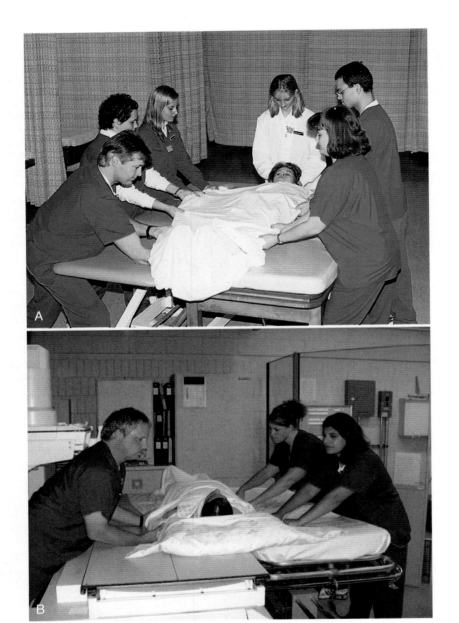

Fig. 1.7 (A) Technique for a six-person transfer of a patient who is unable to move from a cart to the procedure table. Note the person holding and supporting the head. (B) Three-person transfer of a patient back onto the cart. Note that two people are always on the side that is pulling the patient and one person is on the opposite side pushing the patient. Note also that the backs of the three people are straight, in accordance with correct lifting and moving practices.

with radiolucent tops that allow severely injured patients to be examined on the stretcher and in the position in which they arrive. A mobile radiographic machine is often taken into the ED, and radiographs are exposed there. When this ideal emergency setup does not exist, trauma patients are often conveyed to the main radiology department. There they must be given precedence over nonemergency patients (see Chapter 12).

AGE-SPECIFIC COMPETENCIES

Age-specific competence is defined as the knowledge, skills, ability, and behaviors that are essential for providing optimal care to defined groups of patients. Examples of defined groups include neonatal, pediatric, adolescent, and geriatric patients. Appropriate staff competence in working with these diverse patient groups is crucial in providing quality patient care. The Joint Commission[3] requires that age-specific competencies be written for all health care personnel who provide direct patient care. Radiographers are considered direct patient care providers. The Joint Commission requires radiology departments to document that radiographers maintain competency in providing radiologic examinations to defined groups of patients.

Age-specific competence is based on the knowledge that different groups of patients have special physical and psychosocial needs. Different types and levels of competence are required for specific patient populations. A radiographer who is obtaining radiographic images on a neonatal or pediatric patient must be skilled at interpreting nonverbal communication. Working with a geriatric patient requires the radiographer to have the knowledge and skills necessary to assess and maintain the integrity of fragile skin.

Health care facilities that provide patient care may classify the different age groups for which age-specific competence is defined. Some hospitals may classify patients by *chronologic* age, some may use *functional* age, and others may use *life stage* groupings.[4,5] Specialty organizations, such as pediatric hospitals, veterans' hospitals, psychiatric hospitals, or long-term care facilities, might use institution-specific criteria, such as premature or newborn, Vietnam veteran, closed ward, or Alzheimer disease.

The principle supporting age-related competencies is that staff involved in direct patient care who are not competent to provide care to patients in specific age or functional groups can alter treatment, increase patient complaints about care, make serious medical errors, and increase operational costs. The Joint Commission looks for evidence of staff development programs that are effective and ongoing and serve to maintain and improve staff competence.

When The Joint Commission surveys organizations, it looks for evidence of competence assessment primarily in personnel records. The Joint Review Committee on Education in Radiologic Technology (JRCERT), the organization that accredits radiography programs, makes site visits of radiography programs and looks for evidence that students not only learn the basic theories supporting age-related competence but also are competent. Table 1.1 shows a checklist that can be used in a radiography program to

TABLE 1.1

Age-specific criteria checklist

This planning tool is an example of a general checklist that can assist organizations in assessing age-specific competencies of staff					
	Neonatal	Pediatric	Adolescent	Adult	Geriatric
Knowledge of growth and development					
Ability to assess age-specific data					
Ability to interpret age-specific data					
Skills/knowledge to perform treatments (i.e., medications, equipment)					
Age-appropriate communication skills					
Knowledge of age-specific community resources					
Family or significant other, or both, involved in plan of care					

Used with permission from The Joint Commission, Oakbrook Terrace, IL, 1998.

document that a student has shown basic competence in several different life stages. Box 1.2 provides examples of age-specific competencies that should be required of a radiographer. Health care facilities are required to prepare age-related competencies for all age groups, including neonates, infants, children, adolescents, adults, and geriatrics.

Merrill's Atlas essentially addresses the normal adult patient in the age group from approximately 18 to 60 years. Although an organization would have published age-specific competencies for this broad age group, this group could be considered the "standard group" for which radiologic procedures are standardized and written. Radiographers must learn the specifics of how to adapt and modify procedures for the extreme groups, such as neonates (see Chapter 22) and geriatric patients (see Chapter 23), and for those in between, such as adolescents.

BOX 1.2

Age-specific competencies that should be required of a radiographer for two selected age groups

Neonate (1-30 days)
Explain examination to the parents if present.
Cover infant with a blanket to conserve body heat.
Cover image receptor with a blanket or sheet to protect the skin from injury.
Collimate to specific area of interest only.
Shield patient and any attendants.

Geriatric (68 years old or older)
Speak clearly and do not raise voice.
Do not rush examination.
Use positioning aids when possible.
Ensure that patient is warm owing to decreased circulation.
Do not leave patient unattended on the x-ray table.

Note: This list is not inclusive for the two age groups listed. Age-related competencies are prepared for other age groups as well.

Clinical History

The radiographer is responsible for performing radiographic examinations according to the standard department procedure except when contraindicated by the patient's condition. The radiologist is a physician who is board certified to read, or interpret, diagnostic images. As the demand for the radiologist's time increases, less time is available to devote to the technical aspects of radiology. This situation makes the radiologist more dependent on the radiographer to perform the technical aspects of patient care. The additional responsibility makes it necessary for the radiographer to know the following:

- Normal anatomy and normal anatomic variations so that the patient can be accurately positioned
- The radiographic characteristics of numerous common abnormalities

Although the radiographer is not responsible for explaining the cause, diagnosis, or treatment of the disease, the radiographer's professional responsibility is to produce an image that clearly shows the abnormality.

When the physician does not see the patient, the radiographer is responsible for obtaining the necessary clinical history and observing any apparent abnormality that might affect the radiographic result (Fig. 1.8). Examples include noting jaundice or swelling, body surface masses possibly casting a density that could be mistaken for internal changes, tattoos that contain ferrous pigment, surface scars that may be visible radiographically, and some decorative or ornamental clothing. The physician should give specific instructions about what information is necessary if the radiographer assumes this responsibility.

The request for an imaging procedure received by the radiographer should clearly identify the exact region to be radiographed and the reason for the procedure. It is the radiographer's responsibility to determine whether the procedure ordered is consistent with the reason for the examination. The patient must be positioned and the exposure factors selected according to the region involved and the radiographic characteristics of the suspected abnormality. Radiographers must understand the rationale behind the examination; otherwise, radiographs of diagnostic value cannot be produced. This may result in a delayed or missed diagnosis. Having the information in advance prevents delay, inconvenience, and, more important, unnecessary radiation exposure for the patient.

With most institutions now using electronic medical records, the radiographer will likely be using the computer system to enter information about the patient. In many of these information systems, the full patient medical record may be accessed. The radiographer needs to observe rules of confidentiality, as required by the Health Insurance and Portability Act of 1996 (HIPAA), restricting access to that part of the patient's protected health information that is relevant to the current procedure.

Diagnosis and the Radiographer

A patient is naturally anxious about procedure results and is likely to ask questions. The radiographer should tactfully advise the patient that the referring physician will receive the report as soon as the radiographs have been interpreted by the radiologist. Referring physicians may also ask the radiographer questions, and they should be instructed to contact the interpreting radiologist. Interpretation of images, beyond assessment of quality, is outside the scope of practice for a radiographer. However, it may be appropriate for a radiographer to notify the radiologist, before the patient is released, if something is seen on a radiograph that may indicate a potentially serious or life-threatening condition.

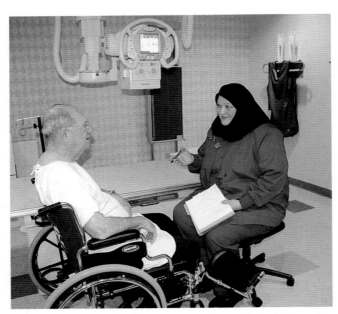

Fig. 1.8 Radiographer is often responsible for obtaining a clinical history from the patient.

Bowel Preparation

Radiologic examinations involving the abdominal organs often require that the entire colon be cleansed before the examination so that diagnostic quality radiographs can be obtained. The patient's colon may be cleansed by one or any combination of the following:

- Limited diet
- Laxatives
- Enemas

The technique used to cleanse the patient's colon generally is selected by the medical facility or physician. The patient should be questioned about any bowel preparation that may have been completed before an abdominal procedure is begun. For additional information on bowel preparation, see Chapter 15.

Patient Clothing, Jewelry, and Surgical Dressings

The patient should be dressed in a gown that allows exposure of limited body regions under examination. A patient is never exposed unnecessarily; a sheet should be used when appropriate. If a region of the body needs to be exposed to complete the examination, only the area under examination should be uncovered while the rest of the patient's body is completely covered for warmth and privacy. When the radiographer is examining parts that must remain covered, disposable paper gowns or cotton cloth gowns without metal or plastic snaps are preferred (Fig. 1.9). If washable gowns are used, they should not be starched; starch is *radiopaque,* which means it cannot be penetrated easily by x-rays. Any folds in the cloth should be straightened to prevent confusing densities on the radiograph. The length of exposure should also be considered. Material that does not cast a density on a heavy exposure, such as that used on an adult abdomen, may show clearly on a light exposure, such as that used on a child's abdomen.

Any radiopaque object should be removed from the region to be radiographed. Zippers, necklaces, snaps, thick elastic, and buttons should be removed when radiographs of the chest and abdomen are produced (Fig. 1.10). When radiographing the skull, the radiographer must make sure that dentures, removable bridgework, earrings, necklaces, and all hairpins are removed.

When the abdomen, pelvis, or hips of an infant are radiographed, the diaper should be removed. Because some diaper rash ointments are radiopaque, the area may need to be cleansed before the procedure.

Surgical dressings, such as metallic salves and adhesive tape, should be examined for radiopaque substances. If permission to remove the dressings has not been obtained or the radiographer does not know how to remove them and the radiology department physician is not present, the surgeon or nurse should be asked to accompany the patient to the radiology department to remove the dressings. When dressings are removed, the radiographer should always ensure that a cover of sterile gauze adequately protects open wounds.

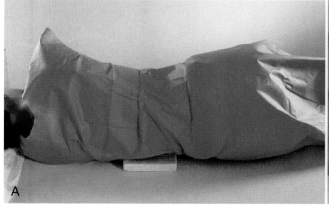 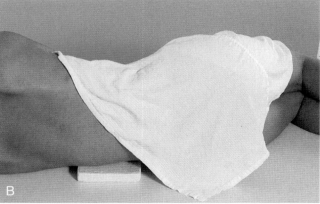

Fig. 1.9 (A) A female patient wearing a disposable paper gown and positioned for a lateral projection of the lumbar spine. Private areas are completely covered. The gown is smoothed around the contour of the body for accurate positioning. (B) The same patient wearing a traditional cloth hospital gown. The gown is positioned for maximal privacy.

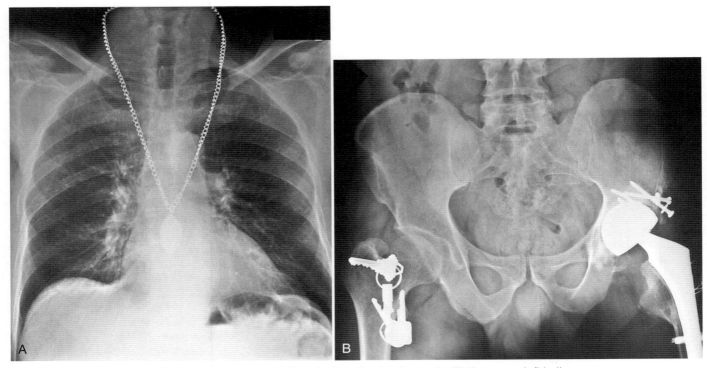

Fig. 1.10 (A) A necklace was left on for this chest radiograph. (B) Keys were left in the pocket of a lightweight hospital robe during the examination of this patient's pelvis. Both radiographs had to be repeated because the metal objects were not removed before the examination.

Motion and Its Control

Patient motion plays a large role in radiography (Fig. 1.11). Because motion is the result of muscle action, the radiographer needs to have some knowledge about the functions of various muscles. The radiographer should use this knowledge to eliminate or control motion for the exposure time necessary to complete a satisfactory examination. The three types of muscular tissue that affect motion are the following:

- Smooth (involuntary)
- Cardiac (involuntary)
- Striated (voluntary)

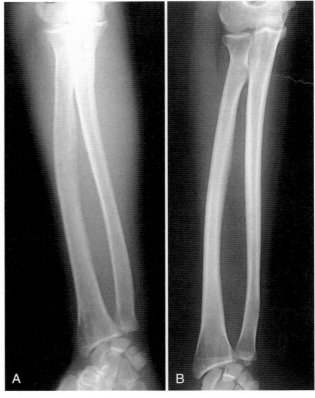

Fig. 1.11 (A) Forearm radiograph of a patient who moved during the exposure. Note the fuzzy appearance of the edges of the bones. (B) Radiograph of patient without motion.

INVOLUNTARY MUSCLES

The visceral (organ) muscles are composed of *smooth* muscular tissue and are controlled partially by the autonomic nervous system and the muscles' inherent characteristics of rhythmic contractility. By their rhythmic contraction and relaxation, these muscles perform the movement of the internal organs. The rhythmic action of the muscular tissue of the alimentary tract, called *peristalsis,* is normally more active in the stomach (approximately three or four waves per minute) and gradually diminishes along the intestine. The specialized *cardiac* muscular tissue functions by contracting the heart to pump blood into the arteries and by expanding or relaxing to permit the heart to receive blood from the veins. The pulse rate of the heart varies with emotions, exercise, diet, size, age, and gender.

Involuntary motion is caused by the following:
- Heart pulsation
- Chill
- Peristalsis
- Tremor
- Spasm
- Pain

The primary method of reducing involuntary motion on radiographic images is to control the length of exposure time—the less exposure time, the better.

VOLUNTARY MUSCLES

The voluntary, or skeletal, muscles are composed of *striated* muscular tissue and are controlled by the central nervous system. These muscles perform the movements of the body initiated by the individual. In radiography the patient's body must be positioned in such a way that the skeletal muscles are relaxed. The patient's comfort level is a good guide in determining the success of the position.

Voluntary motion resulting from lack of control is caused by the following:
- Nervousness
- Discomfort
- Excitability
- Mental illness
- Fear
- Age
- Breathing

The radiographer can control voluntary patient motion on images by doing the following:
- Giving clear instructions
- Providing patient comfort
- Adjusting support devices
- Applying immobilization

Decreasing the length of exposure time is the best way to control voluntary motion for patients who are unable to cooperate, such as young children, the elderly, and those with mental illness. Immobilization for limb radiography can often be obtained for the duration of the exposure by having the patient phonate an *mmm* sound with the mouth closed or an *ahhh* sound with the mouth open. The radiographer should always be watching the patient during the exposure to ensure that the patient has complied with breathing instructions when an exposure is made. Radiolucent positioning sponges and sandbags are commonly used as immobilization devices (Fig. 1.12A). A leg holder is used to stabilize the opposite leg for lateral radiographs of the legs, knee, femur, and hip (Fig. 1.12B). A thin radiolucent mattress, called a *table pad,* may be placed on the radiographic table to reduce movement related to patient discomfort caused by lying on the hard surface. These table pads should not be used when the increased object–to–image receptor distance (OID) would result in unacceptable magnification, such as in radiography of the limbs. If possible, radiographers should use table pads under the patient in the body areas where the projections are not made.

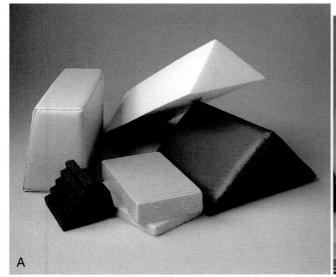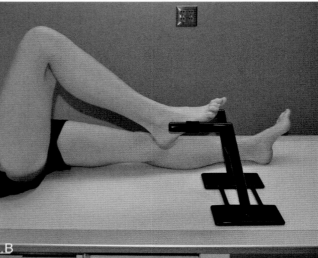

Fig. 1.12 (A) Positioning sponges and sandbags are commonly used as immobilization devices. (B) Ferlic leg holder and immobilization device.

(B, Courtesy Ferlic Filter Company, LLC, White Bear Lake, MN.)

Preexposure Instructions

The radiographer should instruct the patient in the appropriate breathing technique and should have the patient practice until the necessary actions are clearly understood. Most, but not all, radiographic projections require a breath hold in some phase of respiration. The most common are breath holds at the end of inspiration and at the end of expiration. The appropriate phase of breath hold or breathing technique is included in the positioning instructions for each projection in the text.

During trunk examination, the patient's phase of breathing is important. *Inspiration* (inhalation, or breathing in) depresses the diaphragm and abdominal viscera, lengthens and expands the lung fields, elevates the sternum and pushes it anteriorly, and elevates the ribs and reduces their angle near the spine. *Expiration* (exhalation, or breathing out) elevates the diaphragm and abdominal viscera, shortens the lung fields, depresses the sternum, and lowers the ribs and increases their angle near the spine. When exposures are to be made during shallow breathing, the patient should practice slow, even breathing, so that only the structures above the one being examined move.

After the patient is in position but before the radiographer leaves to make the exposure, the radiographer should have the patient practice the appropriate breath hold once more. This step requires a few minutes, but it may prevent a repeat exposure. The eyes of the radiographer should always be on the patient when the exposure is made to ensure that an exposure is not made if the patient moves or breathes. This is particularly important when pediatric, trauma, unconscious, and some geriatric patients undergo radiography.

Image Receptor

In radiography the *image receptor* is the device that receives the energy of the x-ray beam and forms the image of the body part.

In diagnostic radiology the IR is one of the following four devices:

1. *Cassette with film:* A device that contains special intensifying screens that emit light when struck by x-rays and imprint the x-ray image on film. Use of a darkroom, where the film is developed in a processor, is required. Afterward, the radiographic film image is ready for viewing on an illuminator or a viewbox (Fig. 1.13A).
2. *Photostimulable storage phosphor image plate* (PSP IP): A device, used for computed radiography (CR), similar in composition to a conventional intensifying screen that is housed in a specially designed cassette. The IP stores much of the x-ray energy it receives for later processing. After exposure, the cassette is inserted into a CR reader device, which scans the IP with a laser to release the stored x-ray energy pattern as light. The emitted light, constituting the radiographic image, is converted to digital format and viewed on a computer monitor or may be printed on film (see Fig. 1.13B).
3. *Solid-state digital detectors:* Often referred to as digital radiography (DR); uses a flat-panel IR to convert x-ray energy into a digital signal. The digital signal converter may be a thin-film transistor (TFT) array or a charge-coupled device (CCD). The image capture system may be indirect, using a light-emitting scintillator coupled to the digital converter, or direct, consisting of a photoconductor integrated with the digital converter. These solid-state detectors may be built into the x-ray table or upright wall unit (see Fig. 1.13C), or they may be housed in a cassette-like portable enclosure. The portable solid-state detectors may be wired, or "tethered," directly to the digital imaging system computer (see Fig. 1.13D) or may be connected wirelessly (see Fig. 1.13E). The image is viewed on a computer monitor or is printed on film. This is the fastest

image acquisition system, with images available in 6 seconds or less.

4. *Fluoroscopic IR:* A fluoroscopic system is designed for "real-time" imaging, to guide procedures, or capture full-motion video. The IR may be a conventional image intensifier tube (see Fig. 1.13F), coupled to a video camera, or a solid-state flat-panel digital detector (see Fig. 1.13G). The resulting images are viewed on a monitor and may be saved as static images, video recordings, or video files.

IR DIMENSIONS

Radiographic IR systems are manufactured in English and metric sizes. CR IPs are commonly manufactured in five sizes (Table 1.2). However, many departments use only the 10 × 12-inch (24 × 30-cm) and 14 × 17-inch (35 × 43-cm) plates for all routine images. The active surfaces of IRs used for DR are manufactured in approximately 10 × 12-inch (24 × 30-cm), 14 × 17-inch (35 × 43-cm), and 17 × 17-inch (43 × 43-cm) dimensions. The outer dimensions of these IRs are larger and vary in size depending on the manufacturer.

IR DIMENSIONS IN THIS ATLAS

IR dimensions recommended in this atlas are for *adults.* These sizes are subject to modification as needed to fit the size of the body part. Both US and metric sizes are used in the atlas, as appropriate.

TABLE 1.2

Most common computed radiography plate sizes

Inches	Centimeters
8 × 10	18 × 24
10 × 12	24 × 30
14 × 14	35 × 35
14 × 17	35 × 43
14 × 36	35 × 91

Some manufacturers build in inches and some in centimeters.

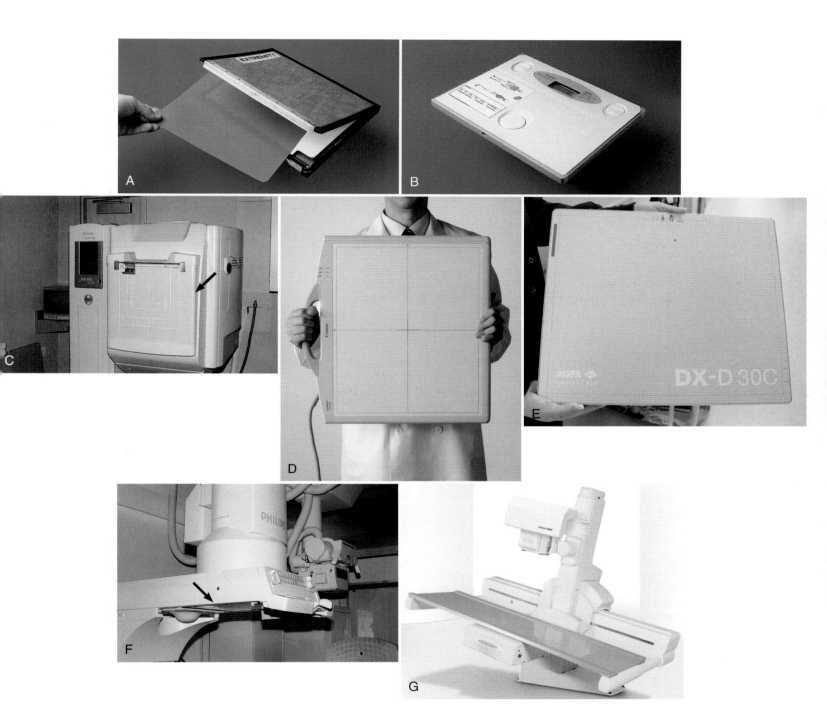

Fig. 1.13 Image receptors. (A) Conventional radiographic cassette, opened and showing a sheet of x-ray film. (B) CR cassette. This contains a photostimulable storage phosphor image plate that stores the x-ray image. (C) DR upright wall unit. A flat-panel digital detector is located behind the front cover *(arrow)*. (D) "Tethered" portable DR IRs. (E) Wireless portable DR IR. (F) Fluoroscopic image intensifier unit located under fluoroscopic tower *(arrow)* transmits x-ray image to a camera and then to a television for real-time viewing. (G) Fluoroscopic solid-state flat-panel digital detector transmits image directly to viewing monitor without the need for an intermediate video camera.

(D, Courtesy Canon USA, Inc. G, Used with permission from Philips Healthcare, Bothell, WA.)

Radiographic Positioning and Procedure

The atlas contains all instructions and recommendations needed to perform any radiographic projection. Updates to this edition reflect changes in current practice. A total of 340 projections are included in Volumes 1 and 2, of which 210 are essential projections. An essential projection, also called a routine projection, is identified in the Summary of Projections in each chapter with the ⚘ symbol.

A procedure or protocol book covering each examination performed in the radiology department is essential. Under the appropriate heading, each procedure should be outlined, and a list of all department-approved projections and positions for each procedure should be listed. For fluoroscopic procedures the protocol should state the staff required and the duties of each team member. A listing of sterile and nonsterile items should also be included. A copy of the sterile instrument requirements should be given to the supervisor of the central sterile supply department to guide preparation of the trays for each procedure.

Initial or Routine Procedure

The radiographs obtained for the initial or routine procedure for each body part are based on the anatomy or function of the part and the type of abnormality indicated by the clinical history. These radiographs are usually the minimum required to detect any demonstrable abnormality in the region and are set by department protocol. They are usually the ones included in the radiology information system (RIS) work list order set for the ordered procedure. Supplemental radiographs, for further investigation, are made as needed. This standard procedure saves time, eliminates unnecessary radiographs, and reduces patient exposure to radiation.

Common Steps for a Radiographic Procedure

Radiographers follow a set of common steps for each radiographic procedure.

TABLE 1.3
Recommended procedural steps

The purpose of these recommended procedural steps is to provide an organizational scheme that will ensure safe and effective performance. The order and details of these steps will vary by anatomy of interest, patient condition, type of equipment available, and department protocol.

Bucky: CR cassette or DR detector	Fixed unit: DR	Tabletop: free cassette or detector
Table or wall unit with an IR tray	IR is built into the unit and cannot be accessed by the radiographer	IR is freely positioned on any surface and in any orientation
Prep room and gather accessory equipment (grid, positioning aids, filter)	**Prep room**—including selection of patient and projection on computer monitor. **Gather accessory equipment** (grid, positioning aids, filter)	**Prep room**—including selection of patient and projection on computer monitor for DR. **Gather accessory equipment** (grid, positioning aids, filter)
Choose IR (size, orientation)	**Choose detector and/or collimation**	**Choose IR** (size, orientation)
Identify patient in HIPAA compliant manner	**Identify patient in HIPAA compliant manner**	**Identify patient in HIPAA compliant manner**
Explain procedure to patient and assess patient (obtain history to determine correct procedure, ability to cooperate, fall risk)	**Explain procedure to patient and assess patient** (obtain history to determine correct procedure, ability to cooperate, fall risk)	**Explain procedure to patient and assess patient** (obtain history to determine correct procedure, ability to cooperate, fall risk)
Prepare patient (remove clothing and potential artifact items, provide a gown, if needed)	**Prepare patient** (remove clothing and potential artifact items, provide a gown, if needed)	**Prepare patient** (remove clothing and potential artifact items, provide a gown, if needed)
Set technical factors	**Set technical factors**	**Set technical factors**
Position patient	**Position patient**	**Position patient**
Set SID	**Set SID**	**Set SID**
Align IR and CR	**Align IR and CR**	**Position part on IR**
Position part	**Position part**	**Align CR to IR/part**
Collimate	**Collimate**	**Collimate**
Place side marker	**Place side marker**	**Place side marker**
Shield patient	**Shield patient**	**Shield patient**
Provide patient instructions (hold still, breathing instructions)	**Provide patient instructions** (hold still, breathing instructions)	**Provide patient instructions** (hold still, breathing instructions)
Expose IR	**Expose IR**	**Expose IR**
Evaluate radiograph (acceptable appearance, centering, positioning, acceptable exposure indicator value)	**Evaluate radiograph** (acceptable appearance, centering, positioning, acceptable exposure indicator value)	**Evaluate radiograph** (acceptable appearance, centering, positioning, acceptable exposure indicator value)
Return or release patient (including exit instructions, follow-up information, postprocedure instructions, if applicable)	**Return or release patient** (including exit instructions, follow-up information, postprocedure instructions, if applicable)	**Return or release patient** (including exit instructions, follow-up information, postprocedure instructions, if applicable)

This improves efficiency, ensures patient safety, reduces mistakes, and minimizes patient radiation exposure. The order of these steps will vary by anatomy of interest, patient condition, type of equipment available, and by department protocol. More complex procedures, involving multiple body parts or fluoroscopy, may require additional steps. Table 1.3 lists recommended procedural steps for a radiographic procedure on a cooperative, uncomplicated patient.

Accessory Equipment

Performance of radiographic procedures may require use of equipment to ensure a body part remains in the appropriate posture during exposure. The most common positioning aids are radiolucent sponges of various shapes and sizes, based on the anatomy of interest. Additional devices may be needed for special purposes by department protocol (see Fig. 1.12).

Other devices may be needed to enhance image quality. These devices are placed between the patient and the IR. These include grids, lead shields, and filters. Grids and lead shields reduce scattered radiation to the IR. For lateral projections of the thoracic and lumbar spine, sacrum, and coccyx, placement of a lead shield on the table posterior to the patient's back will reduce the amount of scattered radiation reaching the IR (Fig. 1.14). Grids reduce scattered and off-focus radiation reaching the IR. They may be attached to the IR (Fig. 1.15) or may be built into the IR holder or Bucky tray (Fig. 1.16).

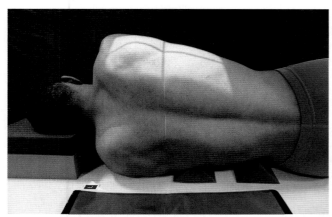

Fig. 1.14 When positioning for a lateral thoracic spine, a lead drape placed on the table in line with the back shadow will reduce the amount of scattered radiation reaching the IR.

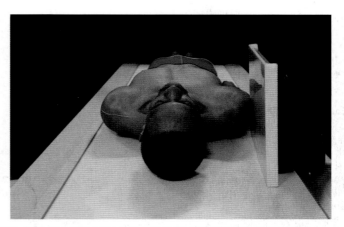

Fig. 1.15 The IR is placed in a grid holder for this cross-table lateral cervical spine radiograph to reduce the amount of scatter radiation reaching the IR.

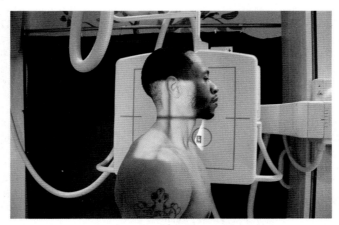

Fig. 1.16 A vertical Bucky unit contains a reciprocating grid to reduce scattered radiation reaching the IR.

Compensating filters are designed to compensate for significantly varied tissue thickness and density within a body part. The filter results in a more uniform image brightness by varying the amount of radiation received by different parts of the anatomy when the filter is placed between the tube and patient. The resulting attenuated beam more appropriately exposes the various tissue densities of the anatomy and reveals greater anatomic detail. Equally important, the filter reduces the entrance skin exposure and thus the absorbed dose to some of the organs in the body (Fig. 1.17). Some of the most common filters currently in use are shown in Fig. 1.18. Without use of filters, radiographs such as the anteroposterior (AP) projection of the thoracic spine (Fig. 1.19), the axiolateral projection (Danelius-Miller method) of

the hip (Fig. 1.20), and the AP shoulder (Fig. 1.21) may demonstrate significant differences in brightness between anatomic structures of widely varying tissue densities, even with DR. Common projections for which filters improve image quality are listed in Table 1.4.

Compensating filters are manufactured in various shapes and are composed of several materials. The shape or material chosen is based on the particular body part to be imaged. The exact placement of the filter also varies, with most placed between the x-ray tube and the skin surface, although some are placed between the anatomy and IR. However, filters placed close to the IR often produce distinct outlines of the filter, which can be objectionable to the radiologist.

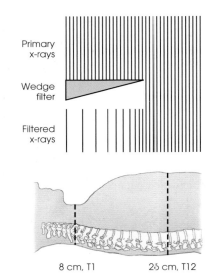

Fig. 1.17 Wedge filter in position for AP projection of thoracic spine. Note how the thick portion of wedge partially attenuates x-ray beam over upper thoracic area while nonfilter area receives full exposure to penetrate thick portion of spine. An even image density results.

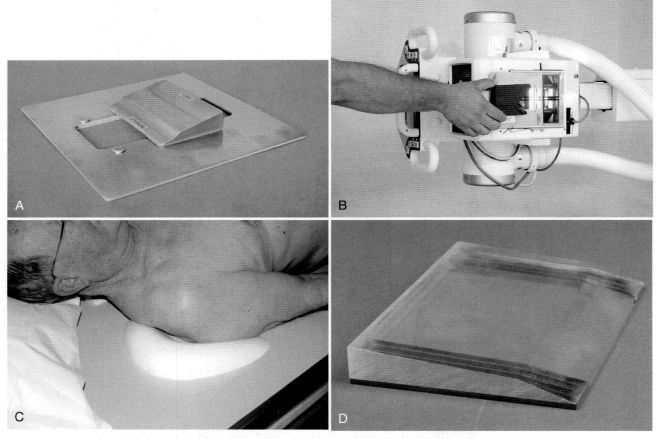

Fig. 1.18 Examples of compensating filters currently in use. (A) Ferlic collimator-mounted filter for AP axial projections of foot. (B) Ferlic collimator-mounted filter positioned on collimator for AP projection of shoulder. (C) Boomerang contact filter in position for AP projection of shoulder. (D) Supertech wedge, collimator-mounted Clear Pb filter.

(B, Courtesy Scott Slinkard, College of Nursing and Health Sciences, Cape Girardeau, MO.)

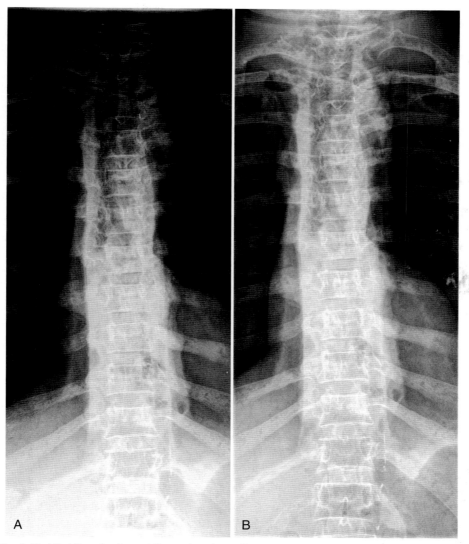

Fig. 1.19 (A) AP projection of thoracic spine without compensating filter. (B) Same projection with Ferlic wedge filter. Note more even brightness of spine, and all vertebrae are shown.

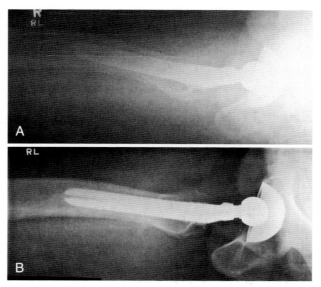

Fig. 1.20 (A) Axiolateral projection of hip (Danelius-Miller method) without compensating filter. (B) Same projection with Ferlic swimmer's filter. Note how acetabulum and end of metal shaft are seen on one image.

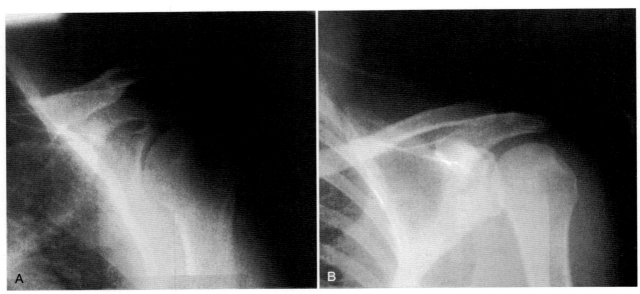

Fig. 1.21 (A) AP projection of shoulder without compensating filter. (B) Same projection using Boomerang contact filter.

TABLE 1.4
Common radiographic projections for which compensating filters improve image quality

Anatomy/projection	Filter	Type	Thick portion oriented to	Improved demonstration of
Mandible/Axiolateral oblique	Ferlic* swimmer's	Collimator	Anterior of mandible	Mandibular symphysis
Nasal bones/Lateral	Wedge	Collimator	Anterior	Nasal bones/cartilage
Facial bones/Lateral	Boomerang†	Contact	Anterior	Anterior facial structures
Cervicothoracic/Lateral	Ferlic* swimmer's	Collimator	Upper cervical	C6-T2
Thoracic spine/AP	Wedge	Collimator	Upper thoracic	Upper thoracic
Shoulder/AP	Boomerang†	Contact and collimator	AC joint	AC joint
	Ferlic* shoulder		AC joint	AC joint
Shoulder/Axial	Ferlic* swimmer's	Collimator	Humerus	Humerus
Shoulder/Oblique	Boomerang†	Contact and collimator	Humeral head	Glenoid fossa
	Ferlic* shoulder		Humeral head	Glenoid fossa
Chest/AP	Supertech‡/trough	Collimator	Sides of chest	Mediastinum
Abdomen/AP upright	Wedge	Collimator	Upper abdomen	Diaphragm
Abdomen/AP decubitus	Wedge	Collimator	Side farthest from table	Abdomen side up
Lateral hip/Axiolateral	Ferlic* swimmer's	Collimator	Distal femur	Proximal femur
Hip/AP (emaciated patient)	Wedge	Collimator	Greater trochanter	Femoral head
Foot/AP	Wedge/gentle slope	Contact and collimator	Toes	Forefoot
Calcaneus/Axial	Ferlic* swimmer's	Collimator	Calcaneus	Posterior calcaneus
Hip-knee-ankle 51 inches/AP	Supertech‡/full-length leg Ferlic* swimmer's	Collimator	Tibia/fibula	Distal tibia-fibula

*Ferlic; Ferlic Filter Company, LLC, White Bear Lake, MN.
†Boomerang; Octostop, Inc., Laval, Canada.
‡Supertech, Elkhart, IN.
This table is not all-inclusive. Other body structures can be imaged, and other filters are available on the market.
AC, Acromioclavicular joint.

The *wedge* is the simplest and most common of the compensating filter shapes. It is used to improve the image quality of a wide variety of body parts. Various filters with more complex shapes, including the *trough, scoliosis, Ferlic,*[6] and *Boomerang,*[7] have been developed for technically challenging anatomic areas.

Compensating filters are composed of a substance of sufficiently high atomic number to attenuate the x-ray beam. The most common filter materials are aluminum and high-density plastics. These are manufactured with varying thickness of material and are generally distributed in a smoothly graduated way that corresponds with the distribution of the different tissue densities of the anatomy (see Fig. 1.18A). Aluminum is an efficient attenuator and a common filter material.

Some manufacturers offer compensating filters made from clear leaded plastic, known as *Clear Pb,*[8] which allows the field light to shine through to the patient but still attenuates the x-ray beam (see Fig. 1.18D). However, this leaded plastic is inappropriate for all filter uses, such as in the extremely dense area of the shoulder during lateral spine radiography, because the thickness required to attenuate the beam sufficiently would result in a prohibitively heavy device. In these cases, aluminum is generally used. The Boomerang (see Fig. 1.18C) filter is composed of an attenuating silicon rubber compound, and some models of this filter have an embedded metal bead chain to mark the filter edge.

Compensating filters are most often placed in the x-ray beam between the x-ray tube and patient. Broadly, filters fall into two categories based on their location during use: *collimator-mounted* filters and *contact* filters. Collimator-mounted filters are mounted on the collimator, using rails installed on both sides of the window on the collimator housing or magnets. Contact compensating filters may be placed directly on the patient or between the anatomy and the IR.

In general, filters placed between the primary beam and the body provide the added benefit of a reduction in radiation exposure to the patient because of the beam-hardening effect of the filter, whereas filters placed between the anatomy and the IR have no effect on patient exposure. Measurements provided with Ferlic filters show radiation exposure reductions of 50% to 80%, depending on the kilovoltage peak (kVp), in the anatomic area covered by the filter. Measurements by Frank et al.[9] show exposure reductions of 20% to 69% to the thyroid, sternum, and breasts. Both types have the same effect on the finished image, which is an appropriate brightness range even though the tissue density varies greatly.

COMPENSATING FILTERS IN THIS ATLAS

Body structures whose radiographic images can be improved through the use of compensating filters are identified throughout the atlas directly on the projection page. The special icon ◣ identifies the use of a filter.

Technical Factors

Variation in electricity delivered to the x-ray tube permits the radiographer to control several prime technical factors: *milliamperage* (mA), *kilovolt peak* (kVp), and *exposure time* (seconds). The radiographer selects the specific factors required to produce a quality radiograph using the generator's control panel after consulting a technique chart. Manual and automatic exposure control (AEC) systems are used to set the factors.

Detailed aspects of each technical factor are presented in radiographic physics and principles courses. Because of the variety of exposure factors and equipment used in clinical practice, exact technical factors are not presented in this atlas. However, each positioning chapter contains a sample exposure technique chart for the essential projections described in the chapter. This chart is accurate for the equipment and IRs used to make the exposures. The exposure techniques listed may not be appropriate for general use because of the variability of x-ray generator output characteristics and because of the energy sensitivities of IR. However, these techniques can be used as a starting point for development of charts for specific radiographic units. In addition, the accompanying radiation dose information can provide a general idea of the relative amount of exposure associated with particular projections. In addition, the companion *Merrill's Pocket Guide to Radiography* contains a recommended kVp for each projection and is designed with a blank table to allow students and radiographers to organize and write in the technical factors used in respective departments with different types of available equipment (Fig. 1.22).

Knee
AP

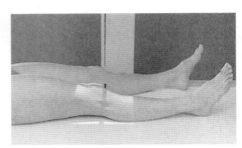

Patient Position
- Position patient supine with leg extended.
- Adjust patient's body so that pelvis is not rotated.

Part Position
- Center knee to IR at level ½ inch (1.3 cm) below patellar apex.
- Adjust leg so that femoral condyles are parallel to IR.

Central Ray
- Enters point ½ inch (1.3 cm) inferior to patellar apex
- Depending on ASIS-to-tabletop measurement, direct central ray as follows:

<19 cm   3 to 5 degrees *caudad* (thin pelvis)
19 to 24 cm   0 degrees
>24 cm   3 to 5 degrees *cephalad* (large pelvis)

Collimation:
Adjust to 10 × 12 inches (24 × 30 cm).

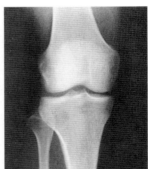

kVp: 70 (non-grid) 85 (grid)   *Reference: 14th edition Atlas, p.344*

Manual Factors

Part Thickness (cm)	mA	kVp	Time	mAs	SID	Image Receptor Size	CR, DR Exposure Indicator	Grid	HF, 1Ø or 3Ø

AEC Factors

Part Thickness (cm)	mA	kVp	AEC Detector	mAs	Density Comp.	Image Receptor Size	CR, DR Exposure Indicator	Grid	HF, 1Ø or 3Ø

Notes: _____ Competency: _____/____/____

_____ Instructor: _____

296

Lower Limb

Fig. 1.22 Exposure technique page from *Merrill's Pocket Guide to Radiography* showing how a specific department's manual techniques and AEC techniques can be written in for reference in setting optimal techniques. Note also patient photograph and radiograph. Quick reference can be made to the exact position of the patient, and the radiograph shows how the final image should appear.

Foundation Exposure Techniques and Charts

An exposure technique chart should be placed in each radiographic room and on mobile units, including machines that use AEC.[10–12] A foundation technique chart is one made for all normal-size adults.

A well-designed chart also includes suggested adjustments for pediatric, emaciated, and obese patients. The chart should be organized to display all radiographic projections performed in the room. Specific exposure factors for each projection should also be indicated (Fig. 1.23). A measuring caliper should be used to ascertain part thickness for accurate technique selection (Fig. 1.24).

A satisfactory technique chart can be established only by the radiographer's familiarity with the characteristics of the particular equipment and accessories used and the radiologist's preference in image quality.

SAMPLE EXPOSURE TECHNIQUE CHART ESSENTIAL PROJECTIONS

These techniques were accurate for the equipment used to produce each exposure. However, use caution when applying them in your department. [1]

This chart was created in collaboration with Dennis Bowman, AS, RT(R), Clinical Instructor, Community Hospital of the Monterey Peninsula, Monterey, CA. http://digitalradiographysolutions.com/.

THORACIC VISCERA

Part	cm	kVp*	SID[†]	Collimation	CR[‡] mAs	CR[‡] Dose (mGy)[ǁ]	DR[§] mAs	DR[§] Dose (mGy)[ǁ]
Chest: Lungs and heart—*PA*[¶]	22	120	72"	14" × 16" (35 × 40 cm)	2.8**	0.188	1.4**	0.089
Chest: Lungs and heart—*lateral*[¶]	33	120	72"	14" × 17" (35 × 43 cm)	7.1**	0.550	3.6**	0.273
Chest: Lungs and heart—*PA oblique*[¶]	25	120	72"	14" × 17" (35 × 43 cm)	3.6**	0.255	1.8**	0.124
Chest: Lungs and heart—*AP*[††]	22	90	40"	16" × 14" (40 × 35 cm)	4.0**	0.655		
Chest: Lungs and heart—*AP*[††]	22	105	40"	16" × 14" (40 × 35cm)			1.6**	0.340
Chest: Lungs and heart—*AP*[¶]	22	120	72"	14" × 16" (35 × 40 cm)	3.2**	0.217	1.6**	0.104
Pulmonary apices—*AP axial*[¶]	23	120	72"	14" × 11" (35 × 28 cm)	4.0**	0.198	2.0**	0.097
Lungs and pleurae—*Lateral decubitus*[¶]	22	120	72"	17" × 14" (43 × 35 cm)	4.0**	0.271	2.0**	0.133
Lungs and pleurae—*Dorsal/ventral decubitus*[¶]	33	120	72"	17" × 14" (43 × 35 cm)	9.0**	0.697	4.5**	0.344

[1]ACR-AAPM-SIMM Practice Parameter for Digital Radiography, revised 2017.
*kVp values are for a high-frequency generator.
[†]40 inch minimum; 44-48 inches recommended to improve spatial resolution (mAs increase needed, but no increase in patient dose will result).
[‡]AGFA CR MD 4.0 General IP, CR 75.0 reader, 400 speed class, with 6:1 (178LPI) grid when needed.
[§]GE Definium 8000, with 13:1 grid when needed.
[ǁ]All doses are skin entrance for average adult (160-200 pound male, 150-190 pound female) at part thickness indicated.
[¶]Bucky/Grid.
**Large focal spot.
[††]Nongrid.

Fig. 1.23 Radiographic exposure technique chart showing manual and AEC technical factors for the examinations identified.

The following primary factors must be taken into account when the correct foundation technique is being established for each unit:

- Milliampere-seconds (mAs)
- kVp
- AECs
- Source-to–image receptor distance (SID)
- Relative patient or part thickness
- Grid
- CR/DR exposure indicators or other digital exposure value estimates

- IR or collimated field dimensions
- Electrical supply characteristics (phase, frequency)

With this information available, the exposure factors can be selected for each region of the body that results in the best possible radiographic quality with minimal radiation exposure.

Modern x-ray generators have anatomic programmers that can store a wide range of radiographic exposure techniques for most body parts (Fig. 1.25). The radiographer simply selects the body part, and the technique is automatically set. However, it is the responsibility of all radiographers to ensure that the programmed techniques are appropriate and optimum for their particular patient.

Adaptation of Exposure Technique to Patients

The radiographer's responsibility is to select the combination of exposure factors that produces the desired quality of radiographs for each region of the body and to minimize radiation exposure to the patient. These foundation factors should be adjusted for every patient's size to maintain uniform radiation exposure to the IR. In addition, congenital and developmental factors, age, and pathologic changes must be considered. Some patients have fine, distinct bony trabecular markings, whereas others do not. Individual differences must be considered when the quality of the radiograph is judged.

Certain conditions require the radiographer to compensate when establishing an exposure technique. Conditions that require a decrease in technical factors include old age, pneumothorax, emphysema, emaciation, degenerative arthritis, and atrophy.

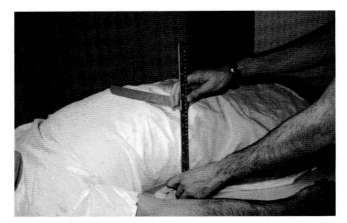

Fig. 1.24 Measuring caliper is used to measure the body part for accurate exposure technique selection.

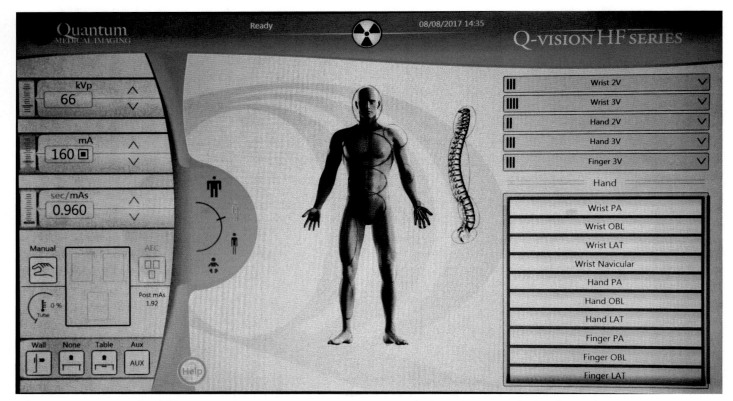

Fig. 1.25 Anatomic programmer on x-ray generator. Technical exposure factors for most body parts are preprogrammed into the computer. The factors on this display are for a PA projection of the hand.

Some conditions require an increase in technical factors to penetrate the part to be examined. These include pneumonia, pleural effusion, hydrocephalus, enlarged heart, edema, and ascites.

Gonad Shielding

The patient's gonads may be irradiated when radiographic examination of the abdomen, pelvis, and hip area is performed. When practical, gonad shielding should always be used to protect the patient. Contact, shadow, and large part area shields are used for radiographic examinations (Figs. 1.26 through 1.28). The Center for Devices of Radiological Health has developed guidelines recommending gonad shielding in the following instances:[13]

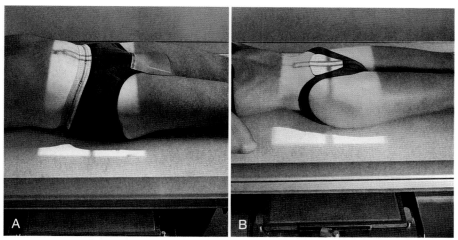

Fig. 1.26 (A) Contact shield placed over the gonads of a male patient. (B) Contact shield placed over the gonads of a female patient.

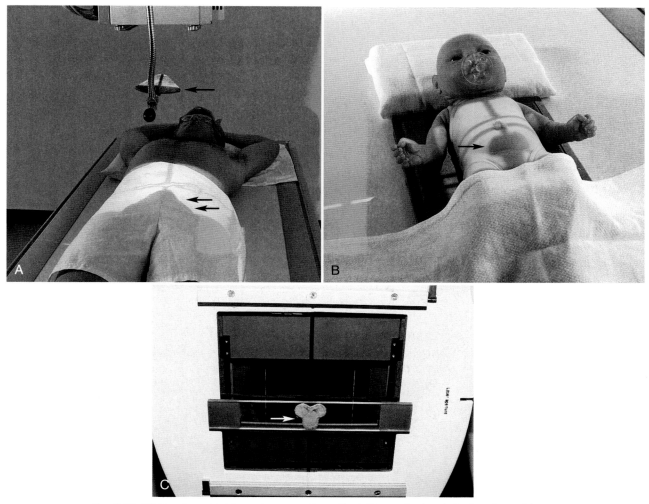

Fig. 1.27 (A) Shadow shield used on a male patient. Triangular lead device *(arrow)* is hung from the x-ray tube and is positioned so that its shadow falls on the gonads *(double arrows)*. (B) Shadow shield used on female infant. Cloverleaf shield is positioned under the collimator with magnets so that its shadow falls over the gonads *(arrow)*. (C) Cloverleaf-shaped shadow shield *(arrow)* positioned under the collimator with magnets.

- When the gonads lie within or close to (approximately 5 cm from) the primary x-ray field despite proper beam limitation
- When the clinical objective of the examination is not compromised
- When the patient has a reasonable reproductive potential

Gonad shielding is often appropriate when limbs are radiographed with the patient seated at the end of the radiographic table (Fig. 1.29). To ensure that shielding is used appropriately, many departments have a policy that states that the gonads must be shielded on every patient and for every projection in which the lead shield would not interfere with the image. Finally, gonad shielding must be considered and used when requested by the patient unless it is contraindicated. Gonad shielding is included in selected illustrations in this atlas.

BONE MARROW DOSE

An organ of particular concern is the bone marrow. Bone marrow dose is used to estimate the population *mean marrow dose* (MMD) as an index of the somatic effect of radiation exposure. Table 1.5 relates the MMD associated with various radiographic examinations. Each of these doses results from partial-body exposure and is averaged over the entire body.

GONAD DOSE

Exposure of the gonads to radiation during diagnostic radiology is of concern because of the possible genetic effects of x-radiation. Table 1.6 indicates average gonad doses received during various radiographic examinations. The large difference between males and females results from shielding of the ovaries by overlying tissue.

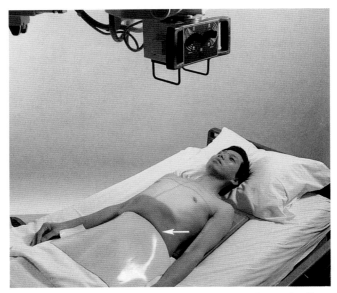

Fig. 1.28 Large piece of flexible lead *(arrow)* is draped over this patient's pelvis to protect the gonads during mobile radiographic examination of the chest.

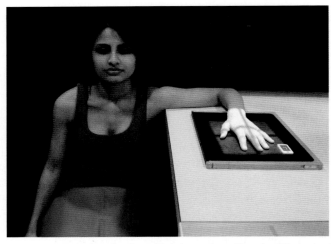

Fig. 1.29 Proper placement of patient and body part position for PA projection of the left hand.

TABLE 1.5

Representative bone marrow dose for selected radiographic examinations

Examination	Mean marrow dose
Skull	0.1 mGy (10 mrad)
Cervical spine	0.2 mGy (20 mrad)
Chest	0.02 mGy (2 mrad)
Stomach and upper gastrointestinal tract	1 mGy (100 mrad)
Gallbladder	0.8 mGy (80 mrad)
Lumbar spine	0.6 mGy (60 mrad)
Intravenous urography	0.25 mGy (25 mrad)
Abdomen	0.3 mGy (30 mrad)
Pelvis	0.2 mGy (20 mrad)
Limb	0.02 mGy (2 mrad)

TABLE 1.6

Approximate gonad dose resulting from various radiographic examinations

Examination	Gonad dose	
	Male	Female
Skull	<0.01 mGy (<1 mrad)	<0.01 mGy (<1 mrad)
Cervical spine	<0.01 mGy (<1 mrad)	<0.01 mGy (<1 mrad)
Full-mouth dental	>0.01 mGy (>1 mrad)	<0.01 mGy (<1 mrad)
Chest	>0.01 mGy (>1 mrad)	<0.01 mGy (<1 mrad)
Stomach and upper gastrointestinal tract	<0.02 mGy (<2 mrad)	0.4 mGy (40 mrad)
Gallbladder	0.01 mGy (1 mrad)	0.2 mGy (20 mrad)
Lumbar spine	1.75 mGy (175 mrad)	4 mGy (400 mrad)
Intravenous urography	1.5 mGy (150 mrad)	3 mGy (300 mrad)
Abdomen	1 mGy (100 mrad)	2 mGy (200 mrad)
Pelvis	3 mGy (300 mrad)	1.5 mGy (150 mrad)
Limb	<0.01 mGy (<1 mrad)	<0.01 mGy (<1 mrad)

Placement and Orientation of Anatomy on the Image Receptor

The part to be examined is usually centered on the center point of the IR or at the position where the angulation of the central ray (CR) projects it to the center. The IR should be adjusted so that its long axis lies parallel to the long axis of the part being examined. Although a long bone angled across the radiograph does not impair the diagnostic value of the image, such an arrangement can be aesthetically distracting. The three general positions of the IR, lengthwise, crosswise, and diagonal, are shown in Fig. 1.30. These positions are named on the basis of their position in relation to the long axis of the body. The lengthwise IR position is used most frequently.

Although the lesion may be known to be at the midbody (central portion) of a long bone, an IR large enough to include at least one joint should be used on all long bone studies (Fig. 1.31). This method

is the only means of determining the precise position of the part and localizing the lesion. Many institutions require that both joints be shown when a long bone is initially radiographed. For tall patients, two exposures may be required—one for the long bone and joint closest to the area of concern and a second to show the joint at the opposite end.

An IR just large enough to cover the region being examined should be used when available. This aids in positioning and encourages proper collimation. This rule does not apply when a department has only one size detector available or for units where the IR is integrated into the housing so it is a fixed size that cannot be changed. Regardless of the IR size, it is the radiographer's responsibility to collimate the exposure field to the body part dimensions, regardless of its location on the detector.

A standard rule in radiography is that the body part must be placed as close to the IR as possible. However, in some situations, this rule is modified. For example,

when lateral images of the middle and ring fingers are obtained, the radiographer increases the OID so that the part lies parallel to the IR. Although magnification is greater, less distortion occurs. The radiographer can increase the SID to compensate for the increase in OID, thereby reducing the magnification. In certain instances, intentional magnification is desirable and can be obtained by positioning and supporting the object between the IR and the focal spot of the tube. This procedure is known as magnification radiography.

Nearly all radiography is currently performed with one exposure for each IR. Multiple images in one image display field are not possible with DR, which captures one image at a time. However, with CR systems, bilateral examinations of small body parts may be placed on a single IR. Many IR cassettes have permanent markings on the edges to assist the radiographer in equally spacing multiple images on one IR. Depending on the size and shape of the body part being radiographed, the IR can be divided transversely or longitudinally.

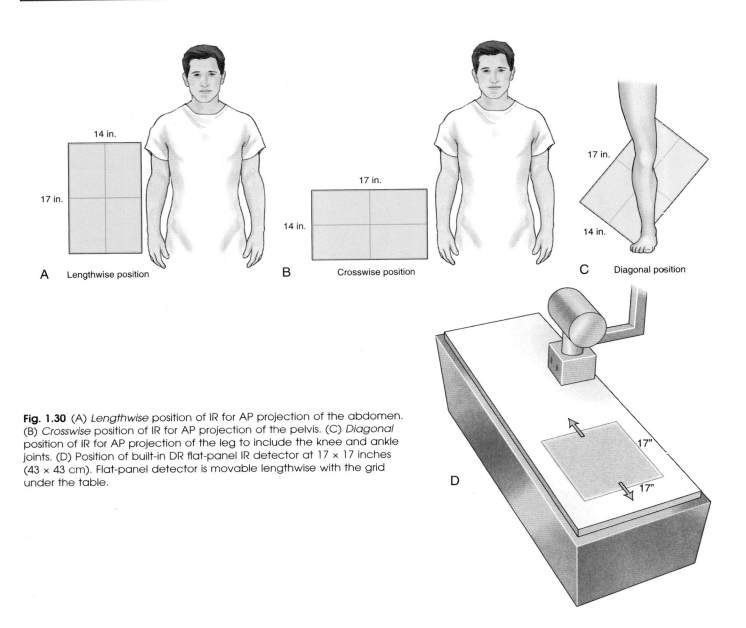

Fig. 1.30 (A) *Lengthwise* position of IR for AP projection of the abdomen. (B) *Crosswise* position of IR for AP projection of the pelvis. (C) *Diagonal* position of IR for AP projection of the leg to include the knee and ankle joints. (D) Position of built-in DR flat-panel IR detector at 17 × 17 inches (43 × 43 cm). Flat-panel detector is movable lengthwise with the grid under the table.

Placement and Direction of the Central Ray

The central or principal beam of rays, simply referred to as the *central ray*, is always centered to the anatomy of interest and usually to the IR, when practical. The CR is angled through the part of interest under the following conditions:

- when overlying or underlying structures must not be superimposed
- when a curved structure, such as the sacrum or coccyx, must not be superimposed on itself

- when projection through angled joints, such as the knee joint and the lumbosacral junction, is necessary
- when projection through angled structures must be obtained without foreshortening or elongation, such as with a lateral image of the neck of the femur

The general goal is to place the CR perpendicular to the structure of interest. Accurate positioning of the part and accurate centering of the CR are of equal importance in obtaining a true structural projection with minimal distortion.

Source-to-Image Receptor Distance

SID is the distance from the anode focal spot inside the x-ray tube to the IR (Fig. 1.32). SID is an important technical consideration in the production of radiographs of optimal quality. This distance is a critical component of each radiograph because it directly affects magnification of the anatomy on the image, the spatial resolution, and the dose to the patient. The greater the SID, the less the anatomy is magnified and the greater the spatial

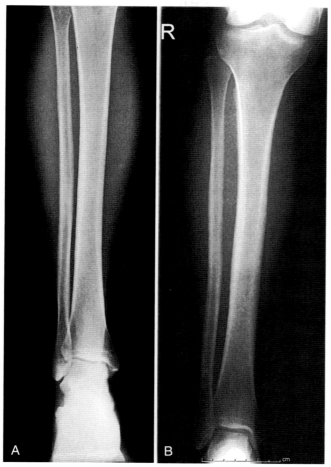

Fig. 1.31 (A) AP projection of the leg showing the ankle joint included on the image. One joint should be shown on all images of long bones. (B) AP projection of the leg showing both the knee and ankle joints on the image.

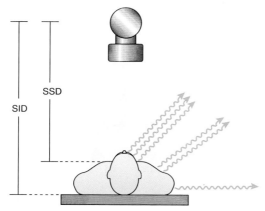

Fig. 1.32 Radiographic tube, patient, and table illustrate SID and SSD.

resolution. An SID of 40 inches (102 cm) has been used traditionally for most conventional examinations. In recent years the SID has increased to 44 to 48 inches (112 to 122 cm) in many departments.[10,11,14–17] It has been determined that an increase in the SID when practical will result in reduced magnification and increased spatial resolution, with a reduction in patient dose of approximately 10%. SID must be established for each radiographic projection, and it must be indicated on the technique chart.

Outside the United States the commonly used SID is 100 cm, instead of our customary 40 inches. For chest radiography, 180 cm is used, instead of the 72 inches we use in the United States. Other intermediate SIDs, such as 120 cm, may also be used.

For a few radiographic projections, a SID less than 40 inches (<102 cm) is desirable. In certain examinations, such as examination of the odontoid in the open mouth position, a short SID of 30 inches (76 cm) may be used. This shorter SID results in differentially greater magnification, in the direction of beam divergence, of the anatomic structures closest to the tube. This results in a greater field of view of the structures closest to the IR. At 30 inches, nearly 0.5 inches more anatomy is seen. The goal of these reduced SID projections is to demonstrate the body part with reduced superimposition of overlying structures. However, a slight increase in patient exposure will occur.

Conversely, a longer than standard SID is used for some radiographic projections. In chest radiography a 72-inch (183-cm) SID is the minimum distance, and in many departments, a distance up to 120 inches (305 cm) is used. These long distances are necessary to ensure that the lungs fit onto the 14-inch (35-cm) width of the IR (via reduced magnification of the body part) and, most important, to ensure that the heart is minimally magnified to allow the diagnosis of cardiac enlargement.

SOURCE-TO-IMAGE RECEPTOR DISTANCE IN THIS ATLAS

When a specific SID is necessary for optimal image quality, it is identified on the page of the specific projection. If not mentioned, it can be assumed that a *minimum* of 40 inches (102 cm) is recommended. Although sample exposure technique charts in each chapter identify the traditional SID of 40 inches (102 cm), this in no way implies that the authors advocate this distance when a greater SID from 44 to 48 inches (112 to 122 cm) may be obtained. Special SID projections vary from 30 inches (76 cm) to 120 inches (305 cm).

Source-to-Skin Distance

The distance between the focal spot of the radiography tube and skin of the patient is termed the *source-to-skin distance* (SSD) (see Fig. 1.32). This distance affects the dose to the patient and is addressed by the National Council on Radiation Protection (NCRP). Current NCRP recommendations state that the SSD *shall not* be less than 12 inches (<30 cm) and *should not* be less than 15 inches (<38 cm).[18] All modern radiographic and fluoroscopic equipment is constructed to prevent an SSD less than 12 inches (30 cm).

Collimation of Radiation Field

The radiation field, also called the exposure field, must be restricted to irradiate only the anatomy of interest. This restriction of the radiation field, called *collimation,* serves two purposes. First, it minimizes the amount of radiation to the patient by restricting exposure to essential anatomy only. Second, it reduces the amount of scatter radiation that can reach the IR, which reduces the potential for a reduction in contrast resolution (Fig. 1.33). Many experts regard collimation as the most important aspect of producing an optimal image. This is true regardless of the type of IR used.

The area of the radiation field is reduced to the required size by using a collimator or a specifically shaped diaphragm constructed of lead or other metal with high radiation absorption capability, attached to the tube housing and placed between the tube and the patient. Because of the metal attenuators of the beam restrictors, the peripheral radiation strikes and is absorbed by the collimator metal, and only x-rays in the exit aperture are transmitted as the exposure field.

For cassette-based or free detector IR systems, positive beam limitation (PBL), also called *automatic collimation,* is possible. The Bucky tray or other IR holder contains a mechanism that senses the dimensions of the IR and automatically collimates the beam to those dimensions. This prevents an exposure field larger than the IR when multiple IR sizes may be used. With fixed detector units that contain an enclosed IR, the system safeguards will

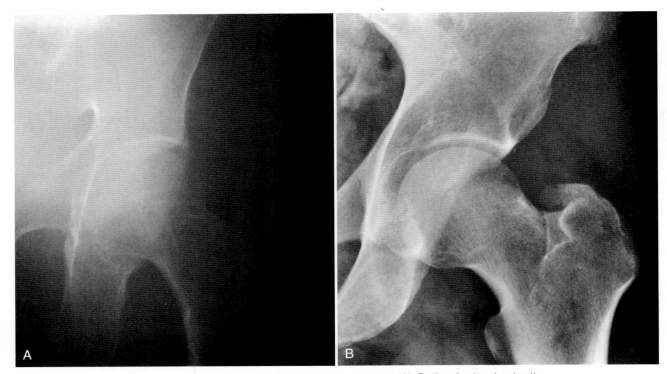

Fig. 1.33 Radiographs of the hip joint and acetabulum. (A) Collimator inadvertently opened to size 14 × 17 inches (35 × 43 cm). Scatter and secondary radiation have reduced radiographic contrast, and poor-quality image results. (B) Collimator set correctly to 8 × 10 inches (18 × 24 cm), improving radiographic contrast and visibility of detail.

not allow the exposure field to exceed the dimensions of the IR, but those dimensions may frequently exceed the dimensions of the anatomy to be imaged. In all cases, PBL is designed to limit only the exposure field to the dimensions of the IR. This does not take the place of proper collimation to the dimensions of the body part.

It is a violation of the ARRT Code of Ethics and ASRT Practice Standards to collimate larger than the required radiation field size. When a larger than required area is exposed, the patient receives unnecessary radiation to areas not needed on the image (Fig. 1.34A). In addition, the increased scatter radiation decreases the contrast resolution and spatial resolution in the image, reducing the ability to ensure an accurate diagnosis. The collimator should be manually adjusted to result in a field size that will include all anatomy pertinent to the radiographic procedure ordered (see Fig. 1.34B). These field dimensions and the extent of collimated field edges in relation to the anatomy of interest are included for all radiographic projections and positions included in the atlas.

The software included in the computers of DR systems allows for shuttering. Shuttering is used in DR to provide a black background around the original collimation edges. This black background eliminates the distracting clear areas and the associated brightness that comes through to the eyes. Radiographers may be tempted to open the collimator larger than is necessary and use the shuttering software to "crop-in" or mask unwanted peripheral image information and create the appearance of proper collimation. This technique irradiates patients unnecessarily, increases scatter radiation, and increases the radiation dose. In addition, the imaging team is exposed to legal liability because captured image information has been masked. *If it is later determined that pathology in this obscured area of the image was missed, causing a missed or delayed diagnosis, the radiographer may be held liable.* Shuttering is an image aesthetic only and should not serve as a substitute for proper and accurate collimation of the body part.

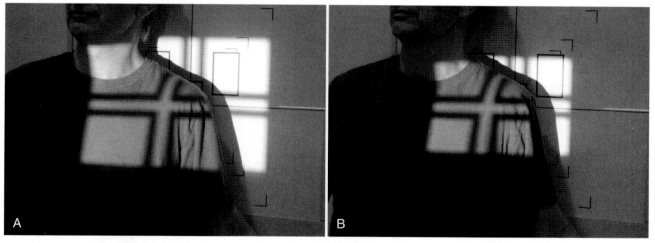

Fig. 1.34 (A) Collimation set too large for AP projection of the shoulder. Note unnecessary radiation of thyroid, sternum, and general thoracic tissues. With this large collimation, more than half of the radiation strikes the table directly, resulting in increased scatter. (B) Collimation set correctly to 10 × 12 inches (24 × 30 cm). Less tissue receives radiation, and less scatter is produced from the radiation striking the table.

Anatomic Markers

Each radiograph must include an appropriate marker that clearly identifies the patient's right (R) or left (L) side. Medicolegal requirements mandate that these markers be present. Radiographers and physicians must see them to determine the correct side of the patient or the correct limb. Markers typically are made of lead and are placed directly on the IR or tabletop. The marker is seen on the image, along with the anatomic part (Fig. 1.35). Box 1.3 presents the specific rules of marker placement.

Basic marker conventions include the following:
- R or L markers must be placed on all radiographs.
- The marker should never obscure anatomy.

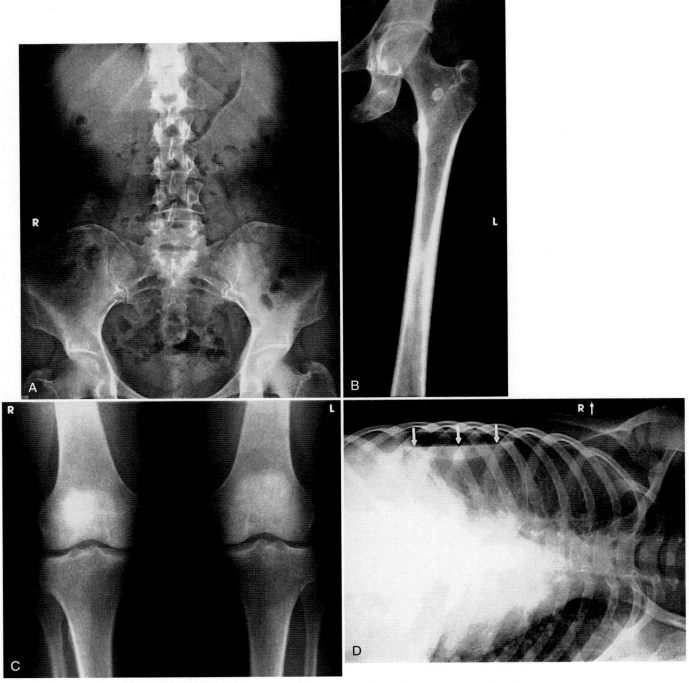

Fig. 1.35 (A) AP projection of the abdomen showing right (R) marker. (B) AP projection of the left limb showing left (L) marker on outer margin of the image. (C) AP projection of the right and left knees on one image showing R and L markers. (D) AP projection of the chest performed in the left lateral decubitus position showing R marker on the "upper" portion of IR.

- The marker should always be placed in The exposure field on the edge of the collimation border.
- The marker should always be placed outside of any lead shielding.
- R and L markers must be used with CR and DR digital imaging.

The development of digital imaging and the use of CR and DR have enabled an environment in which the R and L markers can be "annotated" or placed on the image electronically after exposure at the computer workstation. *This is not recommended* because of the great potential for error, which has legal implications related to side identification. This practice is especially problematic when patients are examined in the prone position. Anatomic markers should be placed directly on the CR cassette or the DR table/wall unit. The

exception to direct marker placement is in sterile (OR), trauma (ED), or infectious environments where marker placement may interfere with proper patient care. In addition, the practice of placing markers directly on the body part is not recommended because the marker is likely to be distorted on the image. This will make side identification difficult, thus defeating the purpose of using a marker.

The Radiograph

The image recorded by exposing any of the IR to x-rays is called a radiograph. Each step in performing a radiographic procedure must be completed accurately to ensure that the maximal amount of information is recorded on the image. The information that is obtained by performing

the radiographic procedure generally shows the presence or absence of abnormality or trauma. This information assists in diagnosis and treatment of the patient.

The radiographer must evaluate each radiograph to determine acceptability of image features, proper radiation safety practices, and whether the objectives for performing the procedure have been met. Additional image evaluation criteria to be considered include presence of patient identification, proper radiographic marker placement, proper collimation, evidence of required patient shielding, and absence of artifacts. This requires an understanding of anatomy, image geometry, image display characteristics, and image appearance of pathology. Figs. 1.36 through 1.39 are radiographs providing examples of image evaluation principles.

BOX 1.3

Specific marker placement recommendations

1. For AP and PA projections that include R and L sides of the body (head, spine, chest, abdomen, and pelvis), R marker is typically used.
2. For lateral projections of the head and trunk (head, spine, chest, abdomen, and pelvis), always mark the side closest to IR. If the left side is closest, use L marker. The marker is typically placed anterior to the anatomy.
3. For oblique projections that include R and L sides of the body (spine, chest, and abdomen), the side down, or nearest IR, is typically marked. For a right posterior oblique (RPO) position, mark R side.
4. For extremity projections, use appropriate R or L marker. The marker must be placed within the edge of the collimated x-ray beam.
5. For extremity projections that are done with two images on one IR, only one of the projections needs to be marked.
6. For extremity projections where R and L sides are imaged side by side on one IR (e.g., R and L, AP knees), R and L markers must be used to identify the two sides clearly.
7. For AP, PA, or oblique chest projections, marker is placed on the upper-outer corner so that the thoracic anatomy is not obscured.
8. For decubitus positions of the chest and abdomen, R or L marker should always be placed on the side up (opposite the side laid on) and away from the anatomy of interest.

Note: No matter which projection is performed, and no matter what position the patient is in, if R marker is used, it must be placed on the "right" side of the patient's body. If L marker is used, it must be placed on the "left" side of the patient's body.

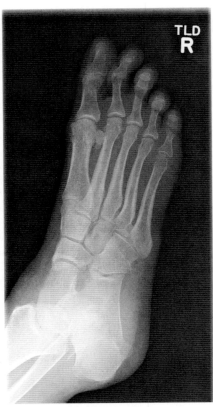

Fig. 1.36 AP oblique foot. All pertinent anatomy is included and demonstrated with good image quality. Optimum appearance and relationships of all important anatomy. Evidence of collimation and appropriately placed side marker. Long axis of foot is slightly angled in relation to the exposure field resulting in a collimated field slightly larger than necessary.

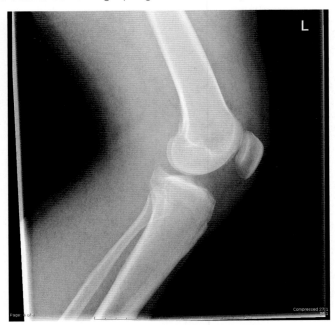

Fig. 1.38 Lateral knee. All pertinent anatomy is included and demonstrated with good image quality. Relationship of femoral condyles indicates slight overrotation of the knee because the medial condyle (identified as the larger, less distinct condyle) is anterior to the lateral condyle. Evidence of collimation. Appearance of side marker indicates it was likely added by annotation rather than placed on the IR prior to exposure, which is not recommended.

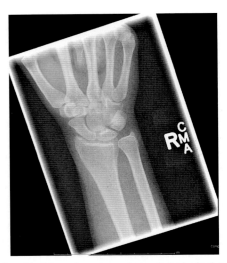

Fig. 1.37 PA wrist. All pertinent anatomy is included cnd demonstrated with good image quality. Optimum appearance and relationships of all important anatomy. Evidence of collimation and appropriately placed side marker. Exposure field and anatomy are angled on the display, which is common with DR but not ideal.

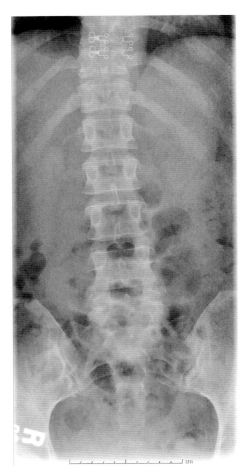

Fig. 1.39 AP lumbar spine. All pertinent anatomy is included and demonstrated with good image quality. Optimum appearance and relationships of all important anatomy. The slight rotation of the lumbar spine is related to a mild scoliosis, so not related to a positioning error. Evidence of collimation. Side marker is appropriately placed but is not oriented correctly. Metallic artifacts, probably bra hooks, are superimposed with the lower thoracic spine.

Display of Radiographs

Radiographs are generally oriented on the display device according to the preference of the interpreting physician. Because methods of displaying radiographic images have developed largely through custom, no fixed rules have been established. However, both the radiologist, who is responsible for making an interpretation on the basis of the radiographic examination, and the radiographer, who performs the examination, follow traditional standards of practice regarding orientation of radiographs on the display monitor.

ANATOMIC POSITION

Radiographs are usually oriented on the display monitor so that the person looking at the image sees the body part as though viewed facing the patient. This is called the *anatomic position*. When in the anatomic position, the patient stands erect with the face and eyes directed forward, arms extended by the sides with the palms of the hands facing forward, heels together, and toes pointing anteriorly (Fig. 1.40). When the radiograph is displayed in this manner, the patient's left side is on the viewer's right side and vice versa (Fig. 1.41). Medical professionals always describe the body, a body part, or a body movement as though it were in the anatomic position.

Posteroanterior and anteroposterior radiographs

Fig. 1.42A illustrates the anterior (front) aspect of the patient's chest placed closest to the IR for a *posteroanterior* (PA) projection. Fig. 1.42B illustrates the posterior (back) aspect of the patient's chest placed closest to the IR for an *anteroposterior* projection. Regardless of whether the anterior or posterior body surface was closest to the IR during the exposure, the radiograph is usually oriented in the anatomic position (Fig. 1.43). (Positioning terminology is fully described in Chapter 3.)

Exceptions to these guidelines include the hands, fingers, wrists, feet, and toes. Hand, finger, and wrist radiographs are routinely displayed with the digits (fingers) pointed to the ceiling. Foot and toe radiographs are placed on the illuminator, with the toes pointed to the ceiling. Hand, finger, wrist, toe, and foot radiographs are viewed from the perspective of the x-ray tube or exactly as the anatomy was projected onto the IR (Figs. 1.29 and 1.44). This perspective means that the individual looking at the radiograph is in the same position as the x-ray tube.

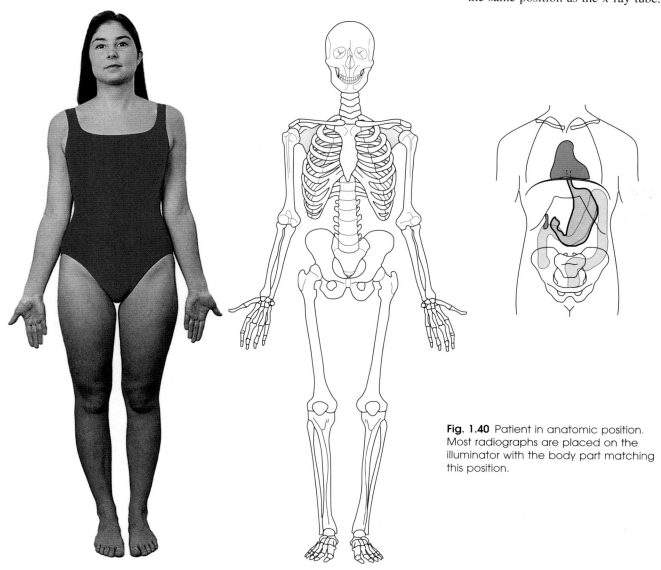

Fig. 1.40 Patient in anatomic position. Most radiographs are placed on the illuminator with the body part matching this position.

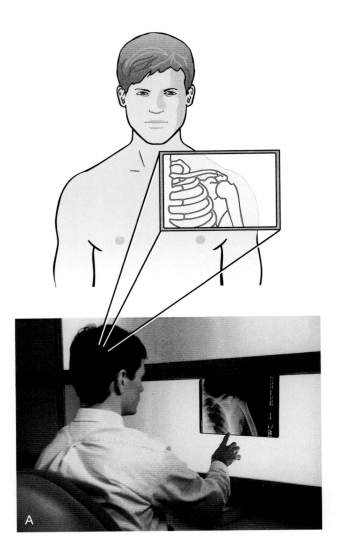

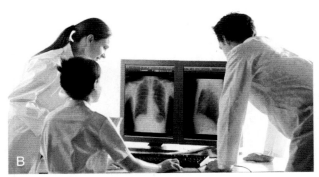

Fig. 1.41 (A) Radiologist interpreting radiograph of a patient's left shoulder. Radiograph is placed on the illuminator with the patient's left side on the viewer's right side. The radiologist spatially pictured the patient's anatomy in the anatomic position and placed the radiograph on the illuminator in that position. (B) Radiographs displayed correctly on a digital display. The same orientation rules apply to digital imaging.

(B, Courtesy Canon USA, Inc.)

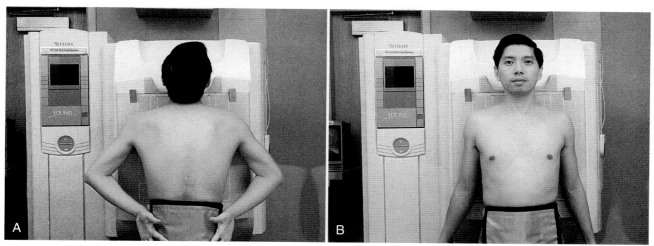

Fig. 1.42 (A) Patient positioned for PA projection of the chest. Anterior aspect of the chest is closest to IRs. (B) Patient positioned for AP projection of the chest. Posterior aspect of the chest is closest to IRs.

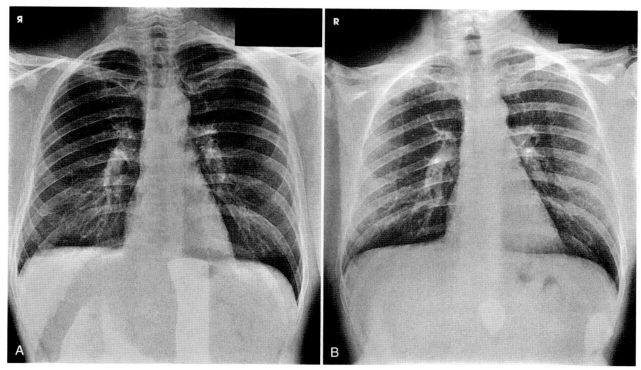

Fig. 1.43 (A) PA projection of the chest. (B) AP projection of the chest. Both radiographs are correctly displayed with the anatomy in the anatomic position even though the patient was positioned differently. Note that the patient's left side is on your right, as though the patient were facing you.

Lateral radiographs

Lateral radiographs are obtained with the patient's right or left side placed against the IR. The patient is generally placed on the illuminator in the same orientation as though the viewer were looking at the patient from the perspective of the x-ray tube at the side where the x-rays first enter the patient—exactly like radiographs of the hands, wrists, feet, and toes. Another way to describe this is to display the radiograph so that the side of the patient closest to the IR during the procedure is also the side in the image closest to the illuminator. A patient positioned for a left lateral chest radiograph is depicted in Fig. 1.45. The resulting left lateral chest radiograph is placed on the illuminator as shown in Fig. 1.46. A right lateral chest position and its accompanying radiograph would be positioned and displayed as the opposite of that shown in Figs. 1.45 and 1.46.

Oblique radiographs

Oblique radiographs are obtained when the patient's body is rotated so that the projection obtained is not frontal, posterior, or lateral (Fig. 1.47). These radiographs are viewed with the patient's anatomy placed in the anatomic position (Fig. 1.48).

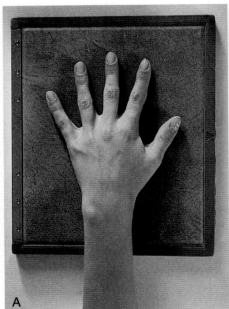
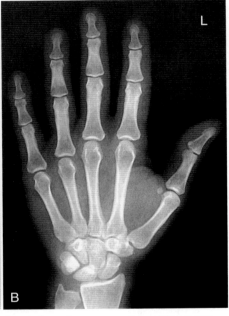

Fig. 1.44 (A) Left hand positioned on IR. This view is from the perspective of the x-ray tube. (B) Radiograph of the left hand is displayed on the monitor in the same manner, with the digits pointed upward.

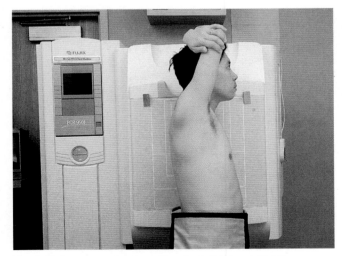

Fig. 1.45 Proper patient position for left lateral chest radiograph. The left side of the patient is placed against the IR.

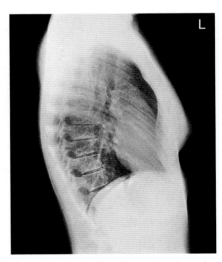

Fig. 1.46 Left lateral chest radiograph placed on illuminator with the anatomy seen from the perspective of the x-ray tube.

Other radiographs

Many other less commonly performed radiographic projections are described throughout this atlas. The most common method of displaying the radiograph that is used in the radiology department and in most clinical practice areas is generally in the anatomic position or from the perspective of the x-ray tube; however, there are exceptions. Some physicians prefer to view all radiographs from the perspective of the x-ray tube rather than in the anatomic position. A neurosurgeon operates on the posterior aspect of the body and does not display spine radiographs in the anatomic position or from the perspective of the x-ray tube. The radiographs are displayed with the patient's right side on the surgeon's right side as though looking at the posterior aspect of the patient. What the surgeon sees on the radiograph is exactly what is seen in the open body part during surgery.

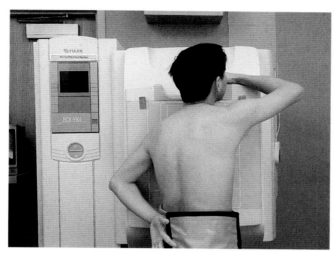

Fig. 1.47 A patient placed in LAO position for PA oblique projection of the chest.

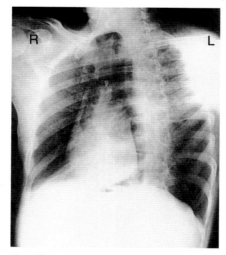

Fig. 1.48 PA oblique chest radiograph is placed on illuminator with the anatomy in the anatomic position. The patient's left side is on your right, as though the patient were facing you.

Identification of Radiographs

All radiographs must include the patient and procedure information required by institutional policy. This information customarily includes (Fig. 1.49A):

- Date
- Patient's name or identification number
- Right or left marker
- Institution identity

Correct identification is vital and should always be confirmed. Identification is absolutely vital in comparison studies, on follow-up examinations, and in medicolegal cases. Radiographers should develop the habit of rechecking the identification side marker just before placing it on the IR. The radiographer associates the patient's identification and other data with each radiograph via the computer workstation (see Fig. 1.49B and C). However, side markers should still be physically placed on the IR. The workstation should not be used to add, or annotate, *right* and *left* markers to the image.

Other patient identification information includes the patient's age or date of birth, the time of day, and the name of the radiographer or attending physician. For certain examinations the radiograph should include such information as cumulative time after introduction of contrast medium (e.g., 5 minutes post injection), the position of the patient (e.g., upright, decubitus), or with other markings specified by the institution. This additional information is usually added by annotation of the completed radiograph during postexposure evaluation.

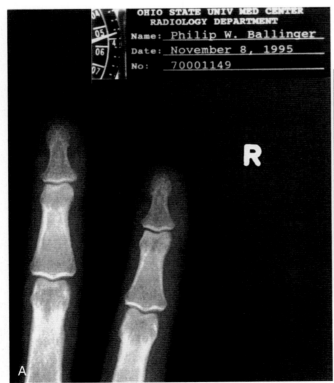

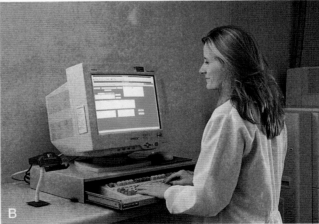

Fig. 1.49 (A) All radiographs must be permanently identified and should contain a minimum of four identification markings. (B) Radiographer using CR system and entering a patient's identification data into a computer in the radiography room. (C) Resulting laser image showing the patient's information.

Working Effectively With Obese Patients

Radiology departments are having a difficult time acquiring and interpreting images of obese patients. One study found that the number of radiology procedures that were difficult to interpret because of obesity doubled over the previous 15 years.[19] According to the CDC, approximately 64% of Americans are overweight, obese, or morbidly obese.[20] More than 72 million adults are obese, and more than 6 million are morbidly obese (Fig. 1.50). The prevalence of obesity in children has been steadily increasing. Over the past 25 years the number of obese children has nearly tripled. Approximately 15% of children 6 to 9 years old are obese.[21] *Obesity* is defined as an increase in body weight caused by excessive accumulation of fat. More specifically, obesity is quantified by the body mass index (BMI).[22] A BMI of 30 to 39.9 is classified as obese.

A BMI greater than 40 is classified as morbidly obese, or approximately 100 lb overweight. The BMI is not of primary importance when radiographic examinations are performed; the patient's *body diameter* and *weight* are the two important considerations. One or both of these factors can determine whether a radiographic examination can be performed.

Obese patients have an effect on the functionality of the imaging equipment, and many obese patients cannot be placed onto radiographic or computed tomography (CT) tables. Patient transportation to the imaging department, as well as transfer to and from imaging equipment, are more challenging. The increased body size and weight of obese patients have a negative impact on image quality and create technical challenges for the imaging professional. However, these challenges must be met because the popularity of bariatric surgery has increased the demand for radiographic procedures in obese patients.

EQUIPMENT

Manufacturers of imaging equipment have defined weight limits. The structural integrity and function of equipment and motors are typically warrantied by manufacturers up to the stated weight only. Radiographic table weight limits cannot be exceeded without voiding the warranty. Fluoroscopy towers have a maximum diameter, and many obese patients cannot fit under the tower of those with undertable units. Over-table IR units have a much greater distance between the tube and the table, making them popular for use with obese patients (Fig. 1.51); CT and magnetic resonance imaging (MRI) scanners have gantry and bore diameters that cannot accommodate some obese patients. Table 1.7 lists the current industry standard weight limits and maximum aperture diameters. For CT and MRI the aperture diameter is accurate in the horizontal plane. The vertical plane must take into consideration the table thickness

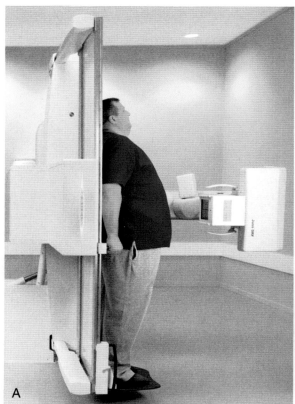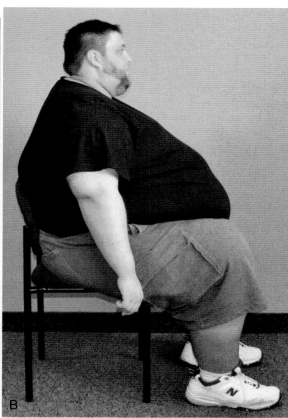

Fig. 1.50 (A) Obese patient. (B) Morbidly obese patient.

entering the gantry or bore. The table takes up 15 to 18 cm of the stated vertical diameter; this limits many obese patients from having CT or MRI examinations. Radiology departments without appropriate equipment cannot perform examinations on patients who weigh more than 350 to 450 lb. Radiographers must be aware of the weight and aperture limits of the radiographic equipment in their department. The radiology department should have a protocol for working with obese patients, and all equipment should be marked with the limits.

To accommodate obese patients, most radiography equipment manufacturers are redesigning their equipment and increasing table weights and aperture dimensions. Table 1.8 shows the limits of the current equipment modified for obese patients. Radiographic and fluoroscopic table weight limits have doubled to 700 lb. CT and MRI table weights and aperture openings have also increased.

TRANSPORTATION

Transportation of obese patients may be difficult with standard equipment. Obese patients require larger wheelchairs (Fig. 1.52) and larger transport beds or stretchers. Some hospitals have installed larger doorways to accommodate larger transportation equipment. The availability of these special chairs and beds may be limited and may affect the scheduling of these patients. One manufacturer[23] has designed a special cart that can hold patients weighing 750 lb; this cart has a 34-inch pad width. Many obese patients, unless they are hospitalized, are able to walk around and access clinics and imaging centers. However, their weight becomes an issue when they have to lie on an imaging table. For this reason, morbidly obese patients who can stand are often imaged in an upright position. If images are to be produced using an upright radiographic-fluoroscopic table, the footboard should be removed, allowing the patient to stand directly on the floor. Under these circumstances, it is recommended that a large, sturdy bench be kept available in case the patient becomes unstable and needs to sit during the radiographic or fluoroscopic procedure.

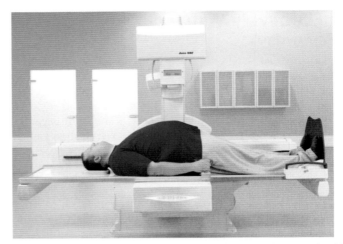

Fig. 1.51 Over-table digital fluoroscopy unit. Note the increased source-to-skin distance achievable with these units.

(Used with permission from Philips Healthcare, Bothell, WA.)

TABLE 1.7

Industry standard weight limit and maximum aperture diameter by imaging technique

Imaging technique	Weight limit	Maximum aperture diameter (cm)
Fluoroscopy	350 lb (159 kg)	45
4- to 16-multidetector CT	450 lb (205 kg)	70*
Cylindrical bore MRI, 1.5-3.0 T	350 lb (159 kg)	60*
Vertical field MRI, 0.3-1.0 T	550 lb (250 kg)	55*

*Aperture is accurate in horizontal plane only. For vertical plane, approximately 15 to 18 cm must be subtracted from diameter to account for table thickness.

TABLE 1.8

Advances in weight limit and maximum aperture diameter by imaging technique

Imaging technique	Weight limit	Maximum aperture diameter (cm)
Fluoroscopy	700 lb (318 kg)	60
16-Multidetector CT	680 lb (308 kg)	90*
Cylindric bore MRI, 1.5 T	550 lb (250 kg)	70*
Vertical field MRI, 0.3-1.0 T	550 lb (250 kg)	55*

*Aperture is accurate in horizontal plane only. For vertical plane, about 15 to 18 cm must be subtracted from diameter to account for table thickness.

An important consideration during transportation and transfer of obese patients is the potential risk of injury to the radiographer and other health care workers during movement and positioning of patients. Radiographic examinations of obese patients who are hospitalized must be coordinated carefully between the radiology department and the patient's nursing section. Appropriate measurements must be made in the patient's room in advance by trained radiology personnel. An obese patient should not be transported to the radiology department and find on arrival that he or she cannot be accommodated.

An appropriate number of staff must be available to ensure that moving assistance is appropriate. Transfer of a patient from the cart to the radiographic table may require a greater number of personnel, up to 8 to 10 individuals, than is specified by department policy. Obese patients are not manually lifted; they are moved by sliding. Although traditional sliding equipment is not sufficiently wide or sturdy, newer sliding technology that rides on a thin film of air is allowing safer and easier movement of obese patients with less personnel (Fig. 1.53). In addition, creative use of high-capacity power lifts is allowing transfer of obese patients in situations where sliding is not practical (Fig. 1.54). Regardless of the transfer method used, it is imperative that proper body mechanics be used by all personnel moving these patients.

In the event that a morbidly obese patient falls or collapses to the floor, procedures must be predetermined to move the patient to a stretcher or cart for transportation to an appropriate location for evaluation and possible treatment. Hospitals treating significant numbers of morbidly obese bariatric surgery patients have developed such procedures. For example, St. Vincent Carmel Hospital, a bariatric center of excellence in Indianapolis, Indiana, has developed a "code lift" process. Appropriate personnel from a variety of departments respond with appropriate equipment to safely move the fallen patient, with minimal risk to staff.

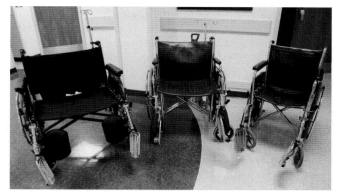

Fig. 1.52 Wheelchairs: extra-large for morbidly obese patients (*left*), large for obese patients (*center*), and standard for smaller patients.

(Courtesy Department of Radiology, St. Vincent Carmel Hospital, Carmel, IN.)

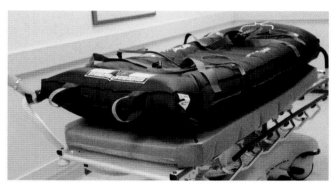

Fig. 1.53 A patient-moving device that rides on a thin film of air. The straps and convenient handholds allow only a few people to securely move very large patients.

(Courtesy Department of Radiology, St. Vincent Carmel Hospital, Carmel, IN.)

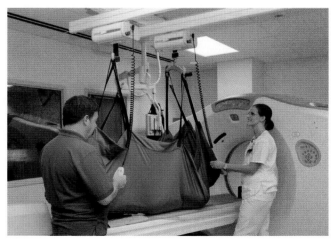

Fig. 1.54 Twin 500-lb capacity power lifts, attached to a ceiling-mounted rail system, allow very large patients to be safety lifted from a bed or a stretcher to the 650-lb capacity CT table. Interdepartmental cooperation is essential because the hoist sling is usually positioned under the patient before transport to the CT suite.

(Courtesy Department of Radiology, St. Vincent Carmel Hospital, Carmel, IN.)

COMMUNICATION

For the most part, communications with obese patients are no different than with nonobese patients. However, communication with obese patients may require personnel to be more aware of the issues of obesity. The radiographer must be able to assess the difficulties created by the limitations of equipment in handling an obese patient and must be able to communicate with the patient without offending him or her. The dignity of the patient must be kept in mind. Sensitivity training should be provided by the hospital or clinic. Reference to the patient's weight should never be made. The radiographer should be sensitive and display compassion. This can be accomplished by clearly explaining the procedure to gain the patient's confidence and trust. After the patient's trust and cooperation have been obtained, it is easier to communicate effectively if any problems or concerns with the examination arise.

There should never be any discussion about the patient in the radiographic room and no discussion within hearing distance of the patient about poor image quality or the difficulty involved in obtaining images. If the radiologist and patient's physician together determine that the patient's weight allows radiographic images to be made, the examination should proceed in the same manner as with any other patient. Although more staff may be needed for transfer or positioning purposes, communications and performance of the examination should remain the same.

IMAGING CHALLENGES

When the patient is on the imaging table, it is imperative that he or she is centered accurately on the table. This is necessary because it may be impossible to palpate traditional landmarks such as the anterior superior iliac spine (ASIS) and the iliac crest (see Chapter 3 for positioning landmarks). One of the most important considerations in positioning an obese patient is the need to recognize that the bony skeleton and most organs have not changed in position and the organs are not larger. Most of what is seen physically on these patients is fat. In Fig. 1.55, although the soft tissue dimensions of patient B are much greater than those of patient A, the skeleton of patient B is approximately the same size as that of patient A. and most organs are located in their normal positions. The only exception would be seen in morbidly obese patients, in whom the width of the thoracic cage and ribs may be expanded by 2 inches, the stomach may be slightly larger, and the colon may be spread out more across the width of the abdomen (Fig. 1.56). Most positioning landmarks used on obese patients will serve as reference points in the midsagittal plane of the patient.

Radiographic projections of the skull, cervical spine, and upper limb are obtainable on all obese patients, as are projections of the lower limb from the knee distally. Shoulder and femur projections

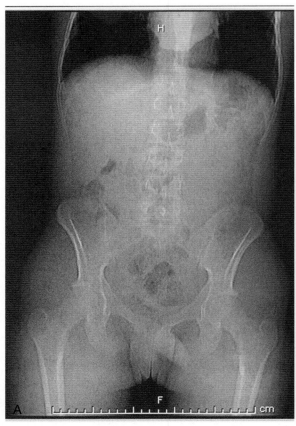
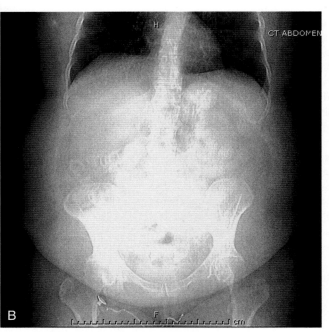

Fig. 1.55 CT abdomen scouts of (A) nonobese patient and (B) obese patient. Note similar skeletal size and organ locations, although patient B has much greater external dimensions.

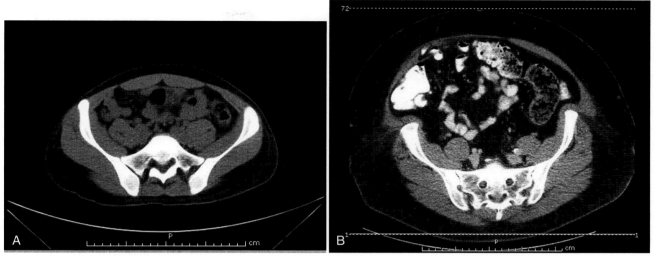

Fig. 1.56 (A) Axial CT image of abdomen on average-size patient. (B) Axial CT image of abdomen on obese patient demonstrating anterior and lateral displacement of colon and small bowel. However, note that the colon is still well within the skin margins.

may be difficult to position but are usually obtainable. All projections of the thorax including lungs, abdomen, thoracic and lumbar spines, pelvis, and hips are very challenging to position and may be impossible to obtain in morbidly obese patients. The patient's lack of mobility makes lateral hip projections virtually impossible. Fig. 1.57 shows that most fat accumulates around the trunk, particularly around the abdomen, pelvis, and hips. Imaging of organs such as the stomach, small bowel, and colon may be very difficult, if not impossible, on morbidly obese patients. CT may be the only imaging alternative if the equipment can support the weight and girth of these patients.

Landmarks

Finding traditional positioning landmarks may be possible in some obese patients and impossible in morbidly obese patients. It is appropriate to enlist the patient's assistance in identifying landmarks if possible. This gives patients a sense of being involved in their examination. In some obese patients the abdominal fat is very soft, movable, and layered in "folds." For these patients the radiographer can gently move or push the folds of skin out of the way to palpate the ASIS or iliac crest. The patient should be informed of what the radiographer is doing every step of the way. The *jugular notch* may be the only palpable landmark on morbidly obese patients. Traditional landmarks such as the xiphoid, ASIS, iliac crest, pubic

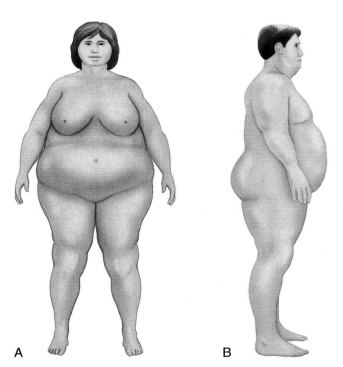

Fig. 1.57 Large amount of body fat that surrounds the abdomen, pelvis, hips, and upper femora on obese patients. Dimensions shown are from actual patient measurements.

symphysis, and greater trochanter may be impossible to palpate. The radiographer should not attempt to push and prod to find these landmarks. Fig. 1.58 illustrates that, although traditional landmarks would be difficult to palpate because of excess body fat, if the patient's chin is raised, the jugular notch can be palpated.

The jugular notch is an essential landmark when obese patients are imaged. Most projections of the thorax, abdomen, and pelvis can be obtained using only this landmark to perform the following localization procedure. Two items should be available in the radiographic room—tongue depressors and a tape measure.

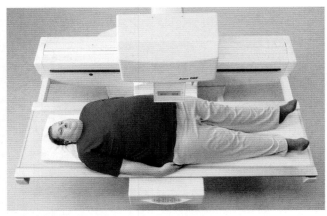

Fig. 1.58 Obese patient. Traditional landmarks would be impossible to palpate. With the chin raised, the jugular notch can be palpated.

(Used with permission from Philips Healthcare, Bothell, WA.)

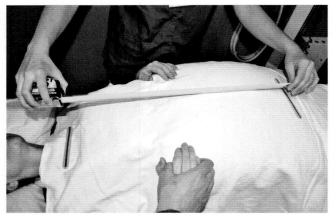

Fig. 1.59 Radiographer measuring jugular notch–to–pubic symphysis plane.

When the jugular notch is found, a tongue depressor should be placed on the notch. With the tape measure kept horizontal, the radiographer measures straight down the midsagittal plane, from the jugular notch point to the pubic symphysis (Fig. 1.59). The pubic symphysis is found at the following distances from the jugular notch:
Patient height: <5 ft: 21 inches
5 to 6 ft: 22 inches
>6 ft: 24 inches

The second tongue depressor is placed at the level of the pubic symphysis. The two depressors present a visual indication of the superior and inferior boundaries of the trunk of the body. Note that the symphysis will not be palpated because of the pendiculum (the fat skirt that hangs down over the symphysis). The indicators above will determine its location. When the radiographer knows where these two anatomic points are, nearly all projections of the trunk can be obtained with moderate accuracy. The bottom edge of a 14 × 17-inch (35 × 43-cm) IR placed lengthwise at the pubic symphysis shows the abdomen and lumbar spine. If the bottom edge of the IR is placed crosswise, it shows the pelvis and hips. The first thoracic vertebra (T1) is located approximately 2 inches (5 cm) above the jugular notch. An understanding of the landmarks related to body structures described in Chapter 3 enables the radiographer to position for nearly all projections of the trunk.

Oblique and lateral projections

Caution should be used when turning patients on their side for oblique and lateral projections. Turning should always be done with the assistance of the patient and with an appropriate number of additional personnel. Positioning aids or equipment should be used to prevent injury to the patient and personnel. Before the patient is turned, measurements should be taken of the body part width to determine whether the exposure technique can be made. Oblique and lateral projections of the hips, lumbar spine, lumbosacral area, sacrum, coccyx, and, in some patients, thoracic spine may be prohibited because of x-ray tube limits. Oblique and lateral projections may be impossible to obtain on a morbidly obese patient. "Crosstable" projections also may be impossible because of the patient's size and the very large amount of scatter radiation produced. Lower grid ratios in grid holders are typically used for these exposures and may not aid in improving image quality. In limited instances, two exposures can be made in rapid succession. However, the patient must be able to hold very still, and this works only on bone projections.

Image receptor sizes and collimation

Based on the exterior dimensions of obese patients, it may seem that larger IRs are needed to image these patients. In most instances, this is not the case. If care is taken to find landmarks, in particular the jugular notch and the pubic symphysis, relatively accurate positioning can be accomplished. Collimation is one of the most important considerations when obese patients are imaged. Setting the collimator to the smallest dimensions possible reduces scatter radiation. The reduced scatter increases contrast, which enables improved visibility of the structures (Fig. 1.60). The use of standard-size IRs and standard collimation settings for DR keeps scatter radiation to low levels, and scatter radiation fog on the image is reduced. *The collimator should never be set larger than the size of the IR.* This requires referring to the field size indicators on the collimator, rather than using the projected light field size as an indicator of size at the IR.

With DR and the availability of the 17 × 17-inch (43 × 43-cm) flat-panel detector built into the table (see Fig. 1.30D),

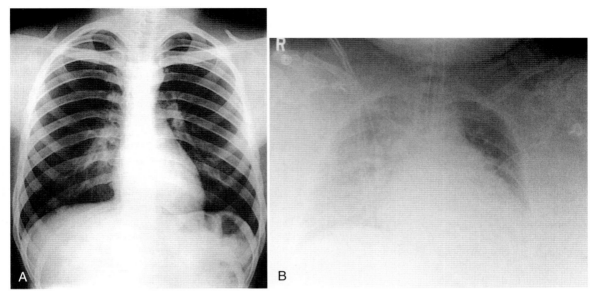

Fig. 1.60 (A) Chest radiograph on 160-lb patient. Note very good contrast and visibility of structures. (B) Chest radiograph on 360-lb patient. Note reduced contrast and fogging on image. However, a reasonable image was obtained.

the radiographer may be tempted to use the maximum size of this field on large patients. *This temptation should be avoided.* This very large collimator setting produces more scatter, which degrades overall image quality. Collimating larger than the traditional 14 × 17 inches (35 × 43 cm) for body parts that require this dimension images only more fat. Recall from Fig. 1.55 that within the large body are a standard-size skeletal frame and organs. A significantly improved diagnostic image is obtained on obese patients when IRs and collimation settings of appropriate size are used. For colon and other abdominal images, it may be necessary to take multiple images on quadrants of the body[22] using smaller collimation settings. When DR is used to image obese patients, radiographers should use collimation settings for the various projections as indicated in this atlas.

Field light size

When the collimator size is set automatically for IRs in the Bucky or manually on the collimator for DR equipment, the field light is visible on a nonobese patient's body relatively close to the actual dimensions of the IR (Fig. 1.61A). This light gives the radiographer an accurate visual indication of where the radiation field falls. On obese patients, in whom the vertical dimension of the thorax and abdomen is very large (see Fig. 1.50B), the field

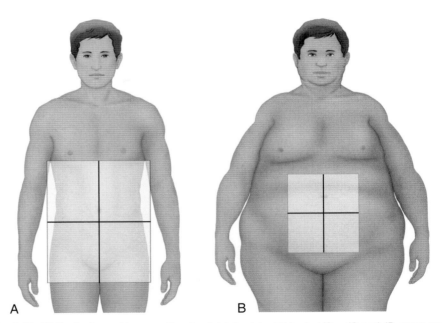

Fig. 1.61 (A) Illustration of how collimator light for 14 × 17-inch (43 × 43-cm) IR appears on normal-size patient with 21-cm abdomen measurement. The light is very close in dimension to IR size. (B) Collimator light shown for same-size IR on obese patient with 45-cm vertical abdomen measurement. Although collimator is set to same dimensions, light field appears small on top of the patient.

light visible on top of the patient appears much smaller than the IR size because the abdomen is closer to the collimator bulb and less light divergence occurs (see Fig. 1.61B). The natural tendency may be to open the collimator when this small field is seen. *The collimator should not*

be opened larger than the size of the IR or the stated collimator dimensions for DR. The radiographer must understand that although the field size visually appears small on top of the patient, the radiation field diverges to expose the entire IR size.

EXPOSURE FACTORS

Modified x-ray exposure techniques need to be used on obese patients. The main factors have to be increased, including mA, kVp, and exposure time. The major limitation in obtaining images of obese patients is inadequate penetration of the body part. This situation results in increased quantum mottle (noise) and decreased contrast resolution. The increased exposure time required for these patients can also contribute to motion artifacts in the image. The most important adjustment that should be made is an increase in the kVp. Increasing the kVp increases the penetration of the x-ray beam. Although mA and exposure time (mAs) have to be increased, caution should be used in increasing the mA. Greater exposures can be obtained safely by using lower mA settings and longer exposure times. (Refer to a tube rating chart in a physics text.)

Body motion is not a major problem in imaging obese patients because the weight of the patient prevents most body parts from moving, and mA settings of approximately 320 can be used. Although this setting may increase exposure time, most obese patients can hold their breath with

an explanation of the importance doing so. With repeated use of high-exposure factors, the x-ray tube can become very hot. Radiographers should ensure that adequate cooling of the anode and tube as a whole occurs; this can be accomplished by simply taking more time between exposures.

Focal spot

The focal spot in the x-ray tube is controlled by the mA that is selected. The mA for obese patient radiographs may be higher than 250 to 320 mA, which may automatically engage the large focus. Use of the small focal spot, which enables greater recorded detail, may be restricted to the distal limbs because of the higher exposure techniques. Radiographers must have a full understanding of the focal spot limits for the machines they use. These should be posted for use with obese patient projections.

Bucky and grid

Use of a Bucky grid or a mobile grid can minimize scatter radiation significantly. The grid is automatically used when standard projections are obtained on the x-ray table and for some cross-table lateral

images of limbs. Although a grid is never used for elbow, ankle, and leg projections on nonobese patients, it can significantly improve image quality on obese patients, in particular on morbidly obese patients (Fig. 1.62). Radiology departments should have a high-ratio mobile grid available for use with obese patients.

Automatic exposure control and anatomically programmed radiography systems

AEC and anatomically programmed radiography (APR) systems are widely used in radiology departments to control technical factors "automatically." Machine-set exposure factors will frequently be inappropriate for obese patients, so kVp, mA, exposure time, AEC detectors, and focal spot should be *manually adjusted*. With AEC the radiographer should ensure that a high kVp and a moderate mA are used. In addition, a backup time greater than the customary 150% of anticipated mAs will likely be required. The radiology department should maintain a special exposure technique chart for obese patients, similar to a special chart used for pediatric patients. When possible, all three AEC detectors should be activated.

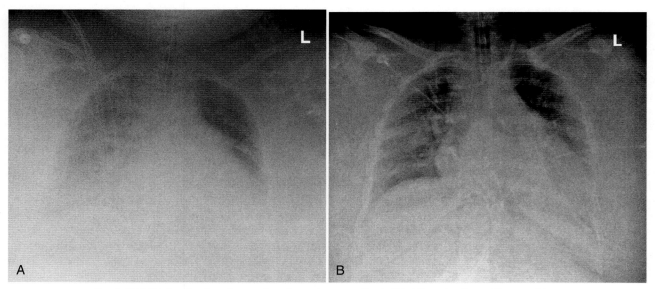

Fig. 1.62 Mobile chest radiographs of an obese patient. (A) AP projection with no grid. (B) AP projection of same patient using a grid. Note increased contrast resolution in image B.

Mobile radiography

Mobile radiography machines may be used for imaging obese patients; however, their use is very limited. Because the x-ray tubes on these machines have limited ratings, exposures high enough to penetrate these patients can be difficult to obtain. However, the greater dynamic range of digital IRs is allowing all but the largest patients to be imaged. Depending on the size of the patient, mobile projections may be restricted to chest and limbs only. The mobile machine should have a special technique chart outlining the technical factors used for this group of patients.

Radiation dose

Radiographers must use caution in all aspects of working with obese patients, including keeping repeat exposures to a minimum. A study of radiation doses to obese patients having bariatric surgery showed a "fourfold" dose increase compared with nonobese patients having the same examinations.[24] Doses to these patients reached 45 mSv (4500 mrem). Precautions must be taken to minimize patient dose. The radiologist should be involved in evaluating the justification of any radiologic procedure on an obese patient. Radiographers should be especially cautious when holding a limb or an IR during an x-ray exposure on an obese patient. The increased exposure techniques prompt increased scatter, which reaches the person holding the patient. If someone has to hold an obese patient, when possible, the person should stand at a right angle (90 degrees) to the CR for maximum scatter protection. (See Chapter 20 for further information.)

Special technical considerations must be followed when working with obese and morbidly obese patients. Box 1.4 summarizes these technical considerations.

BOX 1.4

Technical considerations for working effectively with obese patients

- Warm up x-ray tube before making any exposures.
- Use lower mA settings (<320).
- Use higher kVp settings.
- Do not make repeated exposures near x-ray tube loading limit.
- Use the large focal spot for all but distal limbs.
- Do not use APR systems to determine exposure technique.
- When using AEC systems, ensure kVp is high enough and mA is moderate.
- Collimate to the size of IR or smaller.
- With DR, collimate to suggested field size for the projection.
- Avoid collimating to the maximum 17 × 17-inch (43 × 43-cm) size of the flat-panel DR detector.
- Maintain special exposure technique chart for obese patient projections.
- Stand at right angles (90 degrees) to the central ray when holding an obese patient.

ABBREVIATIONS USED IN CHAPTER 1

AEC	automatic exposure control
ALARA	as low as reasonably achievable
AP	anteroposterior
APR	anatomically programmed radiography
ARRT	American Registry of Radiologic Technologists
ASIS	anterior superior iliac spine
ASRT	American Society of Radiologic Technologists
BMI	body mass index
CAMRT	Canadian Association of Medical Radiation Technologists
CCD	charge-coupled device
CDC	Centers for Disease Control and Prevention
cm	centimeter
CR[a]	central ray
CR[a]	computed radiography
CT	computed tomography
DR	digital radiography
ED	emergency department
IP	image plate
IR	image receptor
JRCERT	Joint Review Committee on Education in Radiologic Technology
kVp	kilovolt peak
L	left
LAO	left anterior oblique
mA	milliamperage
mAs	milliampere second
MMD	mean marrow dose
MRI	magnetic resonance imaging
NCRP	National Council on Radiation Protection
OID	object-to-image receptor distance
OR	operating room
PA	posteroanterior
PBL	positive beam limitation
PPE	personal protective equipment
PSP	photostimulable storage phosphor
R	right
RA	radiologist assistant
RPA	radiology practitioner assistant
RPO	right posterior oblique
SID	source-to–image receptor distance
SSD	source-to-skin distance
TFT	thin-film transistor

[a]Note that there are two different abbreviations for CR.
See Addendum A for a summary of all abbreviations used in Volume 1.

References

1. American Registry of Radiologic Technologists Standards of Ethics, September 1, 2016.
2. Centers for Disease Control and Prevention. cdc.gov.
3. The Joint Commission, Oakbrook Terrace, IL.
4. *Age-specific competence*, Oakbrook Terrace, IL, 1998, The Joint Commission.
5. *Assessing hospital staff competence*, Oakbrook Terrace, IL, 2002, The Joint Commission.
6. Ferlic; Ferlic Filter Company LLC, White Bear Lake, MN.
7. Boomerang; Octostop, Inc., Laval, Canada.
8. ClearPb; Nuclear Associates, Hicksville, NY.
9. Frank ED, Stears JG, Gray JE, et al: Use of the posterioanterior projection: a method of reducing x-ray exposure to specific radiosensitive organs, *Radiol Technol* 54(5): 343-347, 1983.
10. Eastman TR: Digital systems require x-ray charts too, *Radiol Technol* 67(4):354, 1996.
11. Gray JE et al: *Quality control in diagnostic imaging*, Rockville, MD, 1983, Aspen.
12. Eastman TR: Get back to the basics of radiography, *Radiol Technol* 68(4):285, 1997.
13. Bureau of Radiological Health: *Gonad shielding in diagnostic radiology*, Pub No. (FDA) 75-8024, Rockville, MD, 1975, The Bureau.
14. Eastman TR: X-ray film quality and national contracts, *Radiol Technol* 69:12, 1997.
15. Kebart RC, James CD: Benefits of increasing focal film distance, *Radiol Technol* 62(6):434-442, 1991.
16. Brennan PC, Nash M: Increasing SID: an effective dose-reducing tool for lateral lumbar spine investigations, *Radiography* 4:251, 1998.
17. Carlton RR, Adler AM: *Principles of radiographic imaging*, ed 5. Albany, NY, Cengage Learning, 2012.
18. National Council on Radiation Protection: *NCRP Report 102*, Bethesda, MD, 1989, The Council.
19. Trenker SW: Imaging of morbid obesity procedures and their complications, *Abdom Imaging* 34(3):335-344, 2008.
20. Department of Health and Human Services, Centers for Disease Control and Prevention: Overweight and obesity: obesity trends: 1991-2001 prevalence of obesity among U.S. adults by state-behavioral risk factor surveillance system 2001. Available at: www.cdc.gov/nccdphp/dnpa/obesity/trend/prev_reg htm.
21. Choudhary AK, Donnelly LF, Racadio JM, Strife JL: Diseases associated with childhood obesity, *AJR Am J Roentgenol* 188(4):1118-1130, 2007.
22. Uppot RN, Sahani DV, Hahn PF, et al: Impact of obesity on medical imaging and image-guided intervention, *AJR Am J Roentgenol* 188(2):433-440, 2007.
23. Pedigo, Vancouver, WA. Available at: www.pedigo.com. Accessed April 1, 2010.
24. Rampado O, Luberto L, Faletti R, et al: Radiation dose evaluations during radiological contrast studies in patients with morbid obesity, *Radiol Med* 113(8): 1229-1240, 2008.

2

GENERAL ANATOMY AND RADIOGRAPHIC POSITIONING TERMINOLOGY

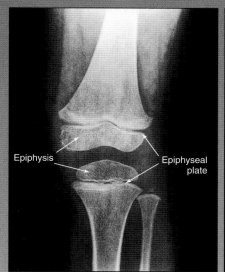

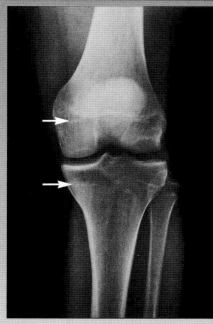

Epiphysis

Epiphyseal plate

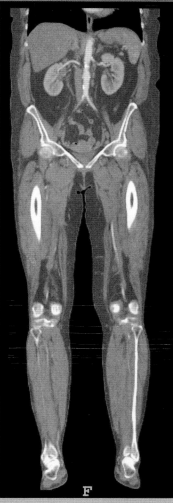

F

General Anatomy

Radiographers must possess a thorough knowledge of anatomy, physiology, and osteology to obtain radiographs that show the desired body part. *Anatomy* is the term applied to the science of the structure of the body. *Physiology* is the study of the function of the body organs. *Osteology* is the detailed study of the body of knowledge related to the bones of the body.

Radiographers also must have a general understanding of all body systems and their functions. Particular attention must be given to gaining a thorough understanding of the skeletal system and the surface landmarks used to locate different body parts. The radiographer must be able to visualize mentally the internal structures that are to be radiographed. By using external landmarks, the radiographer should be able to properly position body parts to obtain the best diagnostic radiographs possible.

BODY PLANES

The full dimension of the human body as viewed in the *anatomic position* (see Chapter 1) can be effectively subdivided through the use of imaginary body planes. These planes slice through the body at designated levels from all directions. The following four fundamental body planes referred to regularly in radiography are illustrated in Fig. 2.1A:

• Sagittal
• Coronal
• Horizontal
• Oblique

Sagittal plane

A sagittal plane divides the entire body or a body part into right and left segments. The plane passes vertically through the body from front to back (see Fig. 2.1A and B). The *midsagittal plane* is a specific sagittal plane that passes through the midline of the body and divides it into equal right and left halves (see Fig. 2.1C).

Coronal plane

A coronal plane divides the entire body or a body part into anterior and posterior segments. The plane passes through the body vertically from one side to the other (see Fig. 2.1A and B). The *midcoronal plane* is a specific coronal plane that passes through the midline of the body, dividing it into equal anterior and posterior halves (see Fig. 2.1C). This plane is sometimes referred to as the *midaxillary plane*.

Horizontal plane

A *horizontal plane* passes crosswise through the body or a body part at right angles to the longitudinal axis. It is positioned at a right angle to the sagittal and coronal planes. This plane divides the body into superior and inferior portions. Often it is referred to as an *axial*, *transverse*, or *cross-sectional plane* (see Fig. 2.1A).

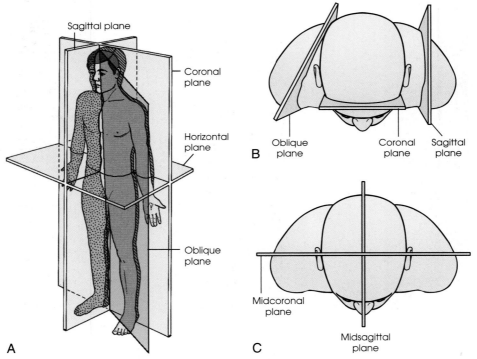

Fig. 2.1 Planes of the body. (A) A patient in anatomic position with four planes identified. (B) Top-down perspective of patient's body showing sagittal plane through left shoulder, coronal plane through anterior head, and oblique plane through right shoulder. (C) Midsagittal plane dividing body equally into right and left halves and midcoronal plane dividing body equally into anterior and posterior halves. Sagittal, coronal, and horizontal planes are always at right angles to one another.

Oblique plane

An oblique plane can pass through a body part at any angle among the three previously described planes (see Fig. 2.1A and B). Planes are used in radiographic positioning to center a body part to the image receptor (IR) or central ray and to ensure that the body part is properly oriented and aligned with the IR. For example, the midsagittal plane may be centered and perpendicular to the IR, with the long axis of the IR parallel to the same plane. Planes can also be used to guide projections of the central ray. The central ray for an anteroposterior (AP) projection passes through the body part parallel to the sagittal plane and perpendicular to the coronal plane. Quality imaging requires attention to all relationships among body planes, the IR, and the central ray.

Body planes are used in computed tomography (CT), magnetic resonance imaging (MRI), and ultrasound (US) to identify the orientation of anatomic cuts or slices shown in the procedure (Fig. 2.2). Imaging in several planes is often used to show large sections of anatomy (Fig. 2.3).

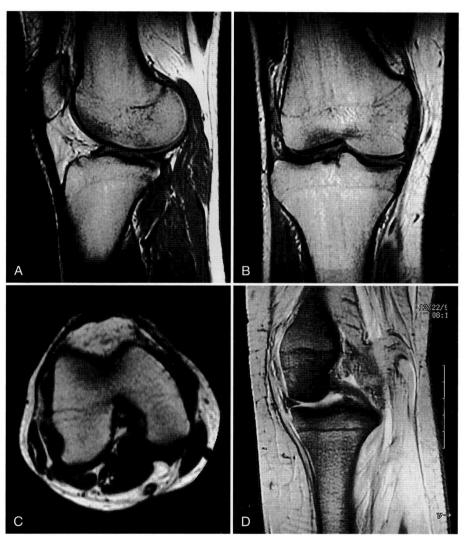

Fig. 2.2 MRI of the knee in four planes. (A) Sagittal. (B) Coronal. (C) Horizontal. (D) Oblique, 45 degrees.

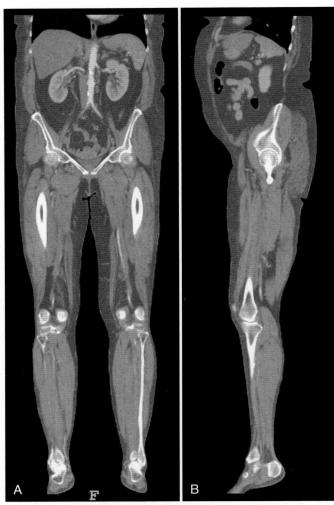

Fig. 2.3 Large sections of anatomy are often imaged in different planes. (A) Coronal plane of abdomen and lower limb. (B) Sagittal plane of abdomen and lower limb at level of left kidney, left acetabulum, and left knee.

SPECIAL PLANES

Two special planes are used in radiographic positioning. These planes are localized to a specific area of the body only.

Interiliac plane

The interiliac plane transects the pelvis at the top of the iliac crests at the level of the fourth lumbar spinous process (Fig. 2.4A). It is used in positioning the lumbar spine, sacrum, and coccyx.

Occlusal plane

The occlusal plane is formed by the biting surfaces of the upper and lower teeth with the jaws closed (see Fig. 2.4B). It is used in positioning of the odontoid process and in some head projections.

BODY CAVITIES

The two great cavities of the torso are the *thoracic* and *abdominal cavities* (Fig. 2.5). The thoracic cavity is subdivided into a pericardial segment and two pleural portions. Although the abdominal cavity has no intervening partition, the lower portion is called the *pelvic cavity*. Some anatomists combine the abdominal and pelvic cavities and refer to them as the *abdominopelvic cavity*. The principal structures located in the cavities are listed on the following page.

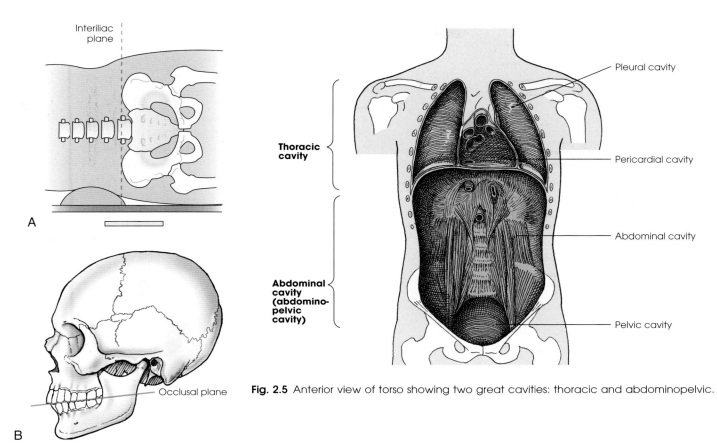

Interiliac plane

A

Occlusal plane

B

Fig. 2.4 Special planes. (A) Interiliac plane transecting trunk at tops of iliac crests. (B) Occlusal plane formed by biting surfaces of teeth.

Pleural cavity

Thoracic cavity

Pericardial cavity

Abdominal cavity (abdomino-pelvic cavity)

Abdominal cavity

Pelvic cavity

Fig. 2.5 Anterior view of torso showing two great cavities: thoracic and abdominopelvic.

Thoracic cavity

- Pleural membranes
- Lungs
- Trachea
- Esophagus
- Pericardium
- Heart and great vessels

Abdominal cavity

- Peritoneum
- Liver
- Gallbladder
- Pancreas
- Spleen
- Stomach
- Intestines
- Kidneys
- Ureters
- Major blood vessels
- **Pelvic portion**—rectum, urinary bladder, and parts of the reproductive system

DIVISIONS OF THE ABDOMEN

The abdomen is the portion of the trunk that is bordered superiorly by the diaphragm and inferiorly by the superior pelvic aperture (pelvic inlet). The location of organs or an anatomic area can be described by dividing the abdomen according to one of two methods: four quadrants or nine regions.

Quadrants

The abdomen is often divided into four clinical divisions called *quadrants* (Fig. 2.6). The midsagittal plane and a horizontal plane intersect at the umbilicus and create the boundaries. The quadrants are named as follows:

- Right upper quadrant (RUQ)
- Right lower quadrant (RLQ)
- Left upper quadrant (LUQ)
- Left lower quadrant (LLQ)

Dividing the abdomen into four quadrants is useful for describing the location of the various abdominal organs. For example, the spleen can be described as being located in the left upper quadrant.

Regions

Some anatomists divide the abdomen into nine regions by using four planes (Fig. 2.7). These anatomic divisions are not used as often as quadrants in clinical practice. The nine regions of the body, divided into three groups, are named as follows:

Superior

- Right hypochondrium
- Epigastrium
- Left hypochondrium

Middle

- Right lateral
- Umbilical
- Left lateral

Inferior

- Right inguinal
- Hypogastrium
- Left inguinal

In the clinical setting, a patient could be described as having "epigastric" pain. A patient with discomfort in the right lower abdomen could be described as having "RLQ" pain. Sometimes a quadrant term is used, and other times a region term is used.

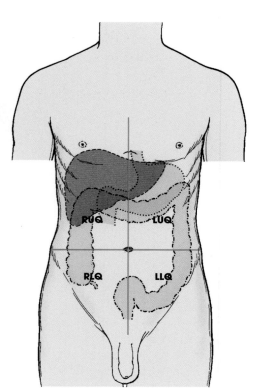

Fig. 2.6 Four quadrants of abdomen.

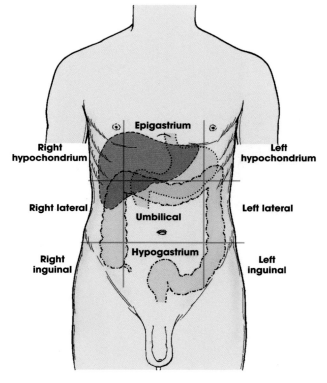

Fig. 2.7 Nine regions of abdomen.

SURFACE LANDMARKS

Most anatomic structures cannot be visualized directly; the radiographer must use various protuberances, tuberosities, and other external indicators to position the patient accurately. These surface landmarks enable the radiographer to obtain radiographs of optimal quality consistently for a wide variety of body types. If surface landmarks are not used for radiographic positioning or if they are used incorrectly, the chance of having to repeat the radiograph greatly increases.

Many commonly used landmarks are listed in Table 2.1 and diagrammed in Fig. 2.8. These landmarks are accepted averages for most patients and should be used only as guidelines. Variations in anatomic build or pathologic conditions may warrant positioning compensation on an individual basis. The ability to compensate is gained through experience. In the Atlas, positioning instructions based on external landmarks are for average-sized adults.

TABLE 2.1
External landmarks related to body structures at the same level

Body structures	External landmarks
Cervical area (see Fig. 2.6)	
C1	Mastoid tip
C2, C3	Gonion (angle of mandible)
C3, C4	Hyoid bone
C5	Thyroid cartilage
C7, T1	Vertebra prominens
Thoracic area	
T1	Approximately 2 inches (5 cm) above level of jugular notch
T2, T3	Level of jugular notch
T4, T5	Level of sternal angle
T7	Level of inferior angles of scapulae
T9, T10	Level of xiphoid process
Lumbar area	
L2, L3	Inferior costal margin
L4, L5	Level of superior-most aspect of iliac crests
Sacrum and pelvic area	
S1, S2	Level of anterior superior iliac spine (ASIS)
Coccyx	Level of pubic symphysis and greater trochanters

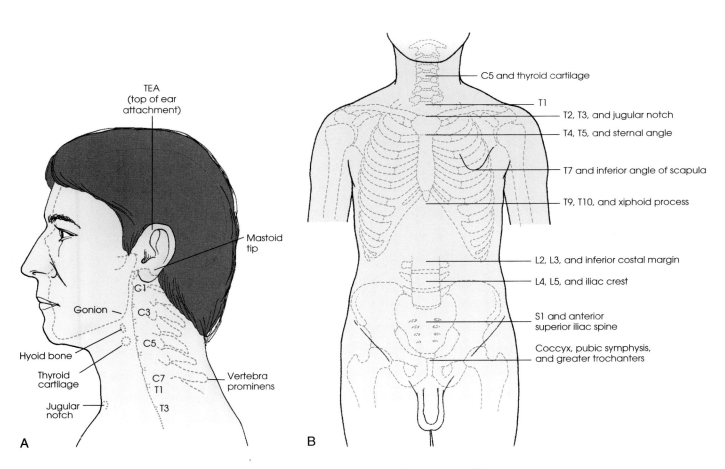

Fig. 2.8 Surface landmarks. (A) Head and neck. (B) Torso.

BODY HABITUS

Common variations in the shape of the human body are termed the *body habitus*. Mills[1] determined the primary classifications of body habitus based on his study of 1000 patients. The specific type of body habitus is important in radiography because it determines the size, shape, and position of the organs of the thoracic and abdominal cavities.

Body habitus directly affects the location of the following:
- Heart
- Lungs
- Diaphragm
- Stomach
- Colon
- Gallbladder

An organ such as the gallbladder may vary in position by 8 inches, depending on the body habitus. The stomach may be positioned horizontally, high, and in the center of the abdomen for one type of habitus and may be positioned vertically, low, and to the side of the midline in another type. Fig. 2.9 shows an example of the placement, shape, and size of the lungs, heart, and diaphragm in patients with four different body habitus types.

Body habitus and placement of the thoracic and abdominal organs are also important in the determination of technical and exposure factors. The standard placement and size of the IR may have to be changed because of body habitus. The selection of kilovolt (peak) and milliampere-second exposure factors may also be affected by the type of habitus because of wide variations in physical tissue density. These technical considerations are described in greater detail in radiography physics and imaging texts.

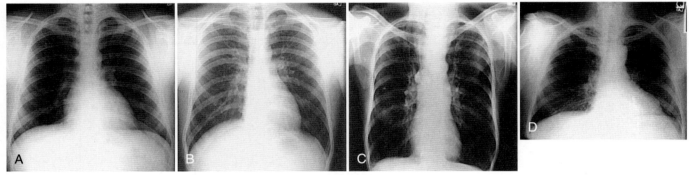

Fig. 2.9 Placement, shape, and size of lungs, heart, and diaphragm in patients with four different body habitus types. (A) Sthenic. (B) Hyposthenic. (C) Asthenic. (D) Hypersthenic.

Box 2.1 describes specific characteristics of the four types of body habitus and outlines their general shapes and variations. The four major types of body habitus and their approximate frequency in the population are identified as follows:
- Sthenic—50%
- Hyposthenic—35%
- Asthenic—10%
- Hypersthenic—5%

More than 85% of the population has either a *sthenic* or *hyposthenic* body habitus. The sthenic type is considered the predominant type of habitus. The relative shape of patients with a sthenic or hyposthenic body habitus and the position of their organs are referred to in clinical practice as *ordinary* or *average*. All standard radiographic positioning and exposure techniques are based on these two groups. Radiographers must become thoroughly familiar with the characteristics and organ placement of these two body types.

BOX 2.1
Four types of body habitus: prevalence, organ placement, and characteristics

Sthenic, 50%

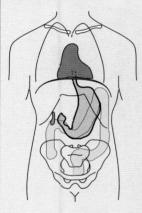

Organs
Heart: Moderately transverse
Lungs: Moderate length
Diaphragm: Moderately high
Stomach: High, upper left
Colon: Spread evenly; slight dip in transverse colon
Gallbladder: Centered on right side, upper abdomen

Characteristics
Build: Moderately heavy
Abdomen: Moderately long
Thorax: Moderately short, broad, and deep
Pelvis: Relatively small

Hyposthenic, 35%

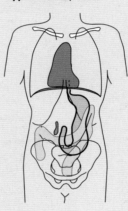

Organs and characteristics for this habitus are intermediate between sthenic and asthenic body habitus types; this habitus is the most difficult to classify.

Asthenic, 10%

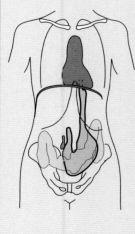

Organs
Heart: Nearly vertical and at midline
Lungs: Long, apices above clavicles, may be broader above base
Diaphragm: Low
Stomach: Low and medial, in the pelvis when standing
Colon: Low, folds on itself
Gallbladder: Low and nearer the midline

Characteristics
Build: Frail
Abdomen: Short
Thorax: Long, shallow
Pelvis: Wide

Hypersthenic, 5%

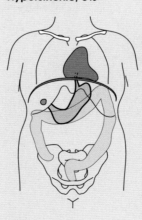

Organs
Heart: Axis nearly transverse
Lungs: Short, apices at or near clavicles
Diaphragm: High
Stomach: High, transverse, and in the middle
Colon: Around periphery of abdomen
Gallbladder: High, outside, lies more parallel

Characteristics
Build: Massive
Abdomen: Long
Thorax: Short, broad, deep
Pelvis: Narrow

Note the significant differences between the two extreme habitus types (i.e., asthenic and hypersthenic). The differences between sthenic and hyposthenic types are less distinct.

Radiographers must also become familiar with the two extreme habitus types: *asthenic* and *hypersthenic*. In these two small groups (15% of the population), placement and size of the organs significantly affect positioning and the selection of exposure factors. Consequently, radiography of these patients can be challenging.

Experience and professional judgment enable the radiographer to determine the correct body habitus and to judge the specific location of the organs.

Body habitus is not an indication of disease or other abnormality, and it is not determined by body fat or by the physical condition of the patient. Habitus is simply a classification of the four general shapes of the *trunk* of the human body. When positioning patients, the radiographer should be conscious that habitus is not associated with height or weight. Four patients of equal height could have four different trunk shapes (Fig. 2.10).

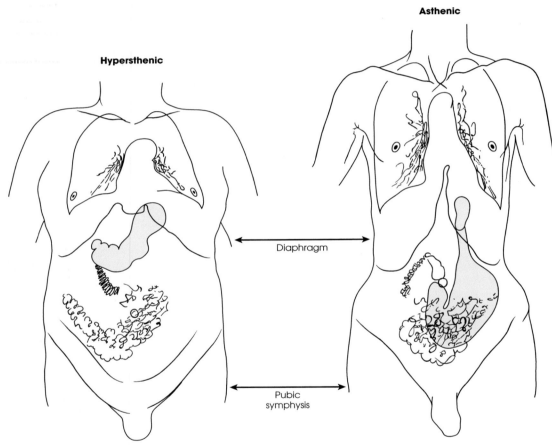

Fig. 2.10 Different trunks are shown for asthenic and hypersthenic habitus, the two extremes. The abdomen is the same length in both patients (diaphragm-to-pubic symphysis). The abdominal organs are in completely different positions. Note high stomach in hypersthenic habitus (*green color*) and low stomach in asthenic habitus.

(Art is based on actual autopsy findings by R. Walter Mills, MD).

Osteology

The adult human skeleton is composed of 206 primary bones. Ligaments unite the bones of the skeleton. Bones provide the following:

- Attachment for muscles
- Mechanical basis for movement
- Protection of internal organs
- A frame to support the body
- Storage for calcium, phosphorus, and other salts
- Production of red and white blood cells

The 206 bones of the body are divided into two main groups:

- Axial skeleton
- Appendicular skeleton

The axial skeleton supports and protects the head and trunk with 80 bones (Table 2.2). The appendicular skeleton allows the body to move in various positions and from place to place with its 126 bones (Table 2.3). Fig. 2.11 identifies these two skeletal areas.

TABLE 2.2

Axial skeleton: 80 bones

Area	Bones	Number
Skull	Cranial	8
	Facial	14
	Auditory ossicles[a]	6
Neck	Hyoid	1
Thorax	Sternum	1
	Ribs	24
Vertebral column	Cervical	7
	Thoracic	12
	Lumbar	5
	Sacrum	1
	Coccyx	1

[a]Auditory ossicles are small bones in the ears. They are not considered official bones of the axial skeleton but are placed here for convenience.

TABLE 2.3

Appendicular skeleton: 126 bones

Area	Bones	Number
Shoulder girdle	Clavicles	2
	Scapulae	2
Upper limbs	Humeri	2
	Ulnae	2
	Radii	2
	Carpals	16
	Metacarpals	10
	Phalanges	28
Lower limbs	Femora	2
	Tibias	2
	Fibulae	2
	Patellae	2
	Tarsals	14
	Metatarsals	10
	Phalanges	28
Pelvic girdle	Hip bones	2

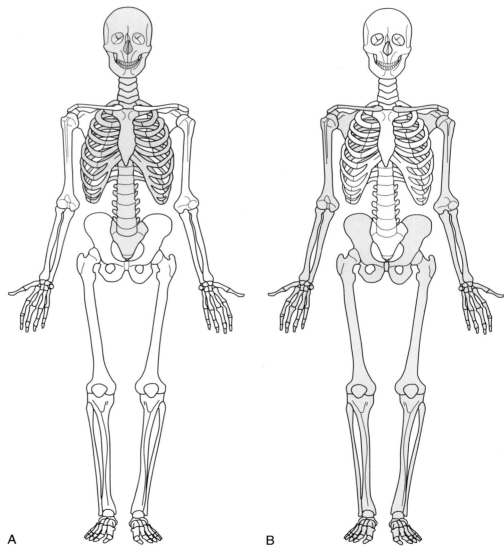

A   B

Fig. 2.11 Two main groups of bones. (A) Axial skeleton. (B) Appendicular skeleton.

GENERAL BONE FEATURES

The general features of most bones are shown in Fig. 2.12. All bones are composed of a strong, dense outer layer called the *compact bone* and an inner portion of less dense *spongy bone*. The hard outer compact bone protects the bone and gives it strength for supporting the body. The softer spongy bone contains a spiculated network of interconnecting spaces called the *trabeculae* (Fig. 2.13). The trabeculae are filled with red and yellow marrow. Red marrow produces red and white blood cells, and yellow marrow stores adipose (fat) cells. Long bones have a central cavity called the *medullary cavity,* which contains trabeculae filled with yellow marrow. In long bones, the red marrow is concentrated at the ends of the bone and not in the medullary cavity.

A tough, fibrous connective tissue called the *periosteum* covers all bony surfaces except the articular surfaces, which are covered by the articular cartilage. The tissue lining the medullary cavity of bones is called the *endosteum.* Bones contain various knoblike projections called *tubercles* and *tuberosities,* which are covered by the periosteum. Muscles, tendons, and ligaments attach to the periosteum at these projections. Blood vessels and nerves enter and exit the bone through the periosteum.

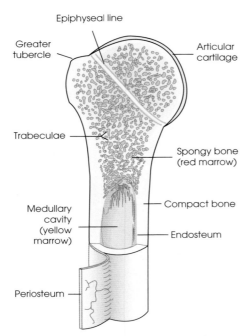

Epiphyseal line

Greater tubercle

Articular cartilage

Trabeculae

Spongy bone (red marrow)

Compact bone

Medullary cavity (yellow marrow)

Endosteum

Periosteum

Fig. 2.12 General bone features and anatomic parts.

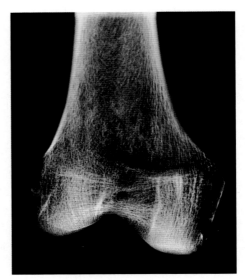

Fig. 2.13 Radiograph of distal femur and condyles showing bony trabeculae within entire bone.

BONE VESSELS AND NERVES

Bones are live organs that must receive a blood supply for nourishment or they die. Bones also contain a supply of nerves. Blood vessels and nerves enter and exit the bone at the same point, through openings called the *foramina*. Near the center of all long bones is an opening in the periosteum called the *nutrient foramen*. The nutrient artery of the bone passes into this opening and supplies the cancellous bone and marrow. The epiphyseal artery separately enters the ends of long bones to supply the area, and periosteal arteries enter at numerous points to supply the compact bone. Veins exiting the bones carry blood cells to the body (Fig. 2.14).

BONE DEVELOPMENT

Ossification is the term given to the development and formation of bones. Bones begin to develop in the second month of embryonic life. Ossification occurs separately by two distinct processes: *intermembranous ossification* and *endochondral ossification*.

Intermembranous ossification

Bones that develop from fibrous membranes in the embryo produce the flat bones—bones of the skull, clavicles, mandible, and sternum. Before birth, these bones are not joined. As flat bones grow after birth, they join and form sutures. Other bones in this category merge and create the various *joints* of the skeleton.

Endochondral ossification

Bones created by endochondral ossification develop from hyaline cartilage in the embryo and produce short, irregular, and long bones. Endochondral ossification occurs from two distinct centers of development called *primary* and *secondary centers of ossification*.

Primary ossification

Primary ossification begins before birth and forms the entire bulk of the short and irregular bones. This process forms the long central shaft in long bones. During development only, the long shaft of the bone is called the *diaphysis* (Fig. 2.15A).

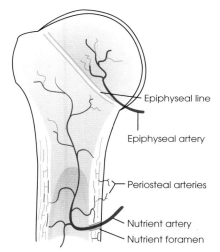

Fig. 2.14 Long bone end showing its rich arterial supply. Arteries, veins, and nerves enter and exit bone at the same point.

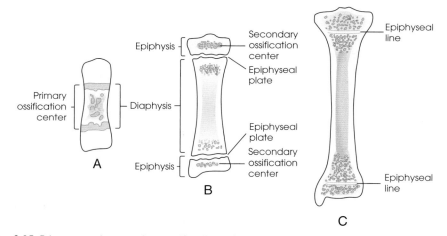

Fig. 2.15 Primary and secondary ossification of bone. (A) Primary ossification of tibia before birth. (B) Secondary ossification, which forms two *epiphyses* after birth. (C) Full growth into single bone, which occurs by age 21 years.

Secondary ossification

Secondary ossification occurs after birth when a separate bone begins to develop at both ends of each long bone. Each end is called the *epiphysis* (see Fig. 2.15B). At first, the diaphysis and the epiphysis are distinctly separate. As growth occurs, a plate of cartilage called the *epiphyseal plate* develops between the two areas (see Fig. 2.15C). This plate is seen on long bone radiographs of all pediatric patients (Fig. 2.16A). The epiphyseal plate is important radiographically because it is a common site of fractures in pediatric patients. Near age 21 years, full ossification occurs, and the two areas become completely joined; only a moderately visible *epiphyseal line* appears on the bone (see Fig. 2.16B).

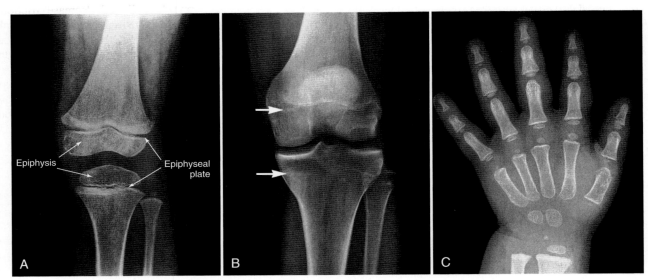

Fig. 2.16 (A) Radiograph of a 6-year-old child. Epiphysis and epiphyseal plate shown on knee radiograph *(arrows)*. (B) Radiograph of same area in a 21-year-old adult. Full ossification has occurred, and only subtle epiphyseal lines are seen *(arrows)*. (C) PA radiograph of hand of a 2½-year-old child. Note early stages of ossification in epiphyses at proximal ends of phalanges and first metacarpal, distal ends of other metacarpals, and radius.

(C, From Standring S: *Gray's anatomy*, ed 40, New York, 2009, Churchill Livingstone.)

CLASSIFICATION OF BONES

Bones are classified by shape, as follows (Fig. 2.17):
- Long
- Short
- Flat
- Irregular
- Sesamoid

Long bones

Long bones are found only in the limbs. They consist primarily of a long cylindric shaft called the *body* and two enlarged, rounded ends that contain a smooth, slippery articular surface. A layer of articular cartilage covers this surface. The ends of these bones all articulate with other long bones. The femur and the humerus are typical long bones. The phalanges of the fingers and toes are also considered long bones. A primary function of long bones is to provide support.

Short bones

Short bones consist mainly of cancellous bone containing red marrow and have a thin outer layer of compact bone. The carpal bones of the wrist and the tarsal bones of the ankles are the only short bones. They are varied in shape and allow minimum flexibility of motion in a short distance.

Flat bones

Flat bones consist largely of two tables of compact bone. The narrow space between the inner and outer tables contains cancellous bone and red marrow, or *diploë,* as it is called in flat bones. The bones of the cranium, sternum, and scapula are examples of flat bones. The flat surfaces of these bones provide protection, and their broad surfaces allow muscle attachment.

Irregular bones

Irregular bones are so termed because their peculiar shapes and variety of forms do not place them in any other category. The vertebrae and the bones in the pelvis and face fall into this category. Similar to other bones, they have compact bone on the exterior and cancellous bone containing red marrow in the interior. Their shape serves many functions, including attachment for muscles, tendons, and ligaments, or they attach to other bones to create joints.

Sesamoid bones

Sesamoid bones are small and oval. They develop inside and beside tendons. Their precise role is not understood. Experts believe that they alter the direction of muscle pull and decrease friction. The largest sesamoid bone is the patella, or the kneecap. Other sesamoids are located beneath the first metatarsophalangeal articulation of the foot and on the palmar aspect of the thumb at the metacarpophalangeal joint of the hand. Two small but prominent sesamoids are located beneath the base of the large toe. Similar to all other bones, they can be fractured.

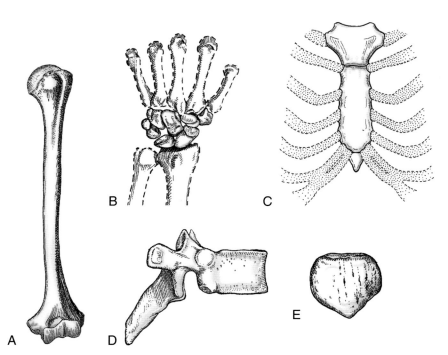

Fig. 2.17 Bones are classified by shape. (A) Humerus is a long bone. (B) Carpals of the wrist are short bones. (C) Sternum is a flat bone. (D) Vertebra is an irregular bone. (E) Patella is a sesamoid bone.

TABLE 2.4
Structural classification of joints

Connective tissue	Classification	Movement
Fibrous	1. Syndesmosis	Slightly movable
	2. Suture	Immovable
	3. Gomphosis	Immovable
Cartilaginous	4. Symphysis	Slightly movable
	5. Synchondrosis	Immovable
Synovial	6. Gliding	Freely movable
	7. Hinge	Freely movable
	8. Pivot	Freely movable
	9. Ellipsoid	Freely movable
	10. Saddle	Freely movable
	11. Ball and socket	Freely movable

Arthrology

Arthrology is the study of the joints, or articulations between bones. Joints make it possible for bones to support the body, protect internal organs, and create movement. Various specialized articulations are necessary for these functions to occur.

The two classifications of joints described in anatomy books are *functional* and *structural*. Studying both classifications can be confusing. The most widely used and primary classification is the structural classification, which is used to describe all the joints in this atlas. This is also the classification recognized by *Nomina Anatomica*. For academic interest, a brief description of the functional classification is provided.

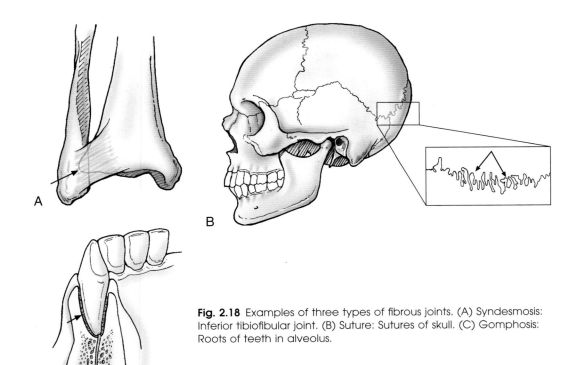

Fig. 2.18 Examples of three types of fibrous joints. (A) Syndesmosis: Inferior tibiofibular joint. (B) Suture: Sutures of skull. (C) Gomphosis: Roots of teeth in alveolus.

FUNCTIONAL CLASSIFICATION

When joints are classified as functional, they are broken down into three classifications. These classifications are based on the mobility of the joint, as follows:
- Synarthroses—immovable joints
- Amphiarthroses—slightly movable
- Diarthroses—freely movable

STRUCTURAL CLASSIFICATION

The structural classification of joints is based on the types of tissues that unite or bind the articulating bones. A thorough study of this classification is easier if radiographers first become familiar with the terminology and breakdown of the structural classification identified in Table 2.4.

Structurally, joints are classified into three distinct groups on the basis of their connective tissues: fibrous, cartilaginous, and synovial. Within these three broad categories are the 11 specific types of joints. They are numbered in the text for easy reference to Table 2.4.

Fibrous joints

Fibrous joints do not have a joint cavity. They are united by various fibrous and connective tissues or ligaments. These are the strongest joints in the body because they are virtually immovable. The three types of fibrous joints are as follows:
1. *Syndesmosis:* An immovable joint or slightly movable joint united by sheets of fibrous tissue. The inferior tibiofibular joint is an example (Fig. 2.18A).
2. *Suture:* An immovable joint occurring only in the skull. In this joint, the interlocking bones are held tightly together by strong connective tissues. The sutures of the skull are an example (see Fig. 2.18B).
3. *Gomphosis:* An immovable joint occurring only in the roots of the teeth. The roots of the teeth that lie in the alveolar sockets are held in place by fibrous periodontal ligaments (see Fig. 2.18C).

Cartilaginous joints

Cartilaginous joints are similar to fibrous joints in two ways: (1) They do not have a joint cavity, and (2) they are virtually immovable. Hyaline cartilage or fibrocartilage unites these joints. The two types of cartilaginous joints are as follows:
4. *Symphysis:* A slightly movable joint. The bones in this joint are separated by a pad of fibrocartilage. The ends of the bones contain hyaline cartilage. A symphysis joint is designed for strength and shock absorbency. The joint between the two pubic bones (pubic symphysis) is an example of a symphysis joint (Fig. 2.19A). Another example of a symphysis joint is the joint between each vertebral body. These joints all contain a fibrocartilaginous pad or disk.
5. *Synchondrosis:* An immovable joint. This joint contains a rigid cartilage that unites two bones. An example is the epiphyseal plate found between the epiphysis and diaphysis of a growing long bone (see Fig. 2.19B). Before adulthood, these joints consist of rigid hyaline cartilage that unites two bones. When growth stops, the cartilage ossifies, making this type of joint a temporary joint.

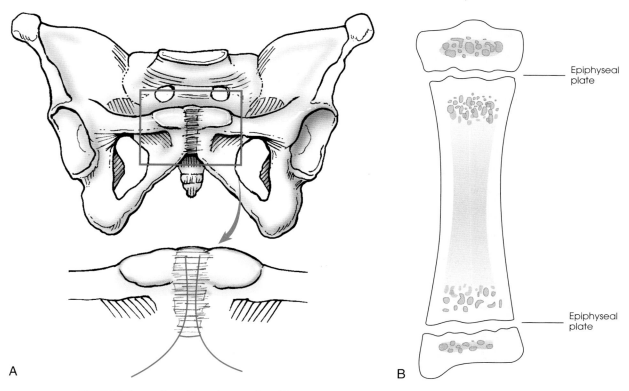

Epiphyseal plate

Epiphyseal plate

A

B

Fig. 2.19 Examples of two types of cartilaginous joints. (A) *Symphysis:* Pubic symphysis. (B) *Synchondrosis:* Epiphyseal plate found between epiphysis and diaphysis of growing long bones.

Synovial joints

Synovial joints permit a wide range of motion, and they all are freely movable. These joints are the most complex joints in the body. Fig. 2.20 shows their distinguishing features.

An articular capsule completely surrounds and enfolds all synovial joints to join the separate bones together. The outer layer of the capsule is called the *fibrous capsule,* and its fibrous tissue connects the capsule to the periosteum of the two bones. The *synovial membrane,* which is the inner layer, surrounds the entire joint to create the joint cavity. The membrane produces a thick, yellow, viscous fluid called *synovial fluid.* Synovial fluid lubricates the joint space to reduce friction between the bones. The ends of the adjacent bones are covered with articular cartilage. This smooth and slippery cartilage permits ease of motion. The two cartilages do not actually touch because they are separated by a thin layer of synovial membrane and fluid.

Some synovial joints contain a pad of fibrocartilage called the *meniscus,* which surrounds the joint. Specific menisci intrude into the joint from the capsular wall. They act as shock absorbers by conforming to and filling in the large gaps around the periphery of the bones. Some synovial joints also contain synovial fluid-filled sacs outside the main joint cavity, which are called the *bursae.* Bursae help reduce friction between skin and bones, tendons and bones, and muscles and bones. Menisci, bursae, and other joint structures can be visualized radiographically by injecting iodine-based contrast medium or air directly into the synovial cavity. This procedure, called *arthrography,* is detailed in Chapter 16.

The six synovial joints complete the 11 types of joints within the structural classification. They are listed in order of increasing movement. The most common name of each joint is identified, and the less frequently used name is given in parentheses.

6. *Gliding (plane):* Uniaxial movement. This is the simplest synovial joint. Joints of this type permit slight movement. They have flattened or slightly curved surfaces, and most glide slightly in only one axis. The intercarpal and intertarsal joints of the wrist and foot are examples of gliding joints (Fig. 2.21A).
7. *Hinge (ginglymus):* Uniaxial movement. A hinge joint permits only flexion and extension. The motion is similar to that of a door. The elbow, knee, and ankle are examples of this type of joint (see Fig. 2.21B).
8. *Pivot (trochoid):* Uniaxial movement. These joints allow only rotation around a single axis. A rounded or pointed surface of one bone articulates within a ring formed partially by the other bone. An example of this joint is the articulation of the atlas and axis of the cervical spine. The atlas rotates around the dens of the axis and allows the head to rotate to either side (see Fig. 2.21C).
9. *Ellipsoid (condyloid):* Biaxial movement, primary. An ellipsoid joint permits movement in two directions at right angles to each other. The radiocarpal joint of the wrist is an example. Flexion and extension occur along with abduction and adduction. Circumduction, a combination of both movements, can also occur (see Fig. 2.21D).
10. *Saddle (sellar):* Biaxial movement. This joint permits movement in two axes, similar to the ellipsoid joint. The joint is so named because the articular surface of one bone is saddle-shaped and the articular surface of the other bone is shaped like a rider sitting in a saddle. The two saddle-like structures fit into each other. The carpometacarpal joint between the trapezium and the first metacarpal is the only saddle joint in the body. The face of each bone end has a concave and a convex aspect. The opposing bones are shaped in a manner that allows side-to-side and up-and-down movement (see Fig. 2.21E).
11. *Ball and socket (spheroid):* Multiaxial movement. This joint permits movement in many axes, including flexion and extension, abduction and adduction, circumduction, and rotation. In a ball-and-socket joint, the round head of one bone rests within the cup-shaped depression of the other bone. The hip and the shoulder are examples (see Fig. 2.21F).

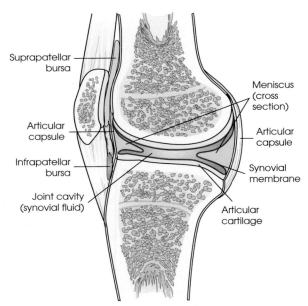

Fig. 2.20 Lateral cutaway view of knee showing distinguishing features of a synovial joint.

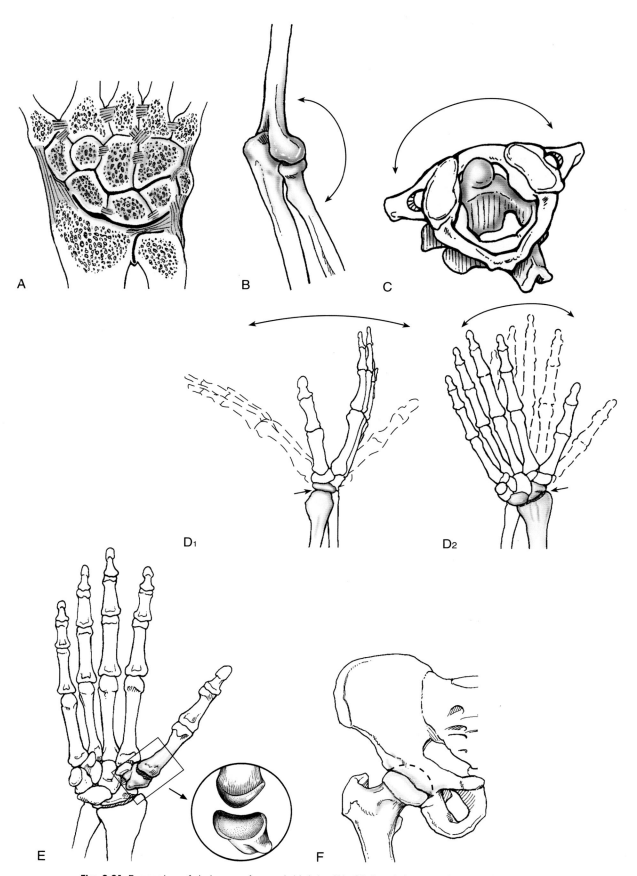

Fig. 2.21 Examples of six types of synovial joints. (A) *Gliding:* Intercarpal joints of wrist. (B) *Hinge:* Elbow joint. (C) *Pivot:* Atlas and axis of cervical spine (viewed from above). (D) *Ellipsoid:* Radiocarpal joint of wrist. (E) *Saddle:* Carpometacarpal joint. (F) *Ball and socket:* Hip joint.

Bone Markings and Features

The following anatomic terms are used to describe either processes or depressions on bones.

PROCESSES OR PROJECTIONS

Processes or projections extend beyond or project out from the main body of a bone and are designated by the following terms:

condyle—rounded process at an articular extremity

coracoid or coronoid—beak-like or crown-like process

crest—ridge-like process

epicondyle—projection above a condyle

facet—small, smooth-surfaced process for articulation with another structure

hamulus—hook-shaped process

head—expanded end of a long bone

horn—horn-like process on a bone

line—less prominent ridge than a crest; a linear elevation

malleolus—club-shaped process

protuberance—projecting part or prominence

spine—sharp process

styloid—long, pointed process

trochanter—either of two large, rounded, and elevated processes (greater or major and lesser or minor) located at junction of neck and shaft of femur

tubercle—small, rounded, and elevated process

tuberosity—large, rounded, and elevated process

DEPRESSIONS

Depressions are hollow or depressed areas and are described by the following terms:

fissure—cleft or deep groove

foramen—hole in a bone for transmission of blood vessels and nerves

fossa—pit, fovea, or hollow space

groove—shallow linear channel

meatus—tube-like passageway running within a bone

notch—indentation into border of a bone

sinus—recess, groove, cavity, or hollow space, such as (1) recess or groove in bone, as used to designate a channel for venous blood on inner surface of cranium; (2) air cavity in bone or hollow space in other tissue (used to designate a hollow space within a bone, as in paranasal sinuses); or (3) fistula or suppurating channel in soft tissues

sulcus—furrow, trench, or fissure-like depression

Fractures

A fracture is a break in the bone. Fractures are classified according to the nature of the break. Several general terms can pertain to them:

closed—fracture that does not break through the skin

displaced—serious fracture in which bones are not in anatomic alignment

nondisplaced—fracture in which bone retains its normal alignment

open—serious fracture in which broken bone or bones project through the skin

Common classifications of fractures are listed as follows and identified in Fig. 2.22:

- Compression
- Open or compound
- Simple
- Greenstick
- Transverse
- Spiral or oblique
- Comminuted
- Impacted

Many fractures fall into more than one category. A fracture could be spiral, closed, *and* nondisplaced.

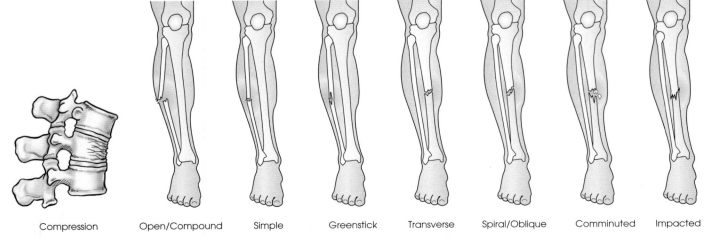

| Compression | Open/Compound | Simple | Greenstick | Transverse | Spiral/Oblique | Comminuted | Impacted |

Fig. 2.22 Common classifications of fractures.

Anatomic Relationship Terms

Various terms are used to describe the relationship of parts of the body in the anatomic position. Radiographers should be thoroughly familiar with these terms, which are commonly used in clinical practice. Most of the following positioning and anatomic terms are paired as opposites. Fig. 2.23 illustrates two commonly used sets of terms.

anterior (ventral) refers to forward or front part of body or forward part of an organ

posterior (dorsal) refers to back part of body or organ (note, however, that the superior surface of the foot is referred to as the dorsal surface)

caudad refers to parts away from the head of the body

cephalad refers to parts toward the head of the body

inferior refers to nearer the feet or situated below

superior refers to nearer the head or situated above

central refers to middle area or main part of an organ

peripheral refers to parts at or near the surface, edge, or outside of another body part

contralateral refers to part or parts on opposite side of body

ipsilateral refers to part or parts on same side of body

lateral refers to parts away from median plane of body or away from the middle of another body part to the right or left

medial refers to parts toward median plane of body or toward the middle of another body part

deep refers to parts far from the surface

superficial refers to parts near skin or surface

distal refers to parts farthest from point of attachment, point of reference, origin, or beginning; away from center of body

proximal refers to parts nearer point of attachment, point of reference, origin, or beginning; toward center of body

external refers to parts outside an organ or on outside of body

internal refers to parts within or on the inside of an organ

parietal refers to the wall or lining of a body cavity

visceral refers to the covering of an organ

dorsum refers to the top or anterior surface of the foot or to the back or posterior surface of the hand

palmar refers to the palm of the hand

plantar refers to the sole of the foot

Radiographic Positioning Terminology

Radiography is the process of recording an image of a body part using one or more types of IRs (PSP plate, digital detector, or fluoroscopic image intensifier). The terminology used to position the patient and to obtain the radiograph was developed through convention. Attempts to analyze usage often lead to confusion because the manner in which the terms are used does not follow one specific rule. During the preparation of this chapter, contact was maintained with the American Registry of Radiologic Technologists (ARRT) and the Canadian Association of Medical Radiation Technologists (CAMRT). The ARRT first distributed the "Standard Terminology for Positioning and Projection" in 1978;[2] it has not been substantially revised since initial distribution.[3] Despite its title, the ARRT document did not actually define selected positioning terms.[4] Terms not defined by the ARRT are defined in this atlas.

Approval of Canadian positioning terminology is the responsibility of the CAMRT Radiography Council on Education. This council provided information used in the development of this chapter and clearly identified terminology differences between the United States and Canada.[5]

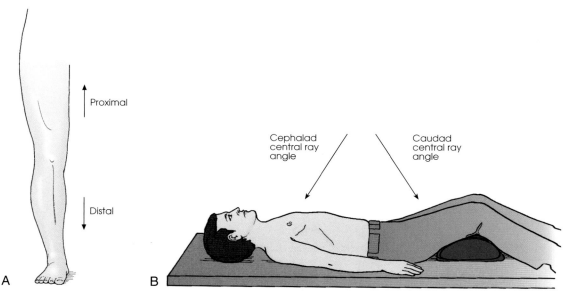

Fig. 2.23 (A) Use of common radiology terms *proximal* and *distal*. (B) Use of common radiology terms *caudad angle* and *cephalad angle*.

BOX 2.2

Primary x-ray projections and body positions

Projections	Positions
Anteroposterior (AP)	**General body positions**
Posteroanterior (PA)	Upright
Lateral	Seated
AP oblique	Supine
PA oblique	Prone
Axial	Recumbent
AP axial	Fowler
PA axial	Trendelenburg
AP axial oblique	
PA axial oblique	**Radiographic body positions**
Axiolateral	Lateral
Axiolateral oblique	Oblique
Transthoracic	Right posterior oblique (RPO)
Craniocaudal	
Tangential	Left posterior oblique (LPO)
Inferosuperior	
Superoinferior	Right anterior oblique (RAO)
Plantodorsal	
Dorsoplantar	Left anterior oblique (LAO)
Lateromedial	
Mediolateral	Decubitus
Submentovertical	Right lateral
Acanthoparietal	Left lateral
Parietoacanthial	Ventral
	Dorsal
	Lordotic

The terminology used by ARRT and CAMRT is consistent overall with that used in this atlas.

The following are the four positioning terms most commonly used in radiology:

- Projection
- Position
- View
- Method

♠ PROJECTION

The term *projection* is defined as the path of the central ray as it exits the x-ray tube and goes through the patient to the IR. Most projections are defined by entrance and exit points in the body and are based on the *anatomic position*. When the central ray enters anywhere in the front (anterior) surface of the body and exits the back (posterior), an *AP projection* is obtained. Regardless of which body position the patient is in (e.g., supine, prone, upright), if the central ray enters the anterior body surface and exits the posterior body surface, the projection is termed an *AP projection* (Fig. 2.24).

Projections can also be defined by the relationship formed between the central ray and the body as the central ray passes through the entire body or body part. Examples include *axial* and *tangential projections*.

All radiographic examinations described in this atlas are standardized and titled by their x-ray projection. The x-ray projection accurately and concisely defines each image produced in radiography. A complete list of the projection terms used in radiology is provided in Box 2.2. The essential radiographic projections follow.

Anteroposterior projection

In Fig. 2.25, a perpendicular central ray enters the anterior body surface and exits the posterior body surface. This is an *AP projection*. The patient is shown in the supine or dorsal recumbent body position. AP projections can also be achieved with upright, seated, or lateral decubitus positions.

Posteroanterior projection

In Fig. 2.26, a perpendicular central ray is shown entering the posterior body surface and exiting the anterior body surface. This illustrates a *posteroanterior (PA) projection* with the patient in the upright body position. PA projections can also be achieved with seated, prone (ventral recumbent), and lateral decubitus positions.

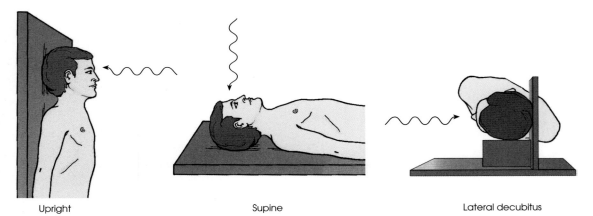

Upright   Supine   Lateral decubitus

Fig. 2.24 Patient's head placed in upright, supine, and lateral decubitus positions for a radiograph. All three body positions produce AP projection of skull.

Axial projection

In an axial projection (Fig. 2.27), there is *longitudinal angulation* of the central ray with the long axis of the body or a specific body part. This angulation is based on the anatomic position and is most often produced by angling the central ray cephalad or caudad. The longitudinal angulation in some examinations is achieved by angling the entire body or body part while maintaining the central ray perpendicular to the IR.

The term *axial,* as used in this atlas, refers to all projections in which the longitudinal angulation between the central ray and the long axis of the body part is *10 degrees or more.* When a range of central ray angles (e.g., 5 to 15 degrees) is recommended for a given projection, the term *axial* is used because the angulation could exceed 10 degrees. Axial projections are used in a wide variety of examinations and can be obtained with the patient in virtually any body position.

Tangential projection

Occasionally the central ray is directed toward the outer margin of a curved body surface to profile a body part just under the surface and project it free of superimposition. This is called a *tangential projection* because of the tangential relationship formed between the central ray and the entire body or body part (Fig. 2.28).

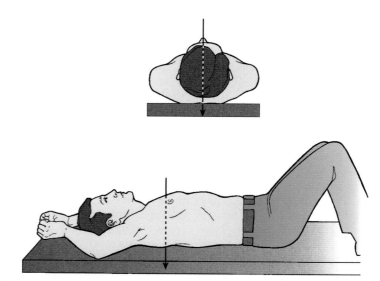

Fig. 2.25 AP projection of chest. Central ray enters anterior aspect and exits posterior aspect.

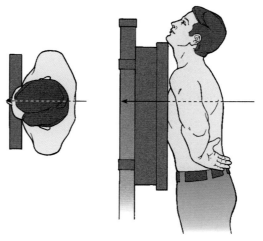

Fig. 2.26 PA projection of chest. Central ray enters posterior aspect and exits anterior aspect. Patient is in upright position.

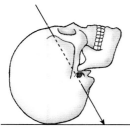
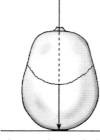

Fig. 2.27 AP axial projection of skull. Central ray enters anterior aspect at an angle and exits posterior aspect.

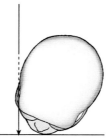
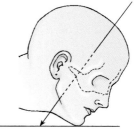

Fig. 2.28 Tangential projection of zygomatic arch. Central ray skims surface of the skull.

Lateral projection

For a lateral projection, a perpendicular central ray enters one side of the body or body part, passes transversely along the coronal plane, and exits on the opposite side. Lateral projections can enter from either side of the body or body part as needed for the examination. This can be determined by the patient's condition or ordered by the physician. When a lateral projection is used for head, chest, or abdominal radiography, the direction of the central ray is described with reference to the associated radiographic position. A left lateral position or right lateral position specifies the *side of the body closest to the IR* and corresponds with the side exited by the central ray (Fig. 2.29). For a right lateral position, the central ray enters the left side of the body and exits the right side (see Fig. 2.29). Lateral projections of the limbs are clarified further by the terms *lateromedial* and *mediolateral* to indicate the sides entered and exited by the central

ray (Fig. 2.30). The *transthoracic projection* is a unique lateral projection used for shoulder radiography and is described in Chapter 6.

Oblique projection

During an oblique projection, the central ray enters the body or body part from a side angle following an oblique plane. Oblique projections may enter from either side of the body and from anterior or posterior surfaces. If the central ray enters the anterior surface and exits the opposite posterior surface, it is an *AP oblique projection;* if it enters the posterior surface and exits anteriorly, it is a *PA oblique projection* (Fig. 2.31).

Most oblique projections are achieved by rotating the patient with the central ray perpendicular to the IR. As in the lateral projection, the direction of the central ray for oblique projections is described with reference to the associated radiographic position. A right posterior oblique position

(RPO) places the right posterior surface of the body closest to the IR and corresponds with an AP oblique projection exiting through the same side. This relationship is discussed later. Oblique projections can also be achieved for some examinations by angling the central ray diagonally along the horizontal plane rather than rotating the patient.

Complex projections

For additional clarity, projections may be defined by entrance and exit points and by the central ray relationship to the body at the same time. In the PA axial projection, the central ray enters the posterior body surface and exits the anterior body surface following an axial or angled trajectory relative to the entire body or body part. Axiolateral projections also use angulations of the central ray, but the ray enters and exits through lateral surfaces of the entire body or body part.

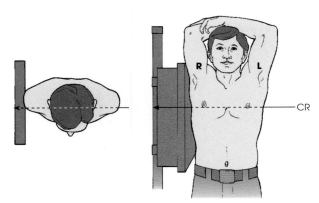

Fig. 2.29 Lateral projection of chest. The patient is placed in right lateral position. Right side of the chest is touching IR. Central ray (CR) enters left or opposite side of body.

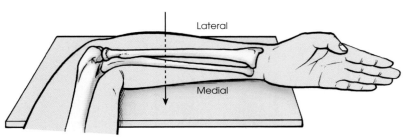

Fig. 2.30 Lateromedial projection of forearm. Central ray enters lateral aspect of forearm and exits medial aspect.

True projections

The term *true (true AP, true PA,* and *true lateral)*[6] is often used in clinical practice. *True* is used specifically to indicate that the body part must be placed exactly in the anatomic position.

A true AP or PA projection is obtained when the central ray is perpendicular to the coronal plane and parallel to the sagittal plane. A true lateral projection is obtained when the central ray is parallel to the normal plane and perpendicular to the sagittal plane. When a body part is rotated for an AP or PA oblique projection, a true AP or PA projection cannot be obtained. In this atlas, the term *true* is used only when the body part is placed in the anatomic position.

In-profile

In-profile is an outlined or silhouette view of an anatomic structure that has a distinctive shape. The distinctive aspect is not superimposed. The view is frequently seen from the side.

POSITION

The term *position* is used in two ways in radiology. One way identifies the overall posture of the patient or the general body position. The patient may be described as upright, seated, or supine. The second use of *position* refers to the specific placement of the body part in relation to the radiographic table or IR during imaging. This is the radiographic position and may be a right lateral, left anterior oblique, or other position depending on the examination and anatomy of interest. A list of all general body positions and radiographic positions is provided in Box 2.2.

During radiography, general body positions are combined with radiographic positions to produce the appropriate image. For clarification of positioning for an examination, it is often necessary to include references to both because a particular radiographic position, such as right lateral, can be achieved in several general body positions (e.g., upright, supine, lateral recumbent) with differing image outcomes. Specific descriptions of general body positions and radiographic positions follow.

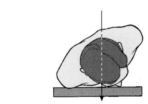

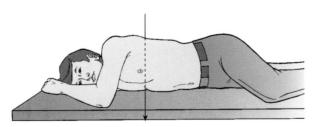

Fig. 2.31 PA oblique projection of chest. Central ray enters posterior aspect of body (even though it is rotated) and exits anterior aspect.

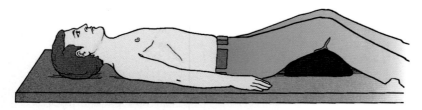

Fig. 2.32 Supine position of body, also termed *dorsal recumbent position*. The patient's knees are flexed for comfort.

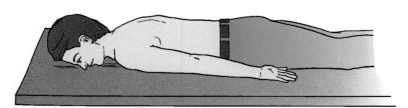

Fig. 2.33 Prone position of body, also termed *ventral recumbent position*.

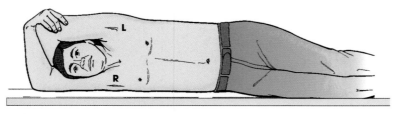

Fig. 2.34 Recumbent position of body, specifically *right lateral recumbent position*.

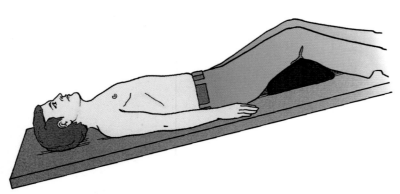

Fig. 2.35 Trendelenburg position of body. Feet are higher than the head.

General body positions

The following list describes the general body positions. All are commonly used in radiography practice.

upright—erect or marked by a vertical position (see Fig. 2.26)

seated—upright position in which the patient is sitting on a chair or stool

recumbent—general term referring to lying down in any position, such as dorsal recumbent (Fig. 2.32), ventral recumbent (Fig. 2.33), or lateral recumbent (Fig. 2.34)

supine—lying on the back (see Fig. 2.32)

prone—lying face down (see Fig. 2.33)

Trendelenburg position—supine position with head tilted downward (Fig. 2.35)

Fowler position—supine position with head higher than the feet (Fig. 2.36)

Sims position—recumbent position with the patient lying on the left anterior side (semiprone) with left leg extended and right knee and thigh partially flexed (Fig. 2.37)

lithotomy position—supine position with knees and hip flexed and thighs abducted and rotated externally, supported by ankle or knee supports (Fig. 2.38)

Lateral position

Lateral radiographic positions are always named according to the side of the patient that is placed closest to the IR (Figs. 2.39 and 2.40). In this atlas, the right and left lateral positions are indicated as subheadings for all lateral x-ray projections of the head, chest, and abdomen in which either the left or the right side of the patient is placed adjacent to the IR. The specific side selected depends on the condition of the patient, the anatomic structure of clinical interest, and the purpose of the examination. In Figs. 2.39 and 2.40, the x-ray projection for the positions indicated is lateral projection.

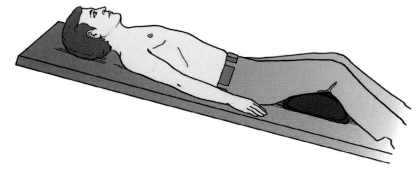

Fig. 2.36 Fowler position of the body. Head is higher than the feet.

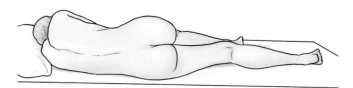

Fig. 2.37 Sims position of body. The patient is on the left side in recumbent oblique position.

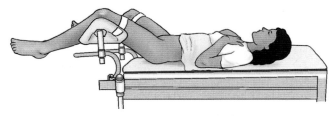

Fig. 2.38 Lithotomy position of body. Knees and hips are flexed, and thighs are abducted and rotated laterally.

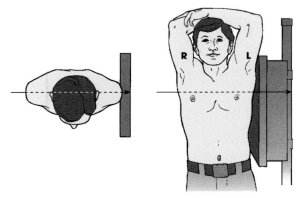

Fig. 2.39 Left lateral radiographic position of chest results in lateral projection.

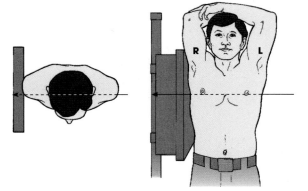

Fig. 2.40 Right lateral radiographic position of chest results in lateral projection.

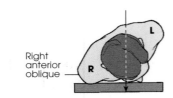

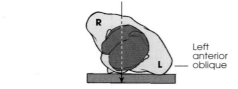

Right
anterior
oblique

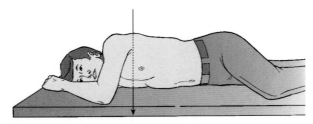

Fig. 2.41 RAO radiographic position of chest results in PA oblique projection.

Oblique position

An oblique radiographic position is achieved when the entire body or body part is rotated so that the coronal plane is not parallel with the radiographic table or IR. The angle of oblique rotation varies with the examination and structures to be shown. In this atlas, an angle is specified for each oblique position (e.g., rotated 45 degrees from the prone position).

Oblique positions, similar to lateral positions, are always named according to the side of the patient that is placed closest to the IR. In Fig. 2.41, the patient is rotated with the right anterior body surface in contact with the radiographic table. This is a *right anterior oblique (RAO) position* because the right side of the anterior body surface is closest to the IR. Fig. 2.42 shows the patient placed in a *left anterior oblique (LAO) position*.

Left
anterior
oblique

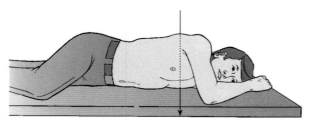

Fig. 2.42 LAO radiographic position of chest results in PA oblique projection.

The relationship between oblique position and oblique projection can be summarized simply. Anterior oblique positions result in PA oblique projections, as shown in Figs. 2.41 and 2.42. Similarly, posterior oblique positions result in AP oblique projections, as illustrated in Figs. 2.43 and 2.44.

The oblique positioning terminology used in this atlas has been standardized using RAO and LAO or RPO and LPO positions along with the appropriate PA or AP oblique projection. For oblique positions of the limbs, the terms *medial rotation* and *lateral rotation* have been standardized to designate the direction in which the limbs have been turned from the anatomic position (Fig. 2.45).

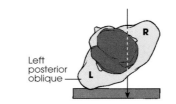

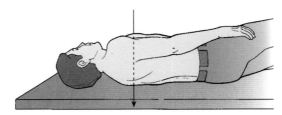

Fig. 2.43 LPO radiographic position of chest results in AP oblique projection.

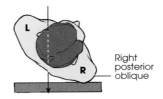

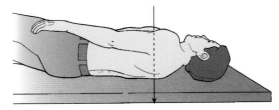

Fig. 2.44 RPO radiographic position of chest results in AP oblique projection.

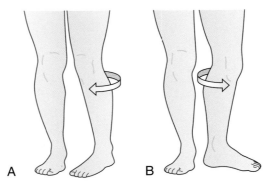

Fig. 2.45 (A) Medial rotation of knee. (B) Lateral rotation of knee.

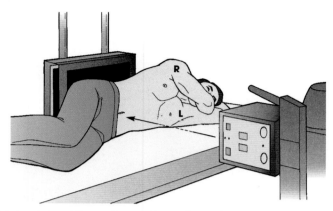

Fig. 2.46 Left lateral decubitus radiographic position of abdomen results in AP projection. Note horizontal orientation of central ray.

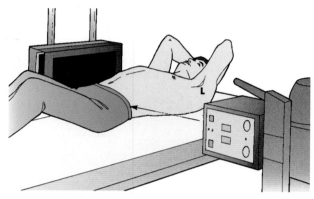

Fig. 2.47 Right dorsal decubitus radiographic position of abdomen results in right lateral projection. Note horizontal orientation of central ray.

Decubitus position

In radiographic positioning terminology, the term *decubitus* indicates that the patient is lying down and that the central ray is horizontal and parallel with the floor. Three primary decubitus positions are named according to the body surface on which the patient is lying: *lateral decubitus (left or right)*, *dorsal decubitus*, and *ventral decubitus*. Of these, the lateral decubitus position is used most often to show the presence of air-fluid levels or free air in the chest and abdomen.

In Fig. 2.46, the patient is placed in the left lateral decubitus radiographic position with the back (posterior surface) closest to the IR. In this position, a horizontal central ray provides an AP projection. Fig. 2.46 is accurately described as an AP projection with the body in the left lateral decubitus position. Alternatively, the patient may be placed with the front of the body (anterior surface) facing the IR, resulting in a PA projection. This would be correctly described as a PA projection of the body in the left lateral decubitus position. Right lateral decubitus positions may be necessary with AP and PA projections, depending on the examination.

In Fig. 2.47, the patient is shown in a dorsal decubitus radiographic position with one side of the body next to the IR. The horizontal central ray provides a lateral projection. This is correctly described as a lateral projection with the patient placed in the dorsal decubitus position. Either side may face the IR, depending on the examination or the patient's condition.

The ventral decubitus radiographic position (Fig. 2.48) also places a side of the body adjacent to the IR, resulting in a lateral projection. Similar to the earlier examples, the accurate terminology is lateral projection with the patient in the ventral decubitus position. Either side may face the IR.

Lordotic position

The lordotic position is achieved by having the patient lean backward while in the upright body position so that only the shoulders are in contact with the IR (Fig. 2.49). An angulation forms between the central ray and the long axis of the upper body, producing an AP axial projection. This position is used for visualization of pulmonary apices (see Chapter 3) and clavicles (see Chapter 6).

Note to educators, students, and clinicians

In clinical practice, the terms *position* and *projection* are often incorrectly used. These are two distinct terms that should not be interchanged. Incorrect use leads to confusion for the student who is attempting to learn the correct terminology of the profession. Educators and clinicians are encouraged to use the term *projection* generally when describing any examination performed. The word *projection* is the only term that accurately describes how the body part is being examined. The term *position* should be used only when referring to placement of the patient's body. Correct examples are, "We are going to perform a PA projection of the chest with the patient in the upright position," and "We are going to perform an AP oblique projection of the lumbar spine in the left posterior oblique (LPO) position."

VIEW

The term *view* is used to describe the body part as seen by the IR. Use of this term is restricted to the general discussion of a finished radiograph or image. *View* and *projection* are exact opposites. For many years, *view* and *projection* were often used interchangeably, which led to confusion. In the United States, *projection* has replaced *view* as the preferred terminology for describing radiographic images. For consistency, this atlas refers to all views as *images* or *radiographs*.

In clinical practice it is common to see the term *view* used in radiology procedure orders. For example, a radiology procedure order pulled from the radiology information system (RIS) worklist may state "3 view shoulder." This should be interpreted as an order for three radiographic projections or positions. The radiology department protocol manual will indicate which three projections are routine for that procedure.

METHOD

Some radiographic projections and procedures are named after individuals (e.g., Waters, Towne) in recognition of their development of a method to show a specific anatomic part. *Method,* which was first described in the fifth edition of this atlas, describes the specific radiographic projection that the individual developed. Most methods are named after an individual; however, a few are named for unique

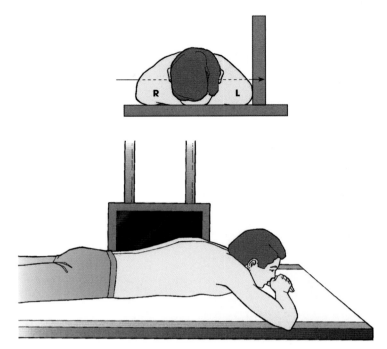

Fig. 2.48 Left ventral decubitus radiographic position of abdomen results in left lateral projection. Note horizontal orientation of central ray.

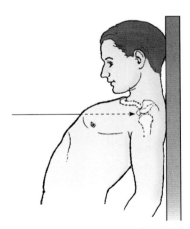

Fig. 2.49 Lordotic radiographic position of chest results in AP axial projection. Central ray is not angled; however, it enters chest axially as a result of body position.

projections. The method specifies the x-ray projection and body position, and it may include specific items such as IR, CR, or other unique aspects. In this atlas, standard projection terminology is used first, and a named method is listed secondarily (e.g., PA axial projection; Towne method). ARRT and CAMRT use standard anatomic projection terminology and list the originator in parentheses.

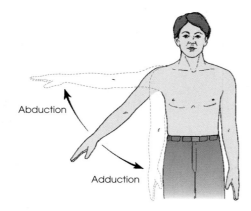

Fig. 2.50 Abduction and adduction of arm.

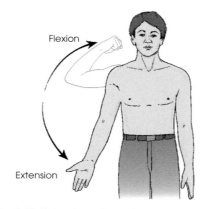

Fig. 2.51 Extension of arm (anatomic position) and flexion (bending).

Body Movement Terminology

The following terms are used to describe movement related to the limbs. These terms are often used in positioning descriptions and in the patient history provided to the radiographer by the referring physician. They must be studied thoroughly.

abduct or abduction—movement of a part away from the central axis of the body or body part

adduct or adduction—movement of a part toward the central axis of the body or body part (Fig. 2.50)

extension—straightening of a joint; when both elements of the joint are in the anatomic position; normal position of a joint (Fig. 2.51)

flexion—act of bending a joint; opposite of extension (Fig. 2.52)

hyperextension—forced or excessive extension of a limb or joints

hyperflexion—forced overflexion of a limb or joints (see Fig. 2.52)

evert/eversion—outward turning of the foot at the ankle

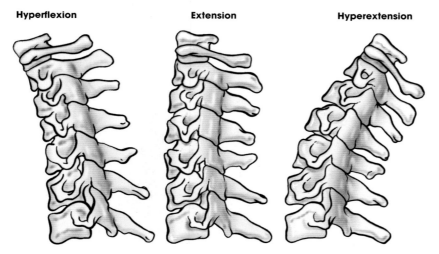

Fig. 2.52 Hyperextension, extension, and hyperflexion of neck.

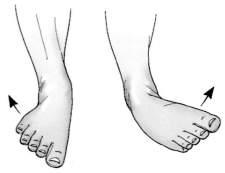

Fig. 2.53 Eversion and inversion of foot at ankle joint.

invert/inversion—inward turning of the foot at the ankle (Fig. 2.53)

pronate/pronation—rotation of the forearm so that the palm is down

supinate/supination—rotation of the forearm so that the palm is up (in the anatomic position) (Fig. 2.54)

rotate/rotation—turning or rotating of the body or a body part around its axis (Fig. 2.55A); rotation of a limb can be medial (toward the midline of the body from the anatomic position [see Fig. 2.55B]) or lateral (away from the midline of the body from the anatomic position [see Fig. 2.55C])

circumduction—circular movement of a limb (Fig. 2.56)

tilt—tipping or slanting a body part slightly; tilt is in relation to the long axis of the body (Fig. 2.57)

deviation—turning away from the regular standard or course (Fig. 2.58)

dorsiflexion—flexion or bending of the foot toward the leg (Fig. 2.59)

plantar flexion—flexion or bending of the foot downward toward the sole (see Fig. 2.59)

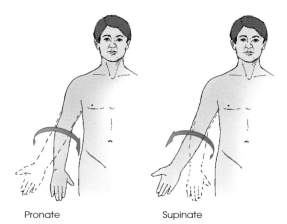

Pronate | Supinate

Fig. 2.54 Pronation and supination of forearm.

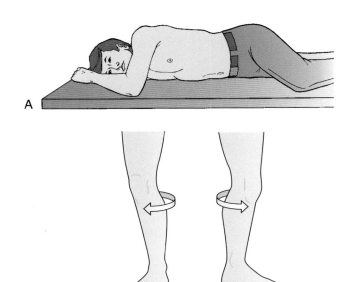

Fig. 2.55 (A) Rotation of chest and abdomen. The patient's arm and knee are flexed for comfort. (B) Medial rotation of left leg. (C) Lateral rotation of left leg.

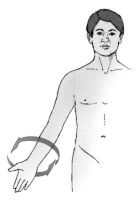

Fig. 2.56 Circumduction of arm.

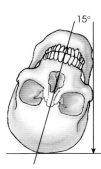

Fig. 2.57 Tilt of skull is 15 degrees from long axis.

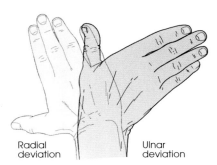

Radial deviation | Ulnar deviation

Fig. 2.58 Radial deviation of hand (turned to radial side) and ulnar deviation (turned to ulnar side).

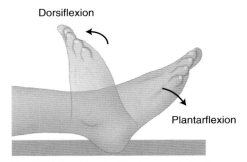

Dorsiflexion | Plantarflexion

Fig. 2.59 Foot in dorsiflexion and plantar flexion. Note movement is at ankle joint.

TABLE 2.5

Greek and Latin nouns: common singular and plural forms

Singular	Plural	Examples: singular—plural
-a	-ae	maxilla—maxillae
-ex	-ces	apex—apices
-is	-es	diagnosis—diagnoses
-ix	-ces	appendix—appendices
-ma	-mata	condyloma—condylomata
-on	-a	ganglion—ganglia
-um	-a	antrum—antra
-us	-i	ramus—rami

Medical Terminology

Single and plural word endings for common Greek and Latin nouns are presented in Table 2.5. Single and plural word forms are often confused. Examples of commonly misused word forms are listed in Table 2.6; the singular form generally is used when the plural form is intended.

TABLE 2.6

Frequently misused single and plural word forms

Singular	Plural	Singular	Plural
adnexus	adnexa	mediastinum	mediastina
alveolus	alveoli	medulla	medullae
areola	areolae	meninx	meninges
bronchus	bronchi	meniscus	menisci
bursa	bursae	metastasis	metastases
calculus	calculi	mucosa	mucosae
coxa	coxae	omentum	omenta
diagnosis	diagnoses	paralysis	paralyses
diverticulum	diverticula	plexus	plexi
fossa	fossae	pleura	pleurae
gingiva	gingivae	pneumothorax	pneumothoraces
haustrum	haustra	ramus	rami
hilum	hila	ruga	rugae
ilium	ilia	sulcus	sulci
labium	labia	thrombus	thrombi
lamina	laminae	vertebra	vertebrae
lumen	lumina	viscus	viscera

ABBREVIATIONS USED IN CHAPTER 2

ARRT	American Registry of Radiologic Technologists
ASIS	Anterior superior iliac spine
CT	Computed tomography
LAO	Left anterior oblique
LLQ	Left lower quadrant
LPO	Left posterior oblique
LUQ	Left upper quadrant
MRI	Magnetic resonance imaging
RAO	Right anterior oblique
RLQ	Right lower quadrant
RPO	Right posterior oblique
RUQ	Right upper quadrant
US	Ultrasound

See Addendum A for a summary of all abbreviations used in Volume 1.

References

1. Mills WR: The relation of bodily habitus to visceral form, position, tonus, and motility, *AJR* 4:155, 1917.
2. *ARRT educator's handbook*, ed 3, 1990, ARRT.
3. *ARRT educator guide*, Spring 2010.
4. ARRT, personal communication and permission, May 2006.
5. CAMRT, Radiography Council on Education, personal communication, July 1993.
6. Bontrager KL: *Textbook of radiographic positioning*, ed 7, St Louis, 2009, Mosby.

3

THORACIC VISCERA: CHEST AND UPPER AIRWAY

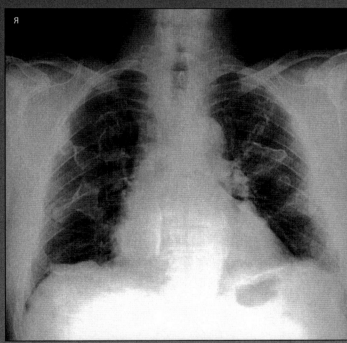

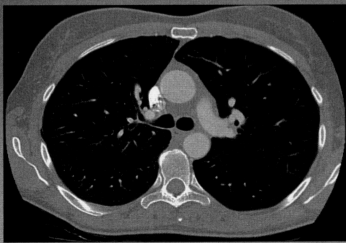

SUMMARY OF PROJECTIONS

PROJECTIONS, POSITIONS, AND METHODS

Page	Essential	Anatomy	Projection	Position	Method
99		Soft tissue neck	AP		
101		Soft tissue neck	Lateral	R or L	
107	♣	Chest: *Lungs and heart*	PA		
110	♣	Chest: *Lungs and heart*	Lateral	R or L	
113	♣	Chest: *Lungs and heart*	PA oblique	RAO and LAO	
117	♣	Chest: *Lungs and heart*	AP oblique	RPO and LPO	
119	♣	Chest	AP		
121	♣	Pulmonary apices	AP axial	Lordotic	LINDBLOM
123		Pulmonary apices	AP axial		
124		Pulmonary apices	PA axial		
125	♣	Lungs and pleurae	AP or PA	R or L lateral decubitus	
127	♣	Lungs and pleurae	Lateral	R or L, ventral or dorsal decubitus	

Icons in the Essential column indicate projections frequently performed in the United States and Canada. Students should be competent in these projections.
AP, Anteroposterior; *L,* left; *LAO,* left anterior oblique; *LPO,* left posterior oblique; *PA,* posteroanterior; *R,* right; *RAO,* right anterior oblique; *RPO,* right posterior oblique.

Body Habitus

The general shape of the human body, or the *body habitus*, determines the size, shape, position, and movement of the internal organs. Fig. 3.1 outlines the general shape of the thorax in the four types of body habitus and shows how each appears on radiographs of the thoracic area.

Thoracic Cavity

The *thoracic cavity* is bounded by the walls of the thorax and extends from the *superior thoracic aperture*, where structures enter the thorax, to the *inferior thoracic aperture*. The *diaphragm* separates the thoracic cavity from the abdominal cavity. The anatomic structures that pass from the thorax to the abdomen go through openings in the diaphragm (Fig. 3.2).

The thoracic cavity contains the *lungs* and *heart*; organs of the *respiratory*, *cardiovascular*, and *lymphatic* systems; the *inferior portion of the esophagus*; and the *thymus gland*. Within the cavity are three separate chambers: a single *pericardial cavity* and the *right* and *left pleural cavities*. These cavities are lined by shiny, slippery, and delicate *serous membranes*. The space between the two pleural cavities is called the *mediastinum*. This area contains all thoracic structures except the lungs and pleurae.

Respiratory System

The *respiratory system* consists of the pharynx, trachea, bronchi, and two lungs. The air passages of these organs communicate with the exterior through the pharynx, mouth, and nose, each of which, in addition to serving other described functions, is considered a part of the respiratory system.

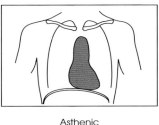
Hypersthenic

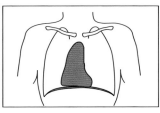
Sthenic

Asthenic

Hyposthenic

Fig. 3.1 Four types of body habitus. Note general shape of thorax, size and shape of lungs, and position of heart. Knowledge of this anatomy is helpful in positioning accurately for projections of the thorax.

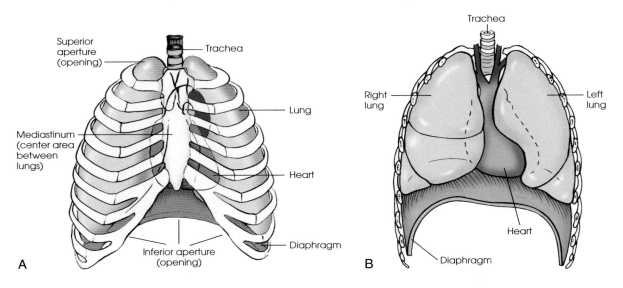

Fig. 3.2 (A) Thoracic cavity. (B) Thoracic cavity with anterior ribs removed.

TRACHEA

The *trachea* is a fibrous, muscular tube with 16 to 20 C-shaped cartilaginous rings embedded in its walls for greater rigidity (Fig. 3.3A). It measures approximately ½ inch (1.3 cm) in diameter and 4½ inches (11 cm) in length, and its posterior aspect is flat. The cartilaginous rings are incomplete posteriorly and extend around the anterior two-thirds of the tube. The trachea lies in the midline of the body, anterior to the esophagus in the neck. In the thorax, the trachea is shifted slightly to the right of the midline as a result of arching of the aorta. The trachea follows the curve of the vertebral column and extends from its junction with the larynx at the level of the sixth cervical vertebra inferiorly through the mediastinum to about the level of the space between the fourth and fifth thoracic vertebrae. The last tracheal cartilage is elongated and has a hooklike process, the *carina*, which extends posteriorly on its inferior surface. At the carina, the trachea divides, or bifurcates, into two lesser tubes—the primary bronchi. One of these bronchi enters the right lung, and the other enters the left lung.

The *primary bronchi* slant obliquely inferiorly to their entrance into the lungs, where they branch out to form the right and left bronchial branches (see Fig. 3.3B). The *right primary bronchus* is shorter, wider, and more vertical than the *left primary bronchus*. Because of the more vertical position and greater diameter of the right main bronchus, foreign bodies entering the trachea are more likely to pass into the right bronchus than the left bronchus.

After entering the lung, each primary bronchus divides, sending branches to each lobe of the lung: three to the right lung and two to the left lung. These *secondary bronchi* divide further and decrease in caliber. The bronchi continue dividing into *tertiary bronchi*, then into smaller *bronchioles*, and end in minute tubes called the *terminal bronchioles* (see Fig. 3.3). The extensive branching of the trachea is commonly referred to as the *bronchial tree*, because it resembles a tree trunk (see box).

SUBDIVISIONS OF THE BRONCHIAL TREE

Trachea
  Primary bronchi
    Secondary bronchi
      Tertiary bronchi
        Bronchioles
          Terminal bronchioles

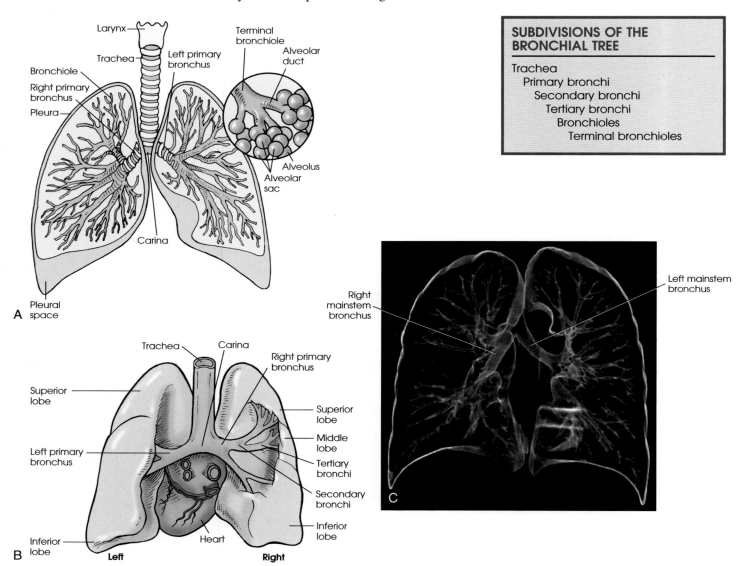

Fig. 3.3 (A) Anterior aspect of respiratory system. (B) Posterior aspect of heart, lungs, trachea, and bronchial trees. (C) Coronal, three-dimensional CT image of central and peripheral airways.

(C, From Kelley LL, Petersen CM: *Sectional Anatomy for Imaging Professionals,* ed 2, St Louis, 2007, Mosby.)

ALVEOLI

The terminal bronchioles communicate with *alveolar ducts*. Each duct ends in several *alveolar sacs*. The walls of the alveolar sacs are lined with *alveoli* (see Fig. 3.3A). Each lung contains millions of alveoli. Oxygen and carbon dioxide are exchanged by diffusion within the walls of the alveoli.

LUNGS

The *lungs* are the organs of respiration (Fig. 3.4). They provide the mechanism for introducing oxygen into the blood and removing carbon dioxide from the blood. The lungs are composed of a light, spongy, highly elastic substance, the *parenchyma,* and they are covered by a layer of serous membrane. Each lung presents a rounded *apex* that reaches above the level of the clavicles into the root of the neck and a broad *base* that, resting on the obliquely placed diaphragm, reaches lower in back and at the sides than in front. The right lung is about 1 inch (2.5 cm) shorter than the left lung because of the large space occupied by the liver, and it is broader than the left lung because of the position

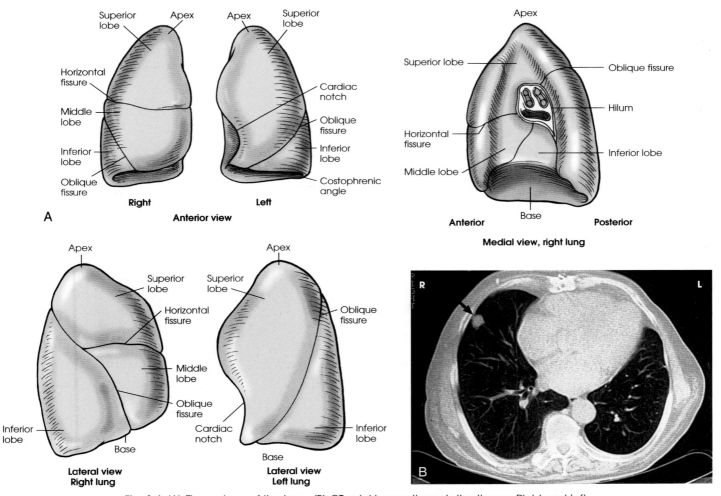

Fig. 3.4 (A) Three views of the lung. (B) CT axial image through the thorax. Right and left lungs are shown in actual position within thorax and in relation to heart. Note nodule in right anterior lung *(arrow)*.

(B, Courtesy Siemens Medical Systems, Iselin, NJ.)

of the heart. The lateral surface of each lung conforms to the shape of the chest wall. The inferior surface of the lung is concave, fitting over the diaphragm, and the lateral margins are thin. During respiration, the lungs move inferiorly for inspiration and superiorly for expiration (Fig. 3.5). During inspiration, the lateral margins descend into the deep recesses of the parietal pleura. In radiology, this recess is called the *costophrenic angle* (see Fig. 3.5B). The mediastinal surface is concave with a depression called the *hilum* that accommodates the bronchi, pulmonary blood vessels, lymph vessels, and nerves. The inferior mediastinal surface of the left lung contains a concavity called the *cardiac notch*. This notch conforms to the shape of the heart.

Each lung is enclosed in a double-walled, serous membrane sac called the *pleura* (see Fig. 3.3A). The inner layer of the pleural sac, called the *visceral pleura*, closely adheres to the surface of the lung, extends into the interlobar fissures, and is contiguous with the outer layer at the hilum. The outer layer, called the *parietal pleura*, lines the wall of the thoracic cavity occupied by the lung and closely adheres to the upper surface of the diaphragm. The two layers are moistened by serous fluid so that they move easily on each other. The serous fluid prevents friction between the lungs and chest walls during respiration. The space between the two pleural walls is called the *pleural cavity*. Although the space is termed a cavity, the layers are actually in close contact.

Each lung is divided into *lobes* by deep fissures. The fissures lie in an oblique plane inferiorly and anteriorly from above, so that the lobes overlap each other in the AP direction. The *oblique fissures* divide the lungs into *superior* and *inferior lobes*. The superior lobes lie above and are anterior to the inferior lobes. The right superior lobe is divided further by a *horizontal fissure*, creating a *right middle lobe* (see Fig. 3.4). The left lung has no horizontal fissure and no middle lobe. The portion of the left lobe that corresponds in position to the right middle lobe is called the *lingula*. The lingula is a tongue-shaped process on the anteromedial border of the left lung. It fills the space between the chest wall and the heart.

Each of the five lobes divides into *bronchopulmonary segments* and subdivides into smaller units called *primary lobules*. The primary lobule is the anatomic unit of lung structure and consists of a terminal bronchiole with its expanded alveolar duct and alveolar sac.

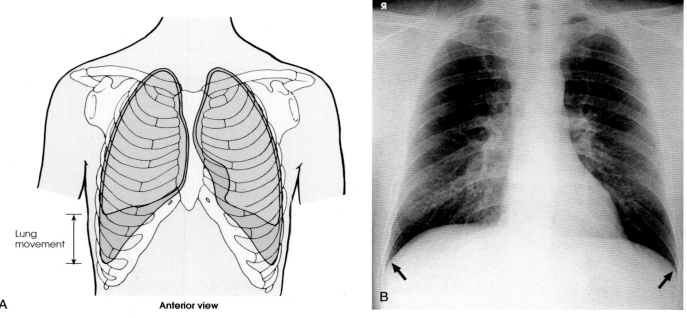

Fig. 3.5 (A) Movement of lungs during inspiration and expiration. (B) Costophrenic angles shown (*arrows*) on PA projection of chest.

Neck

The *neck* occupies the region between the skull and the thorax (Figs. 3.6 and 3.7). For radiographic purposes, the neck is divided into posterior and anterior portions in accordance with tissue composition and function of the structures. The procedures that are required to show the osseous structures occupying the posterior division of the neck are described in the discussion of the cervical vertebrae in Chapter 9. The portions of the central nervous system and circulatory system that pass through the neck are described in Chapters 14 and 27.

The portion of the neck that lies in front of the vertebrae is composed of largely soft tissues. The upper parts of the respiratory and digestive systems are the principal structures. The thyroid and parathyroid glands, and the larger part of the submandibular glands, are also located in the anterior portion of the neck.

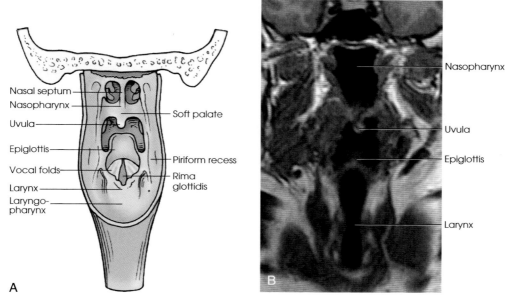

Fig. 3.6 (A) Interior posterior view of neck. (B) Coronal MRI of neck.

(B, Courtesy J. Louis Rankin, BS, RT(R)(MR).)

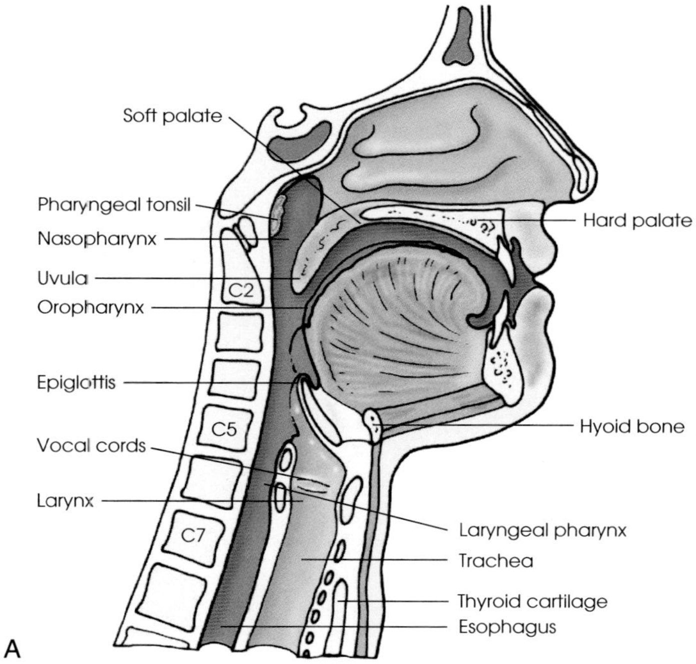

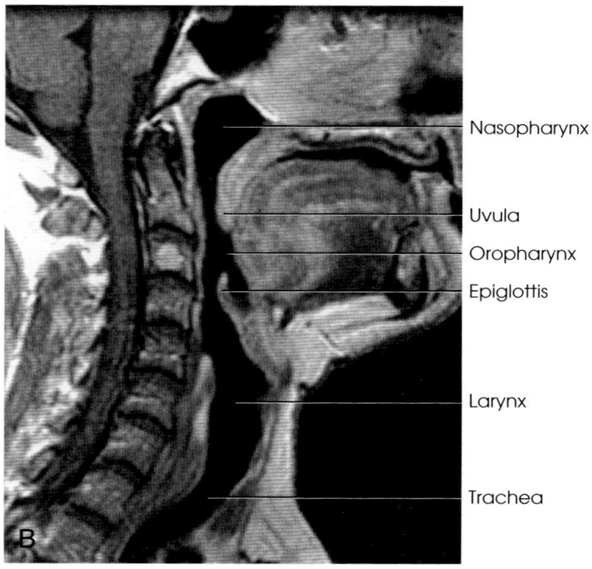

Fig. 3.7 (A) Sagittal section of face and neck. (B) Sagittal MRI of neck.

(B, Courtesy J. Louis Rankin, BS, RT(R)(MR).)

THYROID GLAND

The *thyroid gland* consists of two lateral lobes connected at their lower thirds by a narrow median portion called the *isthmus* (Fig. 3.8). The lobes are approximately 2 inches (5 cm) long, 1¼ inches (3.2 cm) wide, and 3/4 inch (1.9 cm) thick. The isthmus lies at the front of the upper part of the trachea, and the lobes lie at the sides. The lobes reach from the lower third of the thyroid cartilage to the level of the first thoracic vertebra. Although the thyroid gland is normally suprasternal in position, it occasionally extends into the superior aperture of the thorax.

PARATHYROID GLANDS

The *parathyroid glands* are small ovoid bodies—two on each side, *superior* and *inferior*. These glands are situated one above the other on the posterior aspect of the adjacent lobe of the thyroid gland.

PHARYNX

The *pharynx* serves as a passage for air and food and is common to the respiratory and digestive systems (see Fig. 3.7). The pharynx is a musculomembranous, tubular structure situated in front of the vertebrae and behind the nose, mouth, and larynx. Approximately 5 inches (13 cm) in length, the pharynx extends from the undersurface of the body of the sphenoid bone and the basilar part of the occipital bone inferiorly to the level of the disk between the sixth and seventh cervical vertebrae, where it becomes continuous with the esophagus. The pharyngeal cavity is subdivided into nasal, oral, and laryngeal portions.

The *nasopharynx* lies posteriorly above the *soft* and *hard* palates. (The upper part of the hard palate forms the floor of the nasopharynx.) Anteriorly, the nasopharynx communicates with the posterior apertures of the nose. Hanging from the posterior aspect of the soft palate is a small conical process, the *uvula*. On the roof and posterior wall of the nasopharynx, between the orifices of the auditory tubes, the mucosa contains a mass of lymphoid tissue known as the *pharyngeal tonsil* (or *adenoids* when enlarged). Hypertrophy of this tissue interferes with nasal breathing and is common in children. This condition is well shown in a lateral radiographic image of the nasopharynx.

The *oropharynx* is the portion extending from the soft palate to the level of the *hyoid bone*. The base, or root, of the tongue forms the anterior wall of the oropharynx. The *laryngeal pharynx* lies posterior to the larynx, its anterior wall being formed by the posterior surface of the larynx. The laryngeal pharynx extends inferiorly and is continuous with the esophagus.

The air-containing nasal and oral pharynges are well visualized in lateral images, except during the act of phonation, when the soft palate contracts and tends to obscure the nasal pharynx. An opaque medium is required to show the lumen of the laryngeal pharynx, although it can be distended with air during the *Valsalva maneuver* (an increase in intrathoracic pressure produced by forcible expiration effort against the closed glottis).

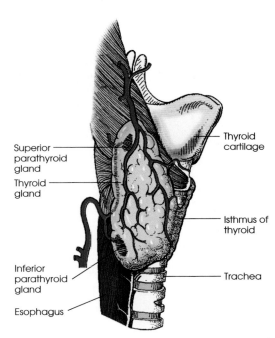

Superior parathyroid gland

Thyroid gland

Inferior parathyroid gland

Esophagus

Thyroid cartilage

Isthmus of thyroid

Trachea

Fig. 3.8 Lateral aspect of laryngeal area showing thyroid gland and isthmus that connects its two lobes.

LARYNX

The larynx is the organ of voice (Figs. 3.9 and 3.10; see Figs. 3.6 through 3.8). Serving as the air passage between the pharynx and the trachea, the larynx is also one of the divisions of the respiratory system.

The larynx is a movable, tubular structure; is broader above than below; and is approximately 1½ inches (3.8 cm) in length. Situated below the root of the tongue and in front of the laryngeal pharynx, the larynx is suspended from the hyoid bone and extends from the level of the superior margin of the fourth cervical vertebra to its junction with the trachea at the level of the inferior margin of the sixth cervical vertebra. The thin, leaf-shaped *epiglottis* is situated behind the root of the tongue and the hyoid bone,

and above the laryngeal entrance. It has been stated that the epiglottis serves as a trap to prevent leakage into the larynx between acts of swallowing. The *thyroid cartilage* forms the laryngeal prominence, or *Adam's apple*.

The inlet of the larynx is oblique, slanting posteriorly as it descends. A pouchlike fossa called the *piriform recess* is located on each side of the larynx and external to its orifice. The piriform recesses are well shown as triangular areas on frontal projections when insufflated with air (Valsalva maneuver) or when filled with an opaque medium.

The entrance of the larynx is guarded superiorly and anteriorly by the epiglottis and laterally and posteriorly by folds of mucous membrane. These folds, which extend around the margin of the laryngeal

inlet from their junction with the epiglottis, function as a sphincter during swallowing. The *laryngeal cavity* is subdivided into three compartments by two pairs of mucosal folds that extend anteroposteriorly from its lateral walls. The superior pairs of folds are the *vestibular folds,* or false vocal cords. The space above them is called the *laryngeal vestibule.* The lower two folds are separated from each other by a median fissure called the *rima glottidis.* They are known as the *vocal folds,* or true vocal folds (see Fig. 3.10). The vocal cords are vocal ligaments that are covered by the vocal folds. The ligaments and the rima glottidis constitute the vocal apparatus of the larynx, and are collectively referred to as the *glottis.*

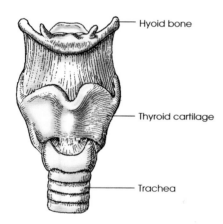

Fig. 3.9 Anterior aspect of larynx.

- Hyoid bone
- Thyroid cartilage
- Trachea

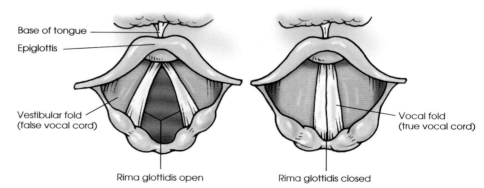

Base of tongue
Epiglottis
Vestibular fold (false vocal cord)
Vocal fold (true vocal cord)
Rima glottidis open
Rima glottidis closed

Fig. 3.10 Superior aspect of larynx (open and closed true vocal folds).

Mediastinum

The *mediastinum* is the area of the thorax bounded by the sternum anteriorly, the spine posteriorly, and the lungs laterally (Fig. 3.11). The structures associated with the mediastinum are as follows:

- Heart
- Great vessels
- Trachea
- Esophagus
- Thymus
- Lymphatics
- Nerves
- Fibrous tissue
- Fat

The *esophagus* is the part of the digestive canal that connects the pharynx with the stomach. It is a narrow, musculomembranous tube about 9 inches (23 cm) in length. Following the curves of the vertebral column, the esophagus descends through the posterior part of the mediastinum and then runs anteriorly to pass through the esophageal hiatus of the diaphragm.

The esophagus lies just in front of the vertebral column, with its anterior surface in close relation to the trachea, aortic arch, and heart. This makes the esophagus valuable in certain heart examinations. When the esophagus is filled with barium sulfate, the posterior border of the heart and the aorta are outlined well in lateral and oblique projections (Fig. 3.12). Frontal, oblique, and lateral images are often used in examinations of the esophagus. Radiography of the esophagus is discussed in Volume 2, Chapter 15.

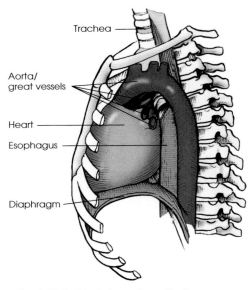

Fig. 3.11 Lateral view of mediastinum, identifying main structures.

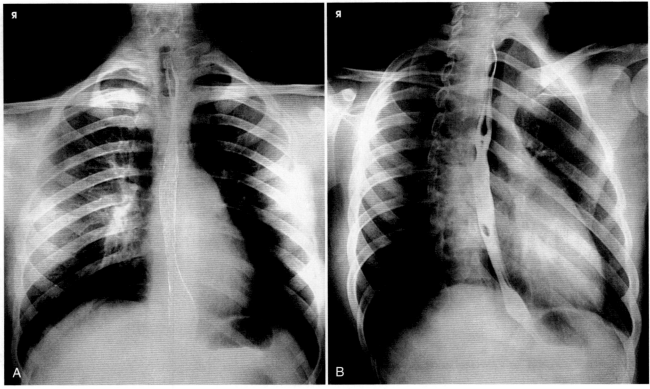

Fig. 3.12 (A) PA projection of esophagus with barium sulfate coating its walls. (B) PA oblique projection with barium-filled esophagus (RAO position).

The *thymus gland* is the primary control organ of the lymphatic system. It is responsible for producing the hormone *thymosin*, which plays a crucial role in the development and maturation of the immune system. The thymus consists of two pyramid-shaped lobes that lie in the lower neck and superior mediastinum, anterior to the trachea and great vessels of the heart, and posterior to the manubrium. The thymus reaches its maximum size at puberty and then gradually undergoes atrophy until it almost disappears (Fig. 3.13).

In older individuals, lymphatic tissue is replaced by fat. At its maximum development, the thymus rests on the pericardium and reaches as high as the thyroid gland. When the thymus is enlarged in infants and young children, it can press on the retrothymic organs, displacing them posteriorly and causing respiratory disturbances. A radiographic examination may be made in the AP and lateral projections. For optimal image contrast, exposures should be made at the end of full inspiration.

COMPUTED TOMOGRAPHY

At the present time, computed tomography (CT) is used almost exclusively to image the anatomic areas of the thorax, including the thymus gland. CT is excellent at showing all thoracic structures (Fig. 3.14).

SUMMARY OF ANATOMY

Body habitus
Sthenic
Asthenic
Hyposthenic
Hypersthenic

Thoracic cavity
Superior thoracic aperture
Inferior thoracic aperture
Diaphragm
Thoracic viscera
  Lungs
  Heart
  Respiratory system
  Cardiac system
  Lymphatic system
  Inferior esophagus
  Thymus gland
  Pericardial cavity
  Pleural cavities
  Serous membranes
  Mediastinum

Respiratory system
Pharynx
Nasopharynx
Soft palate
Hard palate
Uvula
Pharyngeal tonsil
Oropharynx
Hyoid bone
Laryngeal pharynx
Larynx
  Epiglottis
  Thyroid cartilage
  Piriform recess
  Laryngeal cavity
  Vestibular folds (false vocal cords)
  Laryngeal vestibule
  Rima glottides
  Vocal folds (true vocal cords)
  Glottis

Trachea
  Carina
Primary bronchi
  Right primary bronchus
  Left primary bronchus
Secondary bronchi
Tertiary bronchi
Bronchioles
Terminal bronchioles
Bronchial tree

Alveoli
Alveolar duct
Alveolar sac
Alveoli

Lungs
Parenchyma
Apex
Base
Costophrenic angles
Hilum
Cardiac notch
Pleura
  Visceral pleura

Parietal pleura
Serous fluid
Pleural cavity
Lobes
  Superior lobes
  Inferior lobes
  Right middle lobe
Interlobar fissures
  Oblique fissures (2)
  Horizontal fissure
Lingula
Bronchopulmonary segments
Primary lobules

Mediastinum
Heart
Great vessels
Trachea
Esophagus
Thymus
Lymphatics
Nerves
Fibrous tissue
Fat

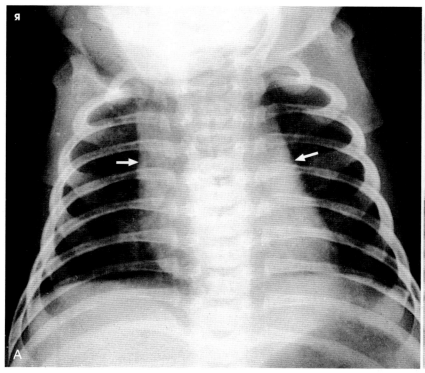

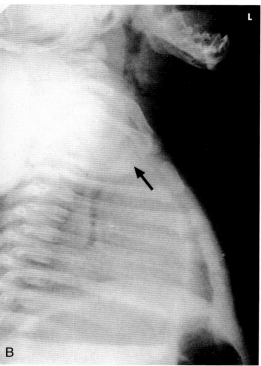

Fig. 3.13 (A) PA chest radiograph showing mediastinal enlargement caused by hypertrophy of thymus *(arrows)*. (B) Lateral chest radiograph showing enlarged thymus *(arrow)*.

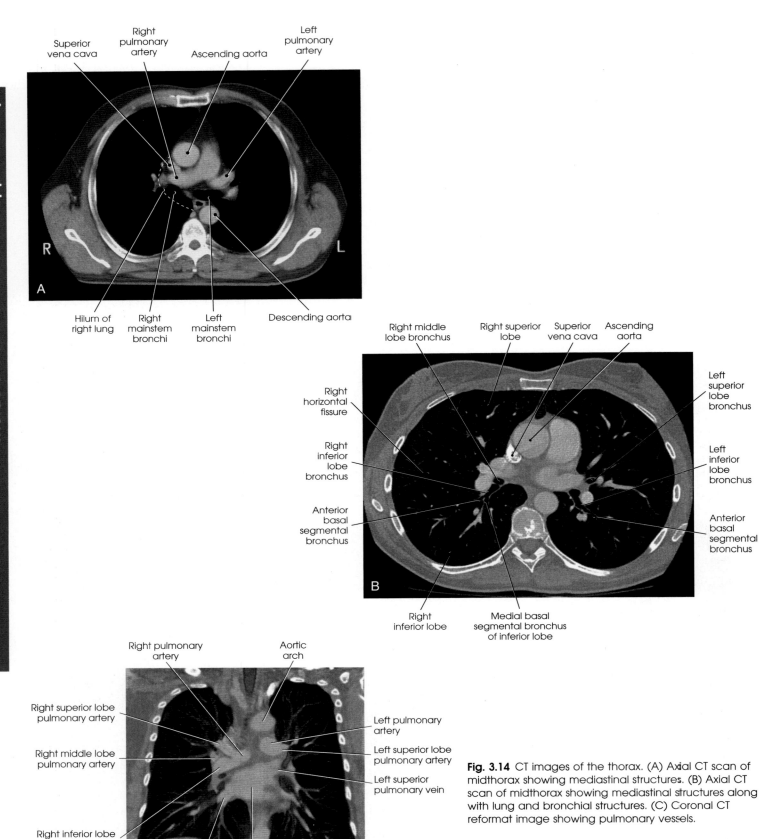

Fig. 3.14 CT images of the thorax. (A) Axial CT scan of midthorax showing mediastinal structures. (B) Axial CT scan of midthorax showing mediastinal structures along with lung and bronchial structures. (C) Coronal CT reformat image showing pulmonary vessels.

SUMMARY OF PATHOLOGY

Condition	Definition
Aspiration/foreign body	Inspiration of a foreign material into the airway
Atelectasis	Collapse of all or part of the lung
Bronchiectasis	Chronic dilation of the bronchi and bronchioles associated with secondary infection
Bronchitis	Inflammation of the bronchi
Chronic obstructive pulmonary disease	Chronic condition of persistent obstruction of bronchial airflow
Cystic fibrosis	Disorder associated with widespread dysfunction of the exocrine glands, abnormal secretion of sweat and saliva, and accumulation of thick mucus in the lungs
Emphysema	Destructive and obstructive airway changes leading to an increased volume of air in the lungs
Epiglottitis	Inflammation of the epiglottis
Fungal disease	Inflammation of the lung caused by a fungal organism
Histoplasmosis	Infection caused by the yeastlike organism *Histoplasma capsulatum*
Granulomatous disease	Condition of the lung marked by formation of granulomas
Sarcoidosis	Condition of unknown origin often associated with pulmonary fibrosis
Tuberculosis	Chronic infection of the lung caused by the tubercle bacillus
Hyaline membrane disease or respiratory distress syndrome	Under-aeration of the lungs caused by lack of surfactant
Metastasis	Transfer of a cancerous lesion from one area to another
Pleural effusion	Collection of fluid in the pleural cavity
Pneumoconiosis	Lung diseases resulting from inhalation of industrial substances
Anthracosis or coal miner lung or black lung	Inflammation caused by inhalation of coal dust (anthracite)
Asbestosis	Inflammation caused by inhalation of asbestos
Silicosis	Inflammation caused by inhalation of silicon dioxide
Pneumonia	Acute infection in the lung parenchyma
Aspiration	Pneumonia caused by aspiration of foreign particles
Interstitial or viral or pneumonitis	Pneumonia caused by a virus and involving the alveolar walls and interstitial structures
Lobar or bacterial	Pneumonia involving the alveoli of an entire lobe without involving the bronchi
Lobular or bronchopneumonia	Pneumonia involving the bronchi and scattered throughout the lung
Pneumothorax	Accumulation of air in the pleural cavity resulting in collapse of the lung
Pulmonary edema	Replacement of air with fluid in the lung interstitium and alveoli
Tumor	New tissue growth where cell proliferation is uncontrolled

Eponymous (ncmed) pathologies are listed in nonpossessive form to conform to the *AMA manual of style: a guide for authors and editors*, ed 10, Oxford, 2009, Oxford University Press.

SAMPLE EXPOSURE TECHNIQUE CHART ESSENTIAL PROJECTIONS

These techniques were accurate for the equipment used to produce each exposure. However, use caution when applying them in your department because "there is considerable variability in image receptor response owing to varying scatter sensitivity, the use of grids with different grid ratios, collimation, beam filtration, the choice of kilovoltage, source-to-image distance, and image receptor size."[1]
This chart was created in collaboration with Dennis Bowman, AS, RT(R), Clinical Instructor, Community Hospital of the Monterey Peninsula, Monterey, CA. http://digitalradiographysolutions.com/.

THORACIC VISCERA

Part	cm	kVp[a]	SID[b]	Collimation	CR[c] mAs	CR[c] Dose (mGy)[e]	DR[d] mAs	DR[d] Dose (mGy)[e]
Chest: Lungs and heart—PA[f]	22	120	72″	14″ × 16″ (35 × 40 cm)	2.8[g]	0.188	1.4[g]	0.089
Chest: Lungs and heart—lateral[f]	33	120	72″	14″ × 17″ (35 ×43 cm)	7.1[g]	0.550	3.6[g]	0.273
Chest: Lungs and heart—PA oblique[f]	25	120	72″	14″ × 17″ (35 × 43 cm)	3.6[g]	0.255	1.8[g]	0.124
Chest: Lungs and heart—AP[h]	22	90	40″	16″ × 14″ (40 × 35 cm)	4.0[g]	0.655		
Chest: Lungs and heart—AP[h]	22	105	40″	16″ × 14″ (40 × 35 cm)			1.6[g]	0.340
Chest: Lungs and heart—AP[f]	22	120	72″	14″ × 16″ (35 × 40 cm)	3.2[g]	0.217	1.6[g]	0.104
Pulmonary apices—AP axial[f]	23	120	72″	14″ × 11″ (35 × 28 cm)	4.0[g]	0.198	2.0[g]	0.097
Lungs and pleurae—lateral decubitus[f]	22	120	72″	17″ ×14″ (43 × 35 cm)	4.0[g]	0.271	2.0[g]	0.133
Lungs and pleurae—dorsal/ventral decubitus[f]	33	120	72″	17″ × 14″ (43 × 35 cm)	9.0[g]	0.697	4.5[g]	0.344

[1]ACR-AAPM-SIMM Practice Parameter for Digital Radiography, revised 2017.
[a]kVp values are for a high-frequency generator.
[b]40 inches minimum; 44 to 48 inches recommended to improve spatial resolution (mAs increase needed, but no increase in patient dose will result).
[c]AGFA CR MD 4.0 General IP, CR 75.0 reader, 400 speed class, with 6:1 (178LPI) grid when needed.
[d]GE Definium 8000, with 13:1 grid when needed.
[e]All doses are skin entrance for average adult (160 to 200 pounds male, 150 to 190 pounds female) at part thickness indicated.
[f]Bucky/Grid.
[g]Large focal spot.
[h]Nongrid.
AP, Anteroposterior; PA, posteroanterior; SID, source-to-image receptor distance.

Radiography of the neck can be used to evaluate the cervical spine or the soft tissues of the anterior neck. Soft tissue neck radiographs can demonstrate foreign bodies, swelling (especially epiglottitis), masses (intrinsic and extrinsic to airway), and fractures of the larynx and hyoid bone. The patient can be positioned either upright or recumbent, depending on physical condition. Radiographs are most commonly made of the upper airway, from the superior oropharynx to the proximal trachea.

AP PROJECTION

Image receptor + grid: Positioned by manufacturer or department protocol for proper anatomy display orientation; CR plate: 10 × 12 inches (24 × 30 cm) lengthwise.

Position of patient

- Performed in either the supine or the upright position, depending on patient condition

Position of part

- Center the midsagittal plane of the body to the midline of the grid.
- Adjust the patient's shoulders to lie in the same transverse plane.
- Extend the patient's neck slightly, and adjust it so that the midsagittal plane is perpendicular to the plane of the IR (Figs. 3.15 and 3.16).
- Center the IR at the level of the laryngeal prominence (for upper airway) or manubrium (for larynx and superior mediastinum).
- *Shield gonads.*

- *Respiration*: Exposure is made during slow inspiration to ensure that the trachea is filled with air.

Central ray

- Perpendicular through the midsagittal plane at the level of the laryngeal prominence (upper airway) or manubrium (larynx and superior mediastinum)

Collimation

- Adjust radiation field to 12 inches (30 cm) lengthwise and 1 inch (2.5 cm) beyond the skin line on the sides, but not more than 10 inches (24 cm). Place a side marker in the collimated exposure field.

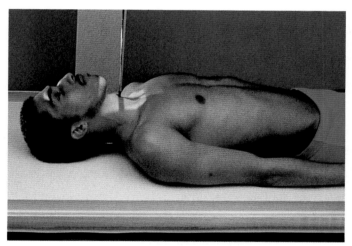

Fig. 3.15 AP soft tissue neck: pharynx and larynx.

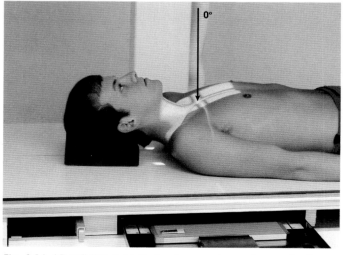

Fig. 3.16 AP soft tissue neck: trachea and superior mediastinum.

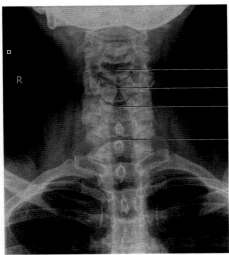

Fig. 3.17 AP soft tissue neck: pharynx and larynx during quiet breathing.

Laryngeal vestibule

Rima glottidis

Infraglottic cavity

Trachea

Structures shown

The resulting image shows the air-filled upper airway or the trachea and superior mediastinum. Under normal conditions, the airway is superimposed on the shadow of the cervical vertebrae (Figs. 3.17 and 3.18).

EVALUATION CRITERIA

The following should be clearly seen:

■ Evidence of proper collimation and presence of a side marker placed clear of anatomy of interest

■ Air-filled upper airway, from the pharynx to the proximal trachea (for upper airway)

■ Air-filled airway, from the midcervical to the midthoracic region (for trachea and superior mediastinum)

■ No rotation, with spinous processes equidistant to the pedicles and aligned with the midline of the cervical bodies

■ Bony trabecular detail and surrounding soft tissues

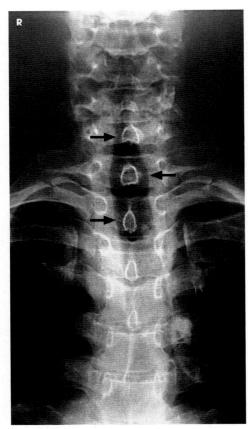

Fig. 3.18 AP soft tissue neck: trachea (*arrows*) and superior mediastinum during quiet breathing.

LATERAL PROJECTION
R or L position

Image receptor + grid: Positioned by manufacturer or department protocol for proper anatomy display orientation; CR plate: 10 × 12 inches (24 × 30 cm) lengthwise.

Position of patient

- Place the patient in a lateral position, either seated or standing, before a vertical grid device. If the standing position is used, the weight of the patient's body must be equally distributed on the feet.

Position of part

- Instruct the patient to clasp the hands behind the body and rotate the shoulders posteriorly as far as possible (Figs. 3.19 and 3.20). This position keeps the superimposed shadows of the arms from obscuring the structures of the superior mediastinum.
- Adjust the patient's position to center the airway to the midline of the IR. The trachea lies in the coronal plane that passes approximately midway between the jugular notch and the midcoronal plane.
- Center the IR at the level of the laryngeal prominence (for upper airway) or manubrium (for larynx and superior mediastinum).
- Readjust the position of the body, being careful to have the midsagittal plane vertical and parallel with the plane of the IR.
- Extend the neck slightly.
- *Shield gonads.*
- *Respiration*: Exposure is made during slow inspiration to ensure that the trachea is filled with air.

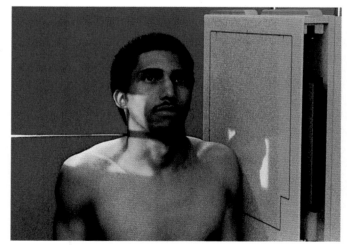

Fig. 3.19 Lateral soft tissue neck: pharynx and larynx.

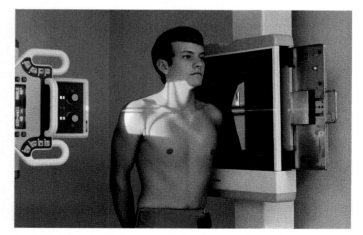

Fig. 3.20 Lateral soft tissue neck: trachea and superior mediastinum.

Central ray

- Horizontal through the midcoronal plane at the level of the laryngeal prominence (for upper airway [Fig. 3.21]) or at the level of the jugular notch through a point midway between the jugular notch and the midcoronal plane (for trachea and superior mediastinum [Fig. 3.22])

Collimation

- Adjust radiation field to 12 inches (30 cm) lengthwise and 1 inch (2.5 cm) beyond the skin line of the anterior and posterior surfaces, but not greater than 10 inches (24 cm). Place a side marker in the collimated exposure field.

Structures shown

The resulting image shows the air-filled upper airway or the trachea and superior mediastinum. The projection for the trachea and superior mediastinum, first described by Eiselberg and Sgalitzer,[1] is used to show retrosternal extensions of the thyroid gland, thymic enlargement in infants (in the recumbent position), the opacified pharynx and upper esophagus, and an outline of the trachea and bronchi. It is also used to locate foreign bodies.

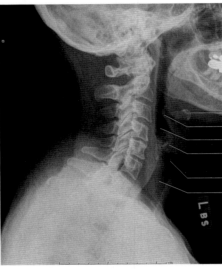

Fig. 3.21 Lateral soft tissue neck: pharynx and larynx during quiet breathing.

Hyoid bone
Epiglottis
Laryngeal vestibule
Thyroid cartilage and laryngeal cavity
Infraglottic cavity
Trachea

EVALUATION CRITERIA

The following should be clearly seen:

- Evidence of proper collimation and presence of a side marker placed clear of anatomy of interest
- Air-filled upper airway, from the pharynx to the proximal trachea (for upper airway)
- Air-filled airway, from the midcervical to the midthoracic region (for trachea and superior mediastinum)
- No rotation or tilt of the cervical spine
  □ Superimposed zygapophyseal joints and open intervertebral joints
  □ Superimposed or nearly superimposed mandibular rami
- Bony trabecular detail and surrounding soft tissues

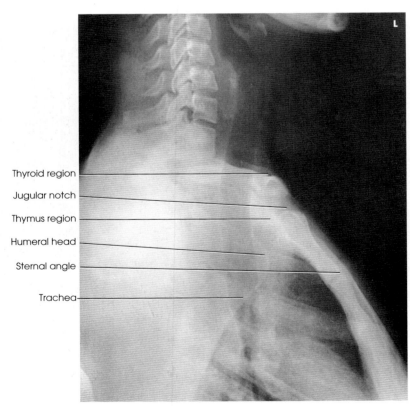

Thyroid region
Jugular notch
Thymus region
Humeral head
Sternal angle
Trachea

Fig. 3.22 Lateral soft tissue neck: trachea and superior mediastinum during quiet breathing.

General Positioning Considerations for the Chest

For radiography of the chest, the patient is placed in an *upright position* whenever possible to prevent engorgement of the pulmonary vessels and to allow gravity to depress the diaphragm. Of equal importance, the upright position shows air and fluid levels. In the recumbent position, gravitational force causes the abdominal viscera and diaphragm to move superiorly; it compresses the thoracic viscera, which prevents full expansion of the lungs. Although the difference in diaphragm movement is not great in hyposthenic individuals, it is marked in hypersthenic individuals. Figs. 3.23 and 3.24 illustrate the effects of body position in the same patient. The left lateral chest position (Fig. 3.25) is most commonly employed because it places the heart closer to the IR, resulting in a less magnified heart image. Left and right lateral chest images are compared in Figs. 3.25 and 3.26.

A *slight amount of rotation* from the PA or lateral projection causes considerable distortion of the heart shadow. To prevent this distortion, the body must be carefully positioned and immobilized.

PA CRITERIA

For PA projections, procedures are as follows:
- Instruct the patient to sit or stand upright. If the standing position is used, the weight of the body must be equally distributed on the feet.
- Position the patient's head upright, facing directly forward.
- Have the patient depress the shoulders and hold them in contact with the grid device to carry the clavicles below the lung apices. Except in the presence of an upper thoracic scoliosis, a faulty body position can be detected by the asymmetric appearance of the sternoclavicular joints. Compare the clavicular margins in Figs. 3.27 and 3.28.

LATERAL CRITERIA

For lateral projections, procedures are as follows:
- Place the side of interest against the IR holder.
- Have the patient stand so that the weight is equally distributed on the feet. The patient should not lean toward or away from the IR holder.
- Raise the patient's arms to prevent the soft tissue of the arms from superimposing the lung fields.
- Instruct the patient to face straight ahead and raise the chin.
- To determine rotation, examine the posterior aspects of the ribs. Radiographs without rotation show superimposed posterior ribs (see Figs. 3.25 and 3.26).

OBLIQUE CRITERIA

In oblique projections, the patient rotates the hips with the thorax and points the feet directly forward. The shoulders should lie in the same transverse plane on all radiographs.

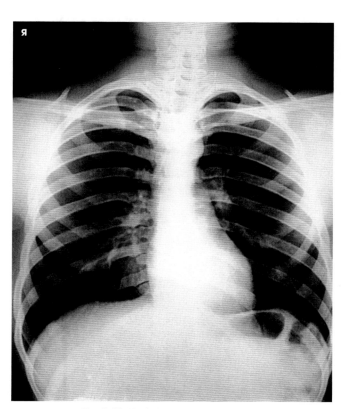

Fig. 3.23 Upright chest radiograph.

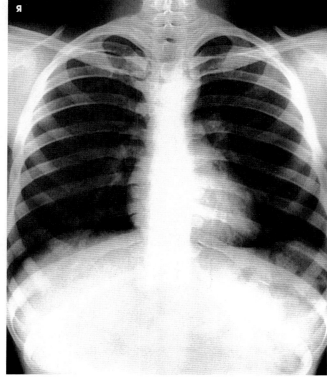

Fig. 3.24 Prone chest radiograph. Diaphragm is superior when compared to Fig. 3.23.

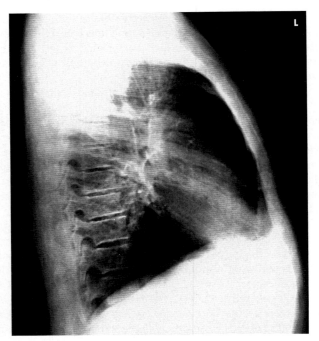

Fig. 3.25 Left lateral chest.

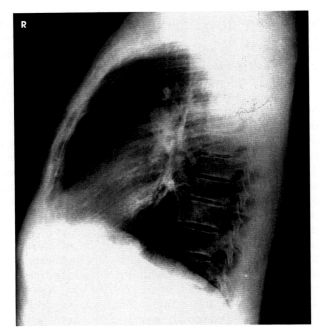

Fig. 3.26 Right lateral chest.

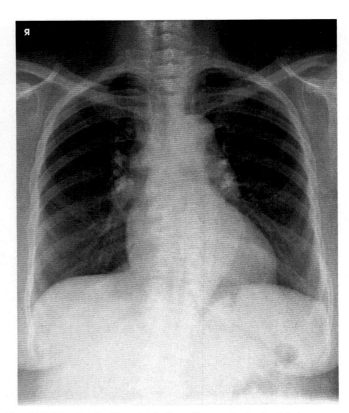

Fig. 3.27 PA chest without rotation. Sternoclavicular joints equidistant from midsagittal plane.

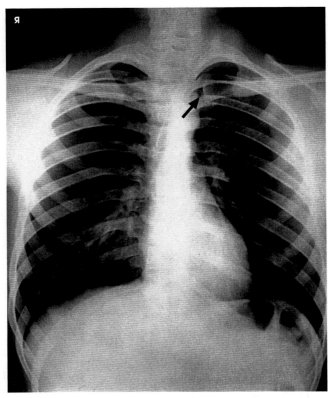

Fig. 3.28 PA chest with rotation. Left sternoclavicular joint *(arrow)* fully visible in pulmonary apex.

Breathing Instructions

During *normal inspiration*, the costal muscles pull the anterior ribs superiorly and, laterally, the shoulders rise, and the thorax expands from front to back and from side to side. These changes in the height and AP dimension of the thorax must be considered when the patient is positioned.

Deep inspiration causes the diaphragm to move inferiorly, resulting in elongation of the heart. Radiographs of the heart should be obtained at the end of normal inspiration to prevent distortion. More air is inhaled during the second breath (and without strain) than during the first breath.

When *pneumothorax* (gas or air in the pleural cavity) is suspected, one exposure is often made at the end of full inspiration and another at the end of full expiration, to show small amounts of free air in the pleural cavity that might be obscured on the inspiration exposure (Figs. 3.29 and 3.30). Inspiration and expiration radiographs are also used to show the movement of the diaphragm, the occasional presence of a foreign body, and atelectasis (absence of air).

Technical Procedure

The projections required to show the thoracic viscera adequately are usually requested by the attending physician and are determined by the clinical history of the patient. The PA projection of the chest is the most common projection, and is used in all lung and heart examinations. The lateral projection is usually ordered in conjunction with the PA. Right and left oblique projections may be employed as required to supplement the PA projection. It is often necessary to improvise variations of the basic positions to project a localized area free of superimposed structures.

The exposure factors and accessories employed in examining the thoracic viscera depend on the radiographic characteristics of the individual patient's pathologic condition. Normally chest radiography uses a high kilovolt (peak; kVp) to penetrate and show all thoracic anatomy on the radiograph. The kVp can be lowered if exposures are made without a grid. An appropriate kVp will penetrate the mediastinum to show a faint image of the spine, as well as demonstrate the pulmonary vascular markings of the lung periphery.

Whenever possible, a minimum source-to-image receptor distance (SID) of 72 inches (183 cm) should be used to minimize magnification of the heart and to obtain greater spatial resolution of the delicate lung structures (Fig. 3.31).

Use of a grid is recommended for opaque areas within the lung fields and to show the lung structure through thickened pleural membranes (Figs. 3.32 and 3.33). This technique allows penetration of these opaque areas while maintain appropriate contrast resolution.

Radiation Protection

Protection of the patient from unnecessary radiation is the professional responsibility of the radiographer (see Chapter 1 for specific guidelines). In this chapter, the *Shield gonads* statement indicates that the patient is to be protected from unnecessary radiation by restricting the radiation beam using proper collimation. In addition, the placement of lead shielding between the gonads and the radiation source is appropriate when the clinical objectives of the examination are not compromised. An example of a properly placed lead shield is shown in Fig. 3.34.

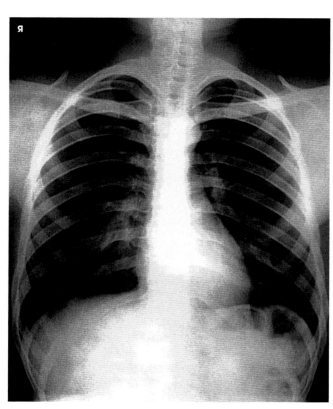

Fig. 3.29 PA chest during inspiration.

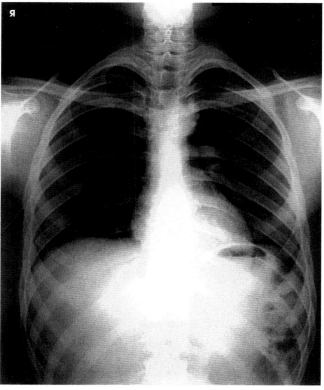

Fig. 3.30 PA chest during expiration. Diaphragm is superior and fewer posterior ribs are visible when compared to Fig. 3.29.

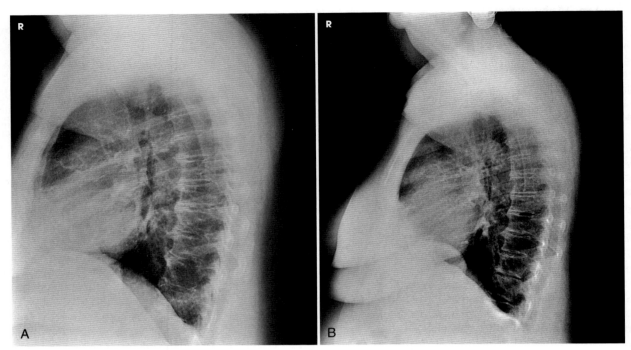

Fig. 3.31 (A) Lateral chest radiograph performed at 44-inch (112-cm) SID. (B) Radiograph in the same patient performed at 72-inch (183-cm) SID. Note decreased magnification and greater recorded detail of lung structures.

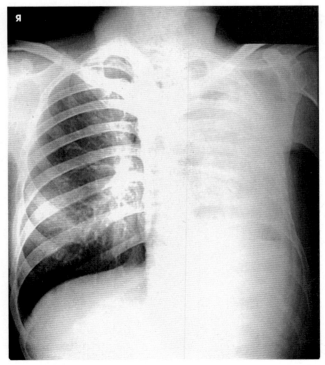

Fig. 3.32 Nongrid radiograph showing fluid-type pathologic condition in same patient as in Fig. 3.33. The left lung is opaque, obscuring lung detail.

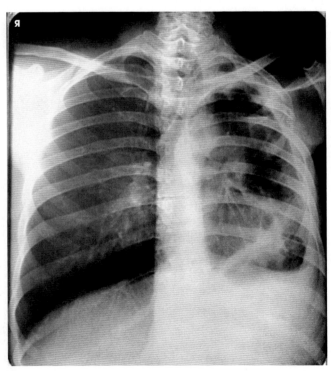

Fig. 3.33 Grid radiograph of the same patient as in Fig. 3.32. Details in the left lung are visible.

🕏 PA PROJECTION

Image receptor + grid: Positioned by a manufacturer or department protocol for proper anatomy display orientation; CR plate: 14×17 inches (35×43 cm) lengthwise, or crosswise for hypersthenic patients.

SID: Minimum SID of 72 inches (183 cm) is recommended to decrease magnification of the heart and increase recorded detail of the thoracic structures.

Position of patient

- If possible, always examine patients in the upright position, either standing or seated, so that the diaphragm is at its lowest position, and air or fluid levels are seen. Engorgement of the pulmonary vessels is also avoided. Patients on a stretcher can be radiographed sitting with the legs dangling over the side of the stretcher, if conditions allow.

Position of part

- Place the patient, with arms hanging at sides, before a vertical grid device.
- Adjust the height of the IR so that its upper border is about 1.5 to 2 inches (3.8 to 5 cm) above the relaxed shoulders.
- Center the midsagittal plane of the patient's body to the midline of the IR.
- Have the patient stand straight, with the weight of the body equally distributed on the feet.
- Extend the patient's chin upward or over the top of the grid device, and adjust the head so that the midsagittal plane is vertical.

- Ask the patient to flex the elbows and to rest the *backs of the hands* low on the hips, below the level of the costophrenic angles. Depress the shoulders and adjust to lie in the same transverse plane. These movements will position the clavicles below the apices of the lungs.
- Rotate the shoulders forward so that both touch the vertical grid device. This movement will rotate the scapulae outward and laterally to reduce superimposition of the scapulae with the lungs (Fig. 3.34).

- If a female patient's breasts are large enough to be superimposed over the lower part of the lung fields, especially the costophrenic angles, ask the patient to pull the breasts upward and laterally. This is especially important when ruling out the presence of fluid. Have the patient hold the breasts in place by leaning against the IR holder (Figs. 3.35 and 3.36).
- *Shield gonads:* Place a lead shield between the x-ray tube and the patient's pelvis (see Fig. 3.34).

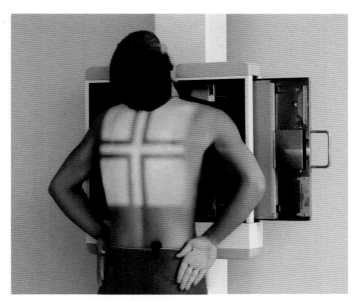

Fig. 3.34 Patient positioned for PA chest.

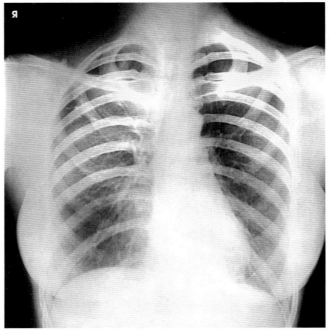

Fig. 3.35 Breasts superimposed over lower lungs.

- *Respiration*: Full inspiration. The exposure is made after the *second* full inspiration to ensure the maximum expansion of the lungs. The lungs expand transversely, anteroposteriorly,

and vertically, with vertical being the greatest dimension.

- For certain conditions, such as pneumothorax and the presence of a foreign body, radiographs are sometimes made

at the end of full inspiration and expiration (Figs. 3.37–3.39). Pneumothorax is shown more clearly on expiration, because collapse of the lung is accentuated.

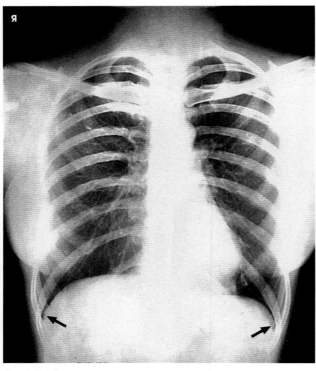

Fig. 3.36 Correct placement of breasts. Costophrenic angles are clearly seen *(arrows)*.

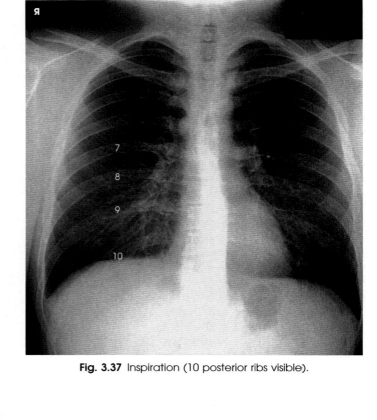

Fig. 3.37 Inspiration (10 posterior ribs visible).

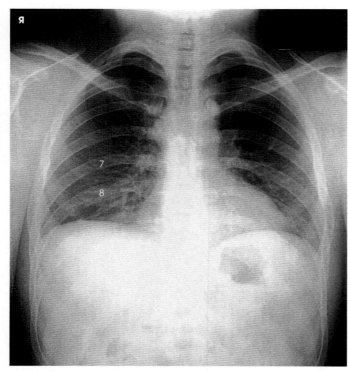

Fig. 3.38 Expiration in the same patient as in Fig. 3.38 (8 posterior ribs visible).

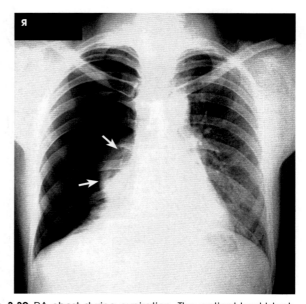

Fig. 3.39 PA chest during expiration. The patient had blunt trauma to the right chest. Left side is normal. Pneumothorax is seen on entire right side, and totally collapsed lung is seen near hilum *(arrows)*.

Central ray

- Perpendicular to the center of the IR. The central ray should enter at the level of T7 (inferior angle of the scapula).

Collimation

- Adjust the radiation field to 17 inches (43 cm) lengthwise and 1 inch (2.5 cm) beyond the lateral shadows, but no more the 14 inches (35 cm). The opposite dimensions are used for a crosswise IR. Vertical dimension may be less for smaller patients. Place a side marker in the collimated exposure field.

Structures shown

PA projection of the thoracic viscera shows the air-filled trachea, the lungs, the diaphragmatic domes, the heart and aortic arch, and if enlarged laterally, the thyroid or thymus gland (Fig. 3.40). The vascular markings are much more prominent on the projection made at the end of expiration. The bronchial tree is shown from an oblique angle. The esophagus is well shown when it is filled with a barium sulfate suspension.

EVALUATION CRITERIA

The following should be clearly seen:
- Evidence of proper collimation and presence of a side marker placed clear of anatomy of interest
- Entire lungs from the apices to the costophrenic angles
- No rotation
  - Sternal ends of the clavicles equidistant from the vertebral column
  - Trachea visible in the midline
  - Equal distance from the vertebral column to the lateral border of the ribs on each side
- Proper anterior shoulder rotation demonstrated by scapulae projected outside the lung fields
- Proper inspiration demonstrated by 10 posterior ribs visible above the diaphragm; at least one less rib visible on expiration
- Sharp outlines of heart and diaphragm
- Faint shadows of the ribs and superior thoracic vertebrae visible through the heart shadow

- Pulmonary vascular markings from the hilar regions to the periphery of the lungs

NOTE: Inferior lobes of both lungs should be carefully checked for adequate penetration in women with large, pendulous breasts.

Cardiac studies with barium

PA chest radiographs may be obtained with the patient swallowing a bolus of barium sulfate to outline the posterior heart and aorta. The barium used in cardiac examinations should be thicker than the barium used for the stomach, so that the contrast medium descends more slowly and adheres to the esophageal walls. The patient should hold the barium in the mouth until just before the exposure is made. Then the patient should take a deep breath and swallow the bolus of barium; the exposure is made at this time (see Fig. 3.12).

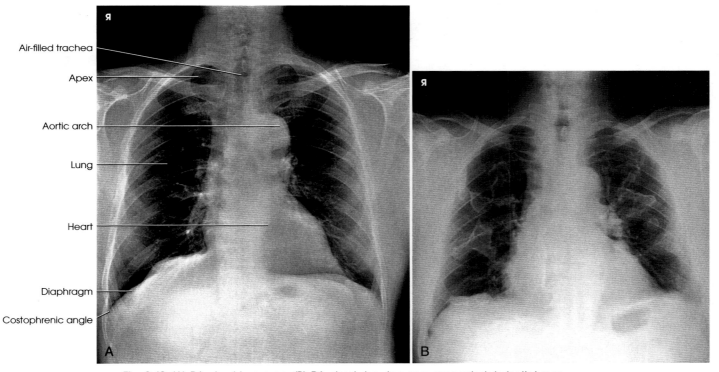

Fig. 3.40 (A) PA chest in a man. (B) PA chest showing pneumoconiosis in both lungs (multiple, irregularly shaped white areas show built-up coal dust).

♠ LATERAL PROJECTION
R or L position

Image receptor + grid: Positioned by manufacturer or department protocol for proper anatomy display orientation; CR plate: 14 × 17 inches (35 × 43 cm) lengthwise.

SID: Minimum SID of 72 inches (183 cm) is recommended to decrease magnification of the heart and increase recorded detail of the thoracic structures.

Position of patient
- If possible, always examine the patient in the upright position, either standing or seated, so that the diaphragm is at its lowest position, and air and fluid levels can be seen. Engorgement of the pulmonary vessels is also avoided.
- Turn the patient to a true lateral position, with arms by the sides.
- To show the heart and left lung, use the left lateral position with the patient's left side against the IR.
- Use the right lateral position to best show the right lung.

Position of part
- Adjust the position of the patient so that the midsagittal plane of the body is parallel with the IR and the adjacent shoulder is touching the grid device.
- Center the thorax to the grid; the midcoronal plane should be perpendicular and centered to the midline of the grid.
- Have the patient extend the arms directly upward, flex the elbows, and with the forearms resting on the head, hold the arms in position (Fig. 3.41).
- Place an intravenous catheter stand in front of an unsteady patient. Have the patient extend the arms and grasp the stand as high as possible for support.
- Adjust the height of the IR so that the upper border is about 1.5 to 2 inches (3.8 to 5 cm) above the shoulders.
- Recheck the position of the body; the midsagittal plane must be vertical. Depending on the width of the shoulders, the lower part of the thorax and hips may be a greater distance from the IR, but this body position is necessary for a true lateral projection. Having the patient *lean* against the grid device (foreshortening) results in distortion of all thoracic structures (Fig. 3.42). *Forward bending* also results in distorted structural outlines (Fig. 3.43).
- *Shield gonads*.

- *Respiration*: Full inspiration. The exposure is made after the *second* full inspiration to ensure the maximum expansion of the lungs.

Central ray
- Perpendicular to the center of the IR. The central ray enters the patient on the midcoronal plane at the level of T7 or at the inferior aspect of the scapula.

Collimation
- Adjust radiation field to 17 inches (43 cm) lengthwise and 1 inch (2.5 cm) beyond the anterior and posterior shadows, but no more the 14 inches (35 cm). Vertical dimension may be less for smaller patients. Place a side marker in the collimated exposure field.

Structures shown
The preliminary left lateral chest position is used to show the heart, the aorta, and left-sided pulmonary lesions (Figs. 3.44 and 3.45). The right lateral chest position is used to show right-sided pulmonary lesions (Fig. 3.46). These lateral projections are employed extensively to show the interlobar fissures, to differentiate the lobes, and to localize pulmonary lesions.

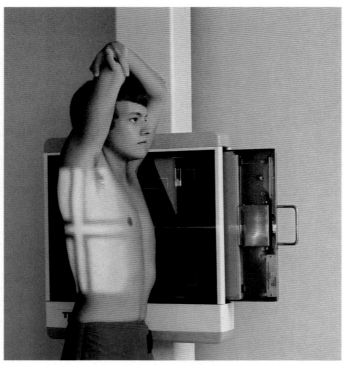

Fig. 3.41 Lateral chest.

EVALUATION CRITERIA

The following should be clearly seen:
- Evidence of proper collimation and presence of a side marker placed clear of anatomy of interest
- Arm or its soft tissues not overlapping the superior lung field
- Costophrenic angles and the portions of the pulmonary apices not obscured by the arms and shoulders

- No rotation
  - ☐ Hila in the approximate center of the radiograph
  - ☐ Superimposition of the ribs posterior to the vertebral column
  - ☐ Sternum in profile
  - ☐ Trachea visible in the midline
- Long axis of the lung fields shown in vertical position, without forward or backward leaning

- Open thoracic intervertebral joint spaces and intervertebral foramina, except in patients with scoliosis
- Sharp outlines of heart and diaphragm
- Pulmonary vascular markings from the hilar regions to the periphery of the lungs

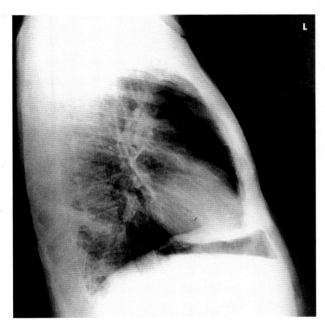

Fig. 3.42 Foreshortening.

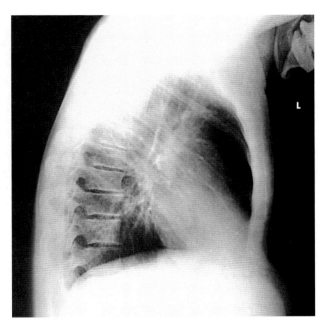

Fig. 3.43 Forward bending.

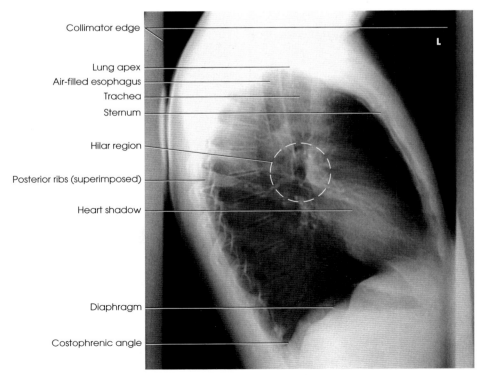

Collimator edge

Lung apex
Air-filled esophagus
Trachea
Sternum

Hilar region

Posterior ribs (superimposed)

Heart shadow

Diaphragm

Costophrenic angle

Fig. 3.44 Left lateral chest.

Cardiac studies with barium

The left lateral position is traditionally used during cardiac studies with barium. The procedure is the same as described for the PA chest projection (see p. 109).

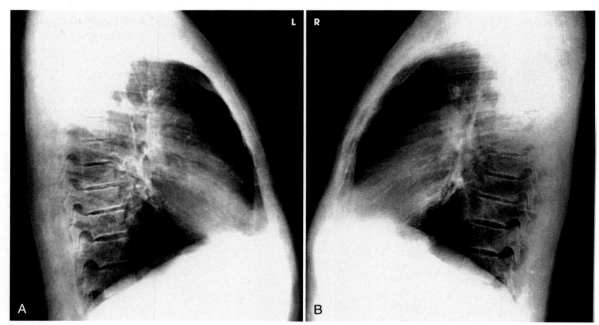

Fig. 3.45 (A) Left lateral chest. (B) Right lateral chest on same patient as in (A). Note the size of the heart shadows.

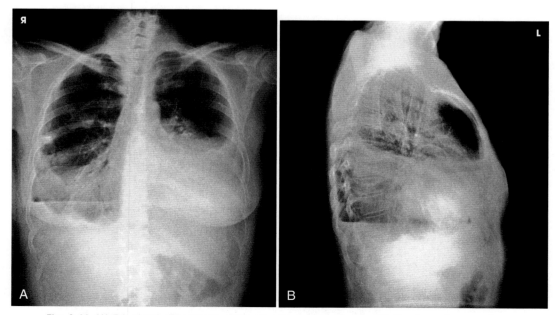

Fig. 3.46 (A) PA chest. (B) Lateral chest on same patient as in (A). The importance of two projections is seen on this patient with multiple chest pathologies, including fluid, air-fluid level, pneumothorax, and enlarged heart.

🦅 PA OBLIQUE PROJECTION
RAO and LAO positions

Image receptor + grid: Positioned by manufacturer or department protocol for proper anatomy display orientation; CR plate: 14 × 17 inches (35 × 43 cm) lengthwise.

SID: Minimum SID of 72 inches (183 cm) is recommended to decrease magnification of the heart and to increase recorded detail of the thoracic structures.

Position of patient
- Maintain the patient in the position (standing or seated upright) used for the PA projection.
- Instruct the patient to let the arms hang free.
- Have the patient turn approximately 45 degrees toward the left side for left anterior oblique (LAO) position and approximately 45 degrees toward the right side for right anterior oblique (RAO) position.

- Ask the patient to stand or sit straight. If the standing position is used, the weight of the patient's body must be equally distributed on the feet to prevent unwanted rotation.
- For PA oblique projections, the side of interest is generally the side *farther* from the IR; however, the lung closer to the IR is also imaged.
- The top of the IR should be placed about 1.5 to 2 inches (3.8 to 5 cm) above the vertebral prominens because the top of the shoulders may not be on the same plane.

Position of part

LAO position

- Rotate the patient 45 degrees to place the left shoulder in contact with the grid device, and center the thorax to the IR. Ensure that the right and left sides of the body are positioned to the IR.
- Instruct the patient to place the left hand on the hip with the palm outward.
- Have the patient raise the right arm to shoulder level and grasp the top of the vertical grid device for support.

- Adjust the patient's shoulders to lie in the same horizontal plane, and instruct the patient not to rotate the head (Fig. 3.47).
- Use a 55- to 60-degree oblique position when the examination is performed for a *cardiac series*. This projection is usually performed with barium contrast medium. The patient swallows the barium just before the exposure.
- *Shield gonads.*
- *Respiration*: Full inspiration. The exposure is made after the *second* full inspiration to ensure the maximum expansion of the lungs.

RAO position

- Reverse the previously described position, placing the patient's right shoulder in contact with the grid device, the right hand on the hip, and the left hand on the top of the vertical grid device (Fig. 3.48).
- *Shield gonads.*
- *Respiration*: Full inspiration. The exposure is made after the second full inspiration to ensure the maximum expansion of the lungs.

Central ray

- Perpendicular to the center of the IR. The central ray should be at the level of T7.

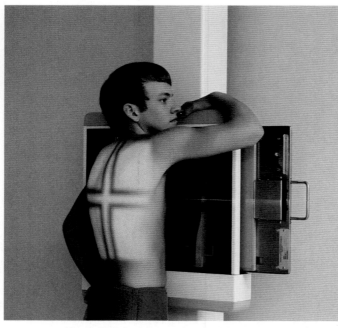

Fig. 3.47 PA oblique chest, LAO position.

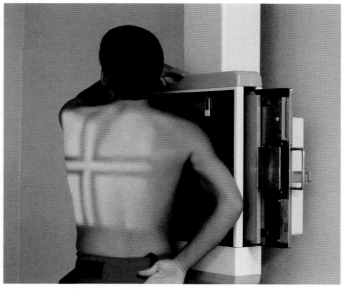

Fig. 3.48 PA oblique chest, RAO position.

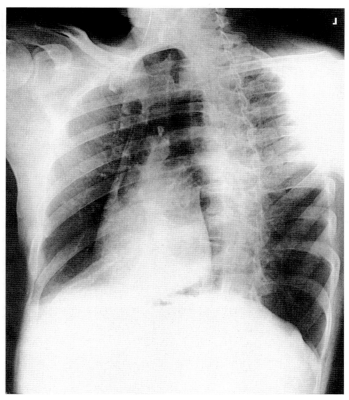

Fig. 3.49 PA oblique chest, LAO position at 45 degrees.

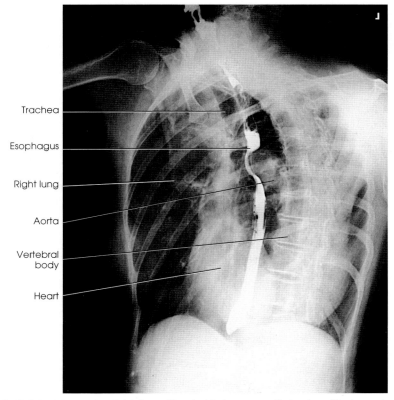

Trachea

Esophagus

Right lung

Aorta

Vertebral body

Heart

Fig. 3.50 PA oblique chest. LAO position is 60 degrees with barium-filled esophagus.

Collimation

- Adjust radiation field to 17 inches (43 cm) lengthwise and 1 inch (2.5 cm) beyond the shadows on both sides, but no more the 14 inches (35 cm). Vertical dimension may be less for smaller patients. Place a side marker in the collimated exposure field.

Structures shown

LAO position. The maximum area of the right lung field (side farther from the IR) is shown along with the thoracic viscera. The anterior portion of the left lung is superimposed by the spine (Figs. 3.49 and 3.50). Also shown are the trachea and its bifurcation (the carina), and the entire right branch of the bronchial tree. The heart, the descending aorta (lying just in front of the spine), and the arch of the aorta are also presented.

RAO position. The maximum area of the left lung field (side farther from the IR) is shown along with the thoracic viscera. The anterior portion of the right lung is superimposed by the spine (Figs. 3.51 and 3.52). Also shown are the trachea and the entire left branch of the bronchial tree. This position gives the best image of the left atrium, the anterior portion of the apex of the left ventricle, and the right retrocardiac space. When filled with barium, the esophagus is shown clearly in the RAO and LAO positions (see Fig. 3.52).

NOTE: The radiographs in this section, similar to the radiographs throughout this text, are printed as though the reader is looking at the patient's anterior body surface (see Chapter 1).

Thoracic Viscera: Chest and Upper Airway

The following should be clearly seen:
- Evidence of proper collimation and presence of a side marker placed clear of anatomy of interest
- Both lungs included from apices to costophrenic angles
- Trachea filled with air
- Heart and mediastinal structures within the lung field of the elevated side in oblique images of 45 degrees
- Right lung best demonstrated on LAO
- Left lung best demonstrated on RAO
- Pulmonary vascular markings from the hilar regions to the periphery of the lung

Barium studies

RAO and LAO positions are routinely used during cardiac studies with barium. Follow the same procedures described in the PA chest section (see p. 109).

NOTE: A slightly oblique position has been found to be of particular value in the study of pulmonary diseases. The patient is turned only slightly (10 to 20 degrees) from the RAO or LAO body position. This slight degree of obliquity rotates the superior segment of the respective lower lobe from behind the hilum and displays the medial part of the right middle lobe or the lingula of the left upper lobe free from the hilum. These areas are not clearly shown in the standard "cardiac oblique" of 45- to 60-degree rotation, largely because of superimposition of the spine.

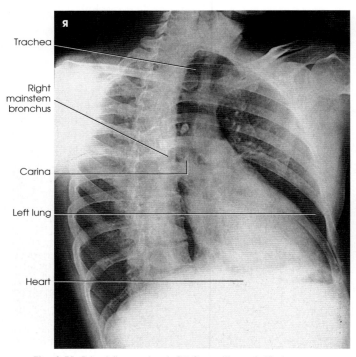

Trachea
Right mainstem bronchus
Carina
Left lung
Heart

Fig. 3.51 PA oblique chest, RAO position at 45 degrees.

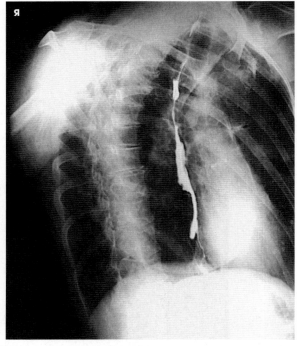

Fig. 3.52 PA oblique chest, RAO position at 60 degrees. Note barium in esophagus.

♠ AP OBLIQUE PROJECTION
RPO and LPO positions

RPO and LPO positions are used when the patient is too ill to be turned to the prone position and sometimes as supplementary positions in the investigation of specific lesions. These positions are also used with the recumbent patient in contrast studies of the heart and great vessels.

For AP oblique projections, the side of interest is generally the side closest to the IR. The resulting image shows the greatest area of the lung closest to the IR. The lung farthest from the IR is also imaged, and diagnostic information is often obtained for that side.

Image receptor + grid: Positioned by manufacturer or department protocol for proper anatomy display orientation; CR plate: 14 × 17 inches (35 × 43 cm) lengthwise.

SID: Minimum SID of 72 inches (183 cm) is recommended to decrease magnification of the heart and increase recorded detail of the thoracic structures.

Position of patient
- With the patient supine or facing the x-ray tube, either upright or recumbent, adjust the IR so that the upper border of the IR is about 1.5 to 2 inches (3.8 to 5 cm) above the vertebral prominens or about 5 inches (12.7 cm) above the jugular notch.

Position of part
- Rotate the patient toward the correct side, adjust the body at a 45-degree angle, and center the thorax to the grid.
- If the patient is recumbent, support the elevated hip and arm. Ensure that both sides of the chest are positioned to the IR.
- Flex the patient's elbows and place the hands on the hips with the palms facing outward, or pronate the hands beside the hips. The arm closer to the IR may be raised as long as the shoulder is rotated anteriorly.
- Adjust the shoulders to lie in the same transverse plane in a position of forward rotation (Figs. 3.53 and 3.54).
- *Shield gonads.*
- *Respiration*: Full inspiration. The exposure is made after the *second* full inspiration to ensure the maximum expansion of the lungs.

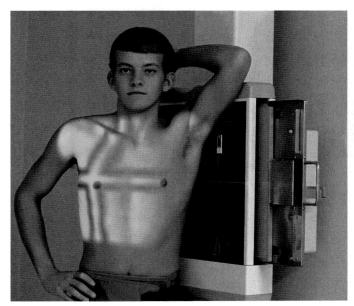

Fig. 3.53 Upright AP oblique chest, LPO position.

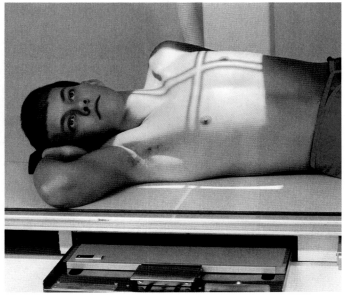

Fig. 3.54 Recumbent AP oblique chest, RPO position.

Central ray

- Perpendicular to the center of the IR at a level 3 inches (7.6 cm) below the jugular notch (central ray exits at T7).

Collimation

- Adjust radiation field to 17 inches (43 cm) lengthwise and 1 inch (2.5 cm) beyond the shadows on both sides, but no more the 14 inches (35 cm). Vertical dimension may be less for smaller patients. Place a side marker in the collimated exposure field.

Structures shown

This radiograph presents an AP oblique projection of the thoracic viscera similar to the corresponding PA oblique projection (Fig. 3.55). The RPO position is comparable with the LAO position. The lung field of the elevated side usually appears shorter, however, because of magnification of the diaphragm. The heart and great vessels also cast magnified shadows as a result of being farther from the IR.

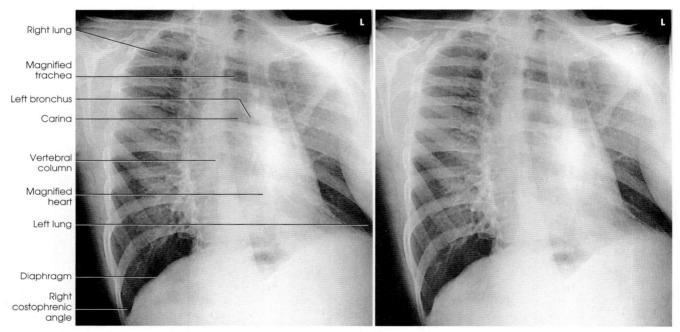

Fig. 3.55 AP oblique chest, LPO position.

🪶 AP PROJECTION[a]

The supine position is used when the patient is too ill to sit or stand. The upright position is used for patients in a wheelchair who cannot stand and must remain in a wheelchair for the radiograph. In addition, patients on a stretcher can be radiographed sitting up with their legs dangling over the side of the stretcher and their back against the upright IR.

Image receptor + grid: Positioned by manufacturer or department protocol for proper anatomy display orientation; CR plate: 14 × 17 inches (35 × 43 cm) lengthwise or crosswise for hypersthenic patients.

SID: SID of 72 inches (183 cm) is recommended. A shorter SID may be required depending on the equipment and space available.

[a]See Chapter 20, Volume 3, for a full description of mobile AP.

Position of patient

- Place the patient in the supine or upright position with the back against the grid.

Position of part

- Center the midsagittal plane of the chest to the IR.
- Adjust the IR so that the upper border is approximately 1.5 to 2 inches (3.8 to 5 cm) above the relaxed shoulders.
- If patient condition allows, flex the patient's elbows, pronate the hands, and place the hands on the hips to draw the scapulae laterally.
- Adjust the shoulders to lie in the same transverse plane (Fig. 3.56).
- *Shield gonads.*
- *Respiration*: Full inspiration. The exposure is made after the *second* full inspiration to ensure the maximum expansion of the lungs.

Central ray

- Perpendicular to the long axis of the sternum and the center of the IR. The central ray should enter about 3 inches (7.6 cm) below the jugular notch.

Collimation

- Adjust radiation field to 17 inches (43 cm) lengthwise and 1 inch (2.5 cm) beyond the shadows on both sides, but no more the 14 inches (35 cm). The opposite dimensions are used for a crosswise IR. Vertical dimension may be less for smaller patients. Place a side marker in the collimated exposure field.

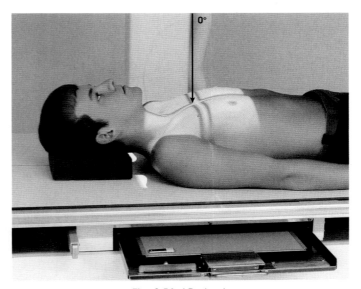

Fig. 3.56 AP chest.

Structures shown

An AP projection of the thoracic viscera (Fig. 3.57) shows an image similar to the PA projection (Fig. 3.58). Being farther from the IR, the heart and great vessels are magnified and engorged, and the lung fields appear shorter because abdominal compression moves the diaphragm to a higher level. The clavicles are projected higher, and the ribs assume a more horizontal appearance.

EVALUATION CRITERIA

The following should be clearly seen:
- Evidence of proper collimation and presence of a side marker placed clear of anatomy of interest
- Entire lungs, from the apices to the costophrenic angles
- No rotation
  - ☐ Sternal ends of the clavicles equidistant from the vertebral column
  - ☐ Trachea visible in the midline
  - ☐ Equal distance from the vertebral column to the lateral border of the ribs on each side
- Clavicles appear more horizontal than in the PA projection.
- Approximately 1 inch of the pulmonary apices should be seen superior to the clavicles.
- Pulmonary vascular markings from the hilar regions to the periphery of the lungs

NOTE: Resnick[2] recommended an angled AP projection to free the basal portions of the lung fields from superimposition by the anterior diaphragmatic, abdominal, and cardiac structures. He reported that this projection also differentiates middle lobe and lingular processes from lower lobe disease. For this projection, the patient may be either upright or supine, and the central ray is directed to the midsternal region at an angle of 30 degrees caudad. Resnick stated that a more suitable angulation may be chosen based on the preliminary films.

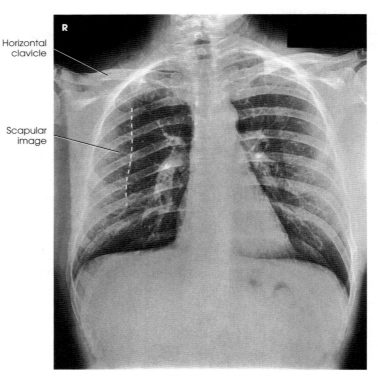

Horizontal clavicle

Scapular image

Fig. 3.57 AP chest.

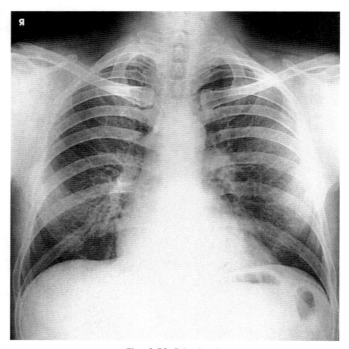

Fig. 3.58 PA chest.

♠ AP AXIAL PROJECTION
LINDBLOM METHOD[3]
Lordotic position

Image receptor + grid: Positioned by manufacturer or department protocol for proper anatomy display orientation; CR plate: 14 × 17 inches (35 × 43 cm) lengthwise.

SID: Minimum SID of 72 inches (183 cm) is recommended to decrease magnification of the heart and to increase recorded details of the thoracic structures.

Position of patient
• Place the patient in the upright position, facing the x-ray tube and standing approximately 1 foot (30.5 cm) in front of the vertical grid device.

Position of part
• Adjust the height of the IR so that the upper margin is about 3 inches (7.6 cm) above the upper border of the shoulders when the patient is adjusted in the lordotic position.
Lordotic position
• Adjust the patient for the AP axial projection, with the coronal plane of the thorax 15 to 20 degrees from the vertical and midsagittal plane centered to the midline of the grid (Fig. 3.59).
Oblique lordotic positions—LPO or RPO
• Rotate the patient's body approximately 30 degrees away from the position used for the AP projection, with the affected side toward and centered to the grid (Fig. 3.60).
• With either of the preceding positions, have the patient flex the elbows and place the hands, palms out, on the hips.
• Have the patient lean backward in a position of extreme lordosis and rest the shoulders against the vertical grid device.
• *Shield gonads.*
• *Respiration:* Full inspiration. The exposure is made after the *second* full inspiration to ensure the maximum expansion of the lungs.

Central ray
• Perpendicular to the center of the IR at the level of the midsternum (3 to 4 inches [7.5 to 10 cm] below jugular notch).

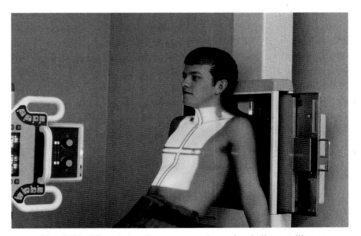

Fig. 3.59 AP axial pulmonary apices, lordotic position.

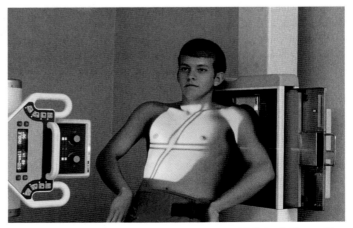

Fig. 3.60 AP axial oblique pulmonary apices, LPO lordotic position.

Pulmonary Apices

Collimation

- Adjust radiation field to 17 inches (43 cm) lengthwise and 1 inch (2.5 cm) beyond the shadows on both sides, but no more the 14 inches (35 cm). Exposure field may be smaller, depending on department protocol. Place a side marker in the collimated exposure field.

Structures shown

AP axial (Fig. 3.61) and AP axial oblique (Fig. 3.62) images of the lungs show the apices and conditions such as interlobar effusions.

EVALUATION CRITERIA

The following should be clearly seen:

- Evidence of proper collimation and presence of a side marker placed clear of anatomy of interest
- Pulmonary vascular markings of the apices

Lordotic position

- Entire apices and appropriate portion of lungs
- Clavicles located superior to the apices
- Sternal ends of the clavicles equidistant from the vertebral column
- Clavicles lying horizontally with their sternal ends overlapping only the first or second ribs
- Ribs distorted with their anterior and posterior portions superimposed

Oblique lordotic position

- Dependent apex and lung of the affected side in its entirety

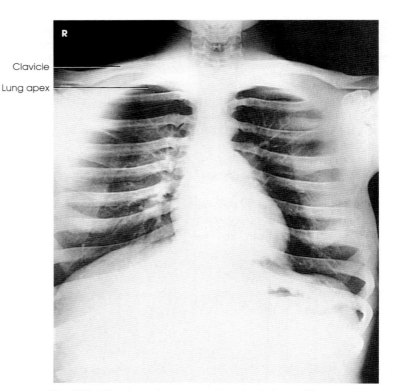

Fig. 3.61 AP axial pulmonary apices, lordotic position.

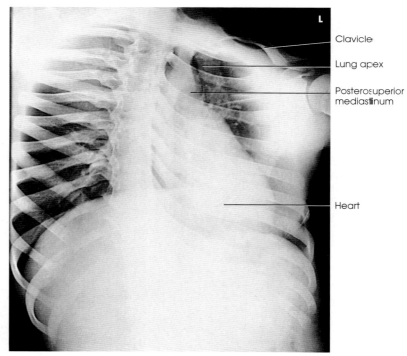

Fig. 3.62 AP axial oblique pulmonary apices, LPO lordotic position.

AP AXIAL PROJECTION

Image receptor + grid: Positioned by manufacturer or department protocol for proper anatomy display orientation; CR plate: 10 × 12 inches (24 × 30 cm) crosswise or 14 × 17 inches (35 × 43 cm)

NOTE: This projection is recommended when the patient cannot be placed in the lordotic position.

SID: Minimum SID of 72 inches (183 cm) is recommended to decrease magnification of the heart and to increase recorded details of the thoracic structures.

Position of patient
- Examine the patient in the upright or supine position.

Position of part
- Center the IR to the midsagittal plane at the level of T2, and adjust the patient's body so that it is not rotated.

- Flex the patient's elbows and place the hands on the hips with the palms out, or pronate the hands beside the hips.
- Place the shoulders back against the grid and adjust them to lie in the same transverse plane (Fig. 3.63).
- *Shield gonads.*
- *Respiration:* Expose at the end of *full inspiration.*

Central ray
- Directed at an angle of 15 or 20 degrees cephalad to the center of the IR and entering the manubrium

Collimation
- Adjust radiation field to 10 × 12 inches (24 × 30 cm). Approximately 1 inch (2.5 cm) of field light should be seen above shadow of the shoulders. Place a side marker in the collimated exposure field.

Structures shown
AP axial projection shows the apices lying below the clavicles (Fig. 3.64).

The following should be clearly seen:
- Evidence of proper collimation and presence of a side marker placed clear of anatomy of interest
- Apices in their entirety
- Superior lung region adjacent to the apices
- Clavicles located superior to the apices and oriented horizontally with the sternal ends overlapping the first or second rib
- Sternal ends of the clavicles equidistant from the vertebral column
- Ribs distorted, with their anterior and posterior portions superimposed
- Pulmonary vascular markings of the apices

NOTE: The AP axial projection is used in preference to the PA axial projection in hypersthenic patients and patients whose clavicles occupy a high position. The AP axial projection makes it possible to separate the apical and clavicular shadows without undue distortion of the apices.

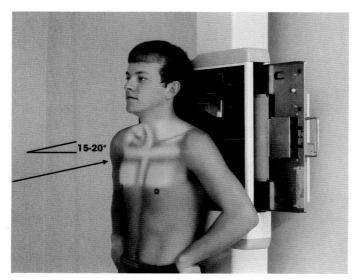

Fig. 3.63 AP axial pulmonary apices.

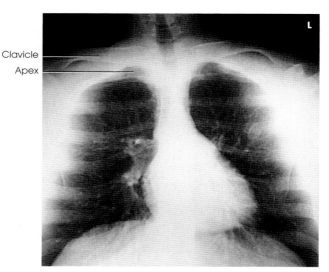

Fig. 3.64 AP axial pulmonary apices.

PA AXIAL PROJECTION

Image receptor + grid: Positioned by manufacturer or department protocol for proper anatomy display orientation; CR plate: 10 × 12 inches (24 × 30 cm) crosswise

SID: Minimum SID of 72 inches (183 cm) is recommended to decrease magnification of the heart and to increase recorded detail of the thoracic structures.

Position of patient

- Position the patient seated or standing before a vertical grid device. If the patient is standing, the weight of the body must be equally distributed on the feet.

Position of part

- Adjust the height of the IR so that it is centered at the level of the jugular notch.
- Center the midsagittal plane of the patient's body to the midline of the IR, and rest the chin against the grid device.
- Adjust the patient's head so that the midsagittal plane is vertical, and then flex the elbows and place the hands, palms out, on the hips.
- Depress the patient's shoulders, rotate them forward, and adjust them to lie in the same transverse plane.
- Instruct the patient to keep the shoulders in contact with the grid device to move the scapulae from the lung fields (Fig. 3.65).
- *Shield gonads.*
- *Respiration:* Make the exposure at the end of *full inspiration* or, as an option, at *full expiration.* The clavicles are elevated by inspiration and depressed by expiration; the apices move little, if at all, during either phase of respiration.

Central ray
Inspiration
- Directed 10 to 15 degrees cephalad through T3 to the center of the IR

Expiration (optional)
- Directed perpendicular to the plane of the IR and centered at the level of T3

Collimation
- Adjust radiation field to 10 × 12 inches (24 × 30 cm). Place a side marker in the collimated exposure field.

Structures shown
The apices are projected above the shadows of the clavicles in the PA axial and PA projections (Fig. 3.66).

The following should be clearly seen:
- Evidence of proper collimation and presence of a side marker placed clear of anatomy of interest
- Entire apices and appropriate portion of lungs
- Clavicles located below the apices
- Sternal ends of the clavicles equidistant from the vertebral column
- Pulmonary vascular markings of the apices

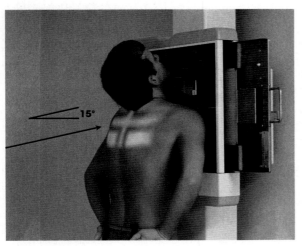

Fig. 3.65 PA axial pulmonary apices (inspiration).

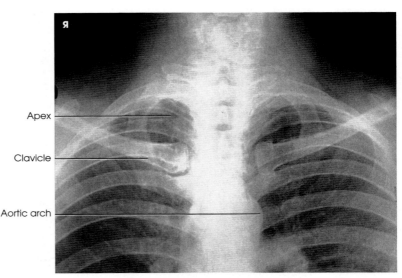

Apex

Clavicle

Aortic arch

Fig. 3.66 PA axial pulmonary apices, inspiration with central ray angled.

♠ AP OR PA PROJECTION[a]
R or L lateral decubitus positions

Image receptor + grid: Positioned by manufacturer or department protocol for proper anatomy display orientation; CR plate:14 × 17 inches (35 × 43 cm) lengthwise.

Position of patient

- Place the patient in a lateral decubitus position, lying on either the affected or the unaffected side, as indicated by the existing condition. A small amount of fluid in the pleural cavity, a pleural effusion, is usually best shown with the patient lying on the affected side. With this positioning, the mediastinal shadows and the fluid do not overlap. A small amount of free air in the pleural cavity, a pneumothorax, is generally best shown with the patient lying on the unaffected side.
- *Exercise care* to ensure that the patient does not fall off the cart. If a cart is used, *lock all wheels* securely in position.
- Achieve the best visualization by allowing the patient to remain in the position for *5 minutes before the exposure.* This allows fluid to settle and air to rise.

---

[a]See Chapter 20, Volume 3, for a full description of mobile AP.

Position of part

- If the patient is lying on the affected side to demonstrate presence of a pleural effusion, elevate the body 2 to 3 inches (5 to 8 cm) on a suitable platform or a firm pad.
- Extend the arms well above the head, and adjust the thorax in a true lateral position (Fig. 3.67).
- Place the anterior or posterior surface of the chest against a vertical grid device.
- Adjust the IR so that it extends approximately 1.5 to 2 inches (3.8 to 5 cm) beyond the shoulders.
- *Shield gonads.*
- *Respiration*: Full inspiration. The exposure is made after the *second* full inspiration to ensure the maximum expansion of the lungs.

Central ray

- *Horizontal* and perpendicular to the center of the IR at a level 3 inches (7.6 cm) below the jugular notch for AP and T7 for PA.

Collimation

- Adjust radiation field to 14 × 17 inches (35 × 43 cm) on the collimator. Place a side marker and decubitus marker in the collimated exposure field.

Structures shown

AP or PA projection obtained using the lateral decubitus position shows the change in fluid position and reveals any previously obscured pulmonary areas or, in the case of suspected pneumothorax, the presence of any free air (Figs. 3.68–3.70).

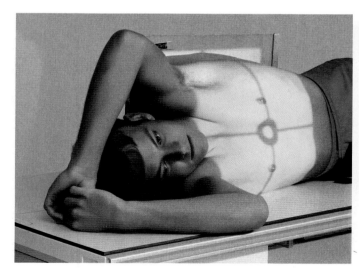

Fig. 3.67 AP projection, right lateral decubitus position. Side up is the affected side, so no table pad was used. This projection would demonstrate free air rising up to the left side.

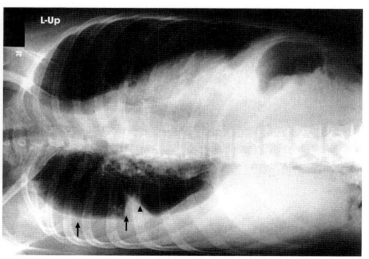

Fig. 3.68 AP projection, right lateral decubitus position, showing a fluid level *(arrows)* on the side that is down. Note the fluid in the lung fissure *(arrowhead)*. Note correct marker placement, with the upper side of the patient indicated.

The following should be clearly seen:

- Evidence of proper collimation and presence of a side marker and decubitus marker placed clear of anatomy of interest
- Affected side in its entirety, from apex to costophrenic angle
- No rotation of the patient, as demonstrated by the sternal ends of the clavicles equidistant from the spine
- Patient's arms not visible in the field of interest
- Faintly visible spine and pulmonary vascular markings from the hilar regions to the periphery of the lungs

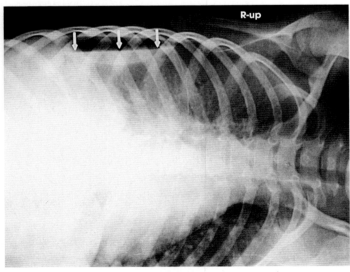

Fig. 3.69 AP projection, left lateral decubitus position, in same patient as in Fig. 3.73. *Arrows* indicate air-fluid level (air on the side up). Note correct marker placement, with upper side of the patient indicated.

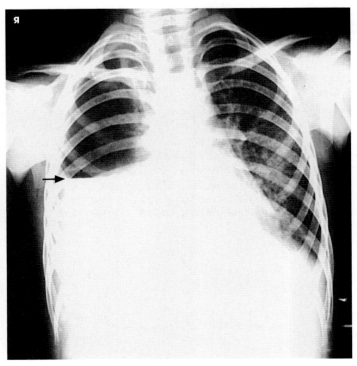

Fig. 3.70 Upright PA chest. *Arrow* indicates air-fluid level.

♠ LATERAL PROJECTION
R or L position
Ventral or dorsal decubitus position

Image receptor + grid: Positioned by manufacturer or department protocol for proper anatomy display orientation; CR plate: 14 × 17 inches (35 × 43 cm) lengthwise.

Position of patient

- With the patient in a prone or supine position, elevate the thorax 2 to 3 inches (5 to 7.6 cm) on folded sheets or a firm pad, centering the thorax to the grid.
- Achieve the best visualization by allowing the patient to remain in the position for *5 minutes before the exposure*. This allows fluid to settle and air to rise.

Position of part

- Adjust the body in a true prone or a supine position, and extend the arms well above the head.
- Place the affected side against a vertical grid device, and adjust it so that the top of the IR extends to the level of the thyroid cartilage (Fig. 3.71).
- *Shield gonads.*
- *Respiration:* Full inspiration. The exposure is made after the *second* full inspiration to ensure the maximum expansion of the lungs.

Central ray

- *Horizontal* and centered to the IR. The central ray enters at the level of the midcoronal plane and 3 to 4 inches (7.6 to 10.2 cm) below the jugular notch for the dorsal decubitus and at T7 for the ventral decubitus.

Collimation

- Adjust radiation field to 14 × 17 inches (35 × 43 cm) on the collimator. Place a side marker in the collimated exposure field.

Structures shown

A lateral projection in the decubitus position shows a change in the position of fluid and reveals pulmonary areas that are obscured by the fluid in standard projections (Figs. 3.72 and 3.73).

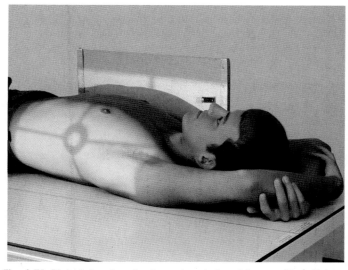

Fig. 3.71 Right lateral projection, dorsal decubitus position. Side up is the affected side, so no table pad was used. This projection would demonstrate free air rising up to the anterior chest.

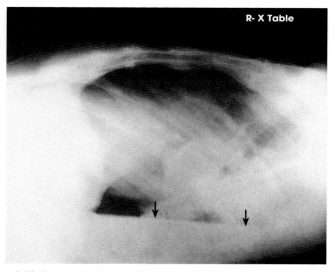

Fig. 3.72 Right lateral projection, dorsal decubitus position. *Arrows* indicate air-fluid level. Note correct marker placement, with upper side of the patient indicated.

EVALUATION CRITERIA

The following should be clearly seen:

- Evidence of proper collimation and presence of side and decubitus markers placed clear of anatomy of interest
- Entire lung fields, including the anterior and posterior surfaces
- Upper lung field not obscured by the arms
- No rotation of the thorax from a true lateral position
- T7 in the center of the IR
- Pulmonary vascular markings from the hilar regions to the periphery of the lungs

References

1. Eiselberg A, Sgalitzer DM: X-ray examination of the trachea and the bronchi, *Surg Gynecol Obstet* 47:53, 1928.
2. Resnick D: The angulated basal view: a new method for evaluation of lower lobe pulmonary disease, *Radiology* 96:204, 1970.
3. Lindblom K: Half-axial projection in accentuated lordosis for roentgen studies of the lungs, *Acta Radiol* 21:119, 1940.

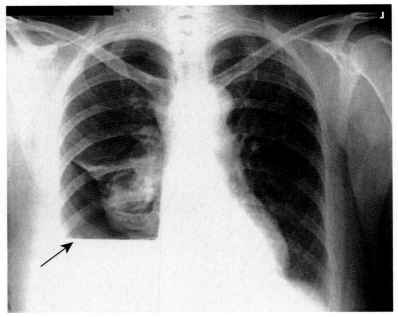

Fig. 3.73 Upright PA chest in same patient as in Fig. 3.72. Note right lung fluid level (*arrow*).

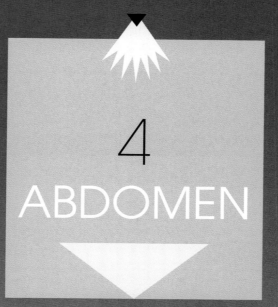

4

ABDOMEN

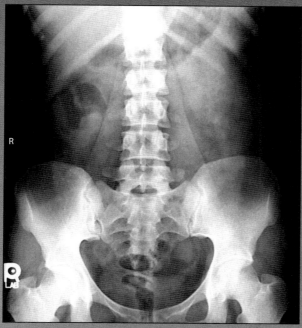

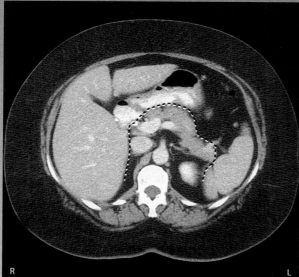

SUMMARY OF PROJECTIONS

PROJECTIONS, POSITIONS, AND METHODS

Page	Essential	Anatomy	Projection	Position	Method
137	✦	Abdomen	AP	Supine; upright	
139	✦	Abdomen	PA	Upright	
139	✦	Abdomen	AP	L lateral decubitus	
141	✦	Abdomen	Lateral	R or L	
142	✦	Abdomen	Lateral	R or L dorsal decubitus	

Icons in the Essential column indicate projections frequently performed in the United States and Canada. Students should be competent in these projections.
AP, Anteroposterior; *L,* left; *PA,* posteroanterior; *R,* right.

Abdominopelvic Cavity

The *abdominopelvic* cavity consists of two parts: (1) a large superior portion, the abdominal cavity; and (2) a smaller inferior part, the pelvic cavity. The *abdominal cavity* extends from the diaphragm to the superior aspect of the bony pelvis. The abdominal cavity contains the stomach, small and large intestines, liver, gallbladder, spleen, pancreas, and kidneys. The *pelvic cavity* lies within the margins of the bony pelvis and contains the rectum and sigmoid of the large intestine, the urinary bladder, and the reproductive organs. Anatomists define the "true pelvis" as that portion of the abdominopelvic cavity inferior to a plane passing through the sacral promontory posteriorly and the superior surface of the pubic bones anteriorly.

The abdominopelvic cavity is enclosed in a double-walled seromembranous sac

called the *peritoneum.* The outer portion of this sac, termed the *parietal peritoneum,* is in close contact with the abdominal wall, the greater (false) pelvic wall, and most of the undersurface of the diaphragm. The inner portion of the sac, known as the *visceral peritoneum,* is positioned over or around the contained organs. The peritoneum forms folds called the *mesentery* and *omenta,* which serve to support the viscera in position. The space

between the two layers of the peritoneum is called the *peritoneal cavity* and contains serous fluid (Fig. 4.1). Because there are no mesenteric attachments of the intestines in the pelvic cavity, pelvic surgery can be performed without entry into the peritoneal cavity.

The *retroperitoneum* is the cavity behind the peritoneum. Organs such as the kidneys and pancreas lie in the retroperitoneum (Fig. 4.2).

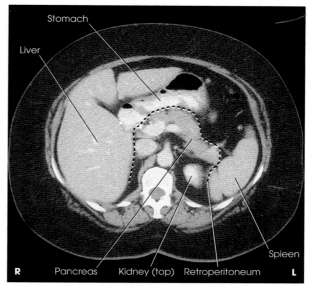

Fig. 4.2 Axial CT image of abdomen showing organs of upper abdomen. Retroperitoneum is posterior and medial to *dashed line.*

(From Kelley LL, Petersen CM: *Sectional anatomy for imaging professionals,* ed 2, St. Louis, 2007, Mosby.)

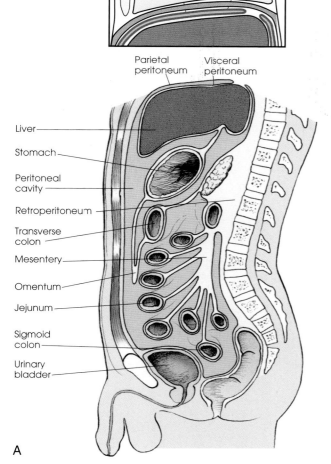

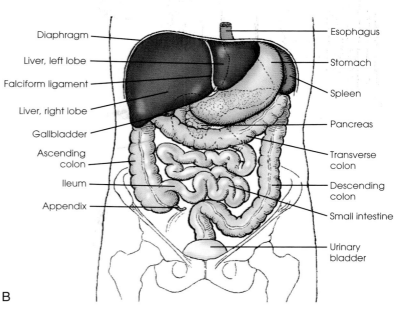

Fig. 4.1 (A) Lateral aspect of abdomen showing peritoneal sac and its components. (B) Anterior aspect of abdominal viscera in relation to surrounding structures.

SUMMARY OF ANATOMY

Abdomen
Abdominopelvic cavity
Abdominal cavity
Pelvic cavity
Peritoneum
Parietal peritoneum
Mesentery
Omenta
Peritoneal cavity
Retroperitoneum
Visceral peritoneum

SUMMARY OF PATHOLOGY

Condition	Definition
Abdominal aortic aneurysm (AAA)	Localized dilation of abdominal aorta
Ascites	Fluid accumulation in the peritoneal cavity
Bowel obstruction	Blockage of bowel lumen
Ileus	Failure of bowel peristalsis
Metastasis	Transfer of a cancerous lesion from one area to another
Pneumoperitoneum	Presence of air in peritoneal cavity
Tumor	New tissue growth where cell proliferation is uncontrolled

SAMPLE EXPOSURE TECHNIQUE CHART ESSENTIAL PROJECTIONS

These techniques were accurate for the equipment used to produce each exposure. However, use caution when applying them in your department because "there is considerable variability in image receptor response owing to varying scatter sensitivity, the use of grids with different grid ratios, collimation, beam filtration, the choice of kilovoltage, source-to-image distance, and image receptor size."[1]

This chart was created in collaboration with Dennis Bowman, AS, RT(R), Clinical Instructor, Community Hospital of the Monterey Peninsula, Monterey, CA. http://digitalradiographysolutions.com/.

ABDOMEN

Part	cm	kVp[a]	SID[b]	Collimation	CR[c] mAs	CR[c] Dose (mGy)[e]	DR[d] mAs	DR[d] Dose (mGy)[e]
AP[f]	21	85	40"	14" × 17" (35 × 43 cm)	25[g]	3.700	10[g]	1.474
PA[f]	21	85	40"	14" × 17" (35 × 43 cm)	22[g]	3.250	9[g]	1.321
AP/lateral decubitus[f]	24	85	40"	17" × 14" (43 × 35 cm)	28[g]	4.480	11[g]	1.753
Lateral[f]	30	90	40"	14" × 17" (35 × 43 cm)	50[g]	10.48	20[g]	4.170
Lateral/dorsal decubitus[f]	30	90	40"	17" × 14" (43 × 35 cm)	65[g]	13.64	25[g]	5.230

[1]ACR-AAPM-SIIMM Practice Parameter for Digital Radiography, revised 2017.
[a]kVp values are for a high-frequency generator.
[b]40 inches minimum; 44 to 48 inches recommended to improve spatial resolution (mAs increase needed, but no increase in patient dose will result).
[c]AGFA CR MD 4.0 General IP, CR 75.0 reader, 400 speed class, with 6:1 (178LPI) grid when needed.
[d]GE Definium 8000, with 13:1 grid when needed.
[e]All doses are skin entrance for average adult (160 to 200 pounds male, 150 to 190 pounds female) at part thickness indicated.
[f]Bucky/Grid.
[g]Large focal spot.
AP, Anteroposterior; CR, central ray; PA, posteroanterior; SID, source-to-image receptor distance.

ABBREVIATIONS USED IN CHAPTER 4

AAA	Abdominal aortic aneurysm
ERCP	Endoscopic retrograde cholangiopancreatography
NPO	Nil per os (nothing by mouth)
PTC	Percutaneous transhepatic cholangiography
RUQ	Right upper quadrant

See Addendum A for a summary of all abbreviations used in Volume 1.

Abdominal Radiographic Procedures

EXPOSURE TECHNIQUE

In examinations without a contrast medium, it is imperative to obtain maximal soft tissue differentiation throughout the different regions of the abdomen. Because of the wide range in the thickness of the abdomen and the delicate differences in physical density between the contained viscera, a proper balance of exposure factors is critical to show both solid organs, as well as adjacent structures, while delivering the lowest possible radiation dose (Fig. 4.3A).

The best criterion for assessing the quality of an abdominal radiographic image is the ability to visualize each of the following (Fig. 4.3B):

- Sharply defined outlines of the psoas muscles
- Lower border of the liver
- Kidneys
- Ribs and transverse processes of the lumbar vertebrae

IMMOBILIZATION

A prime requisite in abdominal examinations is to prevent voluntary and involuntary movement. The following steps are observed:

- To prevent muscle contraction caused by tension, adjust the patient in a comfortable position so that he or she can relax.
- Explain the breathing procedure, and ensure that the patient understands exactly what is expected.

- Do not start the exposure for 1 to 2 seconds after suspension of respiration to allow the patient to come to rest and involuntary movement of the viscera to subside.

Voluntary motion produces a blurred outline of the structures that do not have involuntary movement, such as the liver, psoas muscles, and spine. Patient breathing during exposure results in blurring of bowel gas outlines in the upper abdomen as the diaphragm moves (Fig. 4.4). Involuntary motion caused by peristalsis may produce localized or generalized haziness of the image. Involuntary contraction of the abdominal wall or the muscles around the spine may cause movement of the entire abdominal area and may produce generalized image haziness.

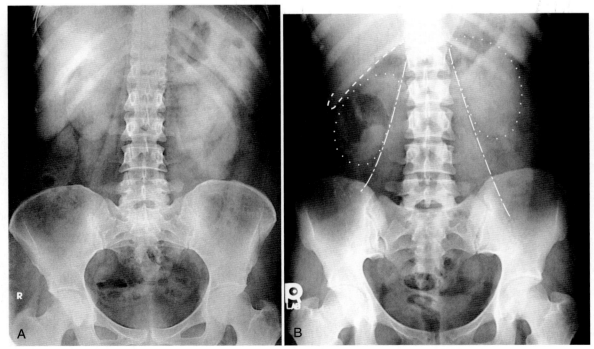

Fig. 4.3 (A) AP abdomen showing proper positioning and collimation. (B) AP abdomen showing kidney shadows *(dotted line)*, margin of liver *(dashed line)*, and psoas muscles *(dot-dash lines)*.

RADIOGRAPHIC PROJECTIONS

Radiographic examination of the abdomen may include one or more projections. The most commonly performed is the supine AP projection, often called a *KUB* because it includes the *kidneys, ureters,* and *bladder.* Projections used to complement the supine AP projection include an upright AP abdomen or an AP or PA projection in the lateral decubitus position (the left lateral decubitus is most often preferred), or both. The AP upright and AP/PA lateral decubitus are useful in assessing the abdomen in patients with free air (pneumoperitoneum) and in determining the presence and location of air-fluid levels. Other abdominal projections include a lateral projection or a lateral projection in the supine (dorsal decubitus) body position. Many institutions also obtain a PA chest image to include the upper abdomen and diaphragm. The upright PA chest is indicated because any air escaping from the gastrointestinal tract into the peritoneal space rises to the highest level, usually just beneath the diaphragm.

POSITIONING PROTOCOLS

The required projections obtained to evaluate the patient's abdomen vary considerably depending on the institution and the physician. Some physicians consider the preliminary evaluation image (often termed a *scout* or *survey*) to consist of only the AP (supine) projection. Others obtain two projections: a supine and an upright AP abdomen (often called a *flat* and an *upright*). A three-way or acute abdomen series may be requested to rule out free air, bowel obstruction, and infection. The three projections usually include (1) AP with the patient supine, (2) AP with the patient upright, and (3) upright PA chest. If the patient cannot stand for the upright AP abdomen projection, the projection is performed using the left lateral decubitus position. The upright PA chest projection can be used to demonstrate free air that may accumulate under the diaphragm.

Positioning for radiographic examination of the abdomen is described in the following pages. (For a description of positioning for the upright PA chest, see Chapter 3.)

Recommended Sequence for Abdominal Radiography

To show small amounts of intraperitoneal gas in acute abdominal cases, Miller[1,2] recommended that the patient be kept in the left lateral position on a stretcher for 10 to 20 minutes before abdominal images are obtained. This position allows gas to rise into the flank area adjacent to the right hemidiaphragm, where the potential pathology would not be superimposed by the gastric air bubble (Fig. 4.5). If larger amounts of free air are present, many radiology departments suggest that the patient lie on the side for a minimum of 5 minutes before the exposure is made.

Projections are taken for a three-way or acute abdomen series as follows:

- Perform an AP or PA projection of the abdomen with the patient in the left lateral decubitus position.
- Maintain the patient in the left lateral decubitus position while the patient is being moved onto a horizontally placed table. Move the patient to the upright position.
- Turn the patient to obtain upright AP or PA projections of the chest (Fig. 4.6) and abdomen (Fig. 4.7).
- Return the patient to the horizontal position for a supine AP projection of the abdomen (Fig. 4.8).

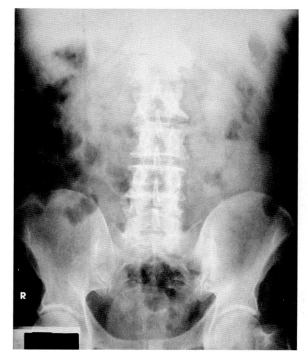

Fig. 4.4 AP abdomen showing blurred bowel gas in right upper quadrant (RUQ), caused by patient breathing during exposure.

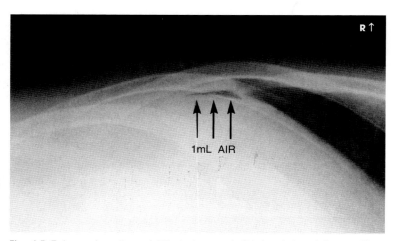

Fig. 4.5 Enlarged portion of AP abdomen, left lateral decubitus position in a patient injected with 1 mL of air into abdominal cavity.

Abdomen

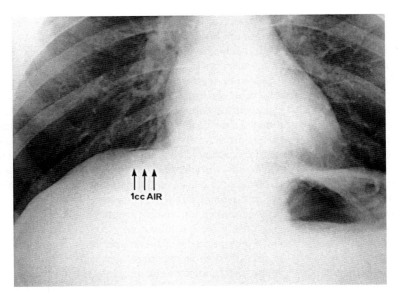

Fig. 4.6 Enlarged portion of upright AP chest showing free air in same patient as in Fig. 4.5.

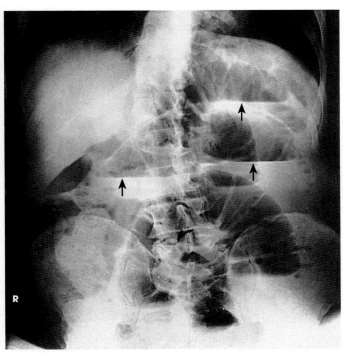

Fig. 4.7 AP abdomen, upright position, showing air-fluid levels (*arrows*) in intestine (same patient as in Fig. 4.8).

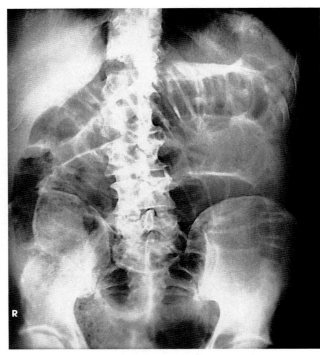

Fig. 4.8 AP abdomen. Supine study showing intestinal obstruction in same patient as in Fig. 4.7.

♠ AP PROJECTION
Supine; upright

Image receptor + grid: Positioned by manufacturer or department protocol for proper anatomy display orientation; CR plate: 14 × 17 inches (35 × 43 cm) lengthwise.

Position of patient
- For the AP abdomen, or KUB, projection, place the patient in either the supine or the upright position. The supine position is preferred for most initial examinations of the abdomen.

Position of part
- Center the midsagittal plane of the body to the midline of the grid device.

- If the patient is upright, distribute the weight of the body equally on the feet.
- Place the patient's arms where they do not cast shadows on the image.
- With the patient supine, place a support under the knees to relieve strain.
- For the *supine position,* center the IR/collimated field at the level of the iliac crests, and ensure that the pubic symphysis is included (Fig. 4.9).
- For the *upright position,* center the IR/collimated field 2 inches (5 cm) above the level of the iliac crests or high enough to include the diaphragm (Fig. 4.10).
- If the bladder is to be included on the upright image, center the IR/collimated field at the level of the iliac crests.

- If a patient is too tall to include the entire pelvic area, obtain a second image to include the bladder, if necessary. A 10 × 12 inches (24 × 30 cm) IR or collimated field is oriented crosswise and is centered 2 to 3 inches (5 to 7.6 cm) above the upper border of the pubic symphysis.
- *Shield gonads:* Use local gonad shielding for examinations of male patients (not shown for illustrative purposes).
- *Respiration:* Suspend at the end of expiration so that the abdominal organs are not compressed.

Central ray
- Perpendicular to the IR at the level of the iliac crests for the supine position.
- Horizontal and 2 inches (5 cm) above the level of the iliac crests to include the diaphragm for the upright position.

Collimation
- Adjust radiation field to 14 × 17 inches (35 × 43 cm) on the collimator. For smaller patients, collimate to within 1 inch (2.5 cm) of shadow of the abdomen flanks. Place side marker in the collimated exposure field.

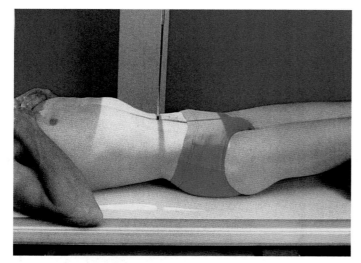

Fig. 4.9 AP Anteroposterior abdomen, supine.

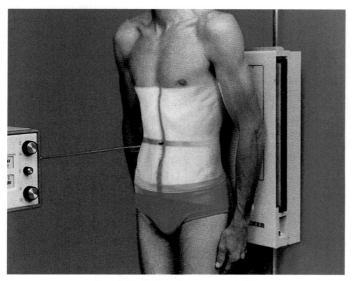

Fig. 4.10 AP abdomen, upright.

Structures shown

AP projection of the abdomen shows the size and shape of the liver, the spleen, and the kidneys and intra-abdominal calcifications or evidence of tumor masses (Fig. 4.11). Additional examples of supine and upright abdomen projections are shown in Figs. 4.7 and 4.8.

The following should be clearly seen:

- Evidence of proper collimation and presence of side marker and upright marker, if appropriate, placed clear of anatomy of interest.
- Area from the pubic symphysis to the upper abdomen (two images may be necessary if the patient is tall or wide)
- Proper patient alignment to IR
  □ Centered vertebral column
  □ Ribs, pelvis, and hips equidistant to the edge of the image or collimated borders on both sides
- No rotation
  □ Spinous processes in the center of the lumbar vertebrae
  □ Ischial spines of the pelvis symmetric, if visible
  □ Alae or wings of the ilia symmetric

- Exposure factors sufficient to demonstrate the following:
  □ Lateral abdominal wall and properitoneal fat layer (flank stripe)
  □ Psoas muscles, lower border of the liver, and kidneys
  □ Inferior ribs
  □ Transverse processes of the lumbar vertebrae
- Diaphragm without motion on upright radiograph (crosswise IR placement/collimated field is appropriate if the patient is large)

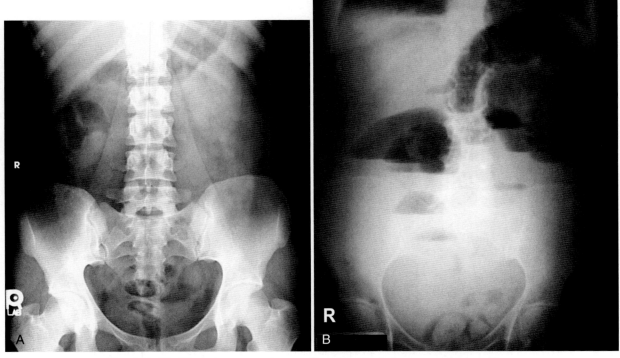

Fig. 4.11 (A) AP abdomen, supine position. (B) AP abdomen, upright position.

♠ PA PROJECTION
Upright

When the kidneys are not of primary interest, the upright PA projection should be considered. Compared with the AP projection, the PA projection of the abdomen greatly reduces patient gonadal dose.

Image receptor + grid: Positioned by manufacturer or department protocol for proper anatomy display orientation; CR plate: 14 × 17 inches (35 × 43 cm) lengthwise.

Position of patient
- With the patient in the upright position, place the anterior abdominal surface in contact with the vertical grid device.
- Center the abdominal midline to the midline of the IR.
- Center the IR/collimated field 2 inches (5 cm) above the level of the iliac crests (Fig. 4.12), as previously described for the upright AP projection. The central ray, structures shown, and evaluation criteria are the same as for the upright AP projection.

♠ AP PROJECTION
Left lateral decubitus position

Image receptor + grid: Positioned by manufacturer or department protocol for proper anatomy display orientation; CR plate: 14 × 17 inches (35 × 43 cm) lengthwise.

Position of patient
- If the patient is too ill to stand, place him or her in a lateral recumbent position lying on a radiolucent pad on a transportation cart. Use a left lateral decubitus position in most situations.
- The radiolucent pad is particularly important to ensure inclusion of the entire dependent side when fluid demonstration is of primary concern.
- When free intraperitoneal air is suspected, have the patient lie on the side for 5 minutes before the exposure to allow air to rise to its highest level within the abdomen.
- Place the patient's arms above the level of the diaphragm so that they are not projected over any abdominal contents.
- Flex the patient's knees slightly to provide stabilization.
- *Exercise care* to ensure that the patient does not fall off the cart; if a cart is used, *lock all wheels* securely in position.

Position of part
- Adjust the height of the vertical grid device so that the long axis of the IR is centered to the midsagittal plane.

- If the abdomen is too wide to include both flanks on one image, adjust patient and IR height to include side down when intraperitoneal fluid is suspected and to include side up when pneumoperitoneum is suspected.
- Position the patient so that the level of the iliac crests is centered to the IR. A slightly higher centering point, 2 inches (5 cm) above the iliac crests, may be necessary to ensure that the diaphragms are included in the image (Fig. 4.13).
- Adjust the patient to ensure that a true lateral position is attained.
- *Shield gonads.*
- *Respiration:* Suspend at the end of expiration.

▼ COMPENSATING FILTER
For patients with a large abdomen, a compensating filter improves image quality by preventing overexposure of the upper-side abdominal area.

Central ray
- Directed *horizontal* and perpendicular to the midpoint of the IR.

Collimation
- Adjust radiation field to 14 × 17 inches (35 × 43 cm) on the collimator. For smaller patients, collimate to within 1 inch (2.5 cm) of shadow of the abdomen flanks. Place side marker and decubitus marker in the collimated exposure field.

NOTE: A right lateral decubitus position is often requested or may be required when the patient cannot lie on the left side.

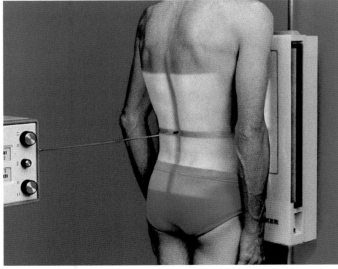

Fig. 4.12 PA abdomen, upright position. This projection is suggested for survey examination of the abdomen when the kidneys are not of primary interest.

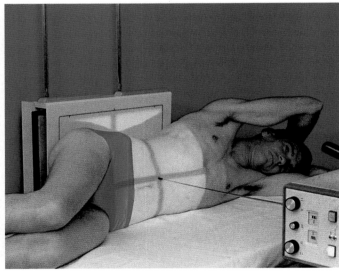

Fig. 4.13 AP abdomen, left lateral decubitus position.

Abdomen

Structures shown

In addition to showing the size and shape of the liver, spleen, and kidneys, the AP abdomen with the patient in the left decubitus position is most valuable for showing free air and air-fluid levels when an upright abdomen projection cannot be obtained (Fig. 4.14).

The following should be clearly seen:
- Evidence of proper collimation and presence of side marker and decubitus marker placed clear of anatomy of interest
- Diaphragm without motion
- Both sides of the abdomen. If abdomen is too wide:
  □ Side down when fluid is suspected (ensure entire dependent side is included in the collimated field)
  □ Side up when free air is suspected
- Abdominal wall, flank structures, and diaphragm
- No rotation
  □ Spinous processes in the center of the lumbar vertebrae
  □ Ischial spines of the pelvis symmetric, if visible
  □ Alae or wings of the ilia symmetric
- Abdominal contents visible without contrast media

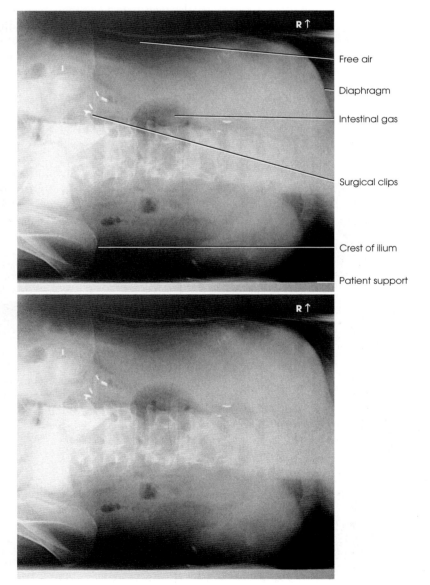

Free air

Diaphragm

Intestinal gas

Surgical clips

Crest of ilium

Patient support

Fig. 4.14 AP abdomen, left lateral decubitus position, showing free air collection along right flank. Note correct marker placement.

🦅 LATERAL PROJECTION
Right or left position

Image receptor + grid: Positioned by manufacturer or department protocol for proper anatomy display orientation; CR plate: 14 × 17 inches (35 × 43 cm) lengthwise.

Position of patient
- Turn the patient to a lateral recumbent position on the right or the left side.

Position of part
- Flex the patient's knees to a comfortable position, and adjust the body so that the midcoronal plane is centered to the midline of the grid.

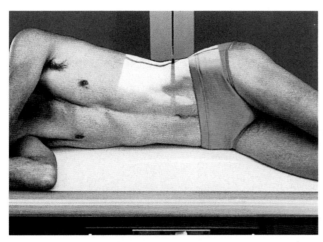

Fig. 4.15 Right lateral abdomen.

- Place supports between the knees and the ankles.
- Flex the elbows, and place the hands under the patient's head (Fig. 4.15).
- Center the IR at the level of the iliac crests or 2 inches (5 cm) above the crests to include the diaphragm.
- *Shield gonads.*
- *Respiration:* Suspend at the end of expiration.

Central ray
- Perpendicular to the IR and entering the midcoronal plane at the level of the iliac crest or 2 inches (5 cm) above the iliac crest if the diaphragm is included.

Collimation
- Adjust radiation field to 14 × 17 inches (35 × 43 cm) on the collimator. For smaller patients, collimate to within 1 inch (2.5 cm) of the anterior and posterior shadows of the abdomen. Place side marker in the collimated exposure field.

Structures shown

A lateral projection of the abdomen shows the prevertebral space occupied by the abdominal aorta and any intra-abdominal calcifications or tumor masses. The lateral abdomen is also used to show proper placement of AAA grafts and other vascular interventional devices (Fig. 4.16).

EVALUATION CRITERIA

The following should be clearly seen:
- Evidence of proper collimation and presence of side marker placed clear of anatomy of interest
- No rotation
  - Superimposed ilia
  - Superimposed lumbar vertebrae pedicles and open intervertebral foramina
- As much of the remaining abdomen as possible when the diaphragm is included
- Abdominal contents visible without contrast media

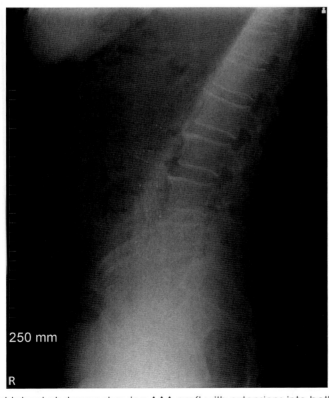

250 mm

R

Fig. 4.16 Right lateral abdomen showing AAA graft with extensions into both common iliac arteries.

(Courtesy NEA Baptist Memorial Hospital, Jonesboro, AR.)

♠ LATERAL PROJECTION
Right or left dorsal decubitus position

Image receptor + grid: Positioned by manufacturer or department protocol for proper anatomy display orientation; CR plate: 14 × 17 inches (35 × 43 cm) lengthwise.

Position of patient
- When the patient cannot stand or lie on the side, place the patient in the supine position on a transportation cart or other suitable support with the right or left side in contact with the vertical grid device.
- Place the patient's arms across the upper chest to ensure that they are not projected over any abdominal contents, or place them behind the patient's head.
- Flex the patient's knees slightly to relieve strain on the back.
- *Exercise care* to ensure that the patient does not fall from the cart or table; if a cart is used, *lock all wheels* securely in position.

Position of part
- Adjust the height of the vertical grid device so that the long axis of the IR is centered to the midcoronal plane.
- Position the patient so that a point approximately 2 inches (5 cm) above the level of the iliac crests is centered to the IR (Fig. 4.17).
- Adjust the patient to ensure that no rotation from the supine position occurs.
- *Shield gonads.*
- *Respiration:* Suspend at the end of expiration.

Central ray
- Directed *horizontal* and perpendicular to the center of the IR, entering the midcoronal plane 2 inches (5 cm) above the level of the iliac crests.

Collimation
- Adjust radiation field to 14 × 17 inches (35 × 43 cm) on the collimator. For smaller patients, collimate to within 1 inch (2.5 cm) of the anterior and posterior shadows of the abdomen. Place side marker in the collimated exposure field.

Structures shown
The lateral projection of the abdomen is valuable in showing the preverterbral space and is useful in determining air-fluid levels in the abdomen (Fig. 4.18).

EVALUATION CRITERIA
The following should be clearly seen:
- ■ Evidence of proper collimation and presence of side marker and decubitus marker placed clear of anatomy of interest
- ■ No rotation
  - □ Superimposed ilia
  - □ Superimposed lumbar vertebrae pedicles and open intervertebral foramina
- ■ As much of the remaining abdomen as possible when the diaphragm is included
- ■ Abdominal contents visible without contrast media

References
1. Miller RE, Nelson SW: The roentgenologic demonstration of tiny amounts of free intraperitoneal gas: experimental and clinical studies, *AJR Am J Roentgenol* 112:574, 1971.
2. Miller RE: The technical approach to the acute abdomen, *Semin Roentgenol* 8:267, 1973.

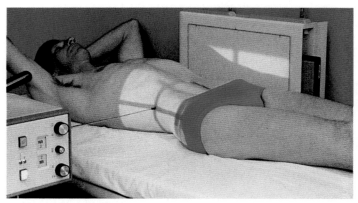

Fig. 4.17 Lateral abdomen, left dorsal decubitus position.

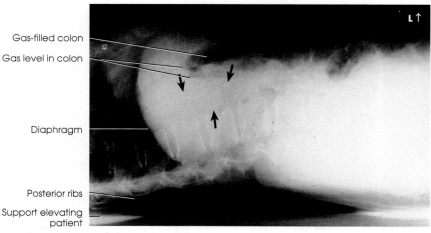

Gas-filled colon

Gas level in colon

Diaphragm

Posterior ribs

Support elevating patient

Fig. 4.18 Lateral abdomen, left dorsal decubitus position, showing calcified aorta *(arrows)*. Note correct marker placement.

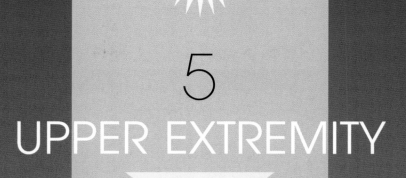

5

UPPER EXTREMITY

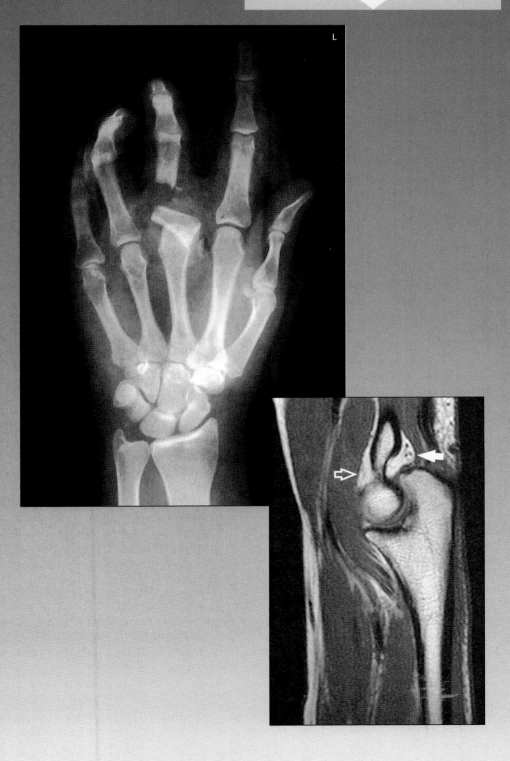

PROJECTIONS, POSITIONS, AND METHODS

Page	Essential	Anatomy	Projection	Position	Method
154	⬥	Digits (second through fifth)	PA		
156	⬥	Digits (second through fifth)	Lateral	Lateromedial, mediolateral	
158	⬥	Digits (second through fifth)	PA oblique	Lateral rotation	
160	⬥	First digit (thumb)	AP		
160		First digit (thumb)	PA		
160	⬥	First digit (thumb)	Lateral		
161	⬥	First digit (thumb)	PA oblique		
162		First digit (thumb): *First carpometacarpal joint*	AP		ROBERT
164		First digit (thumb): *First carpometacarpal joint*	AP		BURMAN
166		First digit (thumb): *First metacarpophalangeal joint*	PA		FOLIO
168	⬥	Hand	PA		
170	⬥	Hand	PA oblique	Lateral rotation	
172	⬥	Hand	Lateral	Extension and fan lateral	
174		Hand	Lateral	Flexion	
174		Hand	AP oblique	Medial rotation	NORGAARD
176	⬥	Wrist	PA		
177		Wrist	AP		
178	⬥	Wrist	Lateral		
180	⬥	Wrist	PA oblique	Lateral rotation	
181		Wrist	AP oblique	Medial rotation	
182	⬥	Wrist	PA	Ulnar deviation	
183		Wrist	PA	Radial deviation	
184	⬥	Wrist: *Scaphoid*	PA axial		STECHER
186		Wrist: *Scaphoid series*	PA, PA axial	Ulnar deviation	RAFERT-LONG
188		Wrist: *Trapezium*	PA axial oblique		CLEMENTS-NAKAYAMA
189		Carpal bridge	Tangential		
190	⬥	Carpal canal	Tangential		GAYNOR-HART
192	⬥	Forearm	AP		
194	⬥	Forearm	Lateral		
195	⬥	Elbow	AP		
196	⬥	Elbow	Lateral		
198	⬥	Elbow	AP oblique	Medial rotation	
199	⬥	Elbow	AP oblique	Lateral rotation	
200	⬥	Elbow: *Distal humerus*	AP	Partial flexion	
201	⬥	Elbow: *Proximal forearm*	AP	Partial flexion	
202		Elbow: *Distal humerus*	AP	Acute flexion	
203		Elbow: *Proximal forearm*	PA	Acute flexion	
204		Elbow: *Radial head*	Lateral		
206	⬥	Elbow: *Radial head, coronoid process*	Axiolateral	Lateral	COYLE
209		Distal humerus	PA axial		
210		Olecranon process	PA axial		
211	⬥	Humerus	AP	Upright	
212	⬥	Humerus	Lateral	Upright	
213	⬥	Humerus	AP	Recumbent	
214	⬥	Humerus	Lateral	Recumbent	
215	⬥	Humerus	Lateral	Recumbent, lateral recumbent	

The icons in the Essential column indicate projections frequently performed in the United States and Canada. Students should demonstrate competence in these projections.

AP, Anteroposterior; *PA*, posteroanterior.

Anatomists divide the bones of the upper extremities into the following main groups:
- Hand
- Forearm
- Arm
- Shoulder girdle

The proximal arm and shoulder girdle are discussed in Chapter 6.

Hand

The *hand* consists of 27 bones, which are subdivided into the following groups:
- Phalanges: Bones of the digits (fingers and thumb)
- Metacarpals: Bones of the palm
- Carpals: Bones of the wrist (Fig. 5.1)

DIGITS

The five *digits* are described by numbers and names; however, description by number is the more correct practice. Beginning at the lateral, or thumb, side of the hand, the numbers and names are as follows:

- First digit (thumb)
- Second digit (index finger)
- Third digit (middle finger)
- Fourth digit (ring finger)
- Fifth digit (small finger)

The digits contain 14 *phalanges* (*phalanx,* singular), which are long bones that consist of a cylindrical body and articular ends. Nine phalanges have two articular ends. The first digit has two phalanges—*proximal* and *distal.* The other digits have three phalanges—*proximal, middle,* and *distal.* The proximal phalanges are the closest to the palm, and the distal phalanges are the farthest from the palm. The distal phalanges are small and flattened, with a roughened rim around their distal anterior end; this gives them a spatula-like appearance. Each phalanx has a *head, body,* and *base.*

METACARPALS

Five *metacarpals,* which are cylindric in shape and slightly concave anteriorly, form the palm of the hand (see Fig. 5.1). They are long bones consisting of a *body* and two articular ends—the *head* distally and the *base* proximally. The area below the head is the *neck,* where fractures often occur. The first metacarpal contains two small *sesamoid* bones on its palmar aspect below the neck (see Fig. 5.1). A single sesamoid is often seen at this same level on the second metacarpal. The metacarpal heads, commonly known as the *knuckles,* are visible on the dorsal hand in flexion. The metacarpals are also numbered 1 to 5, beginning from the lateral side of the hand.

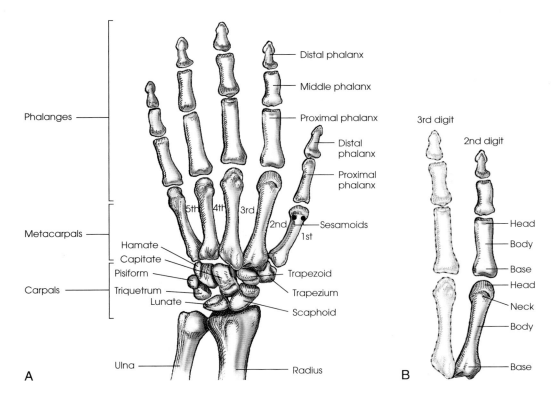

Fig. 5.1 (A) Anterior aspect of right hand and wrist. (B) Second metacarpal and phalanges showing head, neck, body, and base on second digit.

WRIST

The *wrist* has eight *carpal* bones, which are fitted closely together and arranged in two horizontal rows (see Fig. 5.1). The carpals are classified as short bones and are composed largely of cancellous tissue with an outer layer of compact bony tissue. The proximal row of carpals, which is nearest the forearm, contains the scaphoid, lunate, triquetrum, and pisiform. The distal row includes the trapezium, trapezoid, capitate, and hamate.

Each carpal contains identifying characteristics. Beginning at the proximal row of carpals on the lateral side, the *scaphoid,* the largest bone in the proximal carpal row, has a tubercle on the anterior and lateral aspect for muscle attachment and is palpable near the base of the thumb. The *lunate* articulates with the radius proximally and is easy to recognize because of its crescent shape. The *triquetrum* is approximately pyramidal and articulates anteriorly with the hamate. The *pisiform* is a pea-shaped bone situated anterior to the triquetrum and is easily palpated.

Beginning at the distal row of carpals on the lateral side, the *trapezium* has a tubercle and groove on the anterior surface. The tubercles of the trapezium and scaphoid constitute the lateral margin of the carpal groove. The *trapezoid* has a smaller surface anteriorly than posteriorly. The *capitate* articulates with the base of the third metacarpal and is the largest and most centrally located carpal. The wedge-shaped *hamate* exhibits the prominent *hook of hamate,* which is located on the anterior surface. The hamate and the pisiform form the medial margin of the carpal groove.

A triangular depression is located on the posterior surface of the wrist and is visible when the thumb is abducted and extended. This depression, known as the *anatomic snuff-box,* is formed by the tendons of the two major muscles of the thumb. The anatomic snuff-box overlies the scaphoid bone and the radial artery, which carries blood to the dorsum of the hand. Tenderness in the snuff-box area is a clinical sign suggesting fracture of the scaphoid—the most commonly fractured carpal bone.

CARPAL SULCUS

The anterior or palmar surface of the wrist is concave from side to side and forms the *carpal sulcus* (Figs. 5.2 and 5.3). The *flexor retinaculum,* a strong fibrous band, attaches medially to the pisiform and the hook of hamate and laterally to the tubercles of the scaphoid and trapezium. The *carpal canal* or *carpal tunnel* is the passageway created between the carpal sulcus and the flexor retinaculum. The *median nerve* and the *flexor tendons* pass through the carpal canal. Carpal tunnel syndrome results from compression of the median nerve inside the carpal tunnel.

Forearm

The *forearm* contains two bones that lie parallel to each other—the *radius* and the *ulna.* Similar to other long bones, they have a body and two articular extremities. The radius is located on the lateral side of the forearm, and the ulna is located on the medial side (Figs. 5.4 and 5.5).

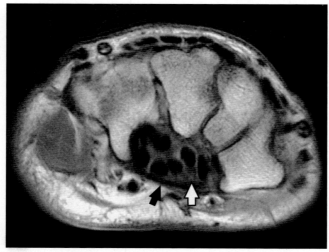

Fig. 5.2 Axial MRI of wrist. Bones in same position as in Fig. 5.3. Note arched position of carpal bones and carpal sulcus protecting tendons of fingers (*black circles* within sulcus) and median nerve (*white arrow*). Flexor retinaculum (*black arrow*) is also seen.

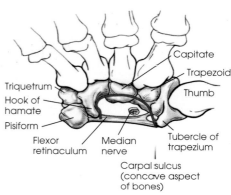

Fig. 5.3 Carpal sulcus.

ULNA

The *body* of the ulna is long and slender and tapers inferiorly. The upper portion of the ulna is large and presents two beak-like processes and concave depressions (Fig. 5.6). The proximal process, or *olecranon process,* concaves anteriorly and slightly inferiorly and forms the proximal portion of the *trochlear notch.* The more distal *coronoid process* projects anteriorly from the anterior surface of the body and curves slightly superiorly. The process is triangular and forms the lower portion of the trochlear notch. A depression called the *radial notch* is located on the lateral aspect of the coronoid process.

The distal end of the ulna includes a rounded process on its lateral side called the *head* and a narrower conic projection on the posteromedial side called the *ulnar styloid process.* An articular disk separates the head of the ulna from the wrist joint.

RADIUS

The proximal end of the radius is small and presents a flat disklike *head* above a constricted area called the *neck.* Just inferior to the neck on the medial side of the *body* of the radius is a roughened process called the *radial tuberosity.* The distal end of the radius is broad and flattened and has a conic projection on its lateral surface called the *radial styloid process.*

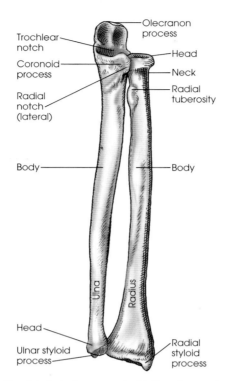

Fig. 5.4 Anterior aspect of left radius and ulna.

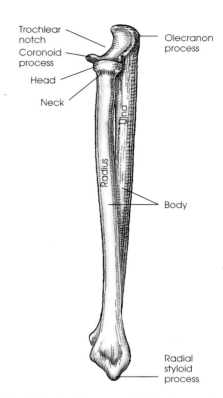

Fig. 5.5 Lateral aspect of left radius and ulna.

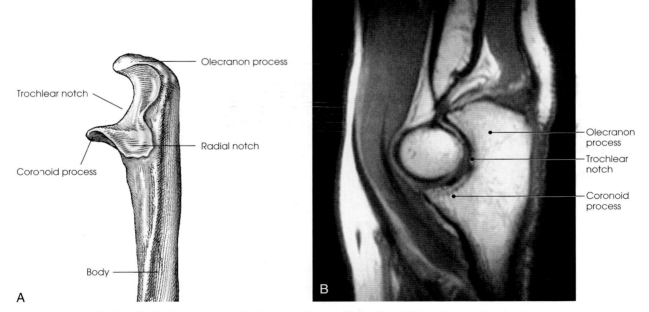

Fig. 5.6 (A) Radial aspect of left proximal ulna. (B) Sagittal MRI of elbow joint showing trochlear notch surrounding trochlea of humerus.

(B, Modified from Kelley LL, Petersen CM: *Sectional anatomy for imaging professionals,* ed 2, St Louis, 2007, Mosby.)

Arm

The arm has one bone called the *humerus,* which consists of a *body* and two articular ends (Fig. 5.7A and B). The proximal part of the humerus articulates with the shoulder girdle and is described further in Chapter 5. The distal humerus is broad and flattened and presents numerous processes and depressions.

The entire distal end of the humerus is called the *humeral condyle* and includes two smooth elevations for articulation with the bones of the forearm—the *trochlea* on the medial side and the *capitulum* on the lateral side. The *medial* and *lateral epicondyles* are superior to the condyle and are easily palpated. On the anterior surface superior to the trochlea, a shallow depression called the *coronoid fossa* receives the coronoid process when the elbow is flexed. The relatively small *radial fossa,* which receives the radial head when the elbow is flexed, is located lateral to the coronoid fossa and proximal to the capitulum. The *olecranon fossa* is a deep depression found immediately behind the coronoid fossa on the posterior surface and accommodates the olecranon process when the elbow is extended (see Fig. 5.7C).

The proximal end of the humerus contains the *head,* which is large, smooth, and rounded and lies in an oblique plane on the superomedial side. Just below the head, lying in the same oblique plane,

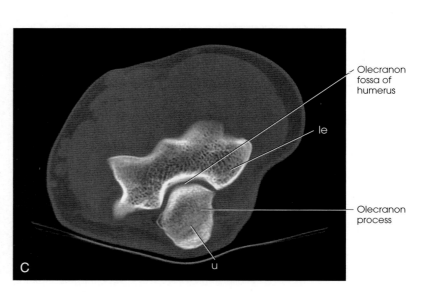

Fig. 5.7 (A) Anterior aspect of left humerus. (B) Medial aspect of left humerus. (C) Axial CT scan of elbow. *le,* Lateral epicondyle; *u,* ulna.

is the narrow, constricted *anatomic neck.* The constriction of the body just below the tubercles is called the *surgical neck,* which is the site of many fractures.

The *lesser tubercle* is situated on the anterior surface of the bone immediately below the anatomic neck. The tendon of the subscapularis muscle inserts at the lesser tubercle. The *greater tubercle* is located on the lateral surface of the bone just below the anatomic neck and is separated from the lesser tubercle by a deep depression called the *intertubercular groove.*

Upper Extremity Articulations

Table 5.1 contains a summary of the joints of the upper extremity. A detailed description of the upper extremity articulations follows.

The *interphalangeal* (IP) articulations between the phalanges are *synovial hinge* type and allow only flexion and extension (Fig. 5.8). The IP joints are named by location and are differentiated as either *proximal interphalangeal* (PIP) or *distal interphalangeal* (DIP), by the digit number, and by right or left hand (e.g., the PIP articulation of the fourth digit of the left hand) (Fig. 5.9A and B). Because the first digit has only two phalanges, the joint between the two phalanges is simply called the IP joint.

The metacarpals articulate with the phalanges at their distal ends and the carpals at their proximal ends. The *metacarpophalangeal* (MCP) articulations are *synovial ellipsoidal* joints and have the movements of flexion, extension, abduction, adduction, and circumduction. Because of the less convex and wider surface of the MCP joint of the thumb, only limited abduction and adduction are possible.

TABLE 5.1
Joints of the upper extremity

| Joint | Structural classification | | |
	Tissue	Type	Movement
Interphalangeal	Synovial	Hinge	Freely movable
Metacarpophalangeal	Synovial	Ellipsoidal	Freely movable
Carpometacarpal			
First digit	Synovial	Saddle	Freely movable
Second to fifth digits	Synovial	Gliding	Freely movable
Intercarpal	Synovial	Gliding	Freely movable
Radiocarpal	Synovial	Ellipsoidal	Freely movable
Radioulnar			
Proximal	Synovial	Pivot	Freely movable
Distal	Synovial	Pivot	Freely movable
Humeroulnar	Synovial	Hinge	Freely movable
Humeroradial	Synovial	Hinge	Freely movable

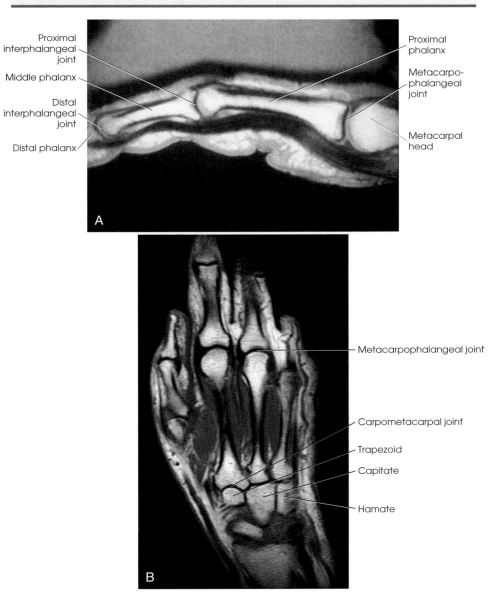

Fig. 5.8 (A) Sagittal MRI of finger showing IP and MCP joints. (B) Coronal MRI of hand and wrist showing same joints.

The carpals articulate with each other, the metacarpals, and the radius of the forearm. In the *carpometacarpal* (CMC) articulations, the first metacarpal and trapezium form a *synovial saddle* joint, which permits the thumb to oppose the fingers (touch the fingertips). The articulations between the second, third, fourth, and fifth metacarpals and the trapezoid, capitate, and hamate form *synovial gliding*

joints. The *intercarpal* articulations are also *synovial gliding* joints. The articulations between the lunate and scaphoid form a gliding joint. The *radiocarpal* articulation is a *synovial ellipsoidal* type. This joint is formed by the articulation of the scaphoid, lunate, and triquetrum, with the radius and the articular disk just distal to the ulna (see Fig. 5.9C).

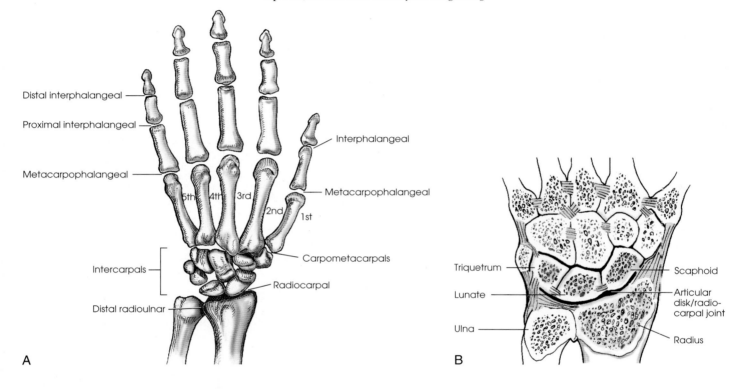

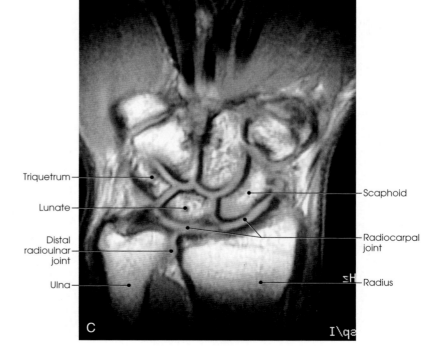

Fig. 5.9 (A) Articulations of hand and wrist. (B) Radiocarpal articulation formed by scaphoid, lunate, and triquetrum with radius. (C) Coronal MRI of wrist showing bones and joints of wrist.

The *distal* and *proximal radioulnar* articulations are synovial pivot joints. The distal ulna articulates with the ulnar notch of the distal radius. The proximal head of the radius articulates with the radial notch of the ulna at the medial side. The movements of supination and pronation of the forearm and hand largely result from the combined rotary action of these two joints. In pronation, the radius turns medially and crosses over the ulna at its upper third, and the ulna makes a slight counter-rotation that rotates the humerus medially.

The elbow joint proper includes the proximal radioulnar articulation and the articulations between the humerus and the radius and ulna. The three joints are enclosed in a common capsule. The trochlea of the humerus articulates with the ulna at the trochlear notch. The capitulum of the humerus articulates with the flattened head of the radius. The *humeroulnar* and *humeroradial* articulations form a *synovial hinge* joint and allow only flexion and extension movement (Figs. 5.10 and 5.11A). The proximal humerus and its articulations are described with the shoulder girdle in Chapter 6.

Fat Pads

The three areas of fat[1,2] associated with the elbow joint can be visualized only in the lateral projection (see Fig. 5.11B and C). The *posterior fat pad* covers the largest area and lies within the olecranon fossa of the posterior humerus. The superimposed coronoid and radial fat pads, which lie in the coronoid and radial fossae of the anterior humerus, form the *anterior fat pad*. The *supinator fat pad* is positioned anterior to and parallel with the anterior aspect of the proximal radius.

When the elbow is flexed 90 degrees for the lateral projection, only the anterior and supinator fat pads are visible and the posterior fat pad is depressed within the olecranon fossa. The anterior fat pad resembles a teardrop, and the supinator fat pad appears as shown in Fig. 5.11B. The fat pads become significant radiographically when an elbow injury causes effusion and displaces the fat pads or alters their shape. Visualization of the posterior fat pad is a reliable indicator of elbow pathology. Exposure factors designed to show soft tissues are extremely important on lateral elbow radiographs because visualization of the fat pads may be the only evidence of injury.

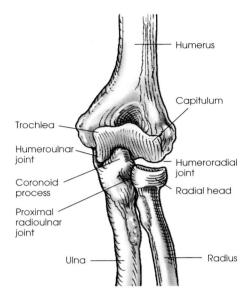

Fig. 5.10 Anterior aspect of left elbow joint.

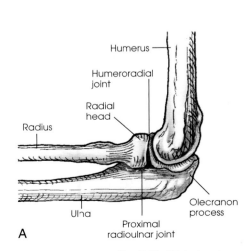

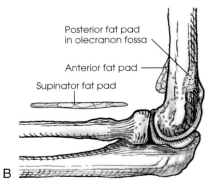

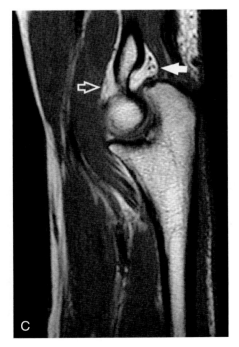

Fig. 5.11 (A) Lateral aspect of elbow. (B) Fat pads of elbow joint. (C) Sagittal MRI of elbow joint showing posterior fat pad *(solid arrow)* and anterior fat pad *(open arrow)*.

SUMMARY OF ANATOMY

Hand
Phalanges (bones of digits)
Digits
 Head
 Body
 Base
Metacarpals
Carpals

Metacarpals
First to fifth metacarpals
 Head
 Neck
 Body
 Base
Sesamoids

Wrist
Scaphoid
Lunate
Triquetrum
Pisiform

Trapezium
Trapezoid
Capitate
Hamate
Hook of hamate
Anatomic snuff-box

Carpal sulcus
Carpal tunnel
Flexor retinaculum
Median nerve
Flexor tendons

Forearm
Ulna
Radius

Ulna
Olecranon process
Trochlear notch
Coronoid process
Radial notch
Body

Head
Ulnar styloid process

Radius
Head
Neck
Radial tuberosity
Body
Radial styloid process

Arm
Humerus

Humerus
Humeral condyle
Trochlea
Capitulum
Medial epicondyle
Lateral epicondyle
Coronoid fossa
Radial fossa
Olecranon fossa
Body

Surgical neck
Lesser tubercle
Greater tubercle
Intertubercular groove
Anatomic neck
Head

Articulations
Interphalangeal
Metacarpophalangeal
Carpometacarpal
Intercarpal
Radiocarpal
Radioulnar
Humeroulnar
Humeroradial

Fat pads
Anterior fat pads
Posterior fat pad
Supinator fat pad

SAMPLE EXPOSURE TECHNIQUE CHART ESSENTIAL PROJECTIONS

These techniques were accurate for the equipment used to produce each exposure. However, use caution when applying them in your department because "there is considerable variability in image receptor response owing to varying scatter sensitivity, the use of grids with different grid ratios, collimation, beam filtration, the choice of kilovoltage, source-to-image distance, and image receptor size."[1]

This chart was created in collaboration with Dennis Bowman, AS, RT(R), Clinical Instructor, Community Hospital of the Monterey Peninsula, Monterey, CA. http://digitalradiographysolutions.com/.

UPPER EXTREMITY

Part	cm	kVp[a]	SID[b]	Collimation	CR[c] mAs	CR[c] Dose (mGy)[e]	DR[d] mAs	DR[d] Dose (mGy)[e]
Digits[f]	1.5	63	40"	2" × 6" (5 × 15 cm)	1.6[g]	0.042	0.6[g]	0.017
Hand—PA[f]	3	66	40"	7" × 8" (18 × 20 cm)	1.6[g]	0.085	0.71[g]	0.035
Hand—Oblique[f]	5	66	40"	7" × 8" (18 × 20 cm)	2.0[g]	0.111	0.8[g]	0.044
Hand—Lateral[f]	7	70	40"	6" × 8" (15 × 20 cm)	2.5[g]	0.166	1.25[g]	0.082
Wrist—PA/AP, Oblique[f]	4	66	40"	4" × 8" (10 × 20 cm)	2.0[g]	0.102	0.9[g]	0.044
Wrist—Lateral[f]	6	70	40"	3" × 8" (8 × 20 cm)	2.5[g]	0.125	1.1[g]	0.054
Carpal canal[f]	6	70	40"	4" × 4" (10 × 10 cm)	2.5[g]	0.134	1.25[g]	0.066
Forearm—AP, lateral[f]	7	70	40"	5" × 15" (13 × 38 cm)	2.2[g]	0.151	1.25[g]	0.084
Elbow—AP, lateral[f]	8	70	40"	5" × 9" (13 × 23 cm)	2.5[g]	0.171	1.4[g]	0.094
Elbow—Distal humerus[f]	9	70	40"	5" × 9" (13 × 23 cm)	3.2[g]	0.224	1.8[g]	0.125
Elbow—Proximal forearm[f]	9	70	40"	5" × 9" (13 × 23 cm)	2.0[g]	0.138	1.25[g]	0.086
Humerus—AP, lateral[f]	12	70	40"	7" × 17" (18 × 43 cm)	4.0[g]	0.314	2.0[g]	0.158
Humerus—AP, lateral[h]	12	75	40"	7" × 17" (18 × 43 cm)	5.6[g]	0.443	2.8[g]	0.222
Cast—Fiberglass[i]	Increase mAs 25% or 4 kVp							
Cast—Plaster medium[i]	Increase mAs 50% or 7 kVp							
Cast—Plaster large[i]	Increase mAs 100% or 10 kVp							

[1]ACR-AAPM-SIMM Practice Parameter for Digital Radiography, revised 2017.
[a]kVp values are for a high-frequency generator.
[b]40-inch minimum; 44–48 inches recommended to improve spatial resolution (mAs increase needed, but no increase in patient dose will result).
[c]AGFA CR MD 4.0 General IP, CR 75.0 reader, 400 speed class, with 6:1 (178LPI) grid when needed.
[d]GE Definium 8000, with 13:1 grid when needed.
[e]All doses are skin entrance for average adult (160- to 200-pound male, 150- to 190-pound female) at part thickness indicated.
[f]Tabletop, nongrid.
[g]Small focal spot.
[h]Bucky/Grid.
[i]Gratale P, Turner GW, Burns CB: Using the same exposure factors for wet and dry casts, *Radiol Technol* 57:328, 1986.

SUMMARY OF PATHOLOGY

Condition	Definition
Bone cyst	Fluid-filled cyst with wall of fibrous tissue
Bursitis	Inflammation of bursa
Dislocation	Displacement of bone from joint space
Fracture	Disruption in continuity of bone
Bennett	Fracture at base of first metacarpal
Boxer	Fracture of metacarpal neck
Colles	Fracture of distal radius with posterior (dorsal) displacement
Smith	Fracture of distal radius with anterior (palmar) displacement
Torus or buckle	Impacted fracture with bulging of periosteum
Gout	Hereditary form of arthritis in which uric acid is deposited in joints
Joint effusion	Accumulation of fluid in joint associated with underlying condition
Metastases	Transfer of cancerous lesion from one area to another
Osteoarthritis or degenerative joint disease	Form of arthritis marked by progressive cartilage deterioration in synovial joints and vertebrae
Osteomyelitis	Inflammation of bone owing to pyogenic infection
Osteopetrosis	Increased density of atypically soft bone
Osteoporosis	Loss of bone density
Rheumatoid arthritis	Chronic, systemic, inflammatory collagen disease
Tumor	New tissue growth where cell proliferation is uncontrolled
Chondrosarcoma	Malignant tumor arising from cartilage cells
Enchondroma	Benign tumor consisting of cartilage
Ewing sarcoma	Malignant tumor of bone arising in medullary tissue
Osteosarcoma	Malignant, primary tumor of bone with bone or cartilage formation

Eponymous (named) pathologies are listed in nonpossessive form to conform to the *AMA manual of style: a guide for authors and editors*, ed 10, Oxford, 2009, Oxford University Press.

ABBREVIATIONS USED IN CHAPTER 5

CMC	Carpometacarpal
DIP	Distal interphalangeal
IP[a]	Interphalangeal
MC	Metacarpal
MCP	Metacarpophalangeal
PIP	Proximal interphalangeal

[a]Note that IP has two different meanings; it is used in Chapter 1 to mean "image plate." See Addendum A for a summary of all abbreviations used in Volume 1.

Digits (Second Through Fifth)

General Procedures

When the upper extremity is radiographed, the following steps should be initiated:

- Remove rings, watches, and other radiopaque objects, and place them in secure storage during the procedure.
- Seat the patient at the side or end of the table to avoid a strained or uncomfortable position.
- Place the IR at a location and angle that allows the patient to be in the most comfortable position. Because the degree of immobilization (particularly of the hand and digits) is limited, the patient must be comfortable to promote relaxation and cooperation in maintaining the desired position.
- Unless otherwise specified, direct the CR at a right angle to the midpoint of the IR. Because the joint spaces of the extremities are narrow, accurate centering is essential to avoid obscuring the joint spaces.
- Radiograph each side separately when performing a bilateral examination of the hands or wrists; this prevents distortion, particularly of the joint spaces.
- Shield gonads from scattered radiation with a sheet of lead-impregnated rubber or a lead apron placed over the patient's pelvis (Fig. 5.12).
- Use close collimation. This technique is recommended for all upper extremity radiographs.
- Use right or left markers and any other identification markers, when appropriate.

Digits (Second Through Fifth)
⬥ PA PROJECTION

Image receptor: Positioned by manufacturer or department protocol for proper anatomy display orientation; CR plate: 10×12 inches (24×30 cm) lengthwise.

Position of patient

- Seat the patient at the end of the radiographic table.

Position of part

When radiographing individual digits (except the first), take the following steps:

- Place the extended digit with the palmar surface down on the IR.
- Separate the digits slightly, and center the digit under examination to the center of the IR.
- Center the PIP joint to the IR (Figs. 5.13–5.15).
- Shield gonads.

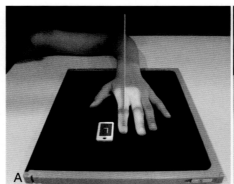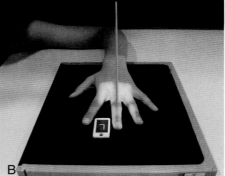

Fig. 5.13 (A) PA second digit. (B) PA third digit.

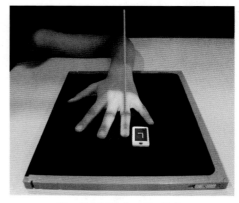

Fig. 5.14 PA fourth digit.

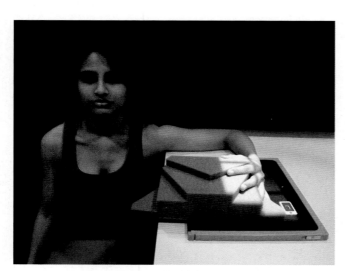

Fig. 5.12 Properly shielded patient.

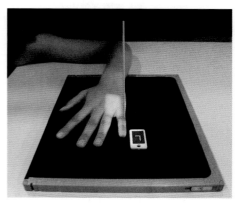

Fig. 5.15 PA fifth digit.

Central ray

- Perpendicular to the PIP joint of the affected digit

Collimation

- Adjust radiation field to 1 inch (2.5 cm) on all sides of the digit, including 1 inch (2.5 cm) proximal to the MCP joint. Place side marker in the collimated exposure field.

COMPUTED RADIOGRAPHY

For all projections, the digit must be centered to the plate or plate section with four collimator margins. Two or more images can be projected on one crosswise IP; however, there should be four collimator margins for each projection. A lead blocker must cover the unexposed side when multiple images are made on one IP.

Structures shown

A PA projection of the appropriate digit (Figs. 5.16 through 5.19).

The following should be clearly seen:
- Evidence of proper collimation and presence of side marker placed clear of anatomy of interest
- Entire digit from fingertip to distal portion of the adjoining metacarpal
- No soft tissue overlap from adjacent digits
- No rotation:
  - □ Equal concavity on both sides of the phalangeal bodies
  - □ Equal amount of soft tissue on both sides of the phalanges
- Fingernail, if seen, centered over the distal phalanx
- Open IP and MCP joint spaces
- Bony trabecular detail and surrounding soft tissues

NOTE: Digits that cannot be extended can be examined in small sections. When joint injury is suspected, an AP projection instead of a PA projection is recommended.

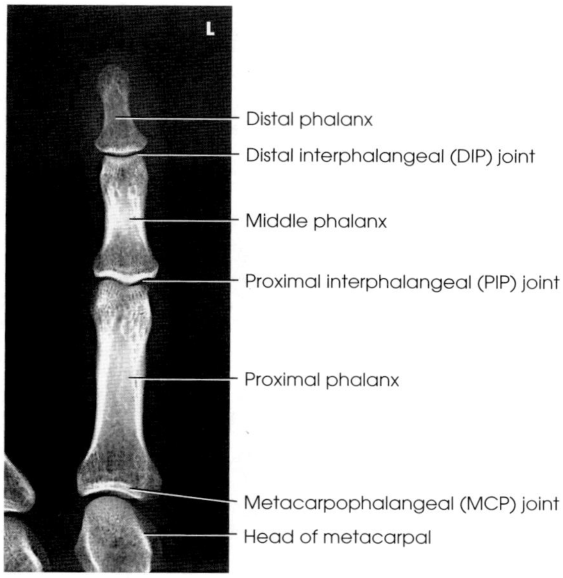

Distal phalanx

Distal interphalangeal (DIP) joint

Middle phalanx

Proximal interphalangeal (PIP) joint

Proximal phalanx

Metacarpophalangeal (MCP) joint

Head of metacarpal

Fig. 5.16 PA second digit.

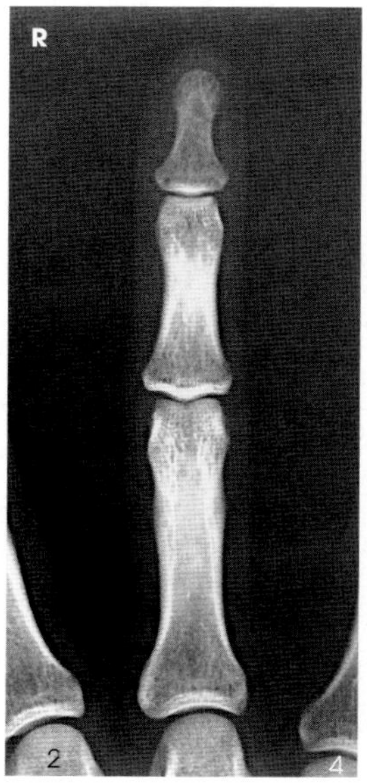

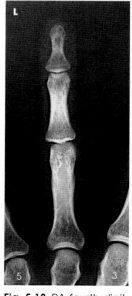

Fig. 5.17 PA third digit.

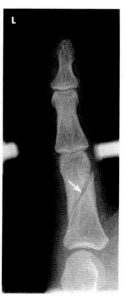

Fig. 5.18 PA fourth digit.

Fig. 5.19 Fractured fifth digit (*arrow*).

⚹ LATERAL PROJECTION
Lateromedial or mediolateral

Image receptor: Positioned by manufacturer or department protocol for proper anatomy display orientation; CR plate: 10×12 inches (24×30 cm) lengthwise.

Position of patient
- Seat the patient at the end of the radiographic table.

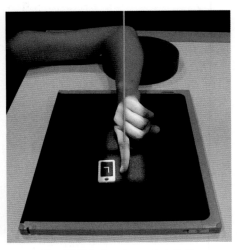

Fig. 5.20 Lateral second digit.

Position of part
- Because lateral digit positions are difficult to hold, tell the patient how the digit is adjusted on the IR and demonstrate with your own finger. Let the patient assume the most comfortable arm position.
- Ask the patient to extend the digit to be examined. Close the rest of the digits into a fist and hold them in complete flexion with the thumb.
- Support the elbow on sandbags or provide other suitable support when the elbow must be elevated to bring the digit into position.
- With the digit under examination extended and other digits folded into a fist, have the patient's hand rest on the lateral, or radial, surface for the second or third digit (Figs. 5.20 and 5.21) or on the medial, or ulnar, surface for the fourth or fifth digit (Figs. 5.22 and 5.23).

- Before making the final adjustment of the digit position, place the IR so that the midline is parallel with the long axis of the digit. Center the IR to the PIP joint.
- Rest the second and fifth digits directly on the IR, but for an accurate image of the bones and joints, elevate the third and fourth digits and place their long axes parallel with the plane of the IR. A radiolucent sponge may be used to support the digits.
- Immobilize the extended digit by placing a strip of adhesive tape, a tongue depressor, or other support against its palmar surface. The patient can hold the support with the opposite hand.
- Adjust the anterior or posterior rotation of the hand to obtain a true lateral position of the digit.
- Shield gonads.

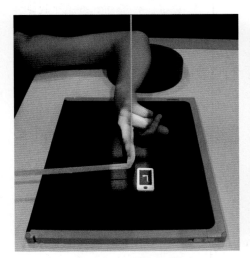

Fig. 5.21 Lateral third digit (adhesive tape).

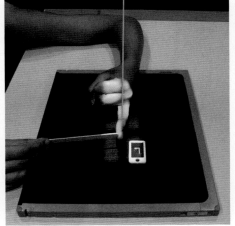

Fig. 5.22 Lateral fourth digit (tongue blade).

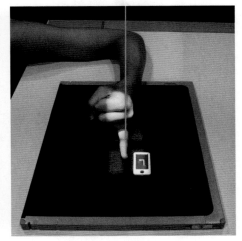

Fig. 5.23 Lateral fifth digit.

Central ray

- Perpendicular to the PIP joint of the affected digit

Collimation

- Adjust radiation field to 1 inch (2.5 cm) on all sides of the digit, including 1 inch (2.5 cm) proximal to the MCP joint. Place side marker in the collimated exposure field.

Structures shown

A lateral projection of the affected digit (Figs. 5.24 through 5.27).

EVALUATION CRITERIA

The following should be clearly seen:

- Evidence of proper collimation and presence of side marker placed clear of anatomy of interest
- Entire digit from fingertip to distal portion of the adjoining metacarpal
- No rotation:
  - ☐ Fingernail in profile, if visualized and normal
  - ☐ Concave, anterior surfaces of the phalanges
- No superimposition of the proximal phalanx or MCP joint by adjacent digits
- Open IP joint spaces
- Bony trabecular detail and surrounding soft tissues

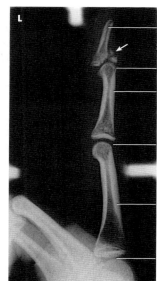

Distal phalanx

Distal interphalangeal (DIP) joint

Middle phalanx

Proximal interphalangeal (PIP) joint

Proximal phalanx

Metacarpophalangeal (MCP) joint

Fig. 5.24 Lateral digit showing chip fracture and dislocation involving DIP joint of second digit *(arrow).*

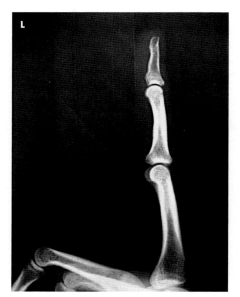

Fig. 5.25 Lateral third digit.

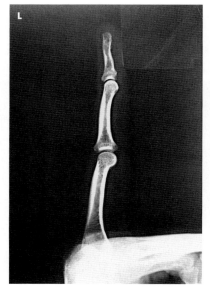

Fig. 5.26 Lateral fourth digit.

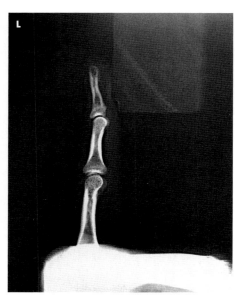

Fig. 5.27 Lateral fifth digit.

Upper Extremity

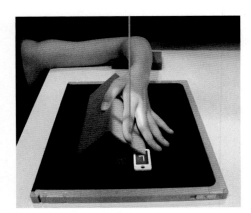

Fig. 5.28 PA oblique second digit.

♠ PA OBLIQUE PROJECTION
Lateral rotation

Image receptor: Positioned by manufacturer or department protocol for proper anatomy display orientation; CR plate: 10 × 12 inches (24 × 30 cm) lengthwise.

Position of patient
- Seat the patient at the end of the radiographic table.

Position of part
- Place the patient's forearm on the table, with the hand pronated and the palm resting on the IR.
- Center the IR at the level of the PIP joint.
- Rotate the hand laterally until the digits are separated and supported on a 45-degree foam wedge. The wedge supports the digits in a position parallel with the IR plane (Figs. 5.28 through 5.31) so that the IP joint spaces are open.
- Shield gonads.

Central ray
- Perpendicular to the PIP joint of the affected digit

Collimation
- Adjust radiation field to 1 inch (2.5 cm) on all sides of the digit, including 1 inch (2.5 cm) proximal to the MCP joint. Place side marker in the collimated exposure field.

Structures shown

A PA oblique projection of the bones and soft tissue of the affected digit (Figs. 5.32 through 5.35).

EVALUATION CRITERIA

The following should be clearly seen:
- Evidence of proper collimation and presence of side marker placed clear of anatomy of interest
- Entire digit, including the distal portion of the adjoining metacarpal
- Digit rotated at 45 degrees, demonstrated by concavity of the elevated side of the phalangeal bodies
- No superimposition of the proximal phalanx or MCP joint by adjacent digits
- Open IP and MCP joint spaces
- Bony trabecular detail and surrounding soft tissues

OPTION: Some radiographers rotate the second digit medially from the pronated position (Fig. 5.36). The advantage of medially rotating the digit is that the part is closer to the IR for improved resolution and increased visibility of certain fractures.[3]

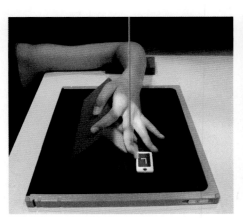

Fig. 5.29 PA oblique third digit.

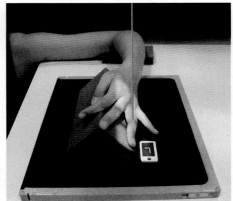

Fig. 5.30 PA oblique fourth digit.

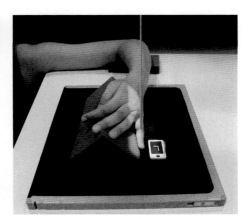

Fig. 5.31 PA oblique fifth digit.

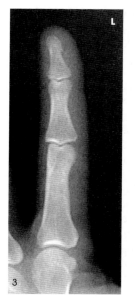

Fig. 5.32 PA oblique second digit.

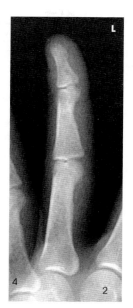

Fig. 5.33 PA oblique third digit.

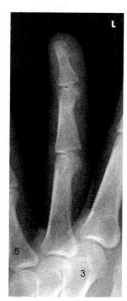

Fig. 5.34 PA oblique fourth digit.

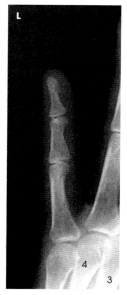

Fig. 5.35 PA oblique fifth digit.

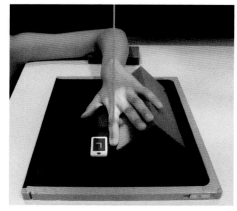

Fig. 5.36 PA oblique second digit (alternative method, medial rotation).

AP, PA, LATERAL, AND PA OBLIQUE PROJECTIONS

Image receptor: Positioned by manufacturer or department protocol for proper anatomy display orientation; CR plate: 10 × 12 inches (24 × 30 cm) lengthwise.

⚕ AP PROJECTION

Position of patient

- Seat the patient at the end of the radiographic table with the arm internally rotated.

Position of part

- Demonstrate how to avoid motion or rotation with the hand. By adjusting the body position on the chair, the patient can place the hand in the correct position with the least amount of strain on the arm.
- Put the patient's hand in a position of extreme medial rotation. Have the patient hold the extended digits back with tape or the opposite hand. Rest the thumb on the IR. If the elbow is elevated, place a support under it and have the patient rest the opposite forearm against the table for support (Fig. 5.37).
- Center the long axis of the thumb parallel with the long axis of the IR. Adjust the position of the hand to ensure a true AP projection of the thumb. Place the fifth metacarpal back far enough to avoid superimposition.
- Lewis[4] suggested directing the CR 10 to 15 degrees along the long axis of the thumb, toward the wrist to show the first metacarpal free of the soft tissue of the palm.
- Shield gonads.

PA PROJECTION

Position of patient

- Seat the patient at the end of the radiographic table with the hand resting on its medial surface.

Position of part

- If a PA projection of the first CMC joint and first digit is to be performed, place the hand in the lateral position. Rest the elevated and abducted thumb on a radiographic support, or hold it up with a radiolucent stick. Adjust the hand to place the dorsal surface of the digit parallel with the IR. This position magnifies the part (Fig. 5.38).
- Center the MCP joint to the center of the IR.
- Shield gonads.

⚕ LATERAL PROJECTION

Position of patient

- Seat the patient at the end of the radiographic table, with the relaxed hand placed on the IR.

Position of part

- Place the hand in its natural arched position, with the palmar surface down and fingers flexed or resting on a sponge.
- Place the midline of the IR parallel with the long axis of the digit. Center the IR to the MCP joint.
- Adjust the arching of the hand until a true lateral position of the thumb is obtained (Fig. 5.39).

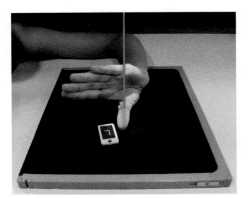

Fig. 5.37 AP first digit.

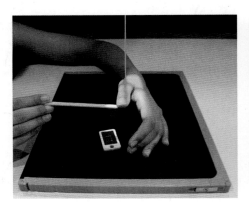

Fig. 5.38 PA first digit (tongue blade).

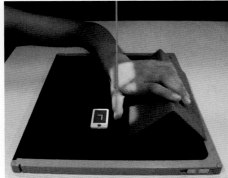

Fig. 5.39 Lateral first digit.

★ PA OBLIQUE PROJECTION

Position of patient
- Seat the patient at the end of the radiographic table, with the palm of the hand resting on the IR.

Position of part
- With the thumb abducted, place the palmar surface of the hand in contact with the IR. Ulnar deviate the hand slightly. This relatively normal placement positions the thumb in the oblique position.
- Align the longitudinal axis of the thumb with the long axis of the IR. Center the IR to the MCP joint (Fig. 5.40).
- Shield gonads.

Central ray
- Perpendicular to the MCP joint for AP, PA, lateral, and oblique projections

Collimation
- Adjust radiation field to 1 inch (2.5 cm) on all sides of the digit, including 1 inch (2.5 cm) proximal to the CMC joint. Place side marker in the collimated exposure field.

Structures shown
AP, PA, lateral, and PA oblique projections of the thumb (Figs. 5.41 through 5.44).

AP and PA Thumb
The following should be clearly seen:
- Evidence of proper collimation and presence of side marker placed clear of anatomy of interest
- Area from the distal tip of the thumb to the trapezium
- No rotation
  - Concavity of the phalangeal and metacarpal bodies
  - Equal amount of soft tissue on both sides of the phalanges
  - Thumbnail, if visualized, in the center of the distal thumb
- Overlap of soft tissue profile of the palm over the midshaft of the first metacarpal
- Open IP and MCP joint spaces without overlap of bones
- Bony trabecular detail and surrounding soft tissues
- PA thumb projection will be magnified compared with AP projection

Lateral thumb
The following should be clearly seen:
- Evidence of proper collimation and presence of side marker placed clear of anatomy of interest
- Area from the distal tip of the thumb to the trapezium
- No rotation
  - Concave anterior surface of the proximal phalanx and metacarpal
  - Thumbnail, if visualized and normal, in profile
- Open IP and MCP joint spaces
- Bony trabecular detail and surrounding soft tissues

Oblique thumb
The following should be clearly seen:
- Evidence of proper collimation and presence of side marker placed clear of anatomy of interest
- Area from the distal tip of the thumb to the trapezium
- Proper rotation, demonstrated by concave surface of elevated side of the proximal phalanx and metacarpal
- Open IP and MCP joint spaces
- Bony trabecular detail and surrounding soft tissues

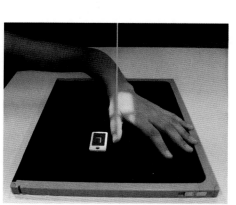

Fig. 5.40 PA oblique first digit.

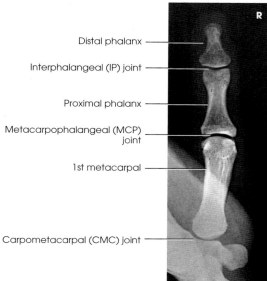

Distal phalanx

Interphalangeal (IP) joint

Proximal phalanx

Metacarpophalangeal (MCP) joint

1st metacarpal

Carpometacarpal (CMC) joint

Fig. 5.41 AP first digit.

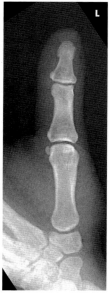

Fig. 5.42 PA first digit.

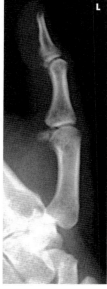

Fig. 5.43 Lateral first digit.

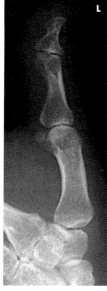

Fig. 5.44 PA oblique first digit.

First Carpometacarpal Joint
AP PROJECTION

ROBERT METHOD

Robert[5] first described the radiographic projection of the first CMC joint in 1936. Lewis[4] modified the CR for this projection in 1988, and Long and Rafert[6] further modified the CR in 1995. This projection is commonly performed to show arthritic changes, fractures, displacement of the first CMC joint, and Bennett fracture. The Robert method does not replace the initial AP or PA thumb projection.

Image receptor: Positioned by manufacturer or department protocol for proper anatomy display orientation; CR plate: 10 × 12 inches (24 × 30 cm) lengthwise.

Position of patient
- Seat the patient sideways at the end of the radiographic table. The patient should be positioned low enough to place the shoulder, elbow, and wrist on the same plane. The entire extremity *must* be on the same plane to prevent elevation of the carpal bones and closing of the first CMC joint (Fig. 5.45A).

Position of part
- Extend the extremity straight out on the radiographic table.
- Rotate the arm internally to place the posterior aspect of the thumb on the IR with the thumbnail down (see Fig. 5.45B).

- Place the thumb in the center of the IR.
- Hyperextend the hand so that the soft tissue over the ulnar aspect does not obscure the first CMC joint (Fig. 5.46). Ensure that the thumb is not oblique.
- Long and Rafert[6] stated that the patient may hold the fingers back with the other hand.
- Steady the hand on a sponge if necessary.
- *Shield gonads.*

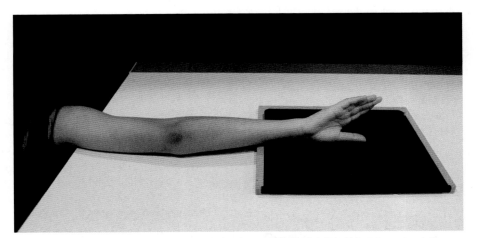

Fig. 5.45 Patient in position for AP thumb to show first CMC joint: Robert method. The patient leans forward to place entire arm on same plane and for ease of maximum internal arm rotation.

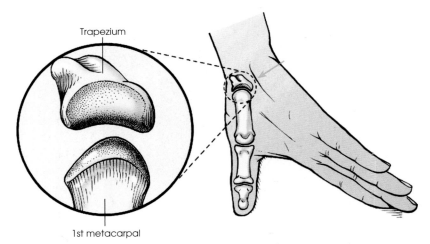

Trapezium

1st metacarpal

Fig. 5.46 Hyperextended hand and thumb position for AP projection of first CMC joint: Robert method. Soft tissue of palm *(arrow)* is positioned out of the way so that joint is clearly seen. *Inset:* First CMC joint is a saddle joint; articular surfaces are shown.

Central ray (Fig. 5.47)

Robert method

- Perpendicular entering at the first CMC joint

Long and Rafert modification

- Angled 15 degrees proximally along the long axis of the thumb and entering the first CMC joint

Lewis modification

- Angled 10 to 15 degrees proximally along the long axis of the thumb and entering the first MCP joint

NOTE: Angulation of the CR serves two purposes: (1) It may help to project the soft tissue of the hand away from the first CMC joint, and (2) it can help to open the joint space when the space is not shown with a perpendicular CR.

Collimation

- Adjust radiation field to 1 inch (2.5 cm) on all sides of the digit, including 1 inch (2.5 cm) proximal to the CMC joint. Place side marker in the collimated exposure field.

Structures shown

The first CMC joint free of superimposition of the soft tissues of the hand (Fig. 5.48).

The following should be clearly seen:

- Evidence of proper collimation and presence of side marker placed clear of anatomy of interest
- First CMC joint free of superimposition of the hand or other bony elements
- First metacarpal with the base in convex profile
- Trapezium
- Bony trabecular detail and surrounding soft tissues

First Digit (Thumb)

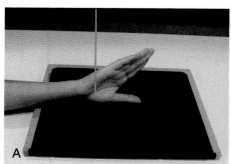
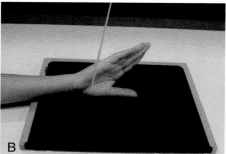
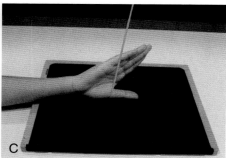

Fig. 5.47 Central ray angulation choices to show first CMC joint. (A) Robert method, 0 degrees to CMC joint. (B) Long-Rafert modification, 15 degrees proximal to CMC joint. (C) Lewis modification, 10 to 15 degrees proximal to MCP joint.

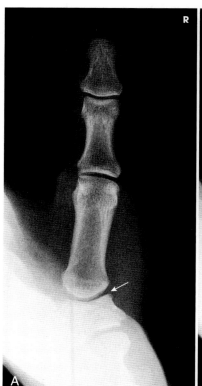
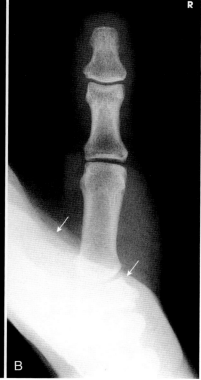

Fig. 5.48 (A) Optimal radiograph of AP first CMC joint *(arrow)*: Robert method. (B) Example of typical repeat radiograph. Soft tissue of palm *(arrows)* obscured first CMC joint. Long-Rafert or Lewis modification of central ray would help to show the joint on this patient.

First Carpometacarpal Joint

AP PROJECTION

BURMAN METHOD

When hyperextension of the wrist is not contraindicated, Burman[7] stated that this projection provides a clearer image of the first CMC joint than is seen on the standard AP projection.

> **Image receptor:** Positioned by manufacturer or department protocol for proper anatomy display orientation; CR plate: 10 × 12 inches (24 × 30 cm) lengthwise.

> **SID:** 18 inches is recommended to produce a magnified image that creates a greater field of view of the concavoconvex aspect of this joint.

Position of patient

- Seat the patient at the end of the radiographic table so that the forearm can be adjusted to lie approximately parallel with the long axis of the IR.

Position of part

- Place the IR under the wrist, and center the first CMC joint to the center of the IR.
- Hyperextend the hand, and have the patient hold the position with the opposite hand or with a bandage looped around the digits.
- Rotate the hand internally, and abduct the thumb so that it is flat on the IR (Fig. 5.49).
- Shield gonads.

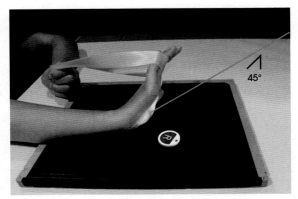

Fig. 5.49 Hyperextended hand and abducted thumb position for AP of first CMC joint: Burman method.

Central ray

• Through the first CMC joint at a 45-degree angle toward the elbow

Structures shown

A magnified concavoconvex outline of the first CMC joint (Fig. 5.50).

EVALUATION CRITERIA

The following should be clearly seen:

■ Evidence of proper collimation and presence of side marker placed clear of anatomy of interest
■ First metacarpal
■ Trapezium in concave profile
■ Base of the first metacarpal in convex profile
■ First CMC joint, unobscured by adjacent carpals
■ Bony trabecular detail and surrounding soft tissues

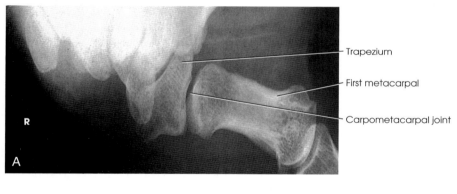

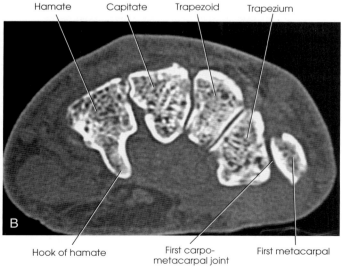

Fig. 5.50 (A) AP thumb to demonstrate the first CMC joint: Burman method. (B) Axial CT scan through distal carpals. Note that CMC joint is well visualized.

(A, Courtesy Michael Burman.)

First Metacarpophalangeal Joint
PA PROJECTION
FOLIO METHOD

This projection is useful for the diagnosis of ulnar collateral ligament (UCL) rupture in the MCP joint of the thumb, also known as "skier's thumb."[8]

Image receptor: Positioned by manufacturer or department protocol for proper anatomy display orientation; CR plate: 10 × 12 inches (24 × 30 cm) crosswise.

Position of patient
- Seat the patient at the end of the radiographic table.

Position of part
- Place the patient's hands on the cassette, resting them on their medial aspects.
- Tightly wrap a rubber band around the distal portion of both thumbs and place a roll of medical tape between the bodies of the first metacarpals.
- Ensure the thumbs remain in the PA plane by keeping the thumbnails parallel to the cassette (Fig. 5.51).
- Before exposure, instruct the patient to pull the thumbs apart and hold.
- *Shield gonads.*

Central ray
- Perpendicular to a point midway between both hands at the level of the MCP joints

NOTE: To avoid motion, have the correct technical factors set on the generator and be ready to make the exposure before instructing the patient to pull the thumbs apart.

Collimation
- Adjust radiation field to include the third metacarpals on the sides, the bases of the thumbs proximally and 1 inch (2.5 cm) distal to the thumbnails. Place side marker in the collimated exposure field.

Structures shown
The MCP joints and MCP angles bilaterally (Fig. 5.52).

EVALUATION CRITERIA

The following should be clearly seen:
- Evidence of proper collimation and presence of side marker placed clear of anatomy of interest
- Thumbs in a PA projection with no rotation
- First metacarpals
- First MCP joint
- Rubber band and medical tape in correct position
- Thumbs centered to the center of the image
- Bony trabecular detail and surrounding soft tissues

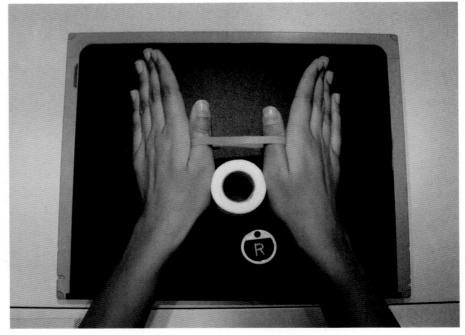

Fig. 5.51 Hands and thumbs in position for PA first MCP joints: Folio method. Note roll of tape between thumbs.

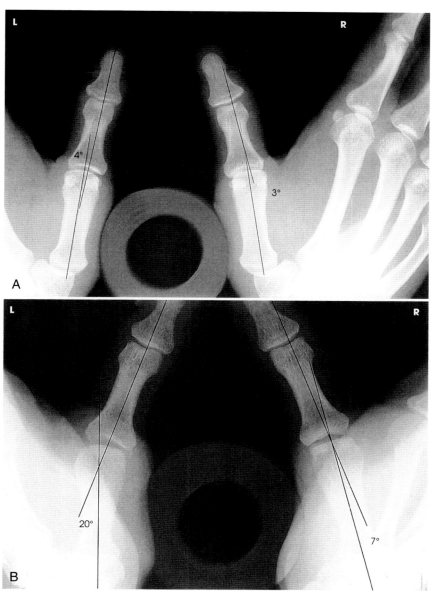

Fig. 5.52 First MCP joint, Folio method. (A) Normal thumbs with acceptable MCP joints bilaterally. Roll of tape between metacarpals and rubber band holding distal aspects of thumbs are visible. (B) Increased angulation of left MCP joint with 13-degree difference compared with right MCP joint. Partially torn left UCL measures 20 degrees between long axis of first metacarpal and proximal phalanx, whereas uninjured side measures 7 degrees.

☀ PA PROJECTION

Image receptor: Positioned by manufacturer or department protocol for proper anatomy display orientation; CR plate: 10 × 12 inches (24 × 30 cm) lengthwise.

Position of patient

- Seat the patient at the end of the radiographic table.
- Adjust the patient's height so that the forearm is resting on the table (Fig. 5.53A).

Position of part

- Rest the patient's forearm on the table, and place the hand with the palmar surface down on the IR.
- Center the IR to the MCP joints, and adjust the long axis of the IR parallel with the long axis of the hand and forearm.
- Spread the fingers slightly (see Fig. 5.53B).
- Ask the patient to relax the hand to avoid motion. Prevent involuntary movement with the use of adhesive tape or positioning sponges. A sandbag may be placed over the distal forearm.
- *Shield gonads.*

Central ray

- Perpendicular to the third MCP joint

Collimation

- Adjust radiation field to 1 inch (2.5 cm) on all sides of the hand, including 1 inch (2.5 cm) proximal to the ulnar styloid. Place side marker in the collimated exposure field.

Structures shown

PA projections of the carpals, metacarpals, phalanges (except the thumb), interarticulations of the hand, and distal radius and ulna are shown in Fig. 5.54. This image also shows a PA oblique projection of the first digit.

The following should be clearly seen:

- Evidence of proper collimation and presence of side marker placed clear of anatomy of interest
- Anatomy from fingertips to distal radius and ulna
- Slightly separate digits with no soft tissue overlap
- No rotation of the hand
  - Equal concavity of the metacarpal and phalangeal bodies on both sides
  - Equal amount of soft tissue on both sides of the phalanges
  - Fingernails, if visualized, in the center of each distal phalanx
  - Equal distance between the metacarpal heads
- Open MCP and IP joints, indicating that the hand is placed flat on the IR
- Bony trabecular detail and surrounding soft tissues

NOTE: When the MCP joints are under examination and the patient cannot extend the hand enough to place its palmar surface in contact with the IR, the position of the hand can be reversed for an AP projection. This position is also used for the metacarpals when the hand cannot be extended because of an injury, a pathologic condition, or the use of dressings.

SPECIAL TECHNIQUES: Clements and Nakayama[9] described a special exposure technique for imaging early rheumatoid arthritis. Lewis[10] described a positioning variation to place the second through fifth metacarpals parallel to the IR, resulting in a true PA projection.

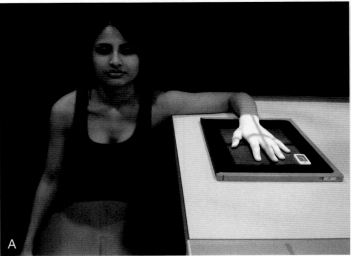
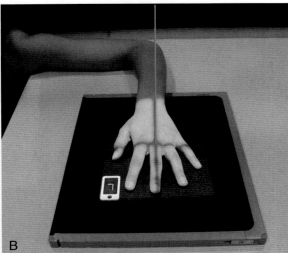

Fig. 5.53 (A) Properly shielded patient in position for PA hand. (B) PA hand.

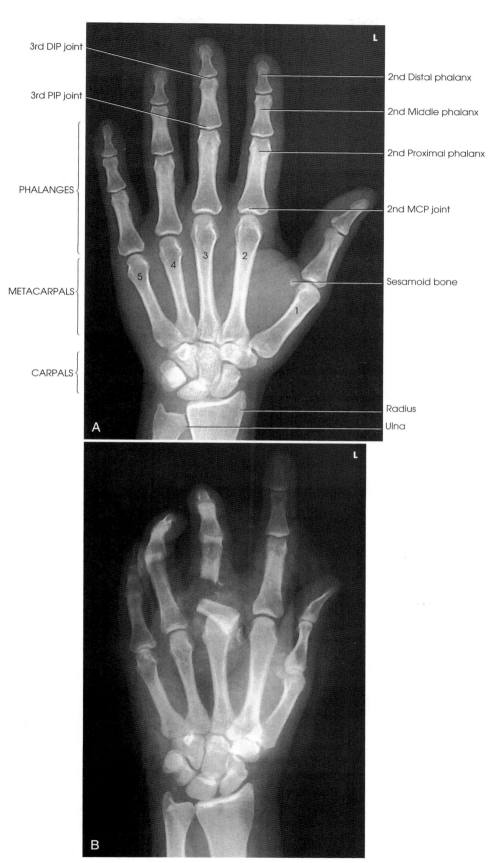

3rd DIP joint

3rd PIP joint

PHALANGES

METACARPALS

CARPALS

2nd Distal phalanx

2nd Middle phalanx

2nd Proximal phalanx

2nd MCP joint

Sesamoid bone

Radius

Ulna

Fig. 5.54 (A) PA hand. (B) PA hand showing closed, displaced, transverse fracture of third proximal phalanx with dislocation of MCP joint. Overall hand was placed in correct position despite trauma. This gives physician accurate information about displacement of bone. *DIP*, Distal interphalangeal; *PIP*, proximal interphalangeal.

🔺 PA OBLIQUE PROJECTION
Lateral rotation

Image receptor: Positioned by manufacturer or department protocol for proper anatomy display orientation; CR plate: 10 × 12 inches (24 × 30 cm) lengthwise.

Position of patient
- Seat the patient at the end of the radiographic table.
- Adjust the patient's height to rest the forearm on the table.

Position of part
- Rest the patient's forearm on the table, with the hand pronated and the palm resting on the IR.
- Adjust the obliquity of the hand so that the MCP joints form an angle of approximately 45 degrees with the IR plane.
- Use a 45-degree foam wedge to support the fingers in the extended position to show the IP joints (Figs. 5.55 and 5.56).

- When examining the metacarpals, obtain a PA oblique projection of the hand by rotating the patient's hand laterally (externally) from the pronated position until the fingertips touch the IR (Fig. 5.57).
- If it is impossible to obtain the correct position with all fingertips resting on the IR, elevate the index finger and thumb on a suitable radiolucent material (see Fig. 5.56). Elevation opens the joint spaces and reduces the degree of foreshortening of the phalanges.
- For either approach, center the IR to the MCP joints and adjust the midline to be parallel with the long axis of the hand and forearm.
- *Shield gonads.*

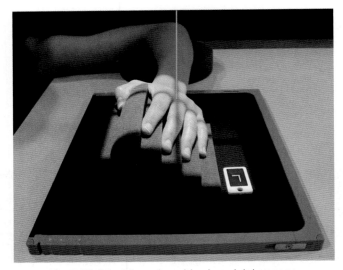

Fig. 5.55 PA oblique hand to show joint spaces.

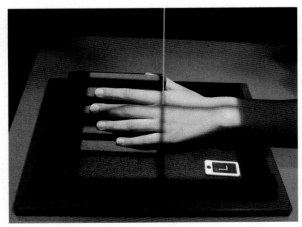

Fig. 5.56 PA oblique hand to show joint spaces.

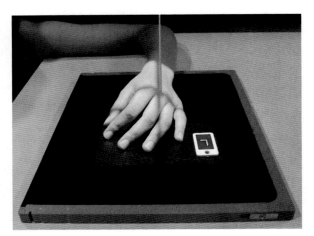

Fig. 5.57 PA oblique hand to show metacarpals.

Central ray

• Perpendicular to the third MCP joint

Collimation

• Adjust radiation field to 1 inch (2.5 cm) on all sides of the hand, including 1 inch (2.5 cm) proximal to the ulnar styloid. Place side marker in the collimated exposure field.

Structures shown

A PA oblique projection of the bones and soft tissues of the hand (Fig. 5.58). This supplemental position is used for investigating fractures and pathologic conditions.

EVALUATION CRITERIA

The following should be clearly seen:
■ Evidence of proper collimation and presence of side marker placed clear of anatomy of interest
■ Anatomy from fingertips to distal radius and ulna

■ Digits separated slightly with no overlap of their soft tissues
■ 45 degrees of rotation of anatomy
  □ Decreasing amounts of separation between metacarpal bodies two through five, with the second and third having the greatest separation.
  □ Partial superimposition of the third, fourth, and fifth metacarpal bases and heads
■ Open MCP joints
■ Open IP joints, when digits are positioned parallel to IR
■ Bony trabecular detail and surrounding soft tissues

NOTE: Lane et al.[11] recommended the inclusion of a reverse oblique projection to better show severe metacarpal deformities or fractures. This projection is accomplished by having the patient rotate the hand 45 degrees medially (internally) from the palm-down position.

Kallen[12] recommended using a tangential oblique projection to show metacarpal head fractures. From the PA hand position, the MCP joints are flexed 75 to 80 degrees with the dorsum of the digits resting on the IR. The hand is rotated 40 to 45 degrees toward the ulnar surface. Then the hand is rotated 40 to 45 degrees forward until the affected MCP joint is projected beyond its proximal phalanx. The perpendicular CR is directed tangentially to enter the MCP joint of interest. Variations of rotation are described to show the second metacarpal head free of superimposition.

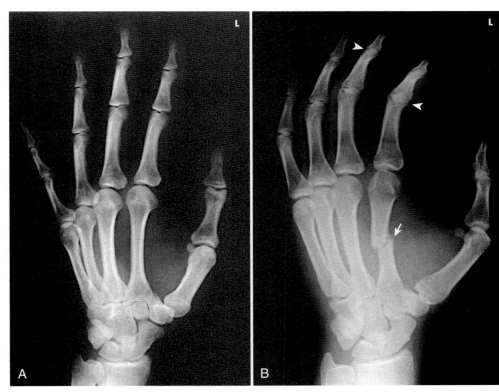

Fig. 5.58 (A) PA oblique hand with digits on sponge to show open joints. (B) PA oblique hand without support sponge, showing fracture *(arrow)*. IP joints *(arrowheads)* are not entirely open, and phalanges are foreshortened.

♠ LATERAL PROJECTION
Mediolateral or lateromedial extension and fan lateral

Image receptor: Positioned by manufacturer or department protocol for proper anatomy display orientation; CR plate: 10 × 12 inches (24 × 30 cm) lengthwise.

Position of patient

- Seat the patient at the end of the radiographic table, with the forearm in contact with the table and the hand in the lateral position with the ulnar aspect down (Fig. 5.59).

- Alternatively, place the radial side of the wrist against the IR (Fig. 5.60). This position is more difficult for the patient to assume.
- If the elbow is elevated, support it with sandbags.

Position of part

- Extend the patient's digits and adjust the first digit at a right angle to the palm.
- Place the palmar surface perpendicular to the IR.

- Center the IR to the MCP joints, and adjust the midline to be parallel with the long axis of the hand and forearm. If the hand is resting on the ulnar surface, immobilization of the thumb may be necessary.
- The two extended digit positions result in superimposition of the phalanges. A modification of the lateral hand is the *fan lateral position,* which eliminates superimposition of all but the proximal phalanges. For the fan lateral position, place the digits on a sponge wedge. Abduct the thumb and place it on the radiolucent sponge for support (Fig. 5.61).
- *Shield gonads.*

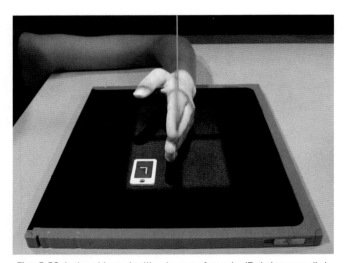

Fig. 5.59 Lateral hand with ulnar surface to IR: lateromedial.

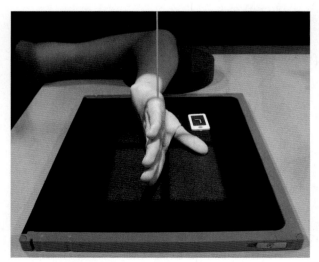

Fig. 5.60 Lateral hand with radial surface to IR: mediolateral.

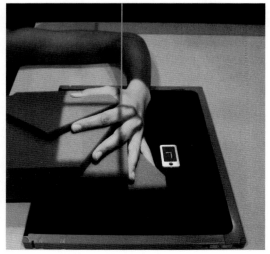

Fig. 5.61 Fan lateral hand.

Central ray

- Perpendicular to the *second digit* MCP joint

Collimation

- Adjust radiation field to 1 inch (2.5 cm) on all sides of the shadow of the hand and thumb, including 1 inch (2.5 cm) proximal to the ulnar styloid. Place side marker in the collimated exposure field.

Structures shown

This image, which shows a lateral projection of the hand in extension (Fig. 5.62), presents the customary position for localizing foreign bodies and metacarpal fracture displacement. The exposure technique depends on the foreign body.

The fan lateral superimposes the metacarpals but shows almost all of the individual phalanges. The most proximal portions of the proximal phalanges remain superimposed (Fig. 5.63).

EVALUATION CRITERIA

The following should be clearly seen:
- Evidence of proper collimation and presence of side marker placed clear of anatomy of interest
- Anatomy from fingertips to distal radius and ulna
- Extended digits
- Hand in a true lateral position
  - □ Superimposed phalanges (individually seen on fan lateral)
  - □ Superimposed metacarpals
  - □ Superimposed distal radius and ulna
- Thumb free of motion and superimposition
- Bony trabecular detail and surrounding soft tissues

NOTE: To show fractures of the fifth metacarpal better, Lewis[4] recommended rotating the hand 5 degrees posteriorly from the true lateral position. This positioning removes the superimposition of the second through fourth metacarpals. The thumb is extended as much as possible, and the hand is allowed to become hollow by relaxation. The central ray is angled so that it passes parallel to the extended thumb and enters the midshaft of the fifth metacarpal.

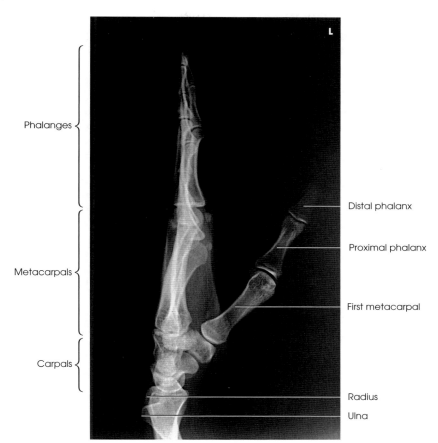

Fig. 5.62 Lateral hand.

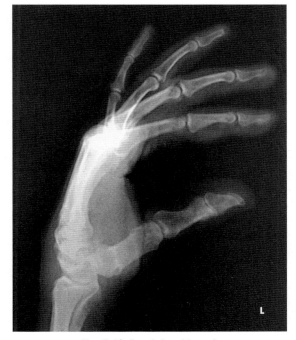

Fig. 5.63 Fan lateral hand.

LATERAL PROJECTION
Lateromedial in flexion

This projection is useful when a hand injury prevents the patient from extending the fingers.

> **Image receptor:** Positioned by manufacturer or department protocol for proper anatomy display orientation; CR plate: 10×12 inches (24×30 cm) lengthwise.

Position of patient

- Seat the patient at the end of the radiographic table.
- Ask the patient to rest the forearm on the table, and place the hand on the IR with the ulnar aspect down.

Position of part

- Center the IR to the MCP joints, and adjust it so that its midline is parallel with the long axis of the hand and forearm.
- With the patient relaxing the digits to maintain the natural arch of the hand, arrange the digits so that they are perfectly superimposed (Fig. 5.64).
- Have the patient hold the thumb parallel with the IR, or, if necessary, immobilize the thumb with tape or a sponge.
- *Shield gonads.*

Central ray

- Perpendicular to the MCP joints, entering MCP joint of the second digit

Structures shown

This projection produces a lateral image of the bony structures and soft tissues of the hand in their normally flexed position (Fig. 5.65). It also shows anterior or posterior displacement in fractures of the metacarpals.

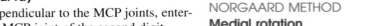

EVALUATION CRITERIA

The following should be clearly seen:

- Evidence of proper collimation and presence of side marker placed clear of anatomy of interest
- Anatomy from fingertips to distal radius and ulna
- Flexed digits
- Superimposed phalanges and metacarpals
- Superimposed distal radius and ulna
- Thumb free of motion and superimposition
- Bony trabecular detail and surrounding soft tissues

AP OBLIQUE PROJECTION
NORGAARD METHOD
Medial rotation

The Norgaard method,[13–15] sometimes referred to as the *ball-catcher's position,* assists in detecting early radiologic changes in the dorsoradial aspects of the second through fifth proximal phalangeal bases that may be associated with rheumatoid arthritis. Norgaard reported that it is often possible to make an early diagnosis of rheumatoid arthritis by using this position before laboratory tests are positive.[15]

In his 1991 article, Stapczynski[15] recommended this projection to show fractures of the base of the fifth metacarpal.

> **Image receptor:** Positioned by manufacturer or department protocol for proper anatomy display orientation; CR plate: 10×12 inches (24×30 cm) crosswise

Position of patient

- Seat the patient at the end of the radiographic table. Norgaard recommended that both hands be radiographed in the half-supinated position for comparison.

Position of part

- Have the patient place the palms of both hands together. Center the MCP joints on the medial aspect of both hands to the IR. Both hands should be in the lateral position.
- Place two 45-degree radiolucent sponges against the posterior aspect of each hand.
- Rotate the patient's hands to a half-supinated position until the dorsal surface of each hand rests against each 45-degree sponge support (Fig. 5.66).
- Extend the patient's fingers, and abduct the thumbs slightly to avoid superimposing them over the second MCP joint.

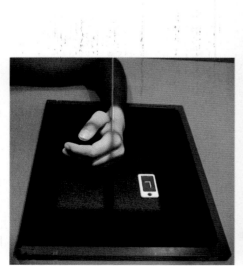

Fig. 5.64 Lateral hand in flexion.

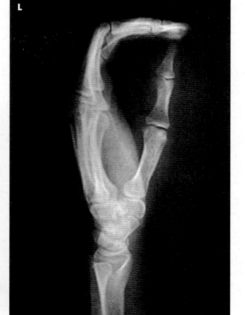

Fig. 5.65 Lateral hand in flexion.

- The original method of positioning the hands is often modified. The patient is positioned similar to the method described, except that the fingers are not extended. Instead the fingers are cupped as though the patient were going to catch a ball (Fig. 5.67). Comparable diagnostic information is provided using either position.
- Shield gonads.

Central ray

- Perpendicular to a point midway between both hands at the level of the MCP joints for either of the two patient positions

Collimation

- Adjust radiation field to 1 inch (2.5 cm) on all sides of the digit, including 1 inch (2.5 cm) proximal to the ulnar styloid. Place side marker in the collimated exposure field.

Structures shown

An AP 45-degree oblique projection of both hands (Fig. 5.68). The early radiologic change significant in making the diagnosis of rheumatoid arthritis is a symmetric, very slight, indistinct outline of the bone corresponding to the insertion of the joint capsule dorsoradial on the proximal end of the first phalanx of the four fingers. In addition, associated demineralization of the bone structure is always present in the area directly below the contour defect.

The following should be clearly seen:
- Evidence of proper collimation and presence of side marker placed clear of anatomy of interest
- Both hands from the carpal area to the tips of the digits
- Metacarpal heads and proximal phalangeal bases free of superimposition
- Bony trabecular detail and surrounding soft tissues

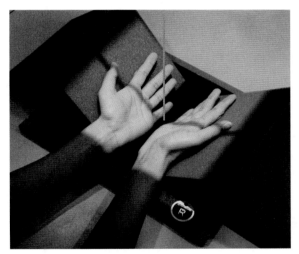

Fig. 5.66 AP oblique hands, semisupinated position.

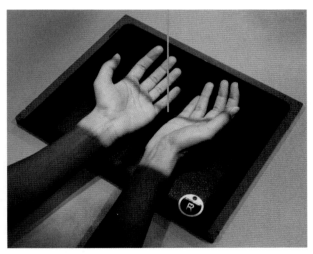

Fig. 5.67 Ball-catcher's position.

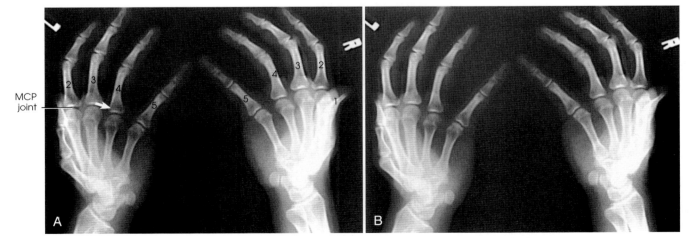

Fig. 5.68 (A) AP oblique hands, ball-catcher's position, showing where indistinct area occurs at dorsoradial aspect of proximal phalangeal base *(arrow)*. (B) Ball-catcher's position. *MCP,* Metacarpophalangeal.

175

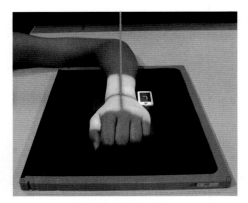

Fig. 5.69 PA wrist.

☀ PA PROJECTION

Image receptor: Positioned by manufacturer or department protocol for proper anatomy display orientation; CR plate: 10×12 inches (24×30 cm) lengthwise.

Position of patient

- Seat the patient low enough to place the axilla in contact with the table, or elevate the extremity to shoulder level on a suitable support. This position places the shoulder, elbow, and wrist joints in the same plane to permit right-angle rotation of the ulna and radius for the lateral position.

Position of part

- Have the patient rest the forearm on the table, and center the wrist joint to the IR area. The wrist (radiocarpal) joint is at a level just distal to the ulnar styloid.
- When it is difficult to determine the exact location of the radiocarpal joint because of a swollen wrist, ask the patient to flex the wrist slightly, and center the IR to the point of flexion. When the wrist is in a cast or splint, the exact point of centering can be determined by comparison with the opposite side.

- Adjust the hand and forearm to lie parallel with the long axis of the IR.
- Slightly arch the hand at the MCP joints by flexing the digits to place the wrist in close contact with the IR (Fig. 5.69).
- When necessary, place a support under the digits to immobilize them.
- *Shield gonads.*

Central ray

- Perpendicular to the midcarpal area

Collimation

- Adjust radiation field to 2.5 inches (6 cm) proximal and distal to the wrist joint and 1 inch (2.5 cm) on the sides. Place side marker in the collimated exposure field.

Structures shown

A PA projection of the carpals, distal radius and ulna, and proximal metacarpals (Fig. 5.70). The projection gives a slightly oblique rotation to the ulna. When the ulna is under examination, an AP projection should be taken.

EVALUATION CRITERIA

The following should be clearly seen:

- Evidence of proper collimation and presence of side marker placed clear of anatomy of interest
- Distal radius and ulna, carpals, and proximal half of metacarpals
- No excessive flexion of digits to overlap and obscure metacarpals
- No rotation in carpals, metacarpals, radius, and ulna
- Open radioulnar joint space
- Bony trabecular detail and surrounding soft tissues

NOTE: To show the scaphoid and capitate better, Daffner et al.[16] recommended angling the central ray when the patient is positioned for a PA radiograph. A central ray angle of 30 degrees toward the elbow elongates the scaphoid and capitate, whereas an angle of 30 degrees toward the fingertips elongates only the capitate.

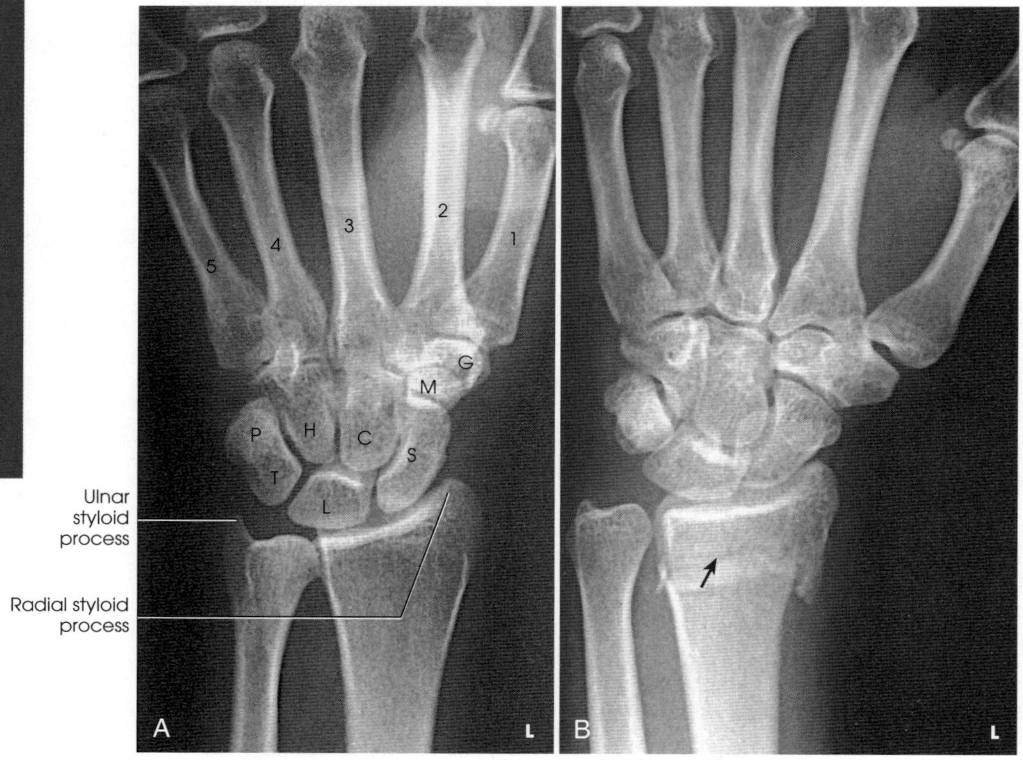

Fig. 5.70 (A) PA wrist. (B) PA wrist showing Smith fracture of distal radius *(arrow)*.
C, Capitate; *G,* trapezium; *H,* hamate; *L,* lunate; *M,* trapezoid; *P,* pisiform; *S,* scaphoid; *T,* triquetrum.

Upper Extremity

Ulnar styloid process

Radial styloid process

AP PROJECTION

Image receptor: Positioned by manufacturer or department protocol for proper anatomy display orientation; CR plate: 10 × 12 inches (24 × 30 cm) lengthwise.

Position of patient

- Seat the patient at the end of the radiographic table.

Position of part

- Have the patient rest the forearm on the table, with the arm and hand supinated.
- Place the IR under the wrist, and center it to the carpals.
- Elevate the digits on a suitable support to place the wrist in close contact with the IR.
- Have the patient lean laterally to prevent rotation of the wrist (Fig. 5.71).
- *Shield gonads.*

Central ray

- Perpendicular to the midcarpal area

Collimation

- Adjust radiation field to 2.5 inches (6 cm) proximal and distal to the wrist joint and 1 inch (2.5 cm) on the sides. Place side marker in the collimated exposure field.

Structures shown

The *carpal interspaces* are better shown in the AP image than in the PA image. Because of the oblique direction of the interspaces, they are more closely parallel with the divergence of the x-ray beam (Fig. 5.72).

The following should be clearly seen:

- Evidence of proper collimation and presence of side marker placed clear of anatomy of interest
- Distal radius and ulna, carpals, and proximal half of the metacarpals
- No excessive flexion of digits to overlap and obscure metacarpals
- No rotation of the carpals, metacarpals, radius, and ulna
- Bony trabecular detail and surrounding soft tissues

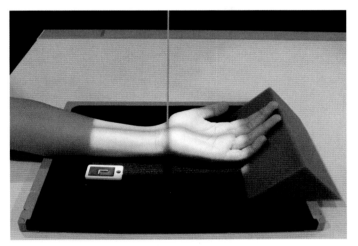

Fig. 5.71 AP wrist.

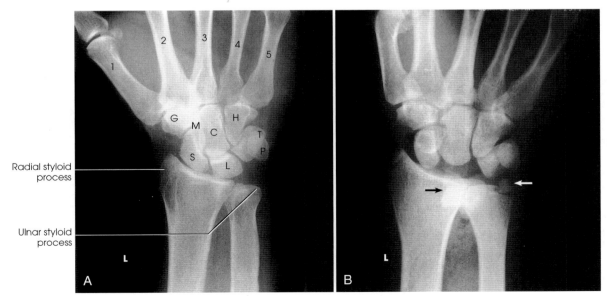

Fig. 5.72 (A) AP wrist. (B) AP wrist showing complete dislocation of lunate *(black arrow)* and fracture of ulnar styloid process *(white arrow)*. *C,* Capitate; *G,* trapezium; *H,* hamate; *L,* lunate; *M,* trapezoid; *P,* pisiform; *S,* scaphoid; *T,* triquetrum.

Upper Extremity

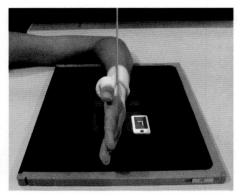

Fig. 5.73 Lateral wrist with ulnar surface to IR.

♠ LATERAL PROJECTION
Lateromedial

Image receptor: Positioned by manufacturer or department protocol for proper anatomy display orientation; CR plate: 10 × 12 inches (24 × 30 cm) lengthwise

Position of patient
- Seat the patient at the end of the radiographic table.
- Have the patient rest the arm and forearm on the table to ensure that the wrist is in a lateral position.

Position of part
- Have the patient flex the elbow 90 degrees to rotate the ulna to the lateral position.
- Center the IR to the wrist (radiocarpal) joint, and adjust the forearm and hand so that the wrist is in a true lateral position (Fig. 5.73).
- *Shield gonads.*

Central ray
- Perpendicular to the wrist joint

Collimation
- Adjust radiation field to 2.5 inches (6 cm) proximal and distal to the wrist joint and 1 inch (2.5 cm) on the palmar and dorsal surfaces. Place side marker in the collimated exposure field.

Structures shown
A lateral projection of the proximal metacarpals, carpals, and distal radius and ulna (Fig. 5.74). An image obtained with the radial surface against the IR (Fig. 5.75) is shown for comparison. This position can also be used to show anterior or posterior displacement in fractures.

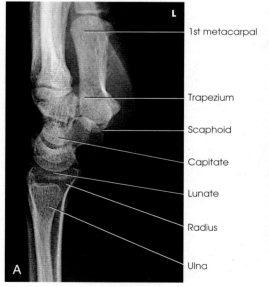
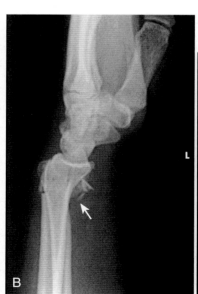
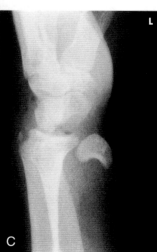

1st metacarpal

Trapezium

Scaphoid

Capitate

Lunate

Radius

Ulna

Fig. 5.74 (A) Lateral wrist with ulnar surface to IR. (B) Lateral with Smith fracture *(arrow)*. This is the same patient as in Fig. 5.70B. (C) Lateral wrist showing obvious complete anterior dislocation of lunate bone. This is the same patient as in Fig. 5.72B.

EVALUATION CRITERIA

The following should be clearly seen:
- Evidence of proper collimation and presence of side marker placed clear of anatomy of interest
- Distal radius and ulna, carpals, and proximal half of metacarpals
- Superimposed distal radius and ulna
- Superimposed metacarpals
- Bony trabecular detail and surrounding soft tissues

NOTE: Burman et al.[17] suggested that the lateral position of the scaphoid should be obtained with the wrist in palmar flexion because this action rotates the bone anteriorly into a dorsovolar position (Fig. 5.76). However, this position is valuable only when sufficient flexion is permitted.

Fiolle[18,19] was the first to describe a small bony growth occurring on the dorsal surface of the third CMC joint. He termed the condition *carpe bossu* (carpal boss) and found that it is shown best in a lateral position with the wrist in palmar flexion (see Fig. 5.76).

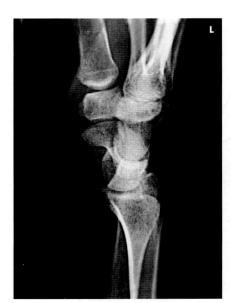

Fig. 5.75 Lateral wrist with radial surface to IR.

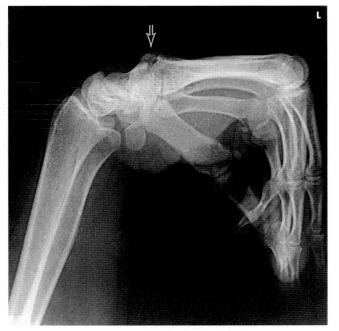

Fig. 5.76 Lateral wrist with palmar flexion of wrist, showing carpal boss *(arrow)*.

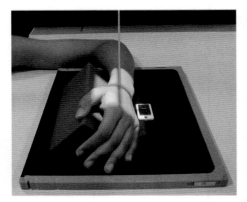

Fig. 5.77 PA oblique wrist: lateral rotation.

▲ PA OBLIQUE PROJECTION
Lateral rotation

Image receptor: Positioned by manufacturer or department protocol for proper anatomy display orientation; CR plate: 10 × 12 inches (24 × 30 cm) lengthwise.

Position of patient

- Seat the patient at the end of the radiographic table, placing the axilla in contact with the table.

Position of part

- Rest the palmar surface of the wrist on the IR.
- Adjust the IR so that its center point is under the scaphoid when the wrist is rotated from the pronated position.
- From the pronated position, rotate the wrist laterally (externally) until the coronal plane forms an angle of approximately 45 degrees with the plane of the IR. For exact positioning and to ensure duplication in follow-up examinations, place a 45-degree foam wedge under the elevated side of the wrist.
- Extend the wrist slightly, and if the digits do not touch the table, support them in place (Fig. 5.77).
- When the scaphoid is under examination, adjust the wrist in ulnar deviation. Place a sandbag across the forearm.
- *Shield gonads.*

Central ray

- Perpendicular to the midcarpal area; it enters just distal to the radius

Collimation

- Adjust radiation field to 2.5 inches (6 cm) proximal and distal to the wrist joint and 1 inch (2.5 cm) on the sides. Place side marker in the collimated exposure field.

Structures shown

The carpals on the lateral side of the wrist, particularly the trapezium and the scaphoid. The scaphoid is superimposed on itself in the direct PA projection (Figs. 5.78 and 5.79).

EVALUATION CRITERIA

The following should be clearly seen:
- Evidence of proper collimation and presence of side marker placed clear of anatomy of interest
- Distal radius and ulna, carpals, and proximal half of metacarpals
- 45-degree rotation of anatomy
  - □ Slight interosseous space between the third, fourth, and fifth metacarpal bodies
  - □ Slight overlap of the distal radius and ulna
- Carpals on lateral side of wrist
- Trapezium and distal half of the scaphoid without superimposition
- Open trapeziotrapezoid and scaphotrapezial joint space
- Bony trabecular detail and surrounding soft tissues

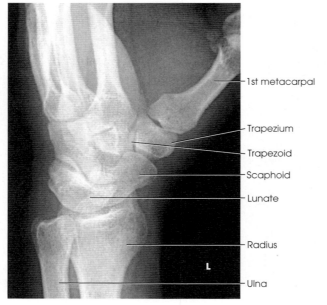

1st metacarpal

Trapezium

Trapezoid

Scaphoid

Lunate

Radius

Ulna

Fig. 5.78 PA oblique wrist.

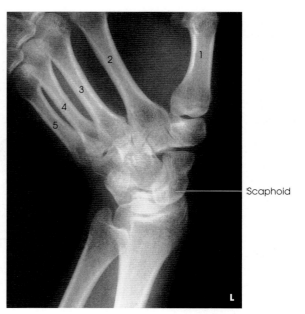

Scaphoid

Fig. 5.79 PA oblique wrist with ulnar deviction.

AP OBLIQUE PROJECTION[20]
Medial rotation

Image receptor: Positioned by manufacturer or department protocol for proper anatomy display orientation; CR plate: 10 × 12 inches (24 × 30 cm) lengthwise.

Position of patient
- Seat the patient at the end of the radiographic table.
- Have the patient rest the forearm on the table in the supine position.

Position of part
- Place the IR under the wrist, and center it at the dorsal surface of the wrist.
- Rotate the wrist medially (internally) until the coronal plane forms an angle of approximately 45 degrees to the plane of the IR (Fig. 5.80).
- *Shield gonads.*

Central ray
- Perpendicular to the midcarpal area; it enters the anterior surface of the wrist midway between its medial and lateral borders

Collimation
- Adjust radiation field to 2.5 inches (6 cm) proximal and distal to the wrist joint and 1 inch (2.5 cm) on the sides. Place side marker in the collimated exposure field.

Structures shown
This position separates the pisiform from adjacent carpal bones. It also provides a more distinct radiograph of the triquetrum and hamate (compare Figs. 5.81 and 5.82).

EVALUATION CRITERIA
The following should be clearly seen:
- Evidence of proper collimation and presence of side marker placed clear of anatomy of interest
- Distal radius and ulna, carpals, and proximal half of metacarpals
- Carpals on medial side of wrist
- Triquetrum, hook of hamate, and pisiform free of superimposition and in profile
- Bony trabecular detail and surrounding soft tissues

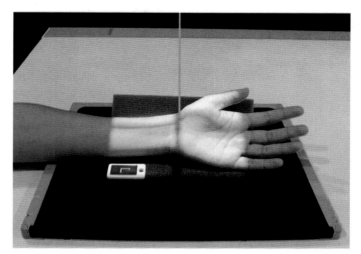

Fig. 5.80 AP oblique wrist: medial rotation.

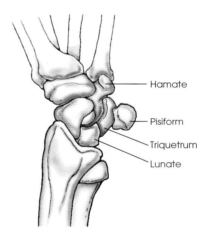

Fig. 5.81 AP oblique wrist.

Hamate
Pisiform
Triquetrum
Lunate

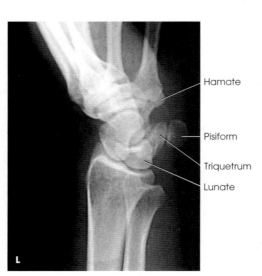
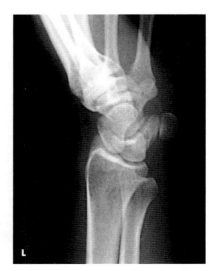

Hamate
Pisiform
Triquetrum
Lunate

Fig. 5.82 AP oblique wrist.

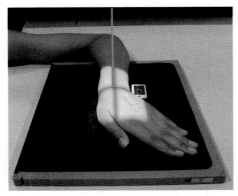

Fig. 5.83 PA wrist in ulnar deviation.

⚹ PA PROJECTION
Ulnar deviation[21]

Image receptor: Positioned by manufacturer or department protocol for proper anatomy display orientation; CR plate: 10×12 inches (24×30 cm) lengthwise.

Position of patient
- Seat the patient at the end of the radiographic table, with the arm and forearm resting on the table. The elbow should be at a 90-degree angle.

Position of part
- Position the wrist on the IR for a PA projection.
- Without moving the forearm, turn the hand outward until the wrist is in extreme ulnar deviation (Fig. 5.83).
- *Shield gonads.*

Central ray
- Perpendicular to the scaphoid
- CR angulation of 10 to 15 degrees proximally or distally sometimes required for clear delineation

Collimation
- Adjust radiation field to 2.5 inches (6 cm) proximal and distal to the wrist joint and 1 inch (2.5 cm) on the sides. Place side marker in the collimated exposure field.

Structures shown
This position reduces foreshortening of the scaphoid, which occurs with a perpendicular CR. It also opens the spaces between adjacent carpals (Fig. 5.84).

EVALUATION CRITERIA
The following should be clearly seen:
- Evidence of proper collimation and presence of side marker placed clear of anatomy of interest
- Distal radius and ulna, carpals, and proximal half of metacarpals
- Scaphoid with adjacent articulations open
- No rotation of wrist
- Maximum ulnar deviation, as revealed by the angle formed between the longitudinal axis of the ulna and the longitudinal axis of the fifth metacarpal
- Bony trabecular detail and surrounding soft tissues

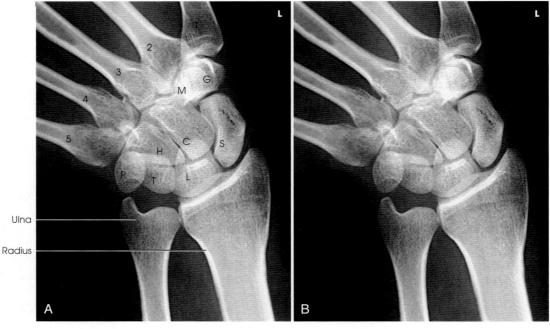

Fig. 5.84 (A) PA wrist in ulnar deviation. (B) Wrist in ulnar deviation. *C,* Capitate; *G,* trapezium; *H,* hamate; *L,* lunate; *M,* trapezoid; *P,* pisiform; *S,* scaphoid; *T,* triquetrum.

PA PROJECTION

Radial deviation[21]

> **Image receptor:** Positioned by manufacturer or department protocol for proper anatomy display orientation; CR plate: 10×12 inches (24×30 cm) lengthwise.

Position of patient

- Seat the patient at the end of the radiographic table, with the arm and forearm resting on the table.

Position of part

- Position the wrist on the IR for a PA projection.
- Without moving the forearm, turn the hand medially until the wrist is in extreme radial deviation (Fig. 5.85).
- *Shield gonads.*

Central ray

- Perpendicular to midcarpal area

Collimation

- Adjust radiation field to 2.5 inches (6 cm) proximal and distal to the wrist joint and 1 inch (2.5 cm) on the sides. Place side marker in the collimated exposure field.

Structures shown

Radial deviation opens the interspaces between the carpals on the medial side of the wrist (Fig. 5.86).

EVALUATION CRITERIA

The following should be clearly seen:
- Evidence of proper collimation and presence of side marker placed clear of anatomy of interest
- Distal radius and ulna, carpals, and proximal half of metacarpals
- Carpals and their articulations on the medial side of the wrist
- No rotation of wrist
- Maximum radial deviation, as revealed by the angle formed between the longitudinal axis of the radius and the longitudinal axis of the first metacarpal
- Bony trabecular detail and surrounding soft tissues

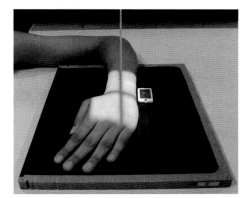

Fig. 5.85 PA wrist in radial deviation.

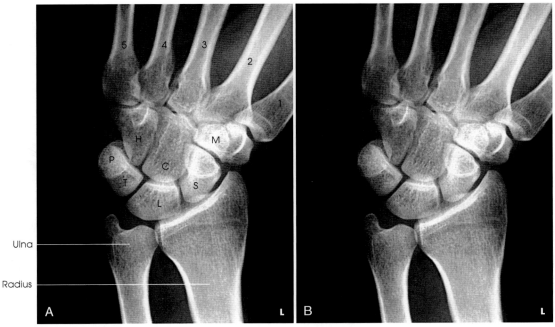

Fig. 5.86 (A) PA wrist in radial deviation. (B) Wrist in radial deviation. *C,* Capitate; *G,* trapezium; *H,* hamate; *L,* lunate; *M,* trapezoid; *P,* pisiform; *S,* scaphoid; *T,* triquetrum.

Scaphoid
⚹ PA AXIAL PROJECTION
STECHER METHOD[22]

Image receptor: Positioned by manufacturer or department protocol for proper anatomy display orientation; CR plate: 10 × 12 inches (24 × 30 cm) lengthwise.

Position of patient
- Seat the patient at the end of the radiographic table, with the arm and axilla in contact with the table.
- Rest the forearm on the table.

Position of part
- Place one end of the IR on a support, and adjust the IR so that the finger end of the IR is elevated 20 degrees (Fig. 5.87).
- Adjust the wrist on the IR for a PA projection, and center the wrist to the IR.
- Bridgman[23] suggested positioning the wrist in ulnar deviation for this radiograph.
- *Shield gonads.*

Central ray
- Perpendicular to the table and directed to enter the scaphoid

Collimation
- Adjust radiation field to 2.5 inches (6 cm) proximal and distal to the wrist joint and 1 inch (2.5 cm) on the sides. Place side marker in the collimated exposure field.

Structures shown
The 20-degree angulation of the wrist places the scaphoid at right angles to the CR, so that it is projected with minimal superimposition (Figs. 5.88 and 5.89).

EVALUATION CRITERIA
The following should be clearly seen:
- Evidence of proper collimation and presence of side marker placed clear of anatomy of interest
- Distal radius and ulna, carpals, and proximal half of the metacarpals
- Scaphoid with adjacent articulations open
- No rotation of wrist
- Bony trabecular detail and surrounding soft tissues

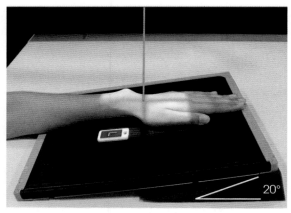

Fig. 5.87 PA axial wrist for scaphoid: Stecher method with IR angled 20 degrees.

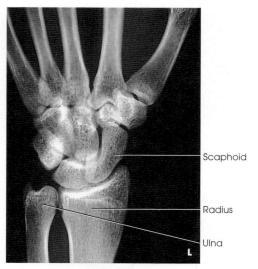

Fig. 5.88 PA axial wrist for scaphoid: Stecher method.

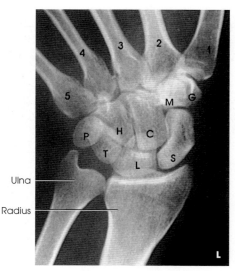

Fig. 5.89 PA axial wrist for scaphoid: Bridgman method, ulnar deviation. *C,* Capitate; *G,* trapezium; *H,* hamate; *L,* lunate; *M,* trapezoid; *P,* pisiform; *S,* scaphoid; *T,* triquetrum.

Variations

Stecher[22] recommended the previous method as preferable; however, a similar position can be obtained by placing the IR and wrist horizontally and directing the CR 20 degrees toward the elbow (Fig. 5.90).

To show a fracture line that angles superoinferiorly, these positions may be reversed. In other words, the wrist may be angled inferiorly, or from the horizontal position the CR may be angled toward the digits.

A third method recommended by Stecher is to have the patient clench the fist. This elevates the distal end of the scaphoid so that it lies parallel with the IR; it also widens the fracture line. The wrist is positioned as for the PA projection, and no CR angulation is used.

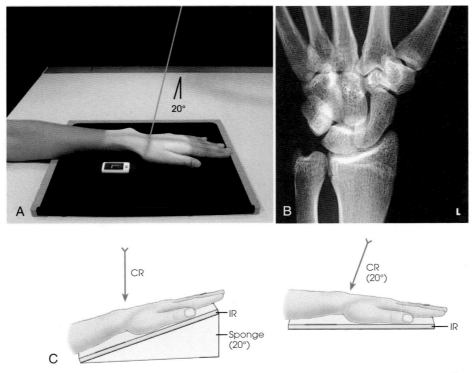

Fig. 5.90 (A) PA axial wrist for scaphoid: Stecher method with 20-degree angulation of CR. (B) PA axial wrist: Stecher method. (C) Angled IR and angled CR methods achieve same projection.

Scaphoid Series
PA AND PA AXIAL PROJECTIONS
RAFERT-LONG METHOD
Ulnar deviation

Scaphoid fractures account for 60% of all carpal bone injuries. In 1991, Rafert and Long[24] described this method of diagnosing scaphoid fractures using a four-image, multiple-angle CR series. The series is performed after routine wrist radiographs do not identify a fracture but symptoms are suspicious for scaphoid fracture.

Image receptor: Positioned by manufacturer or department protocol for proper anatomy display orientation; CR plate: 10 × 12 inches (24 ×× 30 cm) lengthwise

Position of patient
- Seat the patient at the end of the radiographic table, with the arm and forearm resting on the table.

Position of part
- Position the wrist on the IR for a PA projection.
- Without moving the forearm, turn the hand outward until the wrist is in extreme ulnar deviation (Fig. 5.91).
- *Shield gonads.*

Central ray
- Perpendicular and with multiple cephalad angles; with the hand and wrist in the same position for each projection, four separate exposures made at 0, 10, 20, and 30 degrees cephalad
- The CR should directly enter the scaphoid bone.

Collimation
- Adjust radiation field to 2.5 inches (6 cm) proximal and distal to the wrist joint and 1 inch (2.5 cm) on the sides. Place side marker in the collimated exposure field.

Structures shown
The scaphoid is shown with minimal superimposition (Fig. 5.92).

The following should be clearly seen:
- Evidence of proper collimation and presence of side marker placed clear of anatomy of interest
- No rotation of the wrist
- Scaphoid with adjacent articular areas open
- Maximum ulnar deviation
- Bony trabecular detail and surrounding soft tissues

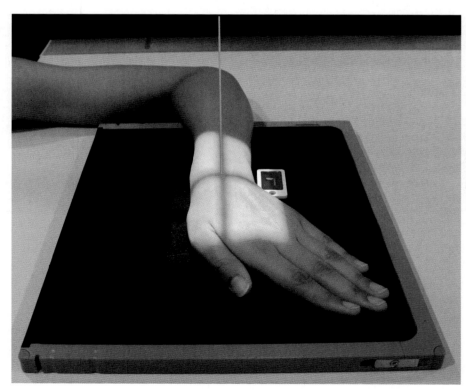

Fig. 5.91 PA wrist in ulnar deviation.

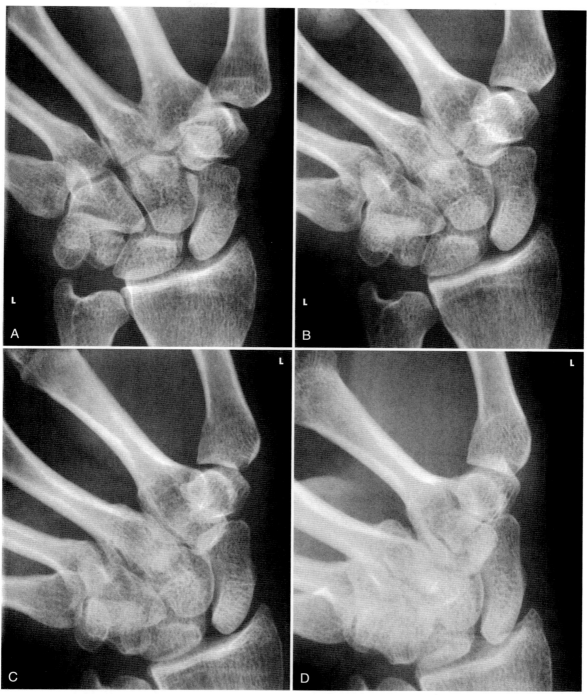

Fig. 5.92 PA and PA axial wrist in ulnar deviation for Rafert-Long method scaphoid series. Radiographs are all from the same patient. (A) PA wrist with 0-degree central ray angle. (B) PA axial wrist with 10-degree cephalad angle. (C) PA axial wrist with 20-degree cephalad angle. (D) PA axial wrist with 30-degree cephalad angle.

(From Rafert JA, Long BW: Technique for diagnosis of scaphoid fractures. *Radiol Technol* 63:16, 1991.)

Trapezium

PA AXIAL OBLIQUE PROJECTION

CLEMENTS-NAKAYAMA METHOD

Fractures of the trapezium are rare; however, if undiagnosed, these fractures can lead to functional difficulties. In certain cases the articular surfaces of the trapezium should be evaluated to treat patients with osteoarthritis.[25]

Image receptor: Positioned by manufacturer or department protocol for proper anatomy display orientation; CR plate: 10×12 inches (24×30 cm) lengthwise.

Position of patient

- With the patient seated at the end of the radiographic table, place the hand on the IR in the lateral position.

Position of part

- Place the wrist in the lateral position, resting on the ulnar surface over the center of the IR.
- Place a 45-degree sponge wedge against the anterior surface, and rotate the hand to come in contact with the sponge.
- If the patient is able to achieve ulnar deviation, adjust the IR so that the long axis of the IR and the forearm align with the CR (Fig. 5.93).
- If the patient is unable to achieve ulnar deviation comfortably, align the straight wrist to the IR, and rotate the elbow end of the IR and arm 20 degrees away from the CR (Fig. 5.94).
- *Shield gonads.*

Central ray

- Angled 45 degrees distally to enter the anatomic snuff-box of the wrist and pass through the trapezium

Collimation

Adjust radiation field to 2.5 inches (6 cm) proximal and distal to the wrist joint and 1 inch (2.5 cm) on the sides. Place side marker in the collimated exposure field.

Structures shown

The trapezium and its articulations with adjacent carpal bones (Fig. 5.95). The articulation of the trapezium and scaphoid is not shown on this image.

EVALUATION CRITERIA

The following should be clearly seen:

- Evidence of proper collimation and presence of side marker placed clear of anatomy of interest
- Trapezium projected free of the other carpal bones with the exception of the articulation with the scaphoid
- Bony trabecular detail and surrounding soft tissues

NOTE: Holly[26] recommended a variation of this method with the hand in ulnar deviation on a 37-degree sponge wedge. The central ray is directed vertically, entering just proximal to the first metacarpal base.

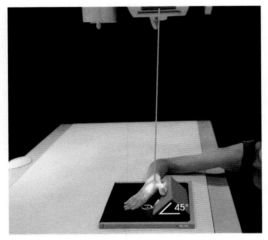

Fig. 5.93 PA axial oblique wrist for trapezium: Clements-Nakayama method; alignment with ulnar deviation.

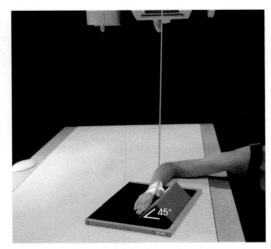

Fig. 5.94 PA axial oblique wrist for trapezium: Clements-Nakayama method; alignment without ulnar deviation.

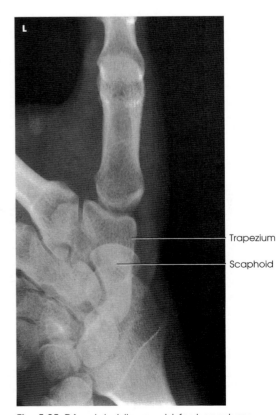

Trapezium

Scaphoid

Fig. 5.95 PA axial oblique wrist for trapezium: Clements-Nakayama method.

Carpal Bridge
TANGENTIAL PROJECTION

Image receptor: Positioned by manufacturer or department protocol for proper anatomy display orientation; CR plate: 10 × 12 inches (24 × 30 cm) lengthwise.

Position of patient
- Seat or stand the patient at the side of the radiographic table to permit the required manipulation of the arm or x-ray tube.

Position of part
- The originators[27] of this projection recommended that the hand lie palm upward on the IR with the hand at right angle to the forearm (Fig. 5.96).

- When the wrist is too painful to be adjusted in the position just described, a similar image can be obtained by elevating the forearm on sandbags or other suitable support. Then with the wrist flexed in right-angle position, place the IR in the vertical position (Fig. 5.97).
- Shield gonads.

Central ray
- Directed to a point approximately $1\frac{1}{2}$ inches (3.8 cm) proximal to the wrist joint at a caudal angle of 45 degrees

Collimation
Adjust radiation field to 2.5 inches (6 cm) proximal and distal to the wrist joint and 1 inch (2.5 cm) on the sides. Place side marker in the collimated exposure field.

Structures shown
The carpal bridge is shown on the image in Figs. 5.98 and 5.99. The originators recommended this procedure to show fractures of the scaphoid, lunate dislocations, calcifications and foreign bodies in the dorsum of the wrist, and chip fractures of the dorsal aspect of the carpal bones.

EVALUATION CRITERIA
The following should be clearly seen:
- Evidence of proper collimation and presence of side marker placed clear of anatomy of interest
- Dorsal surface of the carpals free of superimposition by the metacarpal bases
- Bony trabecular detail and surrounding soft tissues

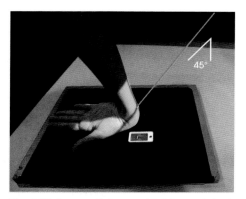

Fig. 5.96 Tangential carpal bridge, original method.

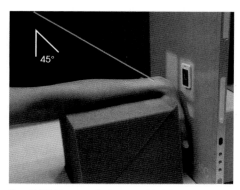

Fig. 5.97 Tangential carpal bridge, modified method.

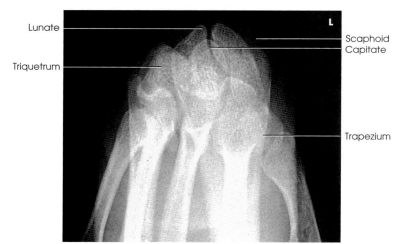

Fig. 5.98 Tangential carpal bridge, original method.

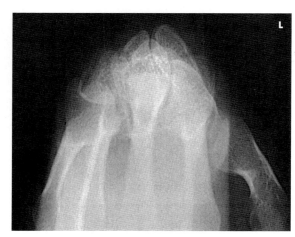

Fig. 5.99 Tangential carpal bridge, modified method.

♠ TANGENTIAL PROJECTION
GAYNOR-HART METHOD[28]

The carpal canal contains the tendons of the flexors of the fingers and the median nerve. Compression of the median nerve results in pain and/or numbness. Radiography is performed to identify abnormality of the bones or soft tissue of the canal.

Fractures of the hook of hamate, pisiform, and trapezium are increasingly seen in athletes. The tangential projection is helpful in identifying fractures of these carpal bones. This projection was added as an essential projection based on the 1997 survey performed by Bontrager.[29]

Image receptor: Positioned by manufacturer or department protocol for proper anatomy display orientation; CR plate: 10 × 12 inches (24 × 30 cm) lengthwise.

Inferosuperior
Position of patient
- Seat the patient at the end of the radiographic table so that the forearm can be adjusted to lie parallel with the long axis of the table.

Position of part
- Hyperextend the wrist, and center the IR to the joint at the level of the radial styloid process.
- For support, place a radiolucent pad approximately 3/4-inch (1.9 cm) thick under the lower forearm.
- Adjust the position of the hand to make its long axis as vertical as possible.
- To prevent superimposition of the shadows of the hamate and pisiform bones, rotate the hand slightly toward the radial side.
- Have the patient grasp the digits with the opposite hand, or use a suitable device to hold the wrist in the extended position (Fig. 5.100).
- *Shield gonads.*

Central ray
- Directed to the palm of the hand at a point approximately 1 inch (2.5 cm) distal to the base of the third metacarpal and at an angle of 25 to 30 degrees to the long axis of the hand
- When the wrist cannot be extended to within 15 degrees of vertical, McQuillen Martensen[30] suggested that the CR first be aligned parallel to the palmar surface, then angled an additional 15 degrees toward the palm.

Collimation
- Adjust radiation field to 1 inch (2.5 cm) on the three sides of the shadow of the wrist. Place side marker in the collimated exposure field.

Structures shown
This image of the carpal canal (carpal tunnel) shows the palmar aspect of the trapezium; the tubercle of the trapezium; and the scaphoid, capitate, hook of hamate, triquetrum, and entire pisiform (Fig. 5.101).

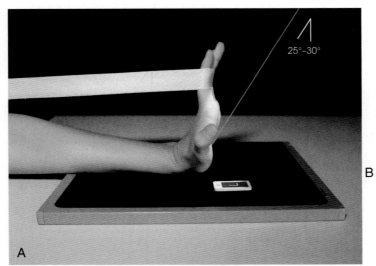

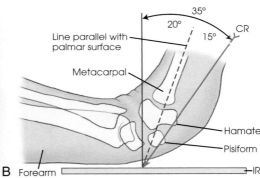

Fig. 5.100 (A) Tangential (inferosuperior) carpal canal: Gaynor-Hart method. (B) Suggested CR alignment when wrist cannot be extended within 15 degrees of vertical. CR is angled 15 degrees more than angle of metacarpals.

(B, Modified from McQuillen Martensen K: *Radiographic image analysis,* ed 3, St Louis, 2010, Saunders.)

Superoinferior

Position of patient

- When the patient cannot assume or maintain the previously described wrist position, a similar image may be obtained.
- Have the patient dorsiflex the wrist as much as is tolerable and lean forward to place the carpal canal tangent to the IR (Fig. 5.102). The canal is easily palpable on the palmar aspect of the wrist as the concavity between the trapezium laterally and hook of hamate and pisiform medially.

Position of part

- When dorsiflexion of the wrist is limited, Marshall[31] suggested placing a 45-degree angle sponge under the palmar surface of the hand. The sponge slightly elevates the wrist to place the carpal canal tangent to the CR. A slight degree of magnification exists because of the increased object-to-IR distance (OID) (Fig. 5.103).

Central ray

- Tangential to the carpal canal at the level of the midpoint of the wrist

Collimation

- Adjust radiation field to include palmar aspect of wrist, proximal one-third of metacarpals, and 1 inch (2.5 cm) on the sides. Place side marker in the collimated exposure field.

EVALUATION CRITERIA

With either approach, the following should be clearly seen:

- Evidence of proper collimation and presence of side marker placed clear of anatomy of interest
- Carpals in an arch arrangement
- Pisiform in profile and free of superimposition
- Hamulus of hamate
- Bony trabecular detail and surrounding soft tissues

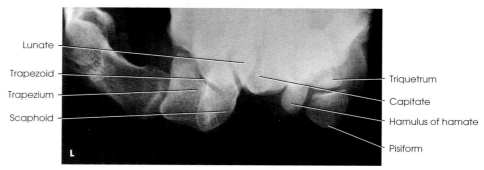

Fig. 5.101 Tangential (inferosuperior) carpal canal: Gaynor-Hart method.

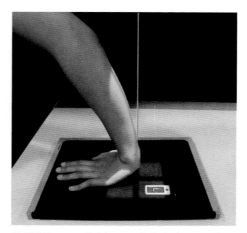

Fig. 5.102 Tangential (superoinferior) carpal canal.

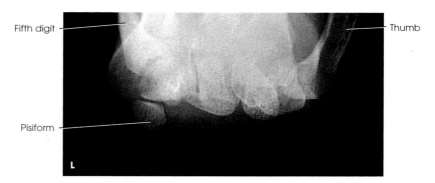

Fig. 5.103 Tangential (superoinferior) carpal canal.

▲ AP PROJECTION

Image receptor: Positioned by manufacturer or department protocol for proper anatomy display orientation; CR plate: 14 × 17 inches (35 × 43 cm) lengthwise.

Position of patient

- Seat the patient close to the radiographic table and low enough to place the entire extremity in the same plane.

Position of part

- Supinate the hand, extend the elbow, and place the dorsal surface of the forearm against the IR. Ensure that the joint of interest is included.
- Adjust the IR so that the long axis is parallel with the forearm.
- Have the patient lean laterally until the forearm is in a true supinated position (Fig. 5.104).
- Because the proximal forearm is commonly rotated in this position, palpate and adjust the humeral epicondyles to be equidistant from the IR.
- Ensure that the hand is supinated (Fig. 5.105). Pronation of the hand crosses the radius over the ulna at its proximal third and rotates the humerus medially, resulting in an oblique projection of the forearm (Fig. 5.106).
- *Shield gonads.*

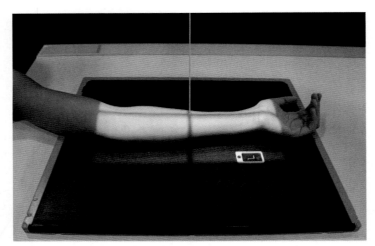

Fig. 5.104 AP forearm.

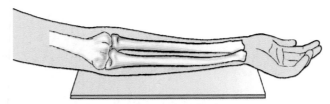

Fig. 5.105 AP forearm with hand supinated.

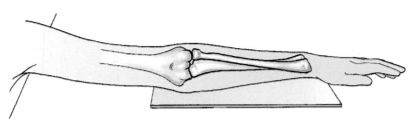

Fig. 5.106 AP forearm with hand pronated—incorrect.

Central ray

- Perpendicular to the midpoint of the forearm

Collimation

- Adjust radiation field to 2 inches (5 cm) distal to the wrist joint and proximal to the elbow joint and 1 inch (2.5 cm) on the sides. Place side marker in the collimated exposure field.

Structures shown

The elbow joint, the radius and ulna, and the proximal row of slightly distorted carpal bones (Fig. 5.107).

EVALUATION CRITERIA

The following should be clearly seen:

- Evidence of proper collimation and presence of side marker placed clear of anatomy of interest
- Entire forearm, including wrist and distal humerus
- Slight superimposition of the radial head, neck, and tuberosity over the proximal ulna
- No elongation or foreshortening of the humeral epicondyles
- Partially open elbow joint if the shoulder was placed in the same plane as the forearm
- Open radioulnar space
- Bony trabecular detail and surrounding soft tissues

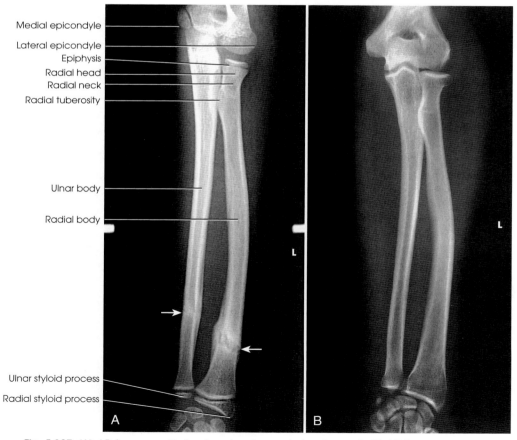

Medial epicondyle
Lateral epicondyle
Epiphysis
Radial head
Radial neck
Radial tuberosity

Ulnar body

Radial body

Ulnar styloid process
Radial styloid process

Fig. 5.107 (A) AP forearm with fractured radius and ulna (*arrows*). (B) AP forearm showing both joints.

☀ LATERAL PROJECTION
Lateromedial

Image receptor: Positioned by manufacturer or department protocol for proper anatomy display orientation; CR plate: 14 × 17 inches (35 × 43 cm) lengthwise.

Position of patient

- Seat the patient close to the radiographic table and low enough that the humerus, shoulder joint, and elbow lie in the same plane.

Position of part

- Flex the elbow 90 degrees, and place the medial aspect of the forearm against the IR. Ensure that the entire joint of interest is included.
- Adjust the IR so that the long axis is parallel with the forearm.
- Adjust the extremity in a true lateral position. The thumb side of the hand must be up (Fig. 5.108).
- *Shield gonads.*

Central ray

- Perpendicular to the midpoint of the forearm

Collimation

- Adjust radiation field to 2 inches (5 cm) distal to the wrist joint and proximal to the elbow joint, and 1 inch (2.5 cm) on the sides. Place side marker in the collimated exposure field.

Structures shown

The elbow joint, the radius and ulna, and the proximal row of superimposed carpal bones (Fig. 5.109).

EVALUATION CRITERIA

The following should be clearly seen:

- ■ Evidence of proper collimation and presence of side marker placed clear of anatomy of interest
- ■ Entire forearm, including wrist and distal humerus in a true lateral position:
  - □ Superimposition of the radius and ulna at their distal end
  - □ Superimposition of the radial head over the coronoid process
  - □ Radial tuberosity facing anteriorly
  - □ Superimposed humeral epicondyles
- ■ Elbow flexed 90 degrees
- ■ Bony trabecular detail and surrounding soft tissues

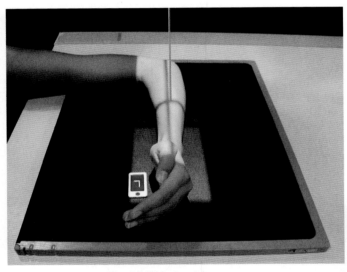

Fig. 5.108 Lateral forearm.

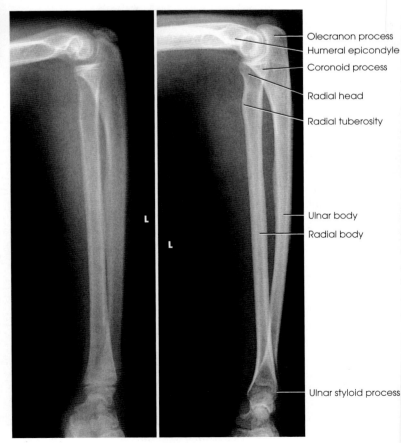

Olecranon process
Humeral epicondyle
Coronoid process
Radial head
Radial tuberosity
Ulnar body
Radial body
Ulnar styloid process

Fig. 5.109 Lateral forearm.

⚕ AP PROJECTION

Image receptor: Positioned by manufacturer or department protocol for proper anatomy display orientation; CR plate: 10 × 12 inches (24 × 30 cm) lengthwise.

Position of patient

- Seat the patient near the radiographic table and low enough to place the shoulder joint, humerus, and elbow joint in the same plane.

Position of part

- Extend the elbow, supinate the hand, and center the IR to the elbow joint.
- Adjust the IR to make it parallel with the long axis of the part (Fig. 5.110).
- Have the patient lean laterally until the humeral epicondyles and anterior surface of the elbow are parallel with the plane of the IR.
- Supinate the hand to prevent rotation of the bones of the forearm.
- *Shield gonads.*

Central ray

- Perpendicular to the elbow joint

Collimation

- Adjust radiation field to 3 inches (8 cm) proximal and distal to the elbow joint and 1 inch (2.5 cm) on the sides. Place side marker in the collimated exposure field.

Structures shown

An AP projection of the elbow joint, distal arm, and proximal forearm (Fig. 5.111).

EVALUATION CRITERIA

The following should be clearly seen:

- Evidence of proper collimation and presence of side marker placed clear of anatomy of interest
- Radial head, neck, and tuberosity slightly superimposed over the proximal ulna
- Elbow joint centered to the exposure field
- Open humeroradial joint
- No rotation of humeral epicondyles (coronoid and olecranon fossae approximately equidistant to epicondyles)
- Bony trabecular detail and surrounding soft tissues

Elbow

Fig. 5.110 AP elbow.

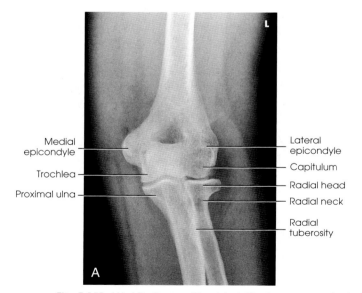
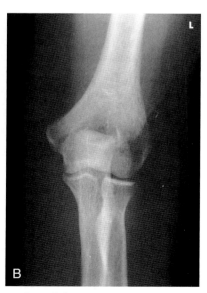

Medial epicondyle
Trochlea
Proximal ulna

Lateral epicondyle
Capitulum
Radial head
Radial neck
Radial tuberosity

Fig. 5.111 (A) AP elbow with wide latitude exposure technique for soft tissue detail. (B) AP elbow with normal exposure technique.

♠ LATERAL PROJECTION
Lateromedial

Griswold[2] gave two reasons for the importance of flexing the elbow 90 degrees: (1) The olecranon process can be seen in profile, and (2) the elbow fat pads are the least compressed. In partial or complete extension, the olecranon process elevates the posterior elbow fat pad and simulates joint pathology.

Image receptor: Positioned by manufacturer or department protocol for proper anatomy display orientation; CR plate: 10 × 12 inches (24 × 30 cm) lengthwise.

Position of patient
- Seat the patient at the end of the radiographic table, low enough to place the humerus and the elbow joint in the same plane.

Position of part
- From the supine position, flex the elbow 90 degrees, and place the humerus and forearm in contact with the table.
- Center the IR to the elbow joint. Adjust the elbow joint so that its long axis is parallel with the long axis of the forearm (Figs. 5.112 and 5.113). On patients with muscular forearms, elevate the wrist to place the forearm parallel with the IR.

- Adjust the IR diagonally to include more of the arm and forearm (Fig. 5.114).
- To obtain a lateral projection of the elbow, adjust the hand in the lateral position and ensure that the humeral epicondyles are perpendicular to the plane of the IR.
- *Shield gonads.*

Central ray
- Perpendicular to the elbow joint, regardless of its location on the IR

Collimation
- Adjust radiation field to 3 inches (8 cm) proximal and distal to the elbow joint. Place side marker in the collimated exposure field.

Structures shown
The lateral projection shows the elbow joint, distal arm, and proximal forearm (see Figs. 5.113 and 5.114).

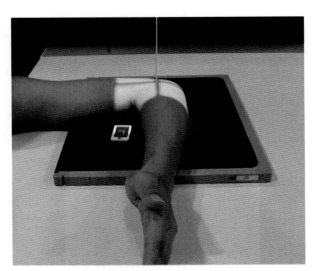

Fig. 5.112 Lateral elbow.

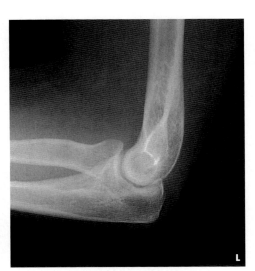

Fig. 5.113 Lateral elbow.

EVALUATION CRITERIA

The following should be clearly seen:

- Evidence of proper collimation and presence of side marker placed clear of anatomy of interest
- Elbow joint centered to the exposure field
- Elbow in a true lateral position:
  - ☐ Superimposed humeral epicondyles
  - ☐ Radial tuberosity facing anteriorly
  - ☐ Radial head partially superimposing the coronoid process
  - ☐ Olecranon process in profile
- Elbow flexed 90 degrees
- Bony trabecular detail and any elevated fat pads in the soft tissue at the anterior and posterior distal humerus and the anterior proximal forearm

NOTE: When injury to the soft tissue around the elbow is suspected, the joint should be flexed only 30 or 35 degrees (Fig. 5.115). This partial flexion does not compress or stretch the soft structures as does the full 90-degree lateral flexion. The posterior fat pad may become visible in this position.

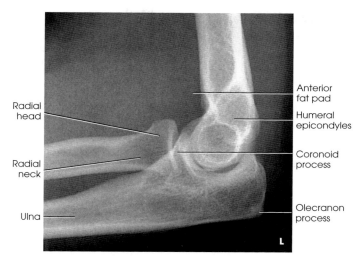

Fig. 5.114 Lateral elbow.

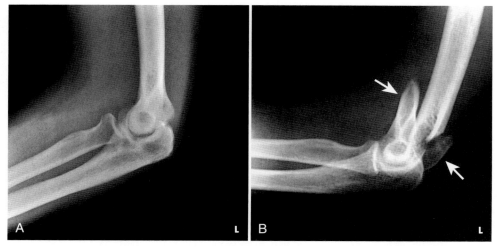

Fig. 5.115 (A) Lateral elbow in partial flexion position for soft tissue image. (B) Lateral elbow of patient who fell from a tree, resulting in impaction fracture *(arrows)* of distal humerus.

▲ AP OBLIQUE PROJECTION
Medial rotation

Image receptor: Positioned by manufacturer or department protocol for proper anatomy display orientation; CR plate: 10 × 12 inches (24 × 30 cm) lengthwise.

Position of patient
- Seat the patient at the end of the radiographic table, with the arm extended and in contact with the table.

Position of part
- Extend the extremity in position for an AP projection, and center the midpoint of the IR to the elbow joint (Fig. 5.116).
- Medially (internally) rotate or pronate the hand, and adjust the elbow to place its anterior surface at an angle of 45 degrees. This degree of obliquity usually clears the coronoid process of the radial head.
- *Shield gonads.*

Central ray
- Perpendicular to the elbow joint

Collimation
- Adjust radiation field to 3 inches (8 cm) proximal and distal to the elbow joint and 1 inch (2.5 cm) on the sides. Place side marker in the collimated exposure field.

Structures shown
An oblique projection of the elbow with the coronoid process projected free of superimposition (Fig. 5.117).

EVALUATION CRITERIA

The following should be clearly seen:
- Evidence of proper collimation and presence of side marker placed clear of anatomy of interest
- Elbow joint centered to the exposure field
- 45-degree medial rotation of elbow:
  - ☐ Coronoid process in profile
  - ☐ Elongated medial humeral epicondyle
  - ☐ Ulna superimposed by the radial head and neck
- Trochlea
- Olecranon process within the olecranon fossa
- Bony trabecular detail and surrounding soft tissues

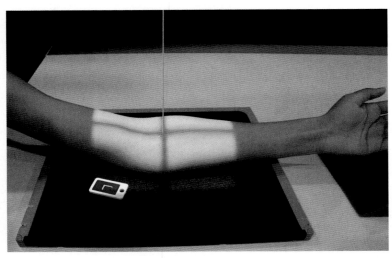

Fig. 5.116 AP oblique elbow: medial rotation.

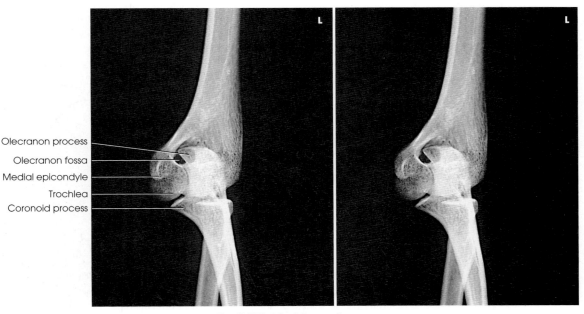

Olecranon process
Olecranon fossa
Medial epicondyle
Trochlea
Coronoid process

Fig. 5.117 AP oblique elbow.

AP OBLIQUE PROJECTION
Lateral rotation

Image receptor: Positioned by manufacturer or department protocol for proper anatomy display orientation; CR plate: 10 × 12 inches (24 × 30 cm) lengthwise.

Position of patient

- Seat the patient at the end of the radiographic table, with the arm extended and in contact with the table.

Position of part

- Extend the patient's arm in position for an AP projection, and center the midpoint of the IR to the elbow joint.
- Rotate the hand laterally (externally) to place the posterior surface of the elbow at a 45-degree angle (Fig. 5.118). When proper lateral rotation is achieved, the patient's first and second digits should touch the table.
- *Shield gonads.*

Central ray

- Perpendicular to the elbow joint

Collimation

- Adjust radiation field to 3 inches (8 cm) proximal and distal to the elbow joint and 1 inch (2.5 cm) on the sides. Place side marker in the collimated exposure field.

Structures shown

An oblique projection of the elbow with the radial head and neck projected free of superimposition of the ulna (Fig. 5.119).

EVALUATION CRITERIA

The following should be clearly seen:
- Evidence of proper collimation and presence of side marker placed clear of anatomy of interest
- Elbow joint centered to the exposure field
- 45-degree lateral rotation of elbow:
  - □ Radial head, neck, and tuberosity projected free of the ulna
  - □ Elongated lateral humeral epicondyle
- Capitulum
- Bony trabecular detail and surrounding soft tissues

Fig. 5.118 AP oblique elbow: lateral rotation.

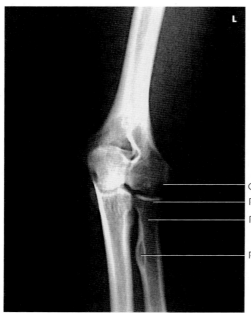
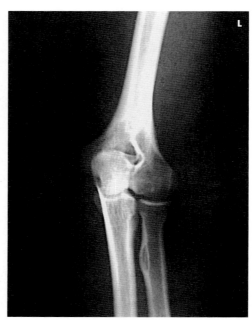

Capitulum

Radial head

Radial neck

Radial tuberosity

Fig. 5.119 AP oblique elbow.

Upper Extremity

Distal Humerus
⚘ AP PROJECTION
Partial flexion

When the patient cannot completely extend the elbow, the lateral position is easily performed; however, two AP projections must be obtained to avoid distortion. Separate AP projections of the distal humerus and proximal forearm are required.

Image receptor: Positioned by manufacturer or department protocol for proper anatomy display orientation;

CR plate: 10 × 12 inches (24 × 30 cm) lengthwise.

Position of patient
• Seat the patient low enough to place the entire humerus in the same plane. Support the elevated forearm.

Position of part
• If possible, supinate the hand. Place the IR under the elbow, and center it to the condyloid area of the humerus (Fig. 5.120).
• *Shield gonads.*

Central ray
• Perpendicular to the humerus, traversing the elbow joint
• Depending on the degree of flexion, angle the CR distally into the joint.

Collimation
• Adjust radiation field to 3 inches (8 cm) proximal and distal to the elbow joint and 1 inch (2.5 cm) on the sides. Place side marker in the collimated exposure field.

Structures shown
The distal humerus when the elbow cannot be fully extended (Figs. 5.121 and 5.122).

EVALUATION CRITERIA
The following should be clearly seen:
■ Evidence of proper collimation and presence of side marker placed clear of anatomy of interest
■ Distal humerus without rotation or distortion
■ Proximal radius superimposed over the ulna
■ Closed elbow joint
■ Greatly foreshortened proximal forearm
■ Bony trabecular detail of the distal humerus and surrounding soft tissues of the elbow

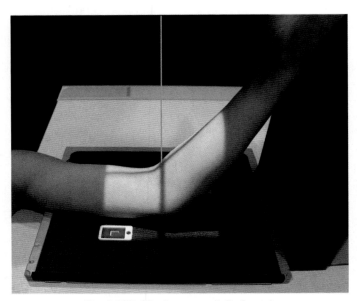

Fig. 5.120 AP elbow, partially flexed.

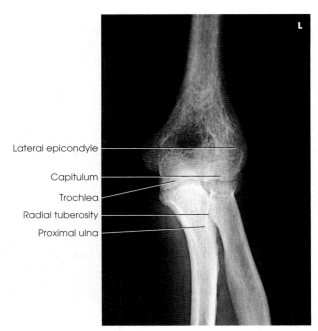

Lateral epicondyle
Capitulum
Trochlea
Radial tuberosity
Proximal ulna

Fig. 5.121 AP elbow, partially flexed, showing distal humerus.

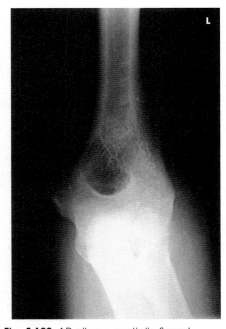

Fig. 5.122 AP elbow, partially flexed, showing distal humerus. White proximal radius and ulna result from overlap of anterior dislocated elbow (see Fig. 5.125).

Proximal Forearm
♠ AP PROJECTION
Partial flexion

Image receptor: Positioned by manufacturer or department protocol for proper anatomy display orientation; CR plate: 10 × 12 inches (24 × 30 cm) lengthwise.

Position of patient
• Seat the patient at the end of the radiographic table, with the hand supinated.

Position of part
• Seat the patient high enough to permit the dorsal surface of the forearm to rest on the table (Fig. 5.123). **Note:** If this position is impossible, elevate the extremity on a support, adjust the extremity in the lateral position, place the IR in the vertical position behind the upper end of the forearm, and direct the CR horizontally.
• *Shield gonads.*

Central ray
• Perpendicular to the elbow joint and long axis of the forearm
• Adjust the IR so that the CR passes to its midpoint.

Collimation
• Adjust radiation field to 3 inches (8 cm) proximal and distal to the elbow joint and 1 inch (2.5 cm) on the sides. Place side marker in the collimated exposure field.

Structures shown
The proximal forearm when the elbow cannot be fully extended (Figs. 5.124 and 5.125).

EVALUATION CRITERIA
The following should be clearly seen:
■ Evidence of proper collimation and presence of side marker placed clear of anatomy of interest
■ Proximal radius and ulna without rotation or distortion
■ Radial head, neck, and tuberosity slightly superimposed over the proximal ulna
■ Partially open elbow joint
■ Foreshortened distal humerus
■ Bony trabecular detail of the proximal radius and ulna, as well as the soft tissues surrounding the elbow

NOTE: Holly[32] described a method of obtaining the AP projection of the radial head. The patient is positioned as described for the distal humerus. The elbow is extended as much as possible, and the forearm is supported. The forearm should be supinated enough to place the horizontal plane of the wrist at an angle of 30 degrees from horizontal.

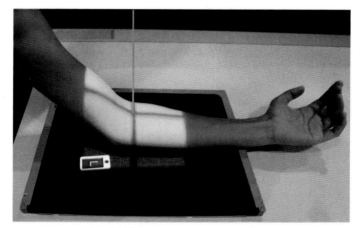

Fig. 5.123 AP elbow, partially flexed.

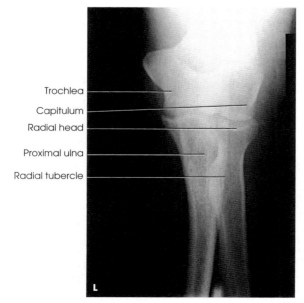

Trochlea
Capitulum
Radial head
Proximal ulna
Radial tubercle

Fig. 5.124 AP elbow, partially flexed, showing proximal forearm. This is a view of the dislocated elbow of the patient shown in Fig. 5.125. White distal humerus is due to dislocated humerus overlapping proximal radius and ulna.

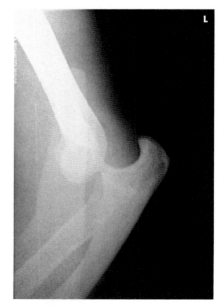

Fig. 5.125 Lateral elbow showing dislocation on same patient as shown in Figs. 5.122 and 5.124.

Distal Humerus
AP PROJECTION
Acute flexion

When fractures around the elbow are being treated using the Jones orthopedic technique (complete flexion), the lateral position offers little difficulty, but the frontal projection must be made through the superimposed bones of the AP arm and PA forearm. This projection is sometimes known as the *Jones method,* although no "Jones" reference has been found.

> **Image receptor:** Positioned by manufacturer or department protocol for proper anatomy display orientation; CR plate: 10 × 12 inches (24 × 30 cm) lengthwise.

Position of patient
- Seat the patient at the end of the radiographic table, with the elbow fully flexed (unless contraindicated).

Position of part
- Center the IR proximal to the epicondylar area of the humerus. The long axis of the arm and forearm should be parallel with the long axis of the IR (Figs. 5.126 and 5.127).
- Adjust the arm or the radiographic tube and IR to prevent rotation.
- *Shield gonads.*

Central ray
- Perpendicular to the humerus, approximately 2 inches (5 cm) superior to the olecranon process

Collimation
- Adjust radiation field to include the proximal half of the forearm and 1 inch (2.5 cm) beyond the olecranon process and sides on the elbow. Place side marker in the collimated exposure field.

Structures shown
This position superimposes the proximal forearm and distal humerus. The olecranon process should be clearly shown (Fig. 5.128).

EVALUATION CRITERIA
The following should be clearly seen:
- Evidence of proper collimation and presence of side marker placed clear of anatomy of interest
- Forearm and humerus superimposed, without rotation
- Olecranon process and distal humerus
- Bony trabecular detail and surrounding soft tissues

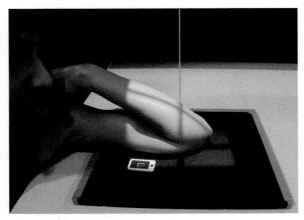

Fig. 5.126 AP distal humerus: acute flexion of elbow.

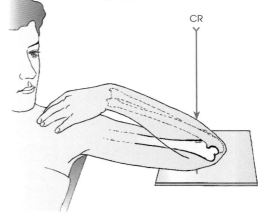

Fig. 5.127 AP distal humerus: acute flexion of elbow.

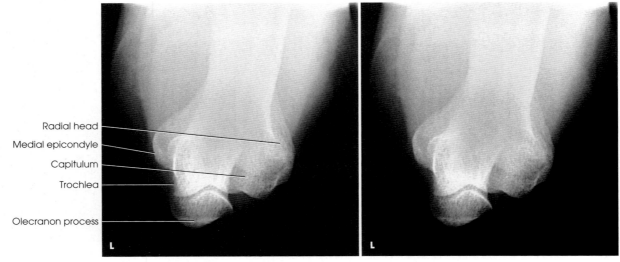

Radial head
Medial epicondyle
Capitulum
Trochlea
Olecranon process

Fig. 5.128 AP distal humerus: acute flexion of elbow.

Proximal Forearm
PA PROJECTION
Acute flexion

Image receptor: Positioned by manufacturer or department protocol for proper anatomy display orientation; CR plate: 10×12 inches (24×30 cm) lengthwise.

Position of patient

- Seat the patient at the end of the radiographic table with the elbow fully flexed.

Position of part

- Center the flexed elbow joint to the center of the IR. The long axis of the superimposed forearm and arm should be parallel with the long axis of the IR (Figs. 5.129 and 5.130).
- Move the IR toward the shoulder so that the CR passes to the midpoint.
- *Shield gonads.*

Central ray

- Angled perpendicular to the flexed forearm, entering approximately 2 inches (5 cm) distal to the olecranon process

Collimation

- Adjust radiation field to include the proximal half of the forearm and 1 inch (2.5 cm) beyond the olecranon process and sides on the elbow. Place side marker in the collimated exposure field.

Structures shown

This position superimposes the proximal forearm and distal humerus (Fig. 5.131). The elbow joint should be more open than for the projection of the distal humerus.

EVALUATION CRITERIA

The following should be clearly seen:
- Evidence of proper collimation and presence of side marker placed clear of anatomy of interest
- Forearm and humerus superimposed, without rotation
- Proximal radius and ulna
- Bony trabecular detail and surrounding soft tissues

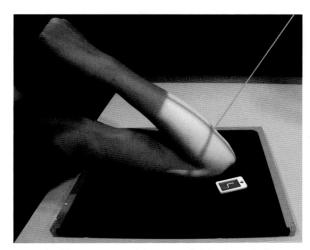

Fig. 5.129 PA proximal forearm: full flexion of elbow.

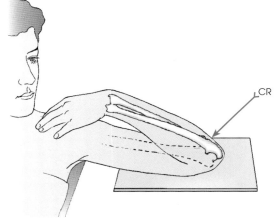

Fig. 5.130 PA proximal forearm: full flexion of elbow.

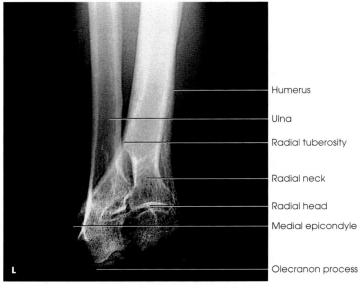
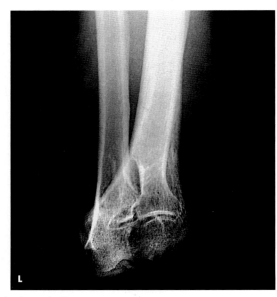

Humerus

Ulna

Radial tuberosity

Radial neck

Radial head

Medial epicondyle

Olecranon process

Fig. 5.131 PA proximal forearm: full flexion of elbow.

Radial Head
LATERAL PROJECTION
Lateromedial
Four-position series

To show the entire circumference of the radial head free of superimposition, four projections with varying positions of the hand are performed.

Image receptor: Positioned by manufacturer or department protocol for proper anatomy display orientation; CR plate: 10 × 12 inches (24 × 30 cm) lengthwise.

Position of patient
- Seat the patient low enough to place the entire arm in the same horizontal plane.

Position of part
- Flex the elbow 90 degrees, center the joint to the unmasked IR, and place the joint in the lateral position.
- Make the first exposure with the hand supinated as much as is possible (Fig. 5.132).

- Replace the IR and make the second exposure with the hand in the lateral position (i.e., with the thumb surface up) (Fig. 5.133).
- Replace the IR, then make the third exposure with the hand pronated (Fig. 5.134).
- Replace the IR, and make the fourth exposure with the hand in extreme internal rotation (i.e., resting on the thumb surface) (Fig. 5.135).
- *Shield gonads.*

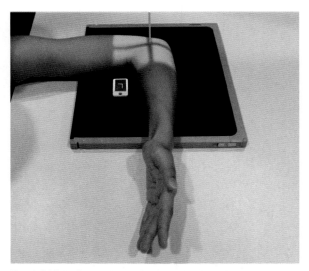

Fig. 5.132 Lateral elbow, radius with hand supinated as much as possible.

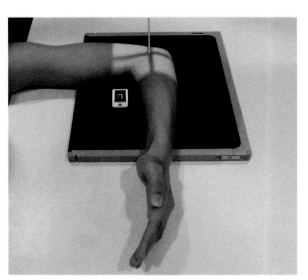

Fig. 5.133 Lateral elbow, radius with hand lateral.

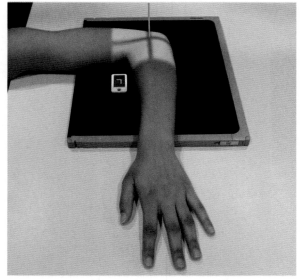

Fig. 5.134 Lateral elbow, radius with hand pronated.

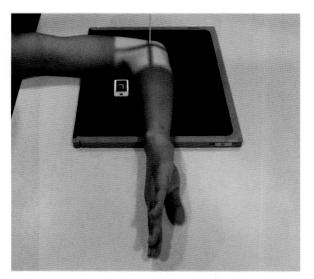

Fig. 5.135 Lateral elbow, radius with hand internally rotated.

Central ray
• Perpendicular to the elbow joint

Collimation
• Adjust radiation field to 3 inches (8 cm) proximal and distal to the elbow joint. Place side marker in the collimated exposure field.

Structures shown
The radial head is projected in varying degrees of rotation (Figs. 5.136 through 5.139).

EVALUATION CRITERIA
The following should be clearly seen:
■ Evidence of proper collimation and presence of side marker placed clear of anatomy of interest
■ Radial tuberosity facing anteriorly for the first and second images and posteriorly for the third and fourth images (see Figs. 5.136 through 5.139)
■ Elbow flexed 90 degrees
■ Radial head partially superimposing the coronoid process but seen in all images
■ Bony trabecular detail and surrounding soft tissues

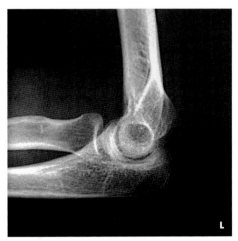

Fig. 5.136 Lateral elbow, radius with hand supinated.

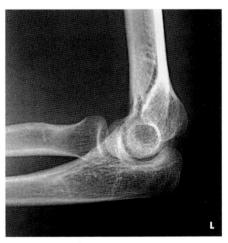

Fig. 5.137 Lateral elbow, radius with hand lateral.

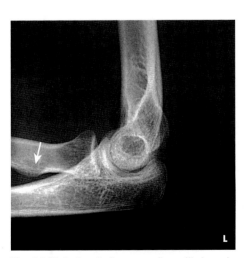

Fig. 5.138 Lateral elbow, radius with hand pronated (radial tuberosity, *arrow*).

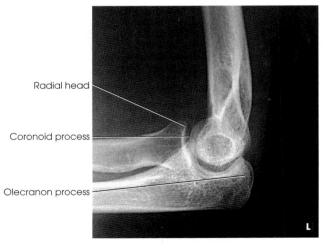

Radial head

Coronoid process

Olecranon process

Fig. 5.139 Lateral elbow, radius with hand internally rotated.

Radial Head and Coronoid Process

⚘ AXIOLATERAL PROJECTION

COYLE METHOD
Lateral

NOTE: This projection was devised for obtaining images of the radial head and coronoid process on patients who cannot fully extend the elbow for medial and lateral oblique projections.[33] It is particularly useful in imaging a traumatized elbow.

Image receptor: Positioned by manufacturer or department protocol for proper anatomy display orientation; CR plate: 10×12 inches (24×30 cm) lengthwise.

Position of patient

- Seat the patient at the end of the radiographic table.
- Position the patient supine for imaging a traumatized elbow.

Position of part
Seated position

- Seat the patient at the end of the radiographic table, low enough to place the humerus, elbow, and wrist joints on the same plane.
- Pronate the hand and flex the elbow 90 degrees to show the radial head or 80 degrees to show the coronoid process.
- Center the IR to the elbow joint. For patients with muscular forearms, elevate the wrist to place the forearm parallel with the IR (Fig. 5.140).

Supine position for trauma

- In most instances of trauma, the patient is lying in the supine position on a cart. The projection is easily performed in this position.
- Elevate the distal humerus on a radiolucent sponge.
- Place the IR in vertical position centered to the elbow joint.
- Epicondyles should be approximately perpendicular to the IR.
- Slowly flex the elbow 90 degrees to show the radial head or 80 degrees for the coronoid process. Turn the hand so that the palmar aspect is facing medially. An assistant may need to hold the hand depending on the severity of trauma (Fig. 5.141).
- *Shield gonads.*

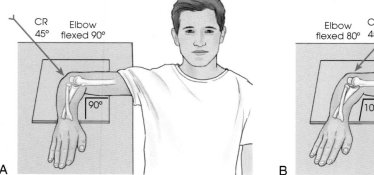
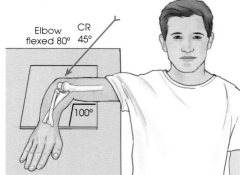

Fig. 5.140 (A) Axiolateral projection of elbow (Coyle method) to show radial head and capitulum. Forearm is 90 degrees, and CR is directed 45 degrees toward shoulder. (B) To show coronoid process and trochlea, forearm is positioned at 80 degrees, and CR is directed 45 degrees away from shoulder.

Central ray

Seated position
Radial head

- Directed toward the shoulder at an angle of 45 degrees to the radial head; CR enters the joint at mid-elbow (see Fig. 5.140A)

Coronoid process

- Directed away from the shoulder at an angle of 45 degrees to the coronoid process; CR enters the joint at mid-elbow (see Fig. 5.140B)

Supine position for trauma
Radial head

- The horizontal CR is directed cephalad at an angle of 45 degrees to the radial head, entering the joint at mid-elbow (see Fig. 5.141A).

Coronoid process

- The horizontal CR is directed caudad at an angle of 45 degrees to the coronoid process, entering the joint at mid-elbow (see Fig. 5.141B).

Collimation

- Adjust radiation field to 3 inches (8 cm) proximal and distal to the elbow joint. Place side marker in the collimated exposure field.

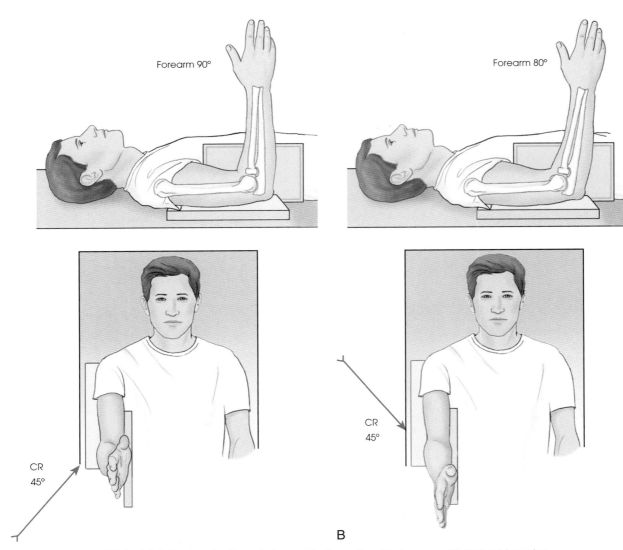

Forearm 90°

Forearm 80°

CR 45°

CR 45°

A

B

Fig. 5.141 Axiolateral projection of elbow (Coyle method) in trauma. (A) Patient is supine with humerus on a block, arm is 90 degrees, and CR is directed cephalad for radial head and capitulum. (B) Arm is 80 degrees, and CR is directed caudad to show coronoid process and trochlea.

Upper Extremity

Structures shown

The resulting projections show an open elbow joint between the radial head and capitulum (Fig. 5.142) or between the coronoid process and trochlea (Fig. 5.143), with the area of interest in profile. These projections are used to show pathologic processes or trauma in the area of the radial head and coronoid process. The value of the projections is evident in the trauma images shown in Fig. 5.144.[34]

The following should be clearly seen:

Radial Head

■ Evidence of proper collimation and presence of side marker placed clear of anatomy of interest
■ Open joint space between radial head and capitulum
■ Radial head, neck, and tuberosity in profile and free from superimposition with the exception of a small portion of the coronoid process
■ Humeral epicondyles distorted owing to CR angulation
■ Radial tuberosity facing posteriorly
■ Elbow flexed 90 degrees

■ Bony trabecular detail and surrounding soft tissues

Coronoid Process

■ Evidence of proper collimation and presence of side marker placed clear of anatomy of interest
■ Open joint space between coronoid process and trochlea
■ Coronoid process in profile and elongated
■ Radial head and neck superimposed by ulna
■ Elbow flexed 80 degrees
■ Bony trabecular detail and surrounding soft tissues

RESEARCH: This projection was researched and standardized for the atlas by Tammy Curtis, MS, RT(R).

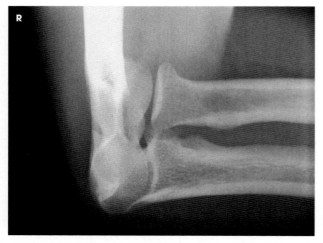

Fig. 5.142 Axiolateral elbow (Coyle method) with radial head and capitulum shown.

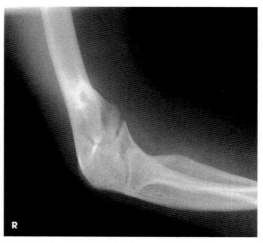

Fig. 5.143 Axiolateral elbow (Coyle method) with coronoid process and trochlea shown.

(From Bontrager KL, Lampignano JP: *Textbook of radiographic positioning and related anatomy*, ed 7, St Louis, 2009, Mosby.)

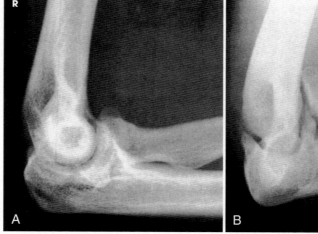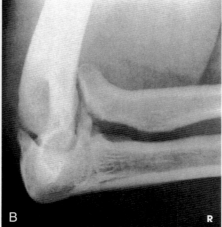

Fig. 5.144 (A) Lateral projection of elbow shows fracture of radial head, but bony overlap prevents exact evaluation of extent of fracture line. (B) Axiolateral projection (Coyle method) clearly shows displaced articular fracture involving posterior third of radial head.

(Used with permission from Greenspan A, Norman A, Rosen H: Radial head capitulum view in elbow trauma: clinical applications and anatomic correlation. *AJR Am J Roentgenol* 143:355, 1984.)

PA AXIAL PROJECTION

Image receptor: Positioned by manufacturer or department protocol for proper anatomy display orientation; CR plate: 10 × 12 inches (24 × 30 cm) lengthwise.

Position of patient

- Seat the patient high enough to enable the forearm to rest on the radiographic table, with the arm in the vertical position. The patient must be seated so that the forearm can be adjusted parallel with the long axis of the table.

Position of part

- Ask the patient to rest the forearm on the table, and then adjust the forearm so that its long axis is parallel with the table.
- Center a point midway between the epicondyles and the center of the IR.

- Flex the patient's elbow to place the arm in a nearly vertical position so that the humerus forms an angle of approximately 75 degrees from the forearm (approximately 15 degrees between the CR and the long axis of the humerus).
- Confirm that the patient is not leaning anteriorly or posteriorly.
- Supinate the hand to prevent rotation of the humerus and ulna, and have the patient immobilize it with the opposite hand (Fig. 5.145).
- *Shield gonads.*

Central ray

- Perpendicular to the ulnar sulcus, entering at a point just medial to the olecranon process

Collimation

- Adjust radiation field to include distal third of humerus and extend 2 inches (5 cm) beyond the olecranon process

and 1 inch (2.5 cm) beyond the sides on the elbow. Place side marker in the collimated exposure field.

Structures shown

The epicondyles, trochlea, ulnar sulcus (groove between the medial epicondyle and the trochlea), and olecranon fossa (Fig. 5.146). The projection is used in radiohumeral bursitis (tennis elbow) to detect otherwise obscured calcifications located in the ulnar sulcus.

NOTE: Long and Rafert[35] describe an AP oblique distal humerus projection that specifically shows the ulnar sulcus.

The following should be clearly seen:

- Evidence of proper collimation and presence of side marker placed clear of anatomy of interest
- Outline of the ulnar sulcus (groove)
- Forearm and humerus superimposed, without rotation
- Bony trabecular detail and surrounding soft tissues

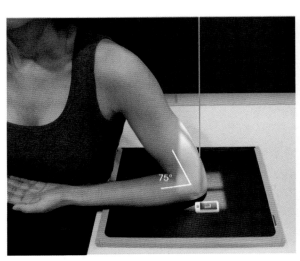

Fig. 5.145 PA axial distal humerus.

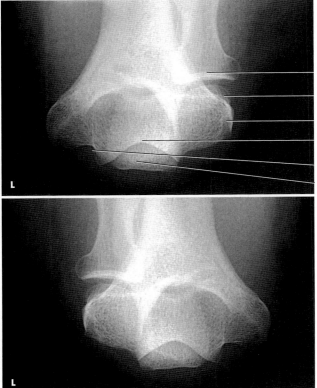

Radial head
Capitulum
Lateral epicondyle
Trochlea
Ulnar sulcus
Olecranon process

Fig. 5.146 PA axial distal humerus.

PA AXIAL PROJECTION

Image receptor: Positioned by manufacturer or department protocol for proper anatomy display orientation; CR plate: 10 × 12 inches (24 × 30 cm) lengthwise.

Position of patient

- Seat the patient at the end of the radiographic table, high enough that the forearm can rest flat on the IR.

Position of part

- Adjust the arm at an angle of 45 to 50 degrees from the vertical position, and ensure that the patient is not leaning anteriorly or posteriorly.
- Supinate the hand, and have the patient immobilize it with the opposite hand.
- Center a point midway between the epicondyles and the center of the IR.
- *Shield gonads.*

Central ray

- Perpendicular to the olecranon process to show the dorsum of the olecranon process and at a 20-degree angle toward the wrist to show the curved extremity and articular margin of the olecranon process (Fig. 5.147)

Collimation

- Adjust radiation field to include distal fourth of humerus and extend 1 inch (2.5 cm) beyond the olecranon process and the sides on the elbow. Place side marker in the collimated exposure field.

Structures shown

The olecranon process and the articular margin of the olecranon and humerus (Figs. 5.148 through 5.150).

EVALUATION CRITERIA

The following should be clearly seen:

- Evidence of proper collimation and presence of side marker placed clear of anatomy of interest
- Olecranon process in profile
- Forearm and humerus superimposed, without rotation
- Bony trabecular detail and surrounding soft tissues

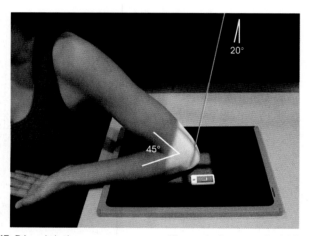

Fig. 5.147 PA axial olecranon process with central ray angled 20 degrees.

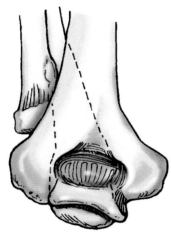

Fig. 5.148 PA axial olecranon process.

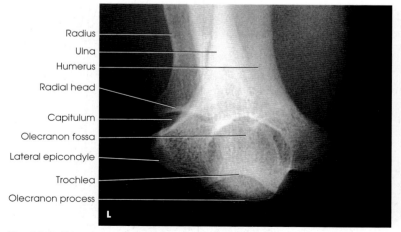

Radius
Ulna
Humerus
Radial head
Capitulum
Olecranon fossa
Lateral epicondyle
Trochlea
Olecranon process

Fig. 5.149 PA axial olecranon process with central ray angulation of 0 degrees.

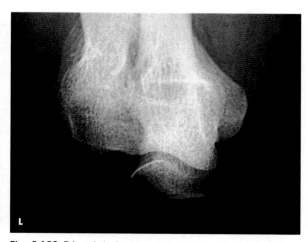

Fig. 5.150 PA axial olecranon process with central ray angulation of 20 degrees.

♠ AP PROJECTION
Upright

Shoulder and arm abnormalities, whether traumatic or pathologic in origin, are extremely painful. For this reason, an upright position, either standing or seated, should be used whenever possible. With rotation of the patient's body as required, the arm can be positioned quickly and accurately with minimal discomfort to the patient.

> **Image receptor + grid:** Positioned by manufacturer or department protocol for proper anatomy display orientation; CR plate: 14 × 17 inches (35 × 43 cm) lengthwise.

Position of patient
- Place the patient in a seated-upright or standing position facing the x-ray tube.
- Fig. 5.151 illustrates the body position used for an AP projection of a freely movable arm. The body position, whether oblique or facing toward or away from the IR, is unimportant as long as an AP radiograph of the arm is obtained.

Position of part
- Adjust the height of the IR to place its upper margin approximately 1½ inches (3.8 cm) above the level of the humeral head.
- Abduct the arm slightly, and supinate the hand.
- A coronal plane passing through the epicondyles should be parallel with the IR plane for the AP (or PA) projection (see Fig. 5.151).
- *Shield gonads.*
- *Respiration:* Suspend.

Central ray
- Perpendicular to the midportion of the humerus and the center of the IR

Collimation
- Adjust radiation field to 2 inches (5 cm) distal to the elbow joint and superior to the shoulder and 1 inch (2.5 cm) on the sides. Place side marker in the collimated exposure field.

Structures shown

The AP projection shows the entire length of the humerus. The accuracy of the position is shown by the epicondyles (Fig. 5.152).

EVALUATION CRITERIA

The following should be clearly seen:
- ■ Evidence of proper collimation and presence of side marker placed clear of anatomy of interest
- ■ Elbow and shoulder joints visible but slightly distorted due to beam divergence
- ■ Humeral epicondyles without rotation
- ■ Humeral head and greater tubercle in profile
- ■ Outline of the lesser tubercle, located between the humeral head and the greater tubercle
- ■ Bony trabecular detail and surrounding soft tissues

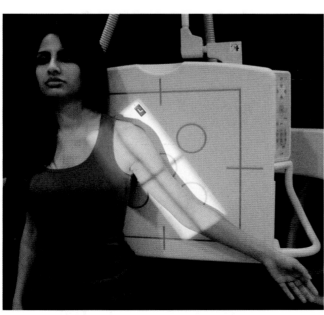

Fig. 5.151 Upright position for AP humerus.

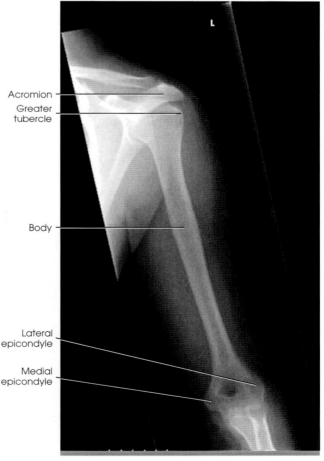

Fig. 5.152 Upright AP humerus.

♠ LATERAL PROJECTION
Lateromedial, mediolateral
Upright

Image receptor + grid: Positioned by manufacturer or department protocol for proper anatomy display orientation; CR plate: 14 × 17 inches (35 × 43 cm) lengthwise.

Position of patient
- Place the patient in a seated-upright or standing position facing the x-ray tube. The body position, whether oblique or facing toward or away from the IR, is not critical as long as a true lateral projection of the arm is obtained.

Position of part
- Place the top margin of the IR approximately 1½ inches (3.8 cm) above the level of the humeral head.

- Unless contraindicated by possible fracture, internally rotate the arm, flex the elbow approximately 90 degrees, and place the patient's anterior hand on the hip. This places the humerus in lateral position. A coronal plane passing through the epicondyles should be perpendicular with the IR plane (Fig. 5.153).
- A patient with a broken humerus may be easier to position by performing a mediolateral projection as shown in Fig. 5.154. Face the sitting or standing patient toward the IR and incline the thorax as necessary to align the humerus for the mediolateral projection. If the patient is not already holding the hand of the broken arm, have the patient do so.
- *Shield gonads.*
- *Respiration:* Suspend.

Central ray
- Perpendicular to the midportion of the humerus and the center of the IR

Collimation
- Adjust radiation field to 2 inches (5 cm) distal to the elbow joint and superior to the shoulder and 1 inch (2.5 cm) on the sides. Place side marker in the collimated exposure field.

Structures shown
The lateral projection shows the entire length of the humerus. A true lateral image is confirmed by superimposed epicondyles (Fig. 5.155).

EVALUATION CRITERIA
The following should be clearly seen:
- Evidence of proper collimation and presence of side marker placed clear of anatomy of interest
- Elbow and shoulder joints visible but slightly distorted due to beam divergence
- Superimposed humeral epicondyles
- Lesser tubercle in profile on medial aspect
- Greater tubercle superimposed over the humeral head
- Bony trabecular detail and surrounding soft tissues

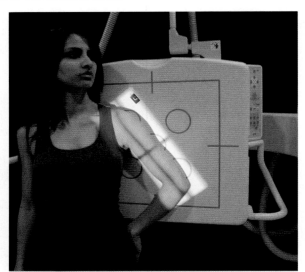

Fig. 5.153 Upright position for lateral (lateromedial) humerus. Note hand placement on hip.

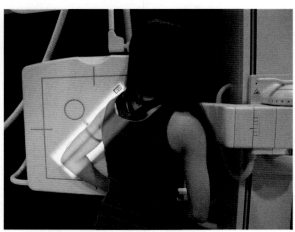

Fig. 5.154 A patient with broken humerus may be easier to position for mediolateral projection as shown.

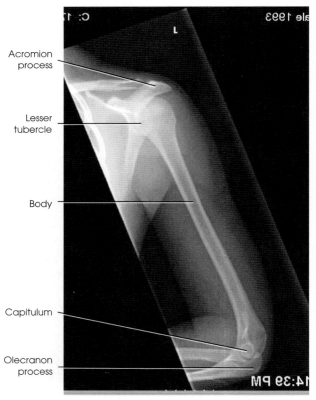

Acromion process

Lesser tubercle

Body

Capitulum

Olecranon process

Fig. 5.155 Upright lateral humerus.

♠ AP PROJECTION
Recumbent

Image receptor + grid: Positioned by manufacturer or department protocol for proper anatomy display orientation; CR plate: 14 × 17 inches (35 × 43 cm) lengthwise.

Position of patient
- With the patient in the supine position, adjust the IR to include the entire length of the humerus.

Position of part
- Place the upper margin of the IR approximately 1½ inches (3.8 cm) above the humeral head.
- Elevate the opposite shoulder on a sandbag to place the affected arm in contact with the IR, or elevate the arm and IR on sandbags.

- Unless contraindicated, supinate the hand, extend the elbow, and rotate the extremity to place the epicondyles parallel with the plane of the IR (Fig. 5.156).
- *Shield gonads.*
- *Respiration:* Suspend.

Central ray
- Perpendicular to the midportion of the humerus and the center of the IR

Collimation
- Adjust radiation field to 2 inches (5 cm) distal to the elbow joint and superior to the shoulder and 1 inch (2.5 cm) on the sides. Place side marker in the collimated exposure field.

Structures shown
The AP projection shows the entire length of the humerus. The accuracy of the position is shown by the epicondyles (see Fig. 5.156).

The following should be clearly seen:
- Evidence of proper collimation and presence of side marker placed clear of anatomy of interest
- Elbow and shoulder joints visible but slightly distorted due to beam divergence
- Humeral epicondyles without rotation
- Humeral head and greater tubercle in profile
- Outline of the lesser tubercle, located between the humeral head and the greater tubercle
- Bony trabecular detail and surrounding soft tissues

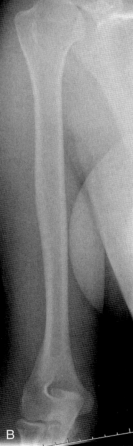

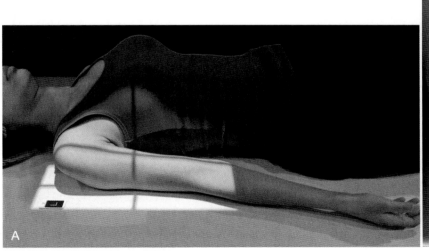

Fig. 5.156 (A) Recumbent position for AP humerus. Note that hand is supinated. (B) AP humerus in correct position.

⚜ LATERAL PROJECTION
Lateromedial
Recumbent

Image receptor + grid: Positioned by manufacturer or department protocol for proper anatomy display orientation; CR plate: 14 × 17 inches (35 × 43 cm) lengthwise.

Position of patient
- Place the patient in the supine position with the humerus centered to the IR, or use a Bucky tray.

Position of part
- Adjust the top of the IR to be approximately 1½ inches (3.8 cm) above the level of the head of the humerus.
- Unless contraindicated by possible fracture, abduct the arm and center the IR under it.
- Rotate the forearm medially to place the epicondyles perpendicular to the plane of the IR, and rest the *posterior aspect* of the hand against the patient's side. This movement turns the epicondyles in the lateral position without flexing the elbow (see Fig. 5.153). (The elbow may be flexed slightly for comfort.)

- Adjust the position of the IR to include the entire length of the humerus (Fig. 5.157).
- *Shield gonads.*
- *Respiration:* Suspend.

Central ray
- Perpendicular to the midportion of the humerus and the center of the IR

Collimation
- Adjust radiation field to 2 inches (5 cm) distal to the elbow joint and superior to the shoulder and 1 inch (2.5 cm) on the sides. Place side marker in the collimated exposure field.

Structures shown
The lateral projection shows the entire length of the humerus. A true lateral image is confirmed by superimposed epicondyles (see Fig. 5.157).

The following should be clearly seen:
- Evidence of proper collimation and presence of side marker placed clear of anatomy of interest
- Elbow and shoulder joints visible but slightly distorted due to beam divergence
- Superimposed humeral epicondyles
- Lesser tubercle in profile
- Greater tubercle superimposed over the humeral head
- Bony trabecular detail and surrounding soft tissues

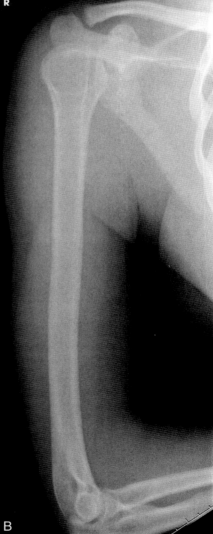

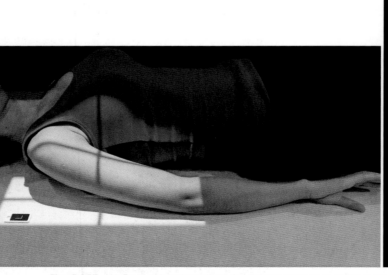

Fig. 5.157 (A) Recumbent position for lateral humerus. Note posterior aspect of the patient's hand against thigh. (B) Lateral humerus, supine position. Note epicondyles are perpendicular to IR. Distal aspect of forearm could not be included because of patient's condition, separate lateral elbow was performed.

☚ LATERAL PROJECTION
Lateromedial
Recumbent or lateral recumbent

Image receptor: Positioned by manufacturer or department protocol for proper anatomy display orientation; CR plate: 10×12 inches (24×30 cm) lengthwise.

Position of patient
- When a known or suspected fracture exists, position the patient in the recumbent or lateral recumbent position, place the IR close to the axilla, and center the humerus to the midline of the IR.
- Unless contraindicated, flex the elbow, turn the thumb surface of the hand up, and rest the humerus on a suitable support (Fig. 5.158).
- Adjust the position of the body to place the lateral surface of the humerus perpendicular to the CR.
- *Shield gonads.*
- *Respiration:* Suspend.

Central ray
Recumbent
- Horizontal and perpendicular to the midportion of the humerus and the center of the IR

Lateral recumbent
- Directed to the center of the IR, which exposes only the distal humerus (see Fig. 5.158)

Collimation
- Adjust radiation field to 2 inches (5 cm) distal to the elbow joint and 1 inch (2.5 cm) on the sides; top collimator margin should extend no farther than edge of the IR

Structures shown
The lateral projection shows the distal humerus (Fig. 5.159).

EVALUATION CRITERIA
The following should be clearly seen:
- Evidence of proper collimation and presence of side marker placed clear of anatomy of interest
- Distal humerus
- Superimposed epicondyles
- Bony trabecular detail and surrounding soft tissues

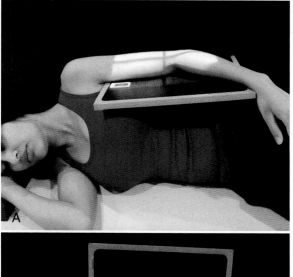

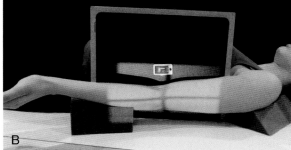

Fig. 5.158 (A) Lateral recumbent body position to show distal lateral humerus. (B) Patient and IR positioned for trauma cross-table lateral projection of humerus.

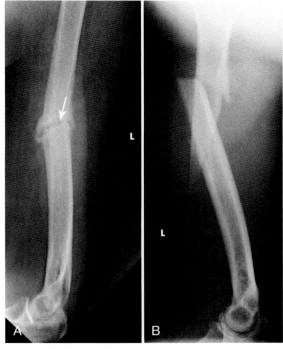

Fig. 5.159 (A) Lateral recumbent humerus, showing healing fracture *(arrow)*. (B) Lateral recumbent humerus showing comminuted fracture. Radiograph had to be obtained using lateral recumbent position owing to the patient's pain.

References

1. McQuillen Martensen K: *Radiographic Image Analysis*, ed 4. St. Louis, 2015, Saunders.

2. Griswold R: Elbow fat pads: a radiography perspective, *Radiol Technol* 53(4): 303–308, 1982.

3. Street JM: Radiographs of phalangeal fractures: importance of the internally rotated oblique projection for diagnosis, *AJR Am J Roentgenol* 160(3):575–576, 1993.

4. Lewis S: New angles on the radiographic examination of the hand—II, *Radiogr Today* 54(618):29, 1988.

5. Robert M: X-ray of trapezo-metacarpal articulation: the arthroses of this joint, *Bulletins et memories de la Societe de Radiologie Medicale de France* 24:687, 1936.

6. Long B, Rafert J: *Orthopaedic radiography*, Philadelphia, 1995, Saunders.

7. Burman M: Anteroposterior projection of the carpometacarpal joint of the thumb by radial shift of the carpal tunnel view, *J Bone Joint Surg Am* 40-A(5):1156–1157, 1958.

8. Folio LR: Patient-controlled stress radiography of the thumb, *Radiol Technol* 70(5):465–469, 1999.

9. Clements RW, Nakayama HK: Technique for detecting early rheumatoid arthritis, *Radiol Technol* 62(6):443–451, 1991.

10. Lewis S: New angles on the radiographic examination of the hand—I, *Radiogr Today* 54(617):44–45, 1988.

11. Lane CS, Kennedy JF, Kuschner SH: The reverse oblique x-ray film: metacarpal fractures revealed, *J Hand Surg Am* 17(3): 504–506, 1992.

12. Kallen MJ: Kallen projection reveals metacarpal head fractures, *Radiol Technol* 65(4):229–233, 1994.

13. Norgaard F: Earliest roentgenological changes in polyarthritis of the rheumatoid type: rheumatoid arthritis, *Radiology* 85: 325–329, 1965.

14. Norgaard F: Earliest roentgen changes in polyarthritis of the rheumatoid type, *Radiology* 92(2):299–303, 1969.

15. Stapczynski JS: Fracture of the base of the little finger metacarpal: importance of the "ball-catcher" radiographic view, *J Emerg Med* 9(3):145–149, 1991.

16. Daffner RH, Emmerling EW, Buterbaugh GA: Proximal and distal oblique radiography of the wrist: value in occult injuries, *J Hand Surg Am* 17(3):499–503, 1992.

17. Burman MS et al: Fractures of the radial and ulnar axes, *AJR Am J Roentgenol* 51:455, 1944.

18. Fiolle J: Le "carpe bossu," *Bull Soc Chir Paris* 57:1687, 1931.

19. Fiolle J et al: Nouvelle observation de "carpe bossu," *Bull Soc Chir Paris* 58:187, 1932.

20. McBride E: Wrist joint injuries, a plea for greater accuracy in treatment, *J Okla Med Assoc* 19:67, 1926.

21. Frank ED et al: Two terms, one meaning, *Radiol Technol* 69:517, 1998.

22. Stecher WR: Roentgenography of the carpal navicular bone, *AJR Am J Roentgenol* 37:704, 1937.

23. Bridgman CF: Radiography of the carpal navicular bone, *Med Radiogr Photogr* 25:104, 1949.

24. Rafert JA, Long BW: Technique for diagnosis of scaphoid fractures, *Radiol Technol* 63:16–20, 1991.

25. Clements R, Nakayama H: Radiography of the polyarthritic hands and wrists, *Radiol Technol* 53(3) 203–217, 1981.

26. Holly EW: Radiography of the greater multangular bone, *Med Radiogr Photogr* 24:79, 1948.

27. Jacobson HG, Lentino W, Lubetsky HW, et al: The carpal bridge view, *J Bone Joint Surg Am* 39-A(1):88–90, 1957.

28. Hart VL, Gaynor V: Roentgenographic study of the carpal canal, *J Bone Joint Surg* 23:382, 1941.

29. Bontrager KL: *Textbook of radiographic positioning and related anatomy*, ed 7, St Louis, 2009, Mosby.

30. McQuillen Martensen K: *Radiographic image analysis*, ed 3, St Louis, 2010, Saunders.

31. Marshall J, Davies R: Imaging the carpal tunnel, *Radiogr Today* 56(633):11–13, 1990.

32. Holly EW: Radiography of the radial head, *Med Radiogr Photogr* 32:13–14, 1956.

33. Coyle GF: *Radiographing immobile trauma patients, Unit 7, Special angled views of joints—elbow, knee, ankle*, Denver, 1980, Multi-Media Publishing.

34. Greenspan A, Norman A, Rosen H: Radial head capitulum view in elbow trauma: clinical applications and anatomic correlation, *AJR Am J Roentgenol* 143(2):355–359, 1984.

35. Long BW, Rafert JA: The elbow. In: *Orthopedic radiography*, Philadelphia, 1995, Saunders.

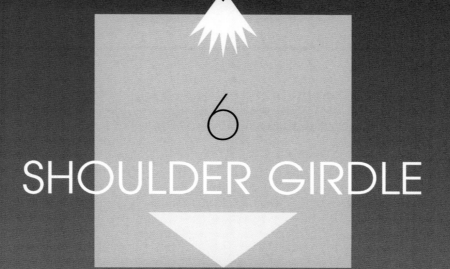

6

SHOULDER GIRDLE

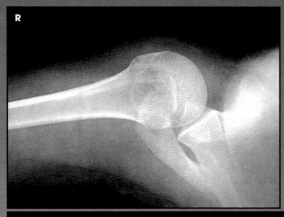

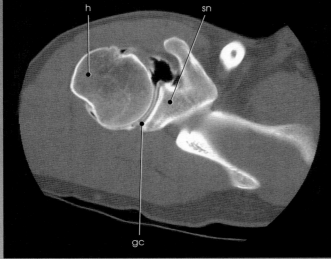

PROJECTIONS, POSITIONS, AND METHODS

Page	Essential	Anatomy	Projection	Position	Method
227	![icon]	Shoulder	AP	External, neutral, internal rotation humerus	
232	![icon]	Shoulder joint: *glenoid cavity*	AP oblique	RPO or LPO	GRASHEY
234		Shoulder joint: *glenoid cavity*	AP oblique	RPO or LPO	APPLE
236	![icon]	Shoulder	Transthoracic lateral	R or L	LAWRENCE
238	![icon]	Shoulder joint	Inferosuperior axial		LAWRENCE
238		Shoulder joint	Inferosuperior axial		RAFERT ET AL. MODIFICATION
240		Shoulder joint	Inferosuperior axial		WEST POINT
242		Shoulder joint	Superoinferior axial		
243	![icon]	Shoulder joint: *scapular Y*	PA oblique	RAO or LAO	
246		Shoulder joint: *supraspinatus "outlet"*	Tangential	RAO or LAO	NEER
247		Shoulder joint	AP axial		
248		Shoulder joint: *proximal humerus*	AP axial		STRYKER "NOTCH"
249		Shoulder joint: *glenoid cavity*	AP axial oblique	RPO or LPO	GARTH
251		Proximal humerus: *intertubercular groove*	Tangential		FISK MODIFICATION
253	![icon]	Acromioclavicular articulations	AP	Bilateral	PEARSON
255		Acromioclavicular articulations	AP axial		ALEXANDER
257	![icon]	Clavicle	AP		
258	![icon]	Clavicle	AP axial	Lordotic	
259	![icon]	Clavicle	PA		
259	![icon]	Clavicle	PA axial		
260	![icon]	Scapula	AP		
262	![icon]	Scapula	Lateral	RAO or LAO	
264		Scapula	AP oblique	RPO or LPO	
266		Scapula: *coracoid process*	AP axial		
268		Scapular spine	Tangential		LAQUERRIÈRE-PIERQUIN

The icons in the Essential column indicate projections frequently performed in the United States and Canada. Students should become competent in these projections.

AP, Anteroposterior; *L,* left; *LAO,* left anterior oblique; *LPO,* left posterior oblique; *PA,* posteroanterior; *R,* right; *RAO,* right anterior oblique; *RPO,* right posterior oblique.

Shoulder Girdle

The *shoulder girdle* is formed by two bones—the *clavicle* and *scapula*. The function of these bones is to connect the upper limb to the trunk. Although the alignment of these two bones is considered a girdle, it is incomplete in back. The girdle is completed in front by the sternum, which articulates with the medial end of the clavicle. The scapulae are widely separated in the back. The proximal portion of the humerus is part of the

upper limb and not the shoulder girdle proper. However, because the proximal humerus is included in the shoulder joint, its anatomy is considered with that of the shoulder girdle (Figs. 6.1 and 6.2).

Clavicle

The *clavicle,* classified as a long bone, has a body and two articular extremities (see Fig. 6.1). The clavicle lies in a horizontal oblique plane just above the first rib

and forms the anterior part of the shoulder girdle. The lateral aspect is termed the *acromial extremity,* and it articulates with the acromion of the scapula. The *medial* aspect, termed the *sternal extremity,* articulates with the manubrium of the sternum and the first costal cartilage. The clavicle, which serves as a fulcrum for the movements of the arm, is doubly curved for strength. The curvature is more acute in males than in females.

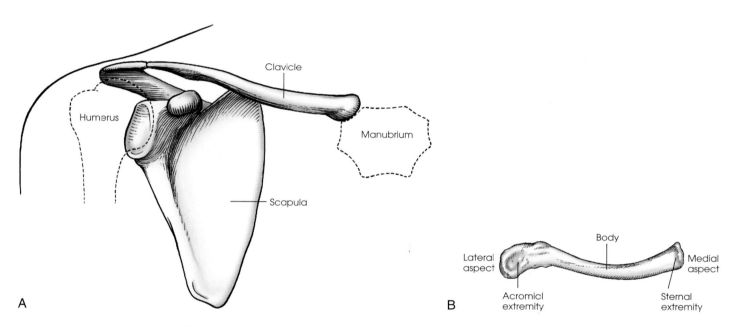

Fig. 6.1 (A) Anterior aspect of shoulder girdle: clavicle and scapula. Girdle attaches to humerus and manubrium of sternum. (B) Superior aspect of right clavicle.

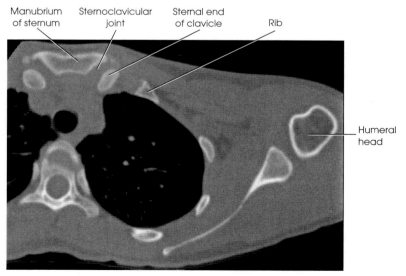

Fig. 6.2 Axial CT scan of shoulder showing relationship of anatomy. Note 45- to 60-degree angle of scapula.

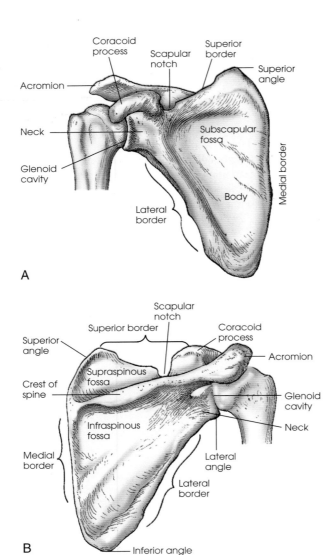

Fig. 6.3 Scapula. (A) Costal surface (anterior aspect). (B) Dorsal surface (posterior aspect).

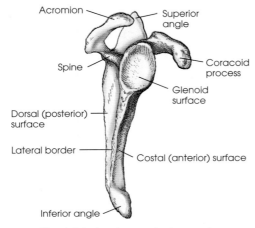

Fig. 6.4 Lateral aspect of scapula.

Scapula

The *scapula,* classified as a flat bone, forms the posterior part of the shoulder girdle (Figs. 6.3 and 6.4). Triangular in shape, the scapula has two surfaces, three borders, and three angles. Lying on the superoposterior thorax between the second and seventh ribs, the *medial border* of the scapula runs parallel with the vertebral column. The body of the bone is arched from top to bottom for greater strength, and its surfaces serve as the attachment sites of numerous muscles. The flat aspect of the bone lies at approximately a 45- to 60-degree angle in relation to the anatomic position (see Fig. 6.2).

The *costal (anterior) surface* of the scapula is slightly concave and contains the *subscapular fossa.* It is filled almost entirely by the attachment of the subscapularis muscle. The anterior serratus muscle attaches to the medial border of the costal surface from the *superior angle* to the *inferior angle.*

The *dorsal (posterior) surface* is divided into two portions by a prominent spinous process. The *crest of spine* arises at the superior third of the medial border from a smooth, triangular area and runs obliquely superior to end in a flattened, ovoid projection called the *acromion.* The area above the spine is called the *supraspinous fossa* and gives origin to the supraspinatus muscle. The infraspinatus muscle arises from the portion below the spine, which is called the *infraspinous fossa.* The teres minor muscle arises from the superior two-thirds of the lateral border of the dorsal surface, and the teres major arises from the distal third and the inferior angle. The dorsal surface of the medial border affords attachment of the levator muscles of the scapulae, greater rhomboid muscle, and lesser rhomboid muscle.

The *superior border* extends from the superior angle to the *coracoid process* and at its lateral end has a deep depression, the *scapular notch.* The *medial border* extends from the superior to the inferior angles. The *lateral border* extends from the *glenoid cavity* to the inferior angle.

The *superior angle* is formed by the junction of the superior and medial borders. The *inferior angle* is formed by the junction of the medial (vertebral) and lateral borders and lies over the seventh rib. The *lateral angle,* the thickest part of the body of the scapula, ends in a shallow, oval depression called the *glenoid cavity.* The constricted region around the glenoid cavity is called the *neck* of the scapula. The coracoid process arises from a thick base that extends from the scapular notch to the superior portion of the neck of the scapula. This process first projects anteriorly and medially and then curves on itself to project laterally. The coracoid process can be palpated just distal and slightly medial to the acromioclavicular (AC) articulation. The acromion, coracoid process, superior angle, and inferior angle are common positioning landmarks for shoulder radiography.

Humerus

The proximal end of the *humerus* consists of a head, an anatomic neck, two prominent processes called the *greater* and *lesser tubercles,* and the surgical neck (Fig. 6.5). The *head* is large, smooth, and rounded, and it lies in an oblique plane on the superomedial side of the humerus. Just below the head, lying in the same oblique plane, is the narrow, constricted *anatomic neck.* The constriction of the body just below the tubercles is called the *surgical neck,* which is the site of many fractures.

The *lesser tubercle* is situated on the anterior surface of the bone, immediately below the anatomic neck (Figs. 6.6 and 6.7; also see Fig. 6.5). The tendon of the subscapular muscle inserts at the lesser tubercle. The *greater tubercle* is located on the lateral surface of the bone, just below the anatomic neck, and is separated from the lesser tubercle by a deep depression called the *intertubercular (bicipital) groove.* The superior surface of the greater tubercle slopes posteriorly at an angle of approximately 25 degrees and has three flattened impressions for muscle insertions. The anterior impression is the highest of the three and affords attachment to the tendon of the supraspinatus muscle. The middle impression is the point of insertion of the infraspinatus muscle. The tendon of the upper fibers of the teres minor muscle inserts at the posterior impression (the lower fibers insert into the *body* of the bone immediately below this point).

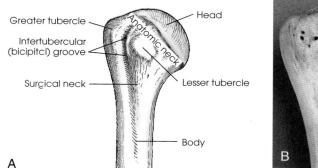 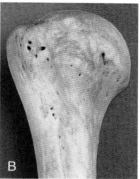

Fig. 6.5 (A) Anterior aspect of right proximal humerus. (B) Photograph of anterior aspect of proximal humerus.

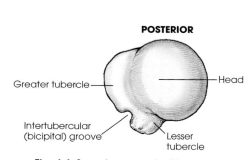

Fig. 6.6 Superior aspect of humerus.

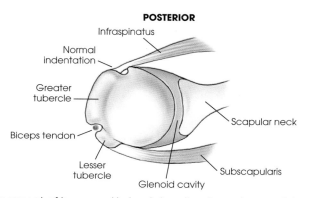

Fig. 6.7 Superior aspect of humerus. Horizontal section through scapulohumeral joint showing normal anatomic relationships.

221

Bursae are small, synovial fluid–filled sacs that relieve pressure and reduce friction in tissue. They are often found between the bones and the skin, and they allow the skin to move easily when the joint is moved. Bursae are found also between bones and ligaments, muscles, or tendons. One of the largest bursae of the shoulder is the *subacromial bursa* (Fig. 6.8). It is located under the acromion and lies between the deltoid muscle and the shoulder joint capsule. The subacromial bursa does not normally communicate with the joint. Other bursae of the shoulder are found superior to the acromion, between the coracoid process and the joint capsule, and between the capsule and the tendon of the subscapular muscle. Bursae become important radiographically when injury or age causes the deposition of calcium.

Shoulder Girdle Articulations

The three joints of the shoulder girdle are summarized in Table 6.1, and a detailed description follows.

SCAPULOHUMERAL ARTICULATION

The *scapulohumeral articulation* between the glenoid cavity and the head of the humerus forms a *synovial ball-and-socket* joint, allowing movement in all directions (Figs. 6.9 and 6.10). This joint is often referred to as the *glenohumeral* joint. Although many muscles connect with, support, and enter into the function of the shoulder joint, radiographers are chiefly concerned with the insertion points of the short rotator cuff muscles (Fig. 6.11). The insertion points of these muscles—the subscapular, supraspinatus, infraspinatus, and teres minor—have already been described.

TABLE 6.1
Joints of the shoulder girdle

| Joint | Structural classification | | Movement |
	Tissue	Type	
Scapulohumeral	Synovial	Ball and socket	Freely movable
Acromioclavicular	Synovial	Gliding	Freely movable
Sternoclavicular	Synovial	Double gliding	Free y movable

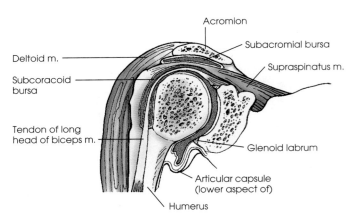

Fig. 6.8 Right shoulder bursae and muscles.

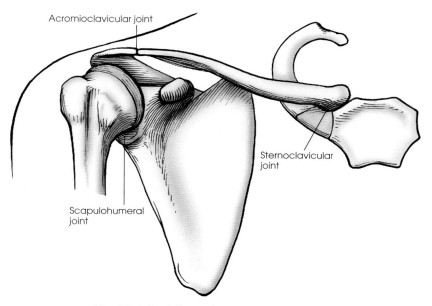

Fig. 6.9 Articulations of scapula and humerus.

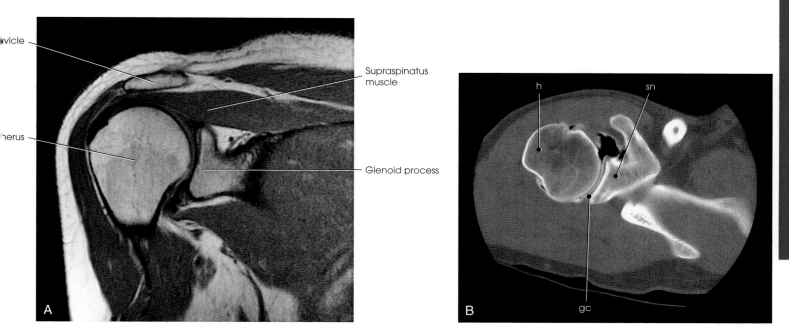

Fig. 6.10 (A) Coronal MRI of shoulder. Note articular cartilage around humeral head and muscles closely surrounding bone. (B) Axial CT of shoulder, midjoint. Note position of bones relative to each other and articular cartilage in glenoid cavity. *gc,* Glenoid cavity; *h,* humerus; *sn,* scapular neck.

(From Kelley LL, Petersen CM: *Sectional anatomy for imaging professionals.* ed 2, St Louis, 2007, Mosby.)

An articular capsule completely encloses the shoulder joint. The tendon of the long head of the biceps brachii muscle, which arises from the superior margin of the glenoid cavity, passes through the capsule of the shoulder joint, goes between its fibrous and synovial layers, arches over the head of the humerus, and descends through the intertubercular (bicipital) groove. The short head of the biceps arises from the coracoid process and, with the long head of the muscle, inserts in the radial tuberosity. Because it crosses with the shoulder and elbow joints, the biceps help to synchronize their action.

The interaction of movement among the wrist, elbow, and shoulder joints makes the position of the hand important in radiography of the upper limb. Any rotation of the hand also rotates the joints. The best approach to the study of the mechanics of joint and muscle action is to perform all movements ascribed to each joint and carefully note the reaction in remote parts.

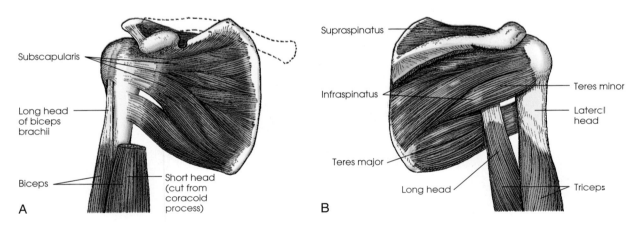

Fig. 6.11 (A) Muscles on costal (anterior) surface of scapula and proximal humerus. (B) Muscles on dorsal (posterior) surface of scapula and proximal humerus.

ACROMIOCLAVICULAR ARTICULATION

The *AC* articulation between the *acromion* of the scapula and the acromial extremity of the *clavicle* forms a *synovial gliding joint* (Fig. 6.12). It permits gliding and rotary (elevation, depression, protraction, and retraction) movement. Because the end of the clavicle rides higher than the adjacent surface of the acromion, the slope of the surfaces tends to favor displacement of the acromion downward and under the clavicle.

STERNOCLAVICULAR ARTICULATION

The *sternoclavicular* (SC) articulation is formed by the sternal extremity of the clavicle with two bones: the manubrium and the first rib cartilage (see Fig. 6.12). The union of the clavicle with the manubrium of the sternum is the only bony union between the upper limb and trunk. This articulation is a *synovial double-gliding* joint. However, the joint is adapted by a fibrocartilaginous disk to provide movements similar to a ball-and-socket joint: circumduction, elevation, depression, and forward and backward movements. The clavicle carries the scapula with it through any movement.

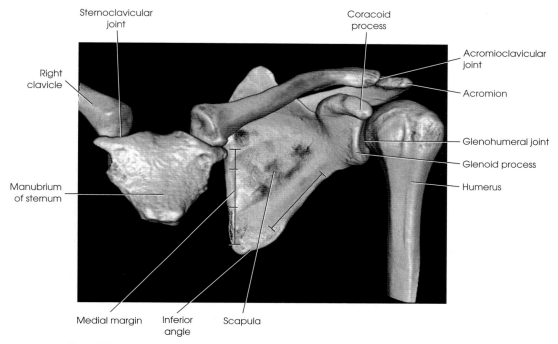

Fig. 6.12 Three-dimensional CT image of shoulder girdle. Note three articulations.

SUMMARY OF ANATOMY

Shoulder girdle	Dorsal surface	**Humerus (proximal**
Clavicle	Crest of spine	**aspect)**
Scapula	Acromion	Head
	Supraspinous fossa	Anatomic neck
Clavicle	Infraspinous fossa	Surgical neck
Body	Superior border	Intertubercular groove
Acromial extremity	Coracoid process	Greater tubercles
Sternal extremity	Scapular notch	Lesser tubercles
	Lateral border	Body
Scapula	Glenoid cavity	Bursae
Medial border	Lateral angle	Subacromial bursa
Body	Neck	
Costal surface		**Shoulder articulations**
Subscapular fossa		Scapulohumeral
Superior angle		Acromioclavicular
Inferior angle		Sternoclavicular

ABBREVIATIONS USED IN CHAPTER 6

AC	Acromioclavicular
SC	Sternoclavicular

See Addendum A for a summary of all abbreviations used in Volume 1.

SUMMARY OF PATHOLOGY

Condition	Definition
Bursitis	Inflammation of the bursa
Dislocation	Displacement of a bone from the joint space
Fracture	Disruption in the continuity of bone
Hill-Sachs defect	Impacted fracture of posterolateral aspect of the humeral head with dislocation
Metastasis	Transfer of a cancerous lesion from one area to another
Osteoarthritis or degenerative joint disease	Form of arthritis marked by progressive cartilage deterioration in synovial joints and vertebrae
Osteopetrosis	Increased density of atypically soft bone
Osteoporosis	Loss of bone density
Rheumatoid arthritis	Chronic, systemic, inflammatory collagen disease
Tendinitis	Inflammation of the tendon and tendon-muscle attachment
Tumor	New tissue growth where cell proliferation is uncontrolled
Chondrosarcoma	Malignant tumor arising from cartilage cells

Eponymous (named) pathologies are listed in nonpossessive form to conform to the AMA manual of style: a guide for authors and editors, ed 10, Oxford, Oxford University Press, 2009.

SAMPLE EXPOSURE TECHNIQUE CHART ESSENTIAL PROJECTIONS

These techniques were accurate for the equipment used to produce each exposure. However, use caution when applying them in your department because "there is considerable variability in image receptor response owing to varying scatter sensitivity, the use of grids with different grid ratios, collimation, beam filtration, the choice of kilovoltage, source-to-image distance, and image receptor size."[1]
This chart was created in collaboration with Dennis Bowman, AS, RT(R), Clinical Instructor, Community Hospital of the Monterey Peninsula, Monterey, CA. http://digitalradiographysolutions.com/.

SHOULDER GIRDLE

Part	cm	kVp[a]	SID[b]	Collimation	CR[c] mAs	CR[c] Dose (mGy)[e]	DR[d] mAs	DR[d] Dose (mGy)[e]
Shoulder—AP[f]	18	85	40"	11" × 9" (28 × 23 cm)	10[g]	1.328	4.5[g]	0.593
Shoulder—transthoracic lateral[f]	40	85	40"	6" × 10" (15 × 25 cm)	56	12.45	28	6.200
Shoulder—inferosuperior axial[f]	18	75	40"	7" × 5" (18 × 13 cm)	5[g]	0.423	2.5[g]	0.234
Shoulder—PA oblique scapular Y[f]	24	85	40"	6" × 6" (15 × 15 cm)	18[g]	2.570	10[g]	1.421
Intertubercular (bicipital) groove[h]	10	70	40"	3" × 3" (8 × 8 cm)	4[g]	0.149	2[g]	0.074
AC articulation—AP[f]	14	81	40"	3.5" × 3.5" (9 × 9 cm)	11[g]	0.692	5.6[g]	0.349
Clavicle—AP, PA[f]	16	81	40"	7" × 4" (18 × 10 cm)	10[g]	0.934	5.0[g]	0.464
Scapula—AP[f]	18	85	40"	7" × 8" (18 × 20 cm)	11[g]	1.422	5.5[g]	0.719
Scapula—lateral[f]	24	85	40"	6" × 8" (15 × 20 cm)	14[g]	2.082	8[g]	1.187

[1]ACR-AAPM-SIMM Practice Parameter for Digital Radiography, Revised 2017.
[a]kVp values are for a high-frequency generator.
[b]40-inch minimum; 44 to 48 inches recommended to improve spatial resolution (mAs increase needed, but no increase in patient dose will result).
[c]AGFA CR MD 4.0 General IP, CR 75.0 reader, 400 speed class, with 6:1 (178LPI) grid when needed.
[d]GE Definium 8000, with 13:1 grid when needed.
[e]All doses are skin entrance for average adult (160- to 200-pound male, 150- to 190-pound female) at part thickness indicated.
[f]Bucky/grid.
[g]Small focal spot.
[h]Tabletop, nongrid.

Radiation Protection

Protection of the patient from unnecessary radiation is a professional responsibility of the radiographer. In this chapter the *Shield gonads* statement at the end of the *Position of part* section indicates that the patient is to be protected from unnecessary radiation by using proper collimation and placing lead shielding between the gonads and the radiation source, when necessary.

Shoulder

🌟 AP PROJECTION

External, neutral, internal rotation humerus

NOTE: Do not have the patient rotate the arm if fracture or dislocation is suspected.

Image receptor + grid: Positioned by manufacturer or department protocol for proper anatomy display orientation; CR plate: 10 × 12 inches (24 × 30 cm); crosswise to include entire clavicle, lengthwise to include more humerus.

Position of patient

- Examine the patient in the upright or supine position, with coronal plane of thorax parallel to the IR. Shoulder and arm lesions, whether traumatic or pathologic in origin, are extremely sensitive to movement and pressure. For this reason, the upright position should be used whenever possible.

Position of part

- Center the shoulder joint to the midline of the grid.
- Adjust the position of the IR so that its center is 1 inch (2.5 cm) inferior to the coracoid process.

Shoulder Girdle

TABLE 6.2
Hand position and its effect on the proximal humerus

Description	Hand position	Proximal humerus position
Supinating hand and adjusting epicondyles parallel to the plane of the IR positions the humerus in *external rotation*	A	B AP shoulder. External rotation humerus. Greater tubercle *(arrow)*
Palm of the hand placed against hip and epicondyles adjusted at approximately a 45-degree angle with the plane of the IR positions the humerus in *neutral rotation*	A	B AP shoulder. Neutral rotation humerus. Greater tubercle *(arrows)*
Posterior aspect of hand may be placed against hip and epicondyles adjusted perpendicular to the plane of the IR to position the humerus in *internal rotation*	A	B AP shoulder. Internal rotation humerus. Greater tubercle *(arrows)*; lesser tubercle in profile *(arrowhead)*

AP, Anteroposterior; *IR,* image receptor.

External rotation humerus

- Ask the patient to supinate the hand, unless contraindicated (Table 6.2).
- Abduct the arm slightly, and rotate it so that the epicondyles are parallel with the plane of the IR. Externally rotating the entire arm from the neutral position places the shoulder and the entire humerus in the true anatomic position (Fig. 6.13).

Neutral rotation humerus

- Ask the patient to rest the palm of the hand against the thigh (see Table 6.2). This position of the arm rolls the humerus slightly internal into a neutral position, placing the epicondyles at an angle of approximately 45 degrees with the plane of the IR.

Internal rotation humerus

- Ask the patient to flex the elbow, rotate the arm internally, and rest the back of the hand on the hip (see Table 6.2).
- Adjust the arm to place the epicondyles perpendicular to the plane of the IR.
- *Shield gonads.*
- *Respiration*: Suspend.

Central ray

- Perpendicular to a point 1 inch (2.5 cm) inferior to the coracoid process, which can be palpated inferior to the clavicle and medial to the humeral head

Collimation

- Adjust radiation field to approximately 10 × 12 inches (24 × 30 cm) on the collimator. If crosswise include 1.5 inches (3.8 cm) above the shoulder, 1 inch (2.5 cm) beyond the lateral aspect of the shoulder, the sternal end of the clavicle and the proximal third of the humerus. If lengthwise, more humerus and less clavicle will be included. Place side marker in the collimated exposure field.

▼ COMPENSATING FILTER

Use of a specially designed compensating filter for the shoulder, called a boomerang, improves the quality of the image. See Chapter 1 for photo. These filters are particularly useful for this projection because all bony and soft tissue structures can be seen without the need to "window."

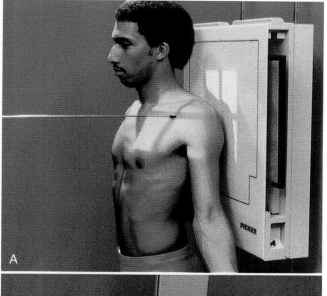
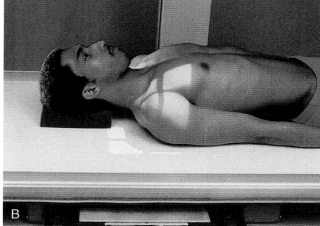

Fig. 6.13 (A) AP shoulder, external rotation humerus, standing position. (B) Same projection in supine position.

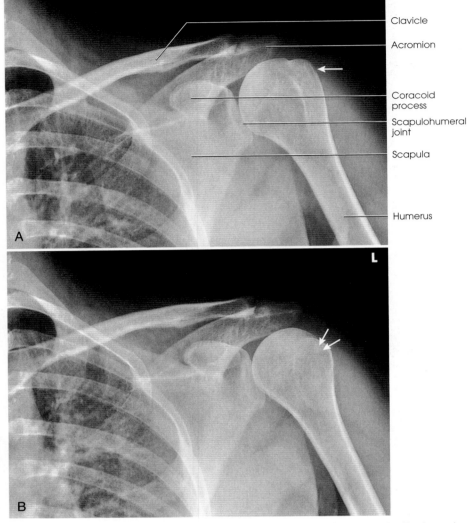

Clavicle

Acromion

Coracoid
process

Scapulohumeral
joint

Scapula

Humerus

Fig. 6.14 (A) AP shoulder, external rotation humerus: greater tubercle in profile *(arrow).*
(B) AP shoulder, neutral rotation humerus: greater tubercle *(arrows).*

Shoulder Girdle

Structures shown

The bony and soft structures of the shoulder and proximal humerus in the anatomic position (Figs. 6.14–6.16). The scapulohumeral joint relationship is seen.

External rotation: The greater tubercle of the humerus and the site of insertion of the supraspinatus tendon are visualized (see Fig. 6.14A).

Neutral rotation: The posterior part of the supraspinatus insertion, which sometimes profiles small calcific deposits not otherwise visualized (see Fig. 6.14B), is seen.

Internal rotation: The proximal humerus is seen in a true lateral position. When the arm can be abducted enough to clear the lesser tubercle from the lateral angle of the scapula, the site of the subscapular tendon insertion is seen (see Fig. 6.15).

EVALUATION CRITERIA

The following should be clearly seen:

- Evidence of proper collimation and presence of side marker placed clear of anatomy of interest
- Superior scapula, clavicle (entire if IR crosswise, lateral half if IR lengthwise), and proximal humerus
- Bony trabecular detail and surrounding soft tissues

External Rotation

- Humeral head in profile
- Greater tubercle in profile on lateral aspect of the humerus
- Scapulohumeral joint visualized with slight overlap of humeral head on glenoid cavity
- Outline of lesser tubercle between the humeral head and greater tubercle

Neutral Rotation

- Greater tubercle partially superimposing the humeral head
- Humeral head in partial profile
- Slight overlap of the humeral head on the glenoid cavity

Internal Rotation

- Lesser tubercle in profile and pointing medially
- Outline of the greater tubercle superimposing the humeral head
- Greater amount of humeral overlap of the glenoid cavity than in external and neutral positions

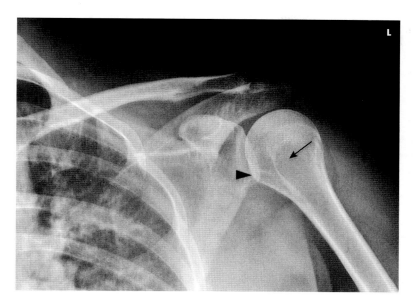

Fig. 6.15 AP shoulder, internal rotation humerus: greater tubercle *(arrow)*; lesser tubercle in profile *(arrowhead)*.

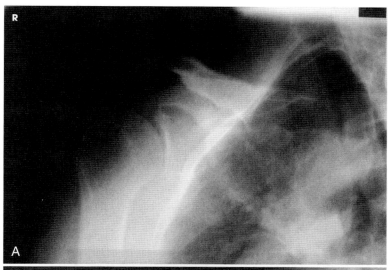

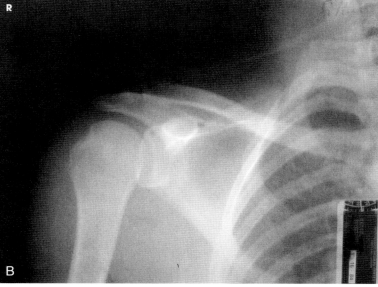

Fig. 6.16 (A) AP oblique projection of right shoulder without use of compensating filter. (B) AP projection of same patient with compensating filter. Note improved visualization of bony and soft tissue areas with filter.

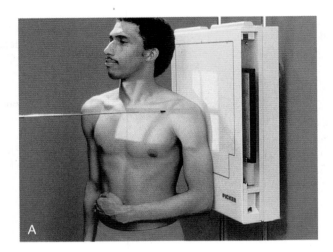

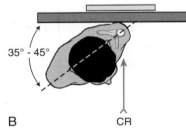

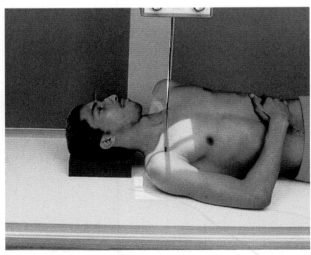

Fig. 6.17 (A) Upright AP oblique glenoid cavity: Grashey method. (B) Note position of shoulder and patient in relationship to IR.

Fig. 6.18 Recumbent AP oblique glenoid cavity: Grashey method.

Glenoid Cavity
AP OBLIQUE PROJECTION
GRASHEY METHOD
RPO or LPO position

Image receptor + grid: Positioned by manufacturer or department protocol for proper anatomy display orientation; CR plate: 10 × 12 inches (24 × 30 cm); crosswise to include entire clavicle, lengthwise to include more humerus.

Position of patient
- Place the patient in the supine or upright position. The upright position is more comfortable for the patient and assists in accurate adjustment of the part.

Position of part
- Center the IR to the scapulohumeral joint. The joint is 2 inches (5 cm) medial and 2 inches (5 cm) inferior to the superolateral border of the shoulder.
- Rotate the body approximately 35 to 45 degrees toward the affected side (Fig. 6.17).
- Adjust the degree of rotation to place the scapula parallel with the plane of the IR. This is accomplished by orienting the plane through the superior angle of the scapula and acromial tip, parallel to the IR.* The head of the humerus is in contact with the IR.
- If the patient is in the recumbent position, the body may need to be rotated more than 45 degrees (up to 60 degrees) to place the scapula parallel to the IR.
- Support the elevated shoulder and hip on sandbags (Fig. 6.18).
- Abduct the arm slightly in internal rotation, and place the palm of the hand on the abdomen. Other arm positions may be dictated by department protocol.
- *Shield gonads.*
- *Respiration:* Suspend.

*NOTE: These landmarks are recommended by Johnston et al.[1] as useful to identify the plane through the scapular body.

Central ray

- Perpendicular to the IR; the CR should be at a point 2 inches (5 cm) medial and 2 inches (5 cm) inferior to the superolateral border of the shoulder

Collimation

- Adjust radiation field to approximately 8 × 10 inches (18 × 24 cm) on the collimator. If crosswise, include 1.5 inches (3.8 cm) above the shoulder, 1 inch (2.5 cm) beyond the lateral aspect of the shoulder, the lateral half of the clavicle, and the proximal third of the humerus. If lengthwise, more humerus and less clavicle will be included. Place side marker in the collimated exposure field.

Structures shown

The joint space between the humeral head and the glenoid cavity (scapulohumeral or glenohumeral joint) (Figs. 6.19 and 6.20).

EVALUATION CRITERIA

The following should be clearly seen:
- Evidence of proper collimation and presence of side marker placed clear of anatomy of interest
- Open joint space between the humeral head and glenoid cavity
- Glenoid cavity in profile
- Bony trabecular detail and surrounding soft tissues

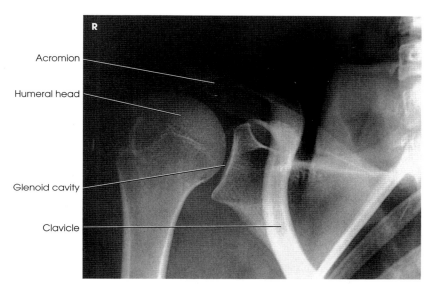

Acromion

Humeral head

Glenoid cavity

Clavicle

Fig. 6.19 AP oblique glenoid cavity: Grashey method.

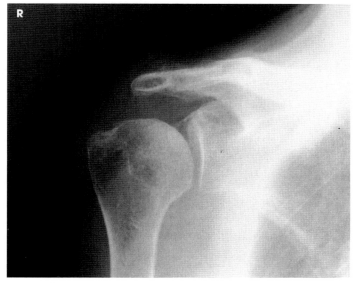

Fig. 6.20 AP oblique glenoid cavity: Grashey method showing moderate deterioration of scapulohumeral joint.

Glenoid Cavity
AP OBLIQUE PROJECTION
APPLE METHOD
RPO or LPO position

The Apple method[2] is similar to the Grashey method but uses weighted abduction to show loss of articular cartilage in the scapulohumeral joint.

Image receptor + grid: Positioned by manufacturer or department protocol for proper anatomy display orientation; CR plate: 10 × 12 inches (24 × 30 cm) crosswise.

Position of patient
- Place the patient in a seated or upright position.

Position of part
- Center the IR to the scapulohumeral joint.
- Rotate the body approximately 35 to 45 degrees toward the affected side.
- The posterior surface of the affected side is closest to the IR.

- The scapula should be positioned parallel to the plane of the IR (see Grashey method for positioning details).
- The patient should hold a 1-lb weight in the hand on the same side as the affected shoulder in a neutral position.
- While holding the weight, the patient should abduct the arm 90 degrees from the midline of the body (Fig. 6.21).
- *Shield gonads.*
- *Respiration:* Suspend.

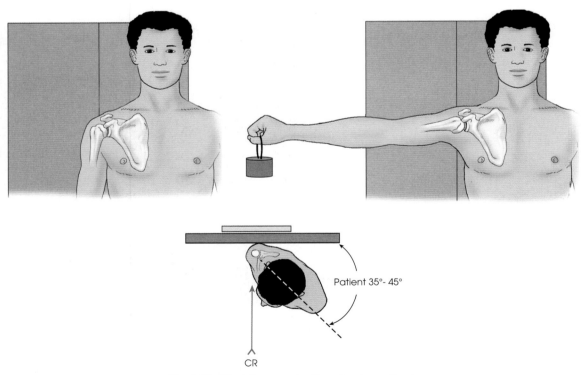

Fig. 6.21 AP oblique projection: Apple method.

Central ray

• Perpendicular to the IR at the level of the coracoid process

Collimation

Adjust radiation field to approximately 8 × 10 inches (18 × 24 cm) on the collimator. Adjust as needed to include 1.5 inches (3.8 cm) above the shoulder, 1 inch (2.5 cm) beyond the lateral aspect of the shoulder, the lateral half of the clavicle, and the proximal third of the humerus. Place side marker in the collimated exposure field.

NOTE: To avoid motion, have the correct technical factors set on the generator and be ready to make the exposure before the patient abducts the arm.

Structures shown

The scapulohumeral joint (Fig. 6.22), with joint space narrowing if present.

EVALUATION CRITERIA

The following should be clearly seen:
■ Evidence of proper collimation and presence of side marker placed clear of anatomy of interest
■ Glenoid cavity in profile
■ The arm in a 90-degree abducted position
■ Open joint space between the humeral head and the glenoid cavity
■ Bony trabecular detail and surrounding soft tissues

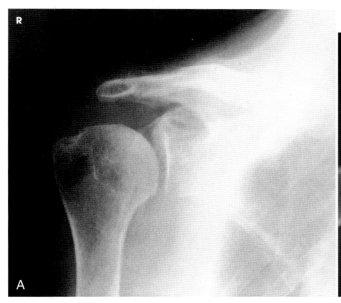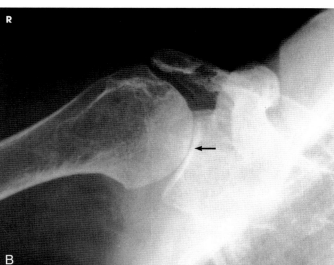

Fig. 6.22 (A) AP oblique projection: Grashey method, with shoulder showing normal scapulohumeral joint space. (B) AP oblique projection: Apple method, with weighted abduction showing loss of articular cartilage *(arrow)*.

TRANSTHORACIC LATERAL PROJECTION

LAWRENCE METHOD

Right or left position

The Lawrence[3] method is used when trauma exists and the arm cannot be rotated or abducted because of an injury. This method results in a projection 90 degrees from the AP projection and shows the relationship between the proximal humerus and the scapula.

Image receptor + grid: Positioned by manufacturer or department protocol for proper anatomy display orientation; CR plate: 10 × 12 inches (24 × 30 cm) lengthwise.

Position of patient

- Although this projection can be carried out with the patient in the upright or supine position, the upright position is much easier on a trauma patient. It also assists accurate adjustment of the shoulder.
- For upright positioning, seat or stand the patient in the lateral position before a vertical grid device (Fig. 6.23).
- If an upright position is impossible, place the patient in a recumbent position on the table with radiolucent pads elevating the head and shoulders (Fig. 6.24).

Position of part

- Have the patient raise the noninjured arm, rest the forearm on the head, and elevate the shoulder as much as possible (see Fig. 6.23). Elevation of the noninjured shoulder drops the injured side, separating the shoulders to prevent superimposition. Ensure that the midcoronal plane is perpendicular to the IR.
- No attempt should be made to rotate or otherwise to move the injured arm.
- Center the IR to the surgical neck area of the affected humerus.
- *Shield gonads.*
- *Respiration:* Full inspiration. Having the lungs full of air improves the contrast and decreases the exposure necessary to penetrate the body.
- If the patient can be sufficiently immobilized to prevent voluntary motion, a breathing technique can be used to blur the pulmonary vasculature In this case, instruct the patient to practice slow, deep breathing. A minimum exposure time of 3 seconds (4 to 5 seconds is desirable) gives excellent results when low milliamperage is used.

Central ray

- Perpendicular to the IR, entering the midcoronal plane at the level of the surgical neck
- If the patient cannot elevate the unaffected shoulder, angle the CR 10 to 15 degrees cephalad to obtain a comparable radiograph.

Collimation

- Adjust radiation field to 10 × 12 inches (24 × 30 cm) on the collimator. The field of light on the skin appears smaller because of the distance from the IR. Do not collimate larger than stated size. Place side marker in the collimated exposure field.

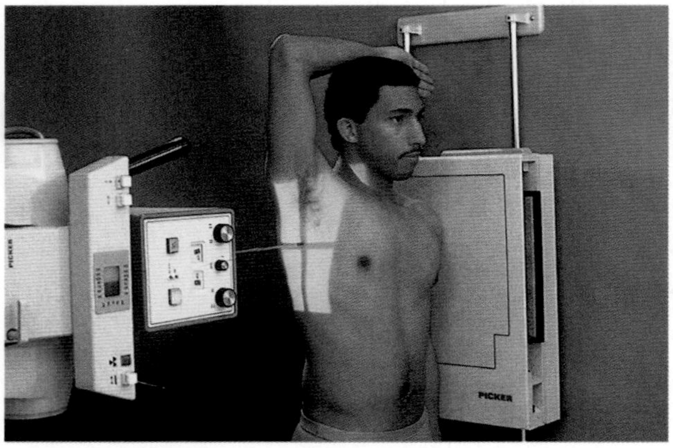

Fig. 6.23 Upright transthoracic lateral shoulder: Lawrence method.

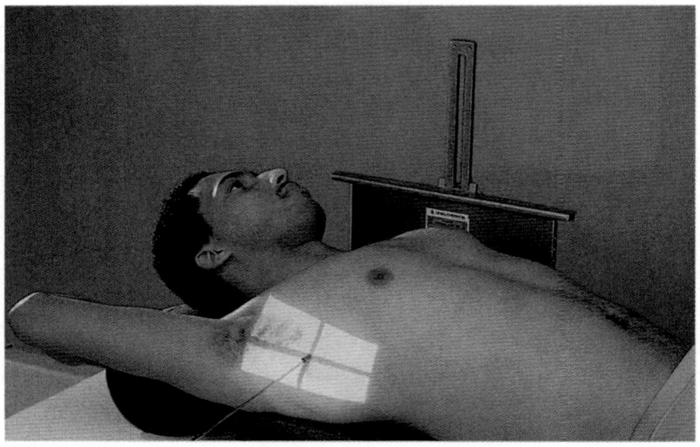

Fig. 6.24 Recumbent transthoracic lateral shoulder: Lawrence method.

Structures shown

A lateral image of the shoulder and proximal humerus is projected through the thorax (Figs. 6.25 and 6.26).

EVALUATION CRITERIA

The following should be clearly seen:

- Evidence of proper collimation and presence of side marker placed clear of anatomy of interest
- Scapula, clavicle, and proximal humerus seen through the lung field
- Scapula superimposed over the thoracic spine
- Unaffected clavicle and humerus projected above the shoulder closest to the IR

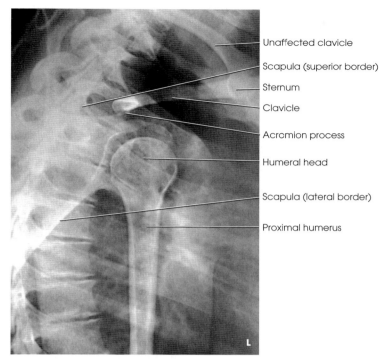

Unaffected clavicle
Scapula (superior border)
Sternum
Clavicle
Acromion process
Humeral head
Scapula (lateral border)
Proximal humerus

Fig. 6.25 Transthoracic lateral shoulder: Lawrence method.

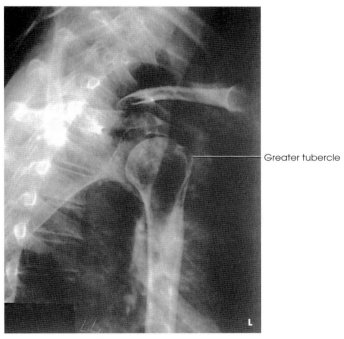

Greater tubercle

Fig. 6.26 Transthoracic lateral shoulder (patient breathing): Lawrence method.

♠ INFEROSUPERIOR AXIAL PROJECTION
LAWRENCE METHOD[4]

INFEROSUPERIOR AXIAL PROJECTION
RAFERT ET AL.[5] MODIFICATION

Image receptor + grid: Positioned by manufacturer or department protocol for proper anatomy display orientation; CR plate: 10 × 12 inches (24 × 30 cm) grid crosswise, placed in the vertical orientation in contact with the superior surface of the shoulder.

Position of patient
- With the patient in the supine position, elevate the head, shoulders, and elbow approximately 3 inches (7.6 cm) on a radiolucent sponge.

Position of part
Lawrence method
- As much as possible, abduct the arm of the affected side at right angles to the long axis of the body. A minimum of 20 degrees is required to prevent superimposition of the arm on the shoulder.
- Keep the humerus in *external rotation,* and adjust the forearm and hand in a comfortable position, grasping a vertical support or extended on sandbags or a firm pillow. Support may be necessary under the forearm and hand. Provide the patient with an extension board for the arm.
- Have the patient turn the head away from the side being examined so that the IR can be placed against the neck.
- Place the IR on the edge against the shoulder and as close as possible to the neck.

- Support the IR in position with sandbags, or use a vertical IR holder (Fig. 6.27).
Rafert modification
- Anterior dislocation of the humeral head can result in a wedge-shaped compression fracture of the articular surface of the humeral head, called the *Hill-Sachs defect.*[6] The fracture is located on the posterolateral humeral head. An *exaggerated external rotation* of the arm may be required to see the defect.
- With the patient in position exactly as for the Lawrence method, externally rotate the extended arm until the hand forms a 45-degree oblique angle. The thumb is pointing downward (Fig. 6.28).
- Assist the patient in rotating the arm to avoid overstressing the shoulder joint.
- *Shield gonads.*
- *Respiration:* Suspend.

Central ray
Lawrence method
- Horizontally through the axilla to the region of the AC articulation. The degree of medial angulation of the CR depends on the degree of abduction of the arm. The degree of medial angulation is often between 15 degrees and 30 degrees. The greater the abduction, the greater the angle.
Rafert modification
- Horizontal and angled approximately 15 degrees medially, entering the axilla and passing through the AC joint.

Collimation
- Adjust radiation field to 12 inches (30 cm) in width on the collimator and to 1 inch (2.5 cm) above the anterior shadow of the shoulder. Place side marker in the collimated exposure field.

Structures shown
An inferosuperior axial image of the proximal humerus, scapulohumeral joint, lateral portion of the coracoid process, and AC articulation. The insertion site of the subscapular tendon on the lesser tubercle of the humerus and the point of insertion of the teres minor tendon on the greater tubercle of the humerus are also shown. A Hill-Sachs compression fracture on the posterolateral humeral head may be seen using the Rafert modification (Figs. 6.29 and 6.30).

EVALUATION CRITERIA
The following should be clearly seen:
- Evidence of proper collimation and presence of side marker placed clear of anatomy of interest
- Scapulohumeral joint with slight overlap
- Coracoid process, pointing anteriorly
- Lesser tubercle in profile and directed anteriorly
- AC joint, acromion, and acromial end of clavicle projected through the humeral head
- Bony trabecular detail and surrounding soft tissues

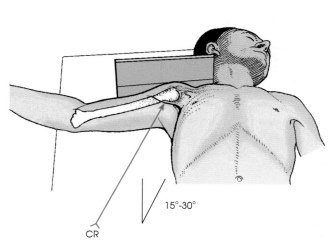

15°-30°

CR

Fig. 6.27 Inferosuperior axial shoulder joint: Lawrence method.

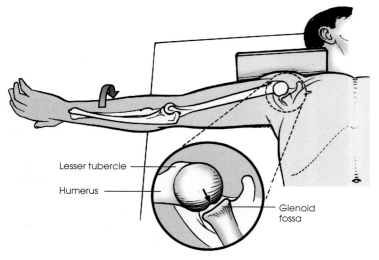

Lesser tubercle

Humerus

Glenoid fossa

Fig. 6.28 Inferosuperior axial shoulder joint: Rafert modification. Note exaggerated external rotation of arm and thumb pointing downward. If present, a Hill-Sachs defect would show as a wedge-shaped depression on posterior aspect of articulating surface of humeral head (*arrow*).

(From Rafert JA, Long BW, Hernandez EM, Kreipke DL: Axillary shoulder with exaggerated rotation: the Hill-Sachs defect. *Radiol Technol* 62:18, 1990.)

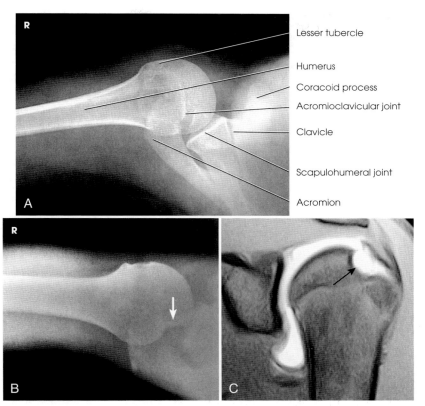

Lesser tubercle

Humerus

Coracoid process

Acromioclavicular joint

Clavicle

Scapulohumeral joint

Acromion

Fig. 6.29 (A) Inferosuperior axial shoulder joint: Lawrence method. (B) Inferosuperior axial shoulder joint: Rafert modification showing Hill-Sachs defect *(arrow)*. (C) Coronal MRI of shoulder joint showing Hill-Sachs defect *(arrow)* after recurrent shoulder dislocation.

(A and B, From Rafert JA, Long BW, Hernandez EM, Kreipke DL: Axillary shoulder with exaggerated rotation: the Hill-Sachs defect. *Radiol Technol* 62:18, 1990. C, From Jackson SA, Thomas RM: *Cross-sectional imaging made easy,* New York, 2004, Churchill Livingstone.)

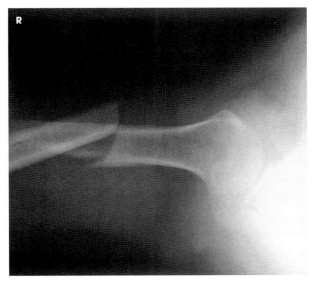

Fig. 6.30 Inferosuperior axial shoulder joint: Lawrence method showing comminuted fracture of humerus. The patient came into emergency department with arm extended out.

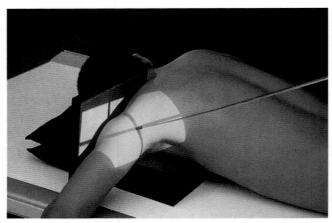

Fig. 6.31 Inferosuperior axial shoulder joint: West Point method.

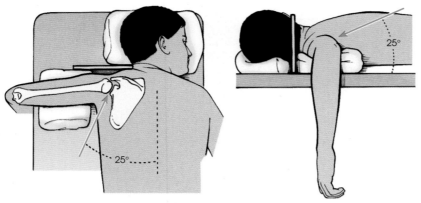

Fig. 6.32 West Point method with anterior and medial central ray angulation.

INFEROSUPERIOR AXIAL PROJECTION

WEST POINT METHOD

The West Point[7] method is used when chronic instability of the shoulder is suspected and to show bony abnormalities of the anterior inferior glenoid rim. Associated Hill-Sachs defect of the posterior lateral aspect of the humeral head is also shown.

> **Image receptor + grid:** Positioned by manufacturer or department protocol for proper anatomy display orientation; CR plate: 10 × 12 inches (24 × 30 cm) crosswise, placed in the vertical orientation in contact with the superior surface of the shoulder.

Position of patient

- Adjust the patient in the prone position with approximately a 3-inch (7.6-cm) pad under the shoulder being examined.
- Turn the patient's head away from the side being examined.

Position of part

- Abduct the arm of the affected side *90 degrees,* and rotate so that the forearm rests over the edge of the table or a Bucky tray, which may be used for support (Figs. 6.31 and 6.32).
- Place a vertically supported IR against the superior aspect of the shoulder with the edge of the IR in contact with the neck.
- Support the IR with sandbags or a vertical IR holder.
- *Shield gonads.*
- *Respiration:* Suspend.

Central ray

- Directed at a dual angle of 25 degrees *anteriorly* from the horizontal and 25 degrees *medially*. The CR enters approximately 5 inches (13 cm) inferior and 1½ inches (3.8 cm) medial to the acromial edge and exits the glenoid cavity.

Collimation

- Adjust radiation field to 12 inches (30 cm) in width on the collimator and to 1 inch (2.5 cm) above the posterior shadow of the shoulder. Place side marker in the collimated exposure field.

Structures shown

Bony abnormalities of the anterior inferior rim of the glenoid and Hill-Sachs defects of the posterolateral humeral head in patients with chronic instability of the shoulder (Fig. 6.33).

EVALUATION CRITERIA

The following should be clearly seen:
- Evidence of proper collimation and presence of side marker placed clear of anatomy of interest
- Scapulohumeral joint with slight overlap
- Humeral head projected free of the coracoid process
- Acromion superimposed over the posterior portion of the humeral head
- Bony trabecular detail and surrounding soft tissues

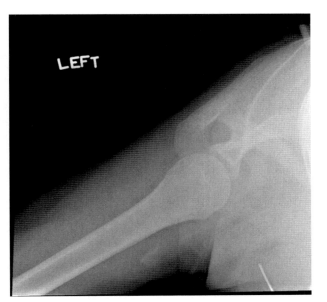

Fig. 6.33 Inferosuperior axial shoulder joint: West Point method.

(Courtesy April S. Apple, RT(R), FASRT.)

SUPEROINFERIOR AXIAL PROJECTION

Image receptor + grid: Positioned by manufacturer or department protocol for proper anatomy display orientation; CR plate: 10 × 12 inches (24 × 30 cm), placed lengthwise for accurate centering to shoulder joint.

Position of patient

- Seat the patient at the end of the table on a stool or chair high enough to enable extension of the shoulder under examination well over the IR.

Position of part

- Place the IR near the end of the table and parallel with its long axis.
- Have the patient lean laterally over the IR until the shoulder joint is over the midpoint of the IR.
- Bring the elbow to rest on the table.
- Flex the patient's elbow 90 degrees, and place the hand in the prone position (Fig. 6.34).
- Have the patient tilt the head toward the unaffected shoulder.
- To obtain direct lateral positioning of the head of the humerus, adjust any anterior or posterior leaning of the body to place the humeral epicondyles in the vertical position.
- *Shield gonads.*
- *Respiration:* Suspend.

Central ray

- Angled 5 to 15 degrees through the shoulder joint and toward the elbow; a greater angle is required when the patient cannot extend the shoulder over the IR.

Collimation

- Adjust radiation field to 10 inches (24 cm) in width on the collimator and to 1 inch (2.5 cm) beyond the anterior and posterior shadows of the shoulder. Place side marker in the collimated exposure field.

Structures shown

A superoinferior axial image shows the joint relationship of the proximal end of the humerus and the glenoid cavity (Fig. 6.35). The AC articulation, the outer portion of the coracoid process, and the points of insertion of the subscapularis muscle (at body of scapula) and teres minor muscle (at inferior axillary border) are shown.

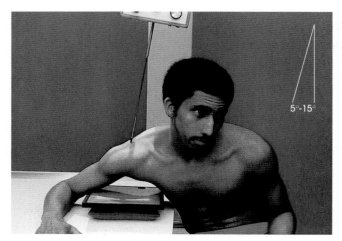

5°-15°

Fig. 6.34 Superoinferior axial shoulder joint: standard IR.

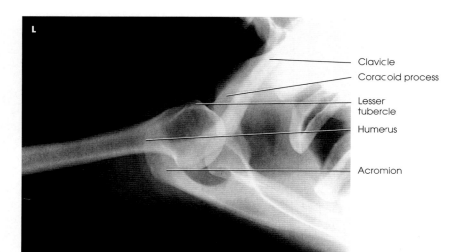

L

Clavicle

Coracoid process

Lesser tubercle

Humerus

Acromion

Fig. 6.35 Superoinferior axial shoulder joint.

EVALUATION CRITERIA

The following should be clearly seen:
- Evidence of proper collimation and presence of side marker placed clear of anatomy of interest
- Scapulohumeral joint (not open on patients with limited flexibility)
- Coracoid process projected above the clavicle
- Lesser tubercle in profile
- AC joint through the humeral head
- Bony trabecular detail and surrounding soft tissues

Scapular Y

♠ PA OBLIQUE PROJECTION
RAO or LAO position

This projection, described by Rubin et al.,[8] obtained its name as a result of the appearance of the scapula. The body of the scapula forms the vertical component of the Y, and the acromion and the coracoid process form the upper limbs. This projection is useful in the evaluation of suspected shoulder dislocations.

Image receptor + grid: Positioned by manufacturer or department protocol for proper anatomy display orientation; CR plate: 10 × 12 inches (24 × 30 cm) lengthwise.

Position of patient
- Radiograph the patient in the upright or recumbent body position; the upright position is preferred.
- When the patient is severely injured and recumbent, modify the anterior oblique position by placing the patient in the posterior oblique position. This position does not require the patient to lie on the injured shoulder.

Position of part
- Position the anterior surface of the shoulder being examined against the upright Bucky.
- Rotate the patient so that the midcoronal plane forms an angle of 45 to 60 degrees to the IR. The position of the arm is not critical because it does not

alter the relationship of the humeral head to the glenoid cavity (Fig. 6.36). Palpate the scapula, and place its flat surface perpendicular to the IR. According to Johnson et al.,[1] this is accomplished by orienting the plane through the superior angle of the scapula and acromial tip, perpendicular to the IR.
- Position the center of the IR at the level of the scapulohumeral joint.
- *Shield gonads.*
- *Respiration:* Suspend.

▼ COMPENSATING FILTER

Use of a specially designed compensating filter for the shoulder, called a boomerang, improves the quality of the image because of the large amount of primary beam radiation striking the IR.

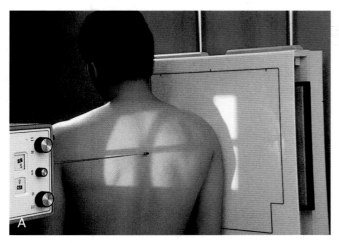
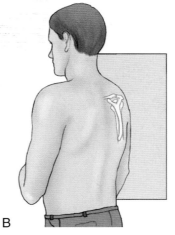
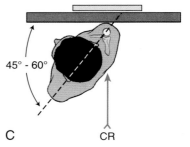

45° - 60°

CR

Fig. 6.36 (A) PA oblique shoulder joint. (B) Perspective from x-ray tube showing scapula centered in true lateral position. (C) Top-down view showing positioning landmarks used for proper orientation of scapular body.

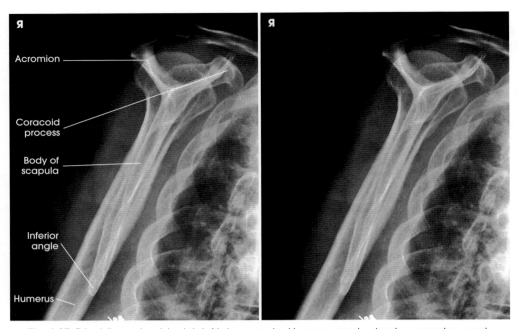

Acromion

Coracoid process

Body of scapula

Inferior angle

Humerus

Fig. 6.37 PA oblique shoulder joint. Note scapular Y components—body, acromion, and coracoid process.

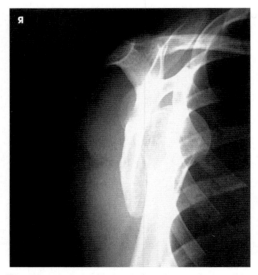

Fig. 6.38 PA oblique shoulder joint showing anterior dislocation (humeral head projected beneath coracoid process).

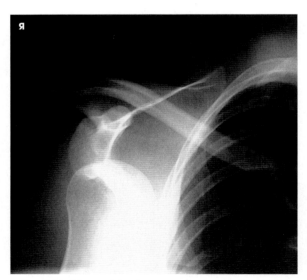

Fig. 6.39 AP shoulder (same patient as in Fig. 6.38).

Central ray

- Perpendicular to the scapulohumeral joint (Table 6.3)

Collimation

- Adjust radiation field to 12 inches (30 cm) in length on the collimator and to 1 inch (2.5 cm) beyond the lateral shadow. Place side marker in the collimated exposure field.

Structures shown

The scapular Y is shown on an oblique image of the shoulder. In the normal shoulder, the humeral head is directly superimposed over the junction of the Y (Fig. 6.37). In anterior (subcoracoid) dislocations, the humeral head is beneath the coracoid process (Fig. 6.38); in posterior (subacromial) dislocations, it is projected beneath the acromion. An AP shoulder projection is shown for comparison (Fig. 6.39).

EVALUATION CRITERIA

The following should be clearly seen:
- Evidence of proper collimation and presence of side marker placed clear of anatomy of interest
- Humeral head and glenoid cavity superimposed
- Humeral shaft and scapular body superimposed
- No superimposition of the scapular body over the bony thorax
- Acromion projected laterally and free of superimposition
- Coracoid possibly superimposed or projected below the clavicle
- Scapula in lateral profile with lateral and vertebral borders superimposed
- Bony trabecular detail and surrounding soft tissues

TABLE 6.3
Similar shoulder projections

Name	Body rotation	Scapula relationship to IR	Central ray angle[a]	Central ray entrance point[a]	Arm position[a]
Shoulder joint: Neer method	45–60 degrees	Perpendicular	10–15 degrees border caudad	Superior humeral	At side
Shoulder joint: scapular Y	45–60 degrees	Perpendicular	0 degrees	Scapulohumeral joint	At side
Scapula lateral	45–60 degrees	Perpendicular	0 degrees	Center of medial border of scapula	Variable

[a]Central ray angles and entrance points and arm positions are the only differences among these three projections.

Supraspinatus "Outlet"
TANGENTIAL PROJECTION
NEER METHOD
RAO or LAO position

This radiographic projection is useful to show tangentially the coracoacromial arch or outlet to diagnose shoulder impingement.[9,10] The tangential image is obtained by projecting the x-ray beam under the acromion and AC joint, which defines the superior border of the coracoacromial outlet.

Image receptor + grid: Positioned by manufacturer or department protocol for proper anatomy display orientation; CR plate: 10 × 12 inches (24 × 30 cm) lengthwise.

Position of patient
- Place the patient in a seated or standing position facing the vertical grid device.

Position of part
- With the patient's affected shoulder centered and in contact with the IR, rotate the patient's unaffected side away from the IR. Palpate the flat aspect of the affected scapula, and place it perpendicular to the IR. The degree of patient obliquity varies from patient to patient. The average degree of patient rotation varies from 45 to 60 degrees from the plane of the IR (Fig. 6.40).
- Place the patient's arm at the patient's side.
- *Shield gonads.*
- *Respiration:* Suspend.

Central ray
- Angled 10 to 15 degrees caudad, entering the superior aspect of the humeral head (see Table 6.3)

Collimation
- Adjust radiation field to 12 inches (30 cm) in length on the collimator and to 1 inch (2.5 cm) beyond the lateral shadow. Place side marker in the collimated exposure field.

Structures shown
The tangential outlet image shows the posterior surface of the acromion and the AC joint identified as the superior border of the coracoacromial outlet (Figs. 6.41 and 6.42).

EVALUATION CRITERIA
The following should be clearly seen:
- Evidence of proper collimation and presence of side marker placed clear of anatomy of interest
- Humeral head projected below the AC joint
- Humeral head and AC joint with bony detail
- Humerus and scapular body, generally parallel
- Bony trabecular detail and surrounding soft tissues

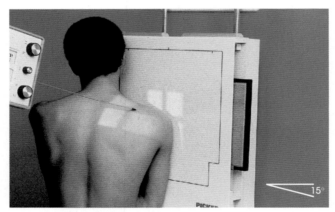

Fig. 6.40 Tangential supraspinatus "outlet" projection.

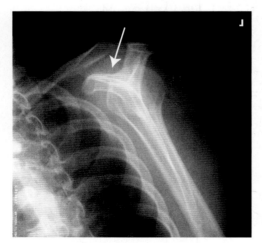

Fig. 6.41 Shoulder joint: Neer method. Supraspinatus outlet *(arrow).*

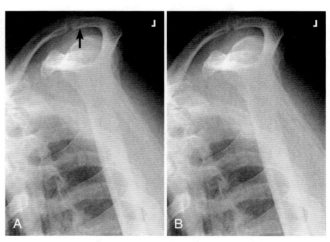

Fig. 6.42 (A) Tangential supraspinatus outlet projection showing impingement of shoulder outlet by subacromial spur *(arrow).* (B) Radiograph of same patient as in Fig. 6.41 after surgical removal of posterolateral surface of clavicle.

AP AXIAL PROJECTION

Image receptor + grid: Positioned by manufacturer or department protocol for proper anatomy display orientation; CR plate: 10 × 12 inches (24 × 30 cm) crosswise.

Position of patient

- Position the patient in the upright or supine position.

Position of part

- Center the scapulohumeral joint of the shoulder being examined to the midline of the grid (Fig. 6.43).
- *Shield gonads.*
- *Respiration:* Suspend.

Central ray

- Directed through the scapulohumeral joint at a cephalic angle of 35 degrees

Collimation

- Adjust radiation field to 10 × 10 inches (24 × 24 cm) on the collimator. Place side marker in the collimated exposure field.

Structures shown

The axial image shows the relationship of the head of the humerus to the glenoid cavity. This is useful in diagnosing cases of posterior dislocation (Fig. 6.44). It also shows the entire coracoid process.

EVALUATION CRITERIA

The following should be clearly seen:
- Evidence of proper collimation and presence of side marker placed clear of anatomy of interest
- Scapulohumeral joint
- Proximal humerus
- Clavicle projected above superior angle of scapula
- Coracoid process
- Bony trabecular detail and surrounding soft tissues

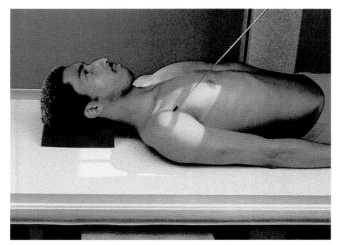

Fig. 6.43 AP axial shoulder joint.

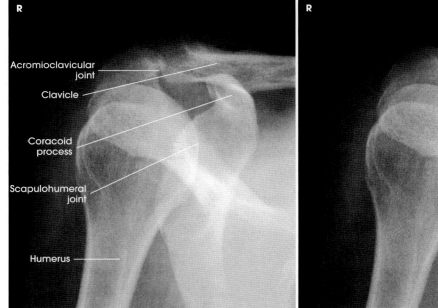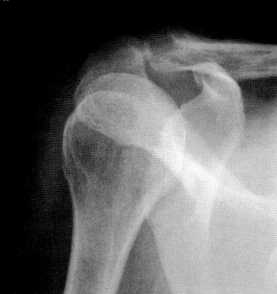

Fig. 6.44 AP axial shoulder joint.

Shoulder Joint

Proximal Humerus
AP AXIAL PROJECTION
STRYKER NOTCH METHOD

Anterior dislocations of the shoulder frequently result in posterior defects involving the posterolateral head of the humerus. Such defects, called *Hill-Sachs defects*,[6] are often not shown using conventional radiographic positions. Hall et al.[11] described the notch projection, from ideas expressed by Stryker, as being useful to show this humeral defect.

> **Image receptor + grid:** Positioned by manufacturer or department protocol for proper anatomy display orientation; CR plate: 10 × 12 inches (24 × 30 cm) lengthwise.

Position of patient

- Place the patient on the radiographic table in the supine position.

Position of part

- With the coracoid process of the affected shoulder centered to the table, ask the patient to flex the arm slightly beyond 90 degrees and place the palm of the hand on top of the head with fingertips resting on the head. (This hand position places the humerus in a slight internal rotation position.) The body of the humerus is adjusted to be vertical so that it is parallel to the midsagittal plane of the body (Fig. 6.45).
- *Shield gonads.*
- *Respiration:* Suspend.

Central ray

- Angled 10 degrees cephalad, entering the coracoid process

Collimation

- Adjust radiation field to 10 × 12 inches (24 × 30 cm) on the collimator. Place side marker in the collimated exposure field.

Structures shown

The posterosuperior and posterolateral areas of the humeral head (Figs. 6.46 and 6.47).

EVALUATION CRITERIA

The following should be clearly seen:

- Evidence of proper collimation and presence of side marker placed clear of anatomy of interest
- Overlapping of coracoid process and clavicle
- Posterolateral lateral aspect of humeral head in profile
- Long axis of the humerus aligned with the long axis of the patient's body
- Bony trabecular detail and surrounding soft tissues

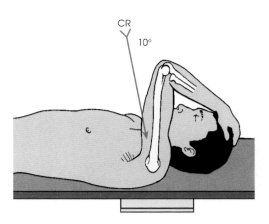

Fig. 6.45 AP axial humeral notch: Stryker notch method.

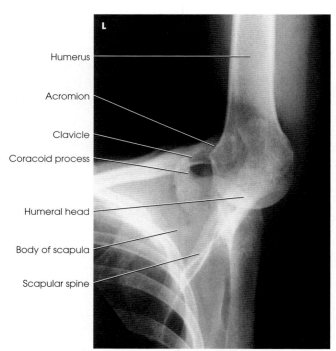

Fig. 6.46 AP axial humeral notch: Stryker notch method.

Humerus

Acromion

Clavicle

Coracoid process

Humeral head

Body of scapula

Scapular spine

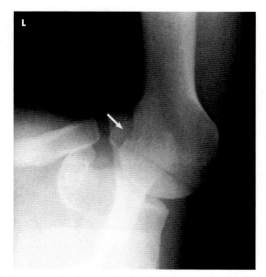

Fig. 6.47 Same projection as in Fig. 6.46 in a patient with small Hill-Sachs defect *(arrow)*.

Glenoid Cavity
AP AXIAL OBLIQUE PROJECTION
GARTH METHOD
RPO or LPO position

This projection is recommended for assessing acute shoulder trauma and for identifying posterior scapulohumeral dislocations, glenoid fractures, Hill-Sachs lesions, and soft tissue calcifications.[12]

> **Image receptor + grid:** Positioned by manufacturer or department protocol for proper anatomy display orientation; CR plate: 10 × 12 inches (24 × 30 cm) lengthwise.

Position of patient

- Place the patient in the supine, seated, or upright position.

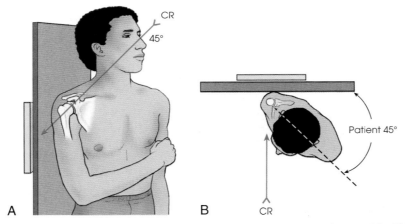

Fig. 6.48 (A) AP axial oblique: Garth method, RPO position. Note 45-degree CR. (B) Top view of same position as in (A). Note 45-degree patient position.

Position of part

- Center the IR to the glenohumeral joint.
- Rotate the body approximately 45 degrees toward the affected side.
- The posterior surface of the affected side is closest to the IR.
- Flex the elbow of the affected arm and place arm across the chest (Fig. 6.48).
- *Shield gonads.*
- *Respiration:* Suspend.

Central ray

- Angled 45 degrees caudad through the scapulohumeral joint

Collimation

- Adjust radiation field to 10 × 12 inches (24 × 30 cm) on the collimator. Adjust as needed to include 1.5 inches (3.8 cm) above the shoulder, 1 inch (2.5 cm) beyond the lateral aspect of the shoulder, the lateral half of the clavicle, and the proximal third of the humerus. Place side marker in the collimated exposure field.

Structures shown

The scapulohumeral joint, humeral head, coracoid process, and scapular head and neck (Fig. 6.49).

EVALUATION CRITERIA

The following should be clearly seen:
- Evidence of proper collimation and presence of side marker placed clear of anatomy of interest
- The scapulohumeral joint, humeral head, lateral angle, and scapular neck free of superimposition
- The coracoid process should be well visualized.
- Posterior dislocations project the humeral head *superiorly* from the glenoid cavity, and anterior dislocations project *inferiorly.*
- Bony trabecular detail and surrounding soft tissues

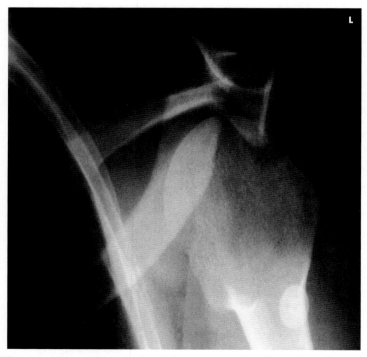

Fig. 6.49 AP axial oblique: Garth method showing anterior dislocation of proximal humerus. Humeral head is shown below coracoid process, a common appearance with anterior dislocation.

(Courtesy Bruce W. Long, MS, RT(R)(CV), and John A. Rafert, MS, RT(R).)

Intertubercular (Bicipital) Groove
TANGENTIAL PROJECTION
FISK MODIFICATION

Various modifications of the intertubercular (bicipital) groove image have been devised. In all cases the CR is aligned to be tangential to the intertubercular (bicipital) groove, which lies on the anterior surface of the humerus.[13]

The x-ray tube head assembly may limit the performance of this examination. Some radiographic units have large collimators or handles, or both, that limit flexibility in positioning. A mobile radiographic unit may be used to reduce this difficulty.

> **Image receptor:** Positioned by manufacturer or department protocol for proper anatomy display orientation; CR plate: 10 × 12 inches (24 × 30 cm) crosswise.

Position of patient

- Place the patient in the supine, seated, or standing position.
- To improve centering, extend the chin or rotate the head away from the affected side.

Position of part

- With the patient supine, palpate the anterior surface of the shoulder to locate the intertubercular (bicipital) groove.
- With the patient's hand in the supinated position, place the IR against the superior surface of the shoulder and immobilize the IR as shown in Fig. 6.50.
- *Shield gonads.*
- *Respiration:* Suspend.

Fisk modification. Fisk first described this position with the patient standing at the end of the radiographic table. This uses a greater object-to-image receptor distance (OID). The following steps are then taken with the Fisk technique:

- Instruct the patient to flex the elbow and lean forward far enough to place the posterior surface of the forearm on the table. The patient supports and grasps the IR as depicted in Fig. 6.51.
- For radiation protection and for reduction of backscatter to the IR from the forearm, place a lead shielding between the IR back and the forearm.
- Place a sandbag under the hand to place the IR horizontal.
- Have the patient lean forward or backward as required to place the vertical humerus at an angle of 10 to 15 degrees.

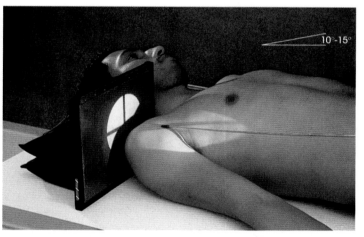

Fig. 6.50 Supine tangential intertubercular groove.

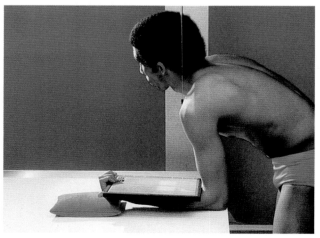

Fig. 6.51 Standing tangential intertubercular groove: Fisk modification.

Central ray

- Angled 10 to 15 degrees posterior (downward from horizontal) to the long axis of the humerus for the supine position (see Fig. 6.50)

  Fisk modification

- Perpendicular to the IR when the patient is leaning forward and the vertical humerus is positioned 10 to 15 degrees (see Fig. 6.51)

Collimation

- Adjust radiation field to 4 × 4 inches (10 × 10 cm) on the collimator. Place side marker in the collimated exposure field.

Structures shown

The tangential image profiles the intertubercular (bicipital) groove free from superimposition of the surrounding shoulder structures (Figs. 6.52 and 6.53).

EVALUATION CRITERIA

The following should be clearly seen:

- Evidence of proper collimation and presence of side marker placed clear of anatomy of interest
- Intertubercular (bicipital) groove in profile
- Bony trabecular detail and surrounding soft tissues

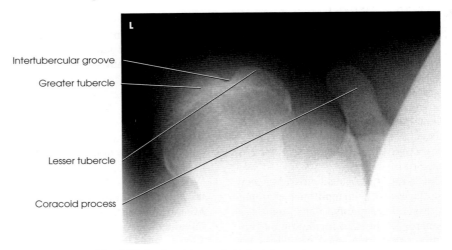

Intertubercular groove
Greater tubercle

Lesser tubercle

Coracoid process

Fig. 6.52 Supine tangential intertubercular groove.

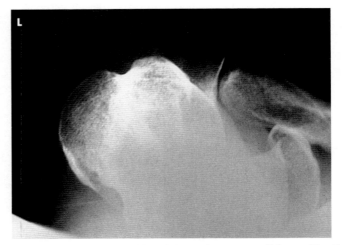

Fig. 6.53 Standing tangential intertubercular groove: Fisk modification.

Shoulder Girdle

♠ AP PROJECTION
Bilateral
PEARSON METHOD

Image receptor + grid: Positioned by manufacturer or department protocol for proper anatomy display orientation; CR plate: 14 × 17 inches (35 × 43 cm) or two 10 × 12 inches (24 × 30 cm), as needed to fit the patient.

SID: 72 inches (183 cm). A longer SID reduces magnification, which enables both joints to be included on one image. It also reduces the distortion of the joint space resulting from beam divergence.

Position of patient
- Place the patient in an upright body position, either seated or standing, because dislocation of the AC joint tends to reduce itself in the recumbent position. The positioning is easily modified to obtain a PA projection.

Position of part
- Place the patient in the upright position before a vertical grid device, and adjust the height of the IR so that the midpoint of the IR lies at the same level as the AC joints (Fig. 6.54).
- Center the midline of the body to the midline of the grid.
- Ensure that the weight of the body is equally distributed on the feet to avoid rotation.
- With the patient's arms hanging by the sides, adjust the shoulders to lie in the same horizontal plane. It is important that the arms hang unsupported.

- Make two exposures: one in which the patient is standing upright *without* weights attached, and a second in which the patient has *equal weights* (5 to 10 lb) affixed to each wrist.[14,15]
- After the first exposure, slowly affix the weights to the patient's wrist, using a band or strap.
- Instruct the patient not to favor (tense up) the injured shoulder.
- *Avoid having the patient hold weights in each hand;* this tends to make the shoulder muscles contract, reducing the possibility of showing a small AC separation (Fig. 6.55).
- *Shield gonads.* Also use a thyroid collar because the thyroid gland is exposed to the primary beam.
- *Respiration:* Suspend.

Central ray
- Perpendicular to the midline of the body at the level of the AC joints for a single projection; directed at each respective AC joint when two separate exposures are necessary for each shoulder in broad-shouldered patients

Collimation
- Adjust radiation field to 6 × 17 inches (15 × 43 cm) on the collimator for both joints with a single exposure
- or to 6 × 8 inches (15 × 20 cm) for separate exposures of each joint on two IRs
- Place side marker in the collimated exposure field.

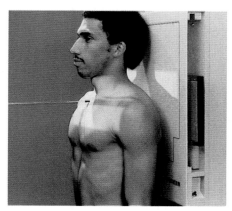

Fig. 6.54 Bilateral AP AC articulations.

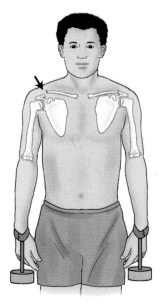

Fig. 6.55 Weights should be attached to wrists as shown and not held in hands. Note how separation of AC joint is shown by pulling of weights.

Structures shown

Bilateral images of the AC joints (Figs. 6.56 and 6.57). This projection is used to show dislocation, separation, and function of the joints.

EVALUATION CRITERIA

The following should be clearly seen:

- Evidence of proper collimation and presence of side markers placed clear of anatomy of interest
- Both AC joints, with and without weights, included on one or two radiographs
- No rotation or leaning by the patient
- AC joint separation, if present, clearly seen on the images with weights
- Bony trabecular detail and surrounding soft tissues

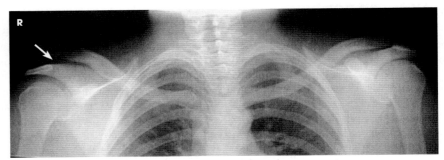

Fig. 6.56 Bilateral AP AC joints showing normal left joint and separation of right joint *(arrow)*.

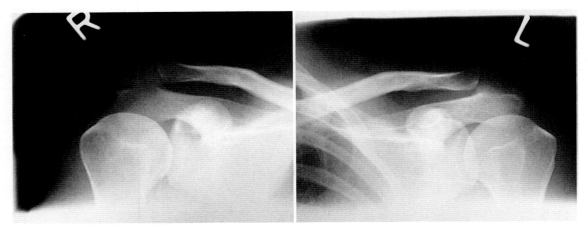

Fig. 6.57 Normal AC joints requiring two separate radiographs.

Shoulder Girdle

AP AXIAL PROJECTION
ALEXANDER METHOD

Alexander[16] suggested that AP and PA axial oblique projections be used in cases of suspected AC subluxation or dislocation. Each side is examined separately.

Image receptor + grid: Positioned by manufacturer or department protocol for proper anatomy display orientation; CR plate: 10 × 12 inches (24 × 30 cm) lengthwise.

Position of patient
- Place the patient in the upright position, either standing or seated.

Position of part
- Have the patient place the back against the vertical grid device and sit or stand upright.
- Center the affected shoulder under examination to the grid.
- Adjust the height of the IR so that the midpoint is at the level of the AC joint.
- Adjust the patient's position to center the coracoid process to the IR (Fig. 6.58).
- *Shield gonads.*
- *Respiration:* Suspend.

Central ray
- Directed to the coracoid process at a cephalic angle of 15 degrees (Fig. 6.59). This angulation projects the AC joint above the acromion.

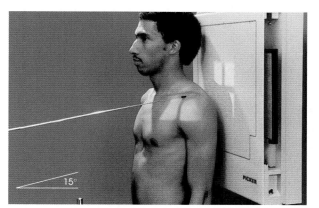

Fig. 6.58 Unilateral AP axial AC articulation: Alexander method.

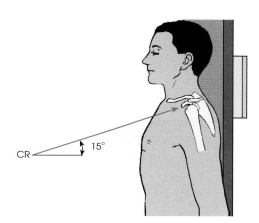

Fig. 6.59 AP axial AC articulation: Alexander method.

Shoulder Girdle

Collimation

- Adjust radiation field to 6 × 8 inches (15 × 20 cm) on the collimator. Place side marker in the collimated exposure field.

Structures shown

The AC joint projected slightly superiorly compared with an AP projection (Fig. 6.60).

The following should be clearly seen:
- Evidence of proper collimation and presence of side marker placed clear of anatomy of interest
- AC joint and clavicle projected above the acromion
- Bony trabecular detail and surrounding soft tissues

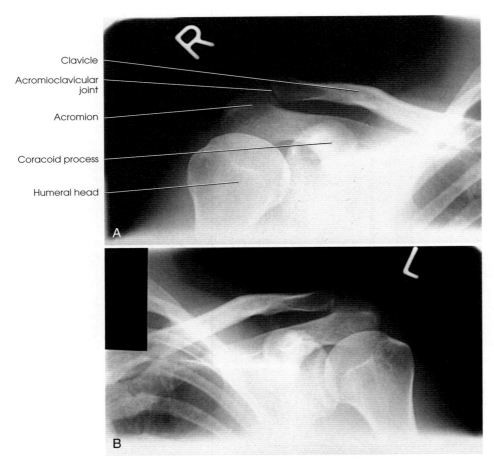

Clavicle
Acromioclavicular joint
Acromion
Coracoid process
Humeral head

Fig. 6.60 (A) and (B) AP axial AC articulation: Alexander method.

♠ AP PROJECTION

Image receptor + grid: Positioned by manufacturer or department protocol for proper anatomy display orientation; CR plate: 10 × 12 inches (24 × 30 cm) crosswise.

Position of patient
- Place the patient in the supine or upright position.
- If the clavicle is being examined for a fracture or a destructive disease, or if the patient cannot be placed in the upright position, use the supine position to reduce the possibility of fragment displacement or additional injury.

Position of part
- Adjust the body to center the clavicle to the midline of the table or vertical grid device.
- Place the arms along the sides of the body, and adjust the shoulders to lie in the same horizontal plane.
- Center the clavicle to the IR (Fig. 6.61).
- *Shield gonads.*
- *Respiration:* Suspend at the end of exhalation to obtain a more uniform-density image.

Central ray
- Perpendicular to the midshaft of the clavicle

Collimation
- Adjust radiation field to 8 × 12 inches (18 × 30 cm) on the collimator. Adjust as needed to include 1.5 inches (3.8 cm) above the shoulder, 1 inch (2.5 cm) beyond the lateral aspect of the shoulder, and the entire clavicle. Place side marker in the collimated exposure field.

Structures shown
An AP image of the entire clavicle (Fig. 6.62).

The following should be clearly see:
- Evidence of proper collimation and presence of side marker placed clear of anatomy of interest
- Entire clavicle centered on the image
- Lateral half of the clavicle above the scapula, with the medial half superimposing the thorax
- Bony trabecular detail and surrounding soft tissues

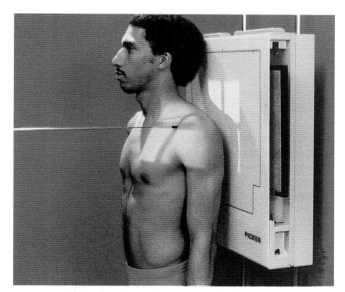

Fig. 6.61 AP clavicle.

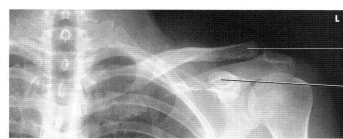

Fig. 6.62 AP clavicle.

Clavicle

Coracoid process

🏕 AP AXIAL PROJECTION

NOTE: If the patient is injured or is unable to assume the lordotic position, a slightly distorted image results when the tube is angled. An optional approach for improved spatial resolution is the PA axial projection.

> **Image receptor + grid:** Positioned by manufacturer or department protocol for proper anatomy display orientation; CR plate: 10 × 12 inches (24 × 30 cm) crosswise.

Position of patient
- Stand or seat the patient with the back against the vertical IR device.
- If the patient cannot stand or sit upright, place the patient supine on the table.

Position of part
Standing position
- Adjust the body to center the clavicle to the vertical grid device.
- Place the arms along the sides of the body, and adjust the shoulders to lie in the same horizontal plane.
- Center the clavicle to the IR (Fig. 6.63A).

Standing lordotic position
- Have the patient step forward about 1 foot, then lean backward in a position of extreme lordosis. Temporarily support the patient in the lordotic position to estimate the required CR angulation, then have the patient reassume the upright position while the equipment is adjusted.
- Return the patient to the lordotic position, with the neck and shoulder resting against the vertical grid device (see Fig. 6.63B).
- Center the clavicle to the center of the IR (see Fig. 6.63B).

Supine position
- Adjust the body to center the clavicle to the table Bucky
- Center the IR to the clavicle (Fig. 6.64).
- *Shield gonads.*
- *Respiration:* Suspend at the end of full inspiration to elevate and angle the clavicle further.

Central ray
- Directed to enter the midshaft of the clavicle.
- Cephalic CR angulation can vary depending on the thickness of the chest;

thinner patients require increased angulation to project the clavicle above the scapula and ribs.
- For the *standing position,* 15 to 30 degrees is recommended
- For the *standing lordotic position,* 0 to 15 degrees is recommended.
- For the *supine position,* 15 to 30 degrees is recommended.

Collimation
- Adjust radiation field to 8 × 12 inches (18 × 30 cm) on the collimator. Place side marker in the collimated exposure field.

Structures shown
An AP axial image of the clavicle is projected above the ribs (Fig. 6.65).

The following should be clearly seen:
- Evidence of proper collimation and presence of side marker placed clear of anatomy of interest
- Entire clavicle along with AC and SC joints
- Lateral two-thirds of the clavicle projected above the ribs and scapula with the medial end superimposing the thorax
- Clavicle in a more horizontal orientation, as compared with the AP projection
- Bony trabecular detail and surrounding soft tissues

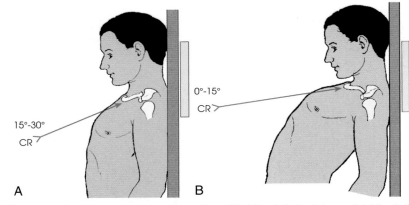

Fig. 6.63 (A) AP axial clavicle, upright position. (B) AP axial clavicle, upright lordotic position.

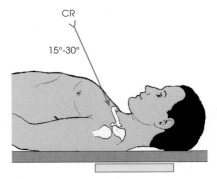

Fig. 6.64 AP axial clavicle, supine position.

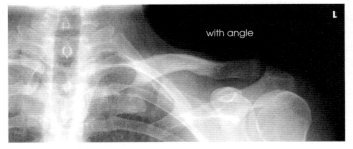

Fig. 6.65 AP axial clavicle. Same patient as Fig. 6.62. Note less superimposition of the clavicle and thorax.

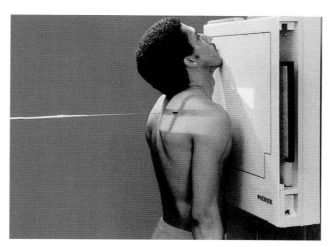

Fig. 6.66 PA clavicle.

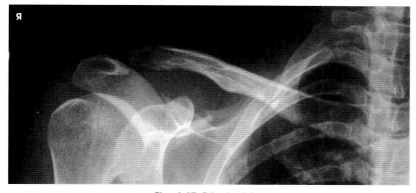

Fig. 6.67 PA clavicle.

☗ PA PROJECTION

The PA projection is generally well accepted by the patient who can stand, and it is most useful when improved spatial resolution is desired. The advantage of the PA projection is that the clavicle is closer to the IR, reducing the OID. Positioning is similar to that of the AP projection. Differences are as follows:

- The patient is standing upright (back toward the x-ray tube) or is prone (Fig. 6.66).
- The perpendicular CR exits the midshaft of the clavicle (Fig. 6.67).

Structures shown and evaluation criteria are the same as for the AP projection.

☗ PA AXIAL PROJECTION

Positioning of the PA axial clavicle is similar to the AP axial projection described previously. The differences are as follows:

- The patient is prone or standing, facing the vertical grid device.
- The CR is angled 15 to 30 degrees caudad (Fig. 6.68).

Structures shown and evaluation criteria are the same as described previously for the AP axial projection.

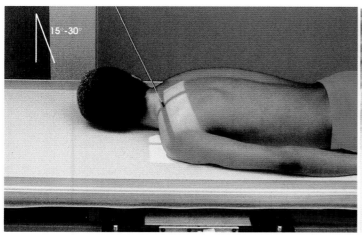

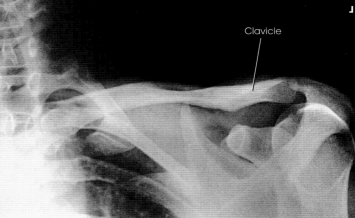

Clavicle

Fig. 6.68 PA axial clavicle.

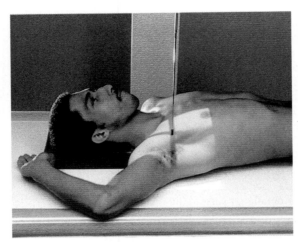

Fig. 6.69 AP scapula.

⚜ AP PROJECTION

Image receptor + grid: Positioned by manufacturer or department protocol for proper anatomy display orientation; CR plate: 10 × 12 inches (24 × 30 cm) lengthwise.

Position of patient

- Place the patient in the upright or supine position. The upright position is usually more comfortable for patients.

Position of part

- Adjust the patient's body, and center the affected scapula to the midline of the grid.
- Abduct the arm to a right angle with the body to draw the scapula laterally. Flex the elbow, and support the hand in a comfortable position.
- For this projection, do not rotate the body toward the affected side because the resultant obliquity would offset the effect of drawing the scapula laterally (Fig. 6.69).
- Position the top of the IR 2 inches (5 cm) above the top of the shoulder.
- *Shield gonads.*
- *Respiration:* Make this exposure during slow breathing to obliterate lung detail.

Central ray

- Perpendicular to the midscapular area at a point approximately 2 inches (5 cm) inferior to the coracoid process

Collimation

- Adjust radiation field to 10 × 12 inches (24 × 30 cm) on the collimator. Include 1.5 inches (3.8 cm) above the shoulder, 2 inches (5 cm) beyond the lateral aspect of the shoulder, the lateral half of the clavicle, and 1 inch (2.5 cm) below the inferior angle of the scapula. Place side marker in the collimated exposure field.

Structures shown

An AP projection of the scapula (Fig. 6.70).

EVALUATION CRITERIA

The following should be clearly seen:
- Evidence of proper collimation and presence of side marker placed clear of anatomy of interest
- Lateral portion of the scapula free of superimposition from the ribs
- Scapula horizontal and not slanted
- Scapular detail through the superimposed lung and ribs (shallow breathing should help to obliterate lung detail)
- Acromion and inferior angle
- Bony trabecular detail and surrounding soft tissues

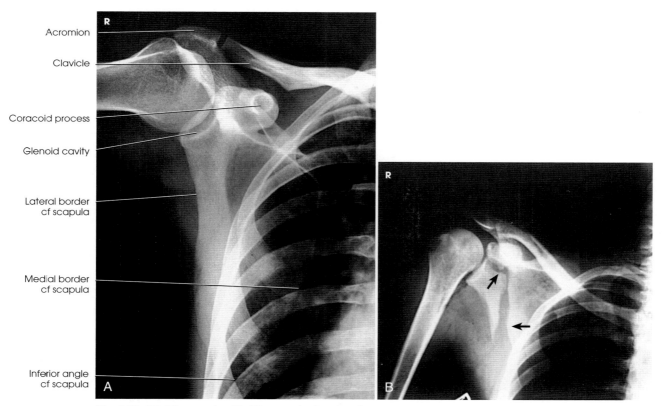

Fig. 6.70 (A) AP scapula. (B) AP scapula showing fracture of scapula through glenoid cavity and extending inferiorly (arrows).

♠ LATERAL PROJECTION
RAO or LAO body position

Image receptor + grid: Positioned by manufacturer or department protocol for proper anatomy display orientation; CR plate: 10 × 12 inches (24 × 30 cm) lengthwise.

Position of patient

- Place the patient in the upright position, standing or seated, facing a vertical grid device.
- The prone position can be used, but the projection is more difficult to perform.

Position of part

- Adjust the patient in RAO or LAO position, with the affected scapula centered to the grid. The average patient requires a 45- to 60-degree rotation from the plane of the IR. According to Johnston et al.,[1] proper patient rotation is accomplished by orienting the plane through the superior angle of the scapula and acromial tip, perpendicular to the IR.
- Position of the arm depends on the area of the scapula to be shown.
  - For delineation of the *acromion* and the *coracoid process* of the scapula, have the patient flex the elbow and place the back of the hand on the posterior thorax at a level sufficient to prevent the humerus from over-lapping the scapula (Figs. 6.71 and 6.72). Mazujian[17] suggested that the patient place the arm across the upper chest by grasping the opposite shoulder, as shown in Fig. 6.73.
  - To show the *body* of the scapula, ask the patient to extend the arm upward and rest the forearm on the head (Fig. 6.74) or alternatively across the upper chest by grasping the opposite shoulder (see Fig. 6.73).
- After placing the arm in any of these positions, grasp the lateral and medial borders of the scapula between the thumb and index finger of one hand. Make a final adjustment of the body rotation, placing the body of the scapula perpendicular to the plane of the IR.
- *Shield gonads.*
- *Respiration:* Suspend.

Central ray

- Perpendicular to the midmedial border of the protruding scapula (see Table 6.3)

Collimation

- Adjust radiation field to 12 inches (30 cm) in length on the collimator, 1.5 inches (3.8 cm) above the shoulder, and 1 inch (2.5 cm) beyond the lateral shadow. Place side marker in the collimated exposure field.

▼ COMPENSATING FILTER

Use of a specially designed compensating filter for the shoulder, called a boomerang, improves the quality of the image because of the large amount of primary beam radiation striking the IR.

Structures shown

A lateral image of the scapula. The placement of the arm determines the portion of the superior scapula that is superimposed over the humerus.

EVALUATION CRITERIA

The following should be clearly seen:
- Evidence of proper collimation and presence of side marker placed clear of anatomy of interest
- Lateral and medial scapular borders superimposed
- No superimposition of the scapular body on the ribs
- No superimposition of the humerus on the area of interest
- Inclusion of the acromion and inferior angle
- Bony trabecular detail and surrounding soft tissues

NOTE: For trauma patients, this projection can be performed using the LPO or RPO position (see Chapter 12 in Volume 2).

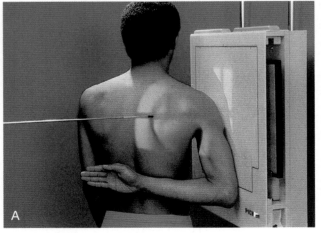
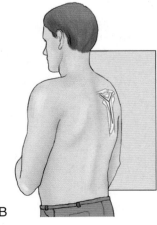

Fig. 6.71 (A) Lateral scapula, RAO body position. (B) Perspective from x-ray tube showing scapula centered in true lateral position.

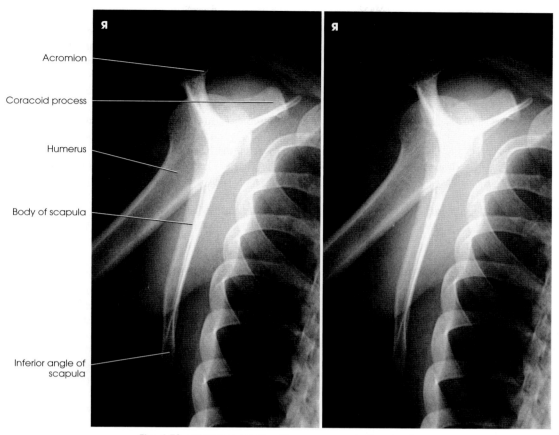

Acromion

Coracoid process

Humerus

Body of scapula

Inferior angle of scapula

Fig. 6.72 Lateral scapula with arm on posterior chest.

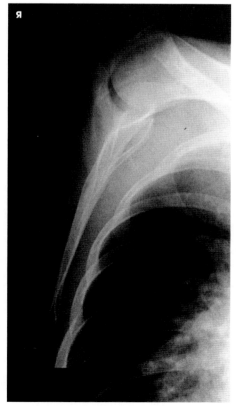

Fig. 6.73 Lateral scapula with arm across upper anterior thorax.

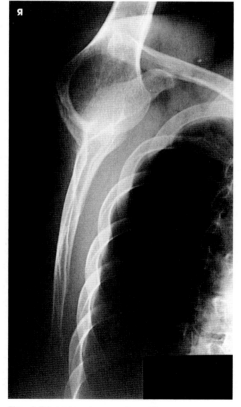

Fig. 6.74 Lateral scapula with arm extended above head.

AP OBLIQUE PROJECTION

RPO or LPO position

Image receptor + grid: Positioned by manufacturer or department protocol for proper anatomy display orientation; CR plate: 10 × 12 inches (24 × 30 cm) lengthwise.

Position of patient

- Place the patient in the supine or upright position.
- Use the upright position when the shoulder is painful unless contraindicated.

Position of part

- Align the body and center the affected scapula to the midline of the grid.
- For moderate AP oblique projection, ask the patient to extend the arm superiorly, flex the elbow, and place the supinated hand under the head, or have the patient extend the affected arm across the anterior chest.
- Have the patient turn away from the affected side enough to rotate the shoulder 15 to 25 degrees (Fig. 6.75).
- For a steeper oblique projection, ask the patient to extend the arm, rest the flexed elbow on the forehead, and rotate the body *away* from the affected side 25 to 35 degrees (Fig. 6.76).
- Grasp the lateral and medial borders of the scapula between the thumb and index finger of one hand, and adjust the rotation of the body to project the scapula free of the rib cage.
- For a direct lateral projection of the scapula using this position, draw the arm across the chest, and adjust the body rotation to place the scapula perpendicular to the plane of the IR as previously described and shown in Figs. 6.71 to 6.74.
- *Shield gonads.*
- *Respiration:* Suspend.

Central ray

- Perpendicular to the lateral border of the rib cage at the midscapular area

Collimation

- Adjust radiation field to 12 inches (30 cm) in length on the collimator, 1.5 inches (3.8 cm) above the shoulder and 1 inch (2.5 cm) beyond the lateral shadow. Place side marker in the collimated exposure field.

Structures shown

An oblique image of the scapula, projected free or nearly free of rib superimposition (Figs. 6.77 and 6.78).

EVALUATION CRITERIA

The following should be clearly seen:
- Evidence of proper collimation and presence of side marker placed clear of anatomy of interest
- Oblique scapula
- Lateral scapular border adjacent to the ribs
- Acromion and inferior angle
- Bony trabecular detail and surrounding soft tissues

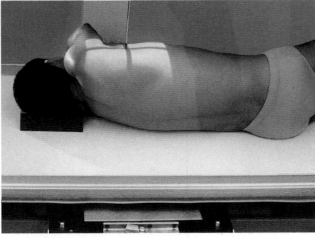

Fig. 6.75 AP oblique scapula, 20-degree body rotation.

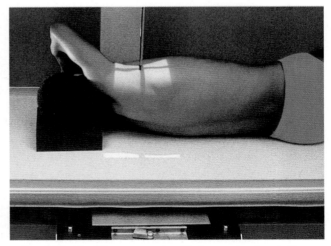

Fig. 6.76 AP oblique scapula, 35-degree body rotation.

Humerus

Acromion

Clavicle

Coracoid process

Scapular spine

Vertebral border
of scapula

Rib cage

Inferior angle of
scapula

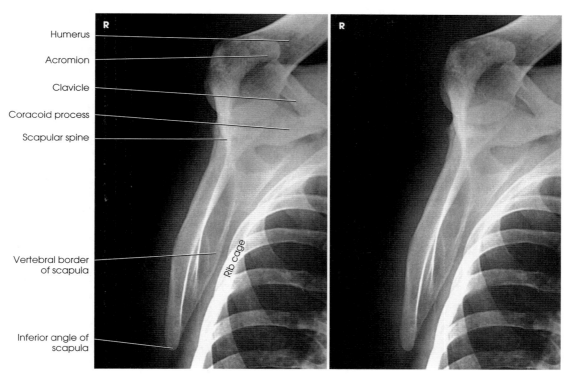

Fig. 6.77 AP oblique scapula, 15- to 25-degree body rotation.

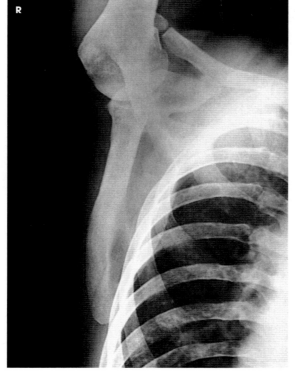

Fig. 6.78 AP oblique scapula, 25- to 30-degree body rotation.

Coracoid Process
AP AXIAL PROJECTION

Image receptor + grid: Positioned by manufacturer or department protocol for proper anatomy display orientation; CR plate: 10 × 12 inches (24 × 30 cm) crosswise

Position of patient

- Place the patient in the supine position with the arms along the sides of the body.

Position of part

- Adjust the position of the body, and center the affected coracoid process to the midline of the grid.
- Position the IR so that the midpoint of the IR coincides with the CR.

- Adjust the shoulders to lie in the same horizontal plane.
- Abduct the arm of the affected side slightly, and supinate the hand, immobilizing it with a sandbag across the palm (Fig. 6.79).
- *Shield gonads.*
- *Respiration:* Suspend at the end of exhalation for a more uniform density.

Central ray

- Directed to enter the coracoid process at an angle of 15 to 45 degrees cephalad. Kwak et al.[18] recommended an angle of 30 degrees. The degree of angulation depends on the shape of the patient's back. Round-shouldered patients require greater angulation than do patients with a straight back (Fig. 6.80).

Collimation

- Adjust radiation field to 8 × 10 inches (18 × 24 cm) on the collimator. Place side marker in the collimated exposure field.

Structures shown

The coracoid process in its entirety with some superimposition by the clavicle (Fig. 6.81).

EVALUATION CRITERIA

The following should be clearly seen:
- Evidence of proper collimation and presence of side marker placed clear of anatomy of interest
- Coracoid process with minimal self-superimposition
- Clavicle slightly superimposing the coracoid process
- Bony trabecular detail and surrounding soft tissues

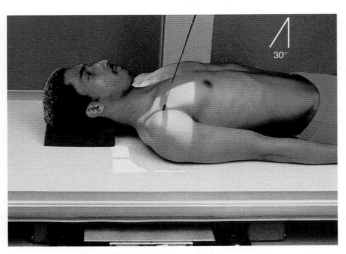

Fig. 6.79 AP axial coracoid process.

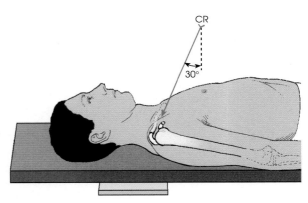

Fig. 6.80 AP axial coracoid process.

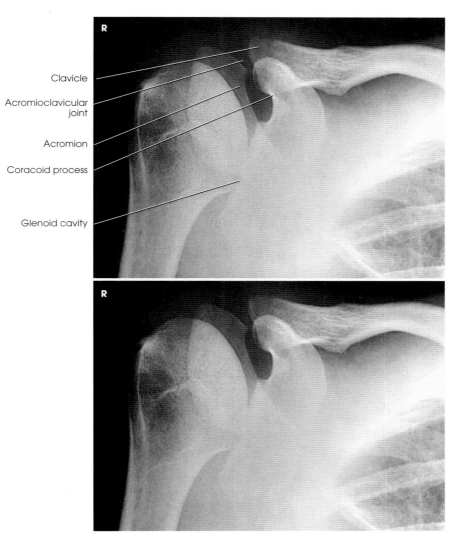

Clavicle

Acromioclavicular
joint

Acromion

Coracoid process

Glenoid cavity

Fig. 6.81 AP axial coracoid process.

Shoulder Girdle

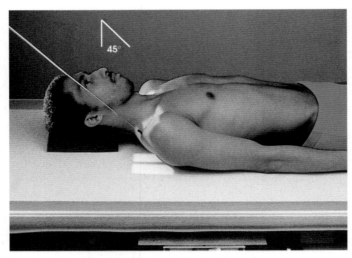

Fig. 6.82 Tangential scapular spine.

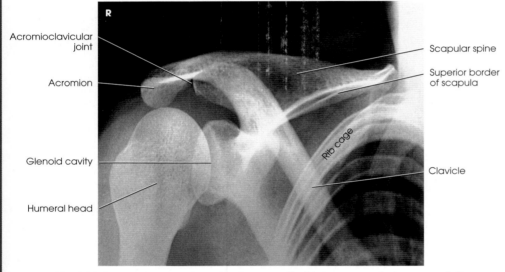

Acromioclavicular joint

Acromion

Glenoid cavity

Humeral head

Scapular spine

Superior border of scapula

Rib cage

Clavicle

Fig. 6.83 Tangential scapular spine image with 45-degree central ray angulation.

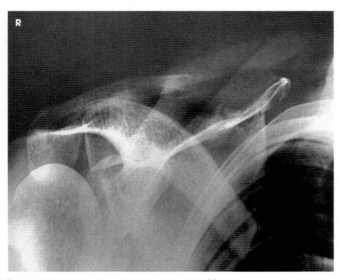

Fig. 6.84 Tangential scapular spine image with 30-degree central ray angulation.

TANGENTIAL PROJECTION
LAQUERRIÈRE-PIERQUIN METHOD

Image receptor + grid: Positioned by manufacturer or department protocol for proper anatomy display orientation; CR plate: 10×12 inches (24×30 cm) crosswise.

Position of patient
- As described by Laquerrière and Pierquin,[19] place the patient in the supine position.

Position of part
- Center the shoulder to the midline of the grid.
- Adjust the patient's rotation to place the body of the scapula in a horizontal position. When this requires elevation of the opposite shoulder, support it on sandbags or radiolucent sponges.
- Turn the head away from the shoulder being examined, enough to prevent superimposition (Fig. 6.82).
- *Shield gonads.*
- *Respiration:* Suspend.

Central ray
- Directed through the posterosuperior region of the shoulder at an angle of 45 degrees caudad. A 35-degree angulation suffices for obese and round-shouldered patients.
- After adjusting the x-ray tube, position the IR so that it is centered to the CR.

Collimation
- Adjust radiation field to 10×10 inches (24×24 cm) on the collimator. Place side marker in the collimated exposure field.

Structures shown
The spine of the scapula in profile and free of bony superimposition except for the lateral end of the clavicle (Figs. 6.83 and 6.84).

EVALUATION CRITERIA

The following should be clearly seen:
- Evidence of proper collimation and presence of side marker placed clear of anatomy of interest
- Scapular spine superior to the scapular body
- Bony trabecular detail and surrounding soft tissues

NOTE: When the shoulder is too painful to tolerate the supine position, this projection can be obtained with the patient in the prone or upright position.

References

1. Johnston J, Killion J, Comello R: Landmarks for lateral scapula and scapular Y positioning, *Radiol Technol* 79:397–404, 2008.
2. Apple AS, Pedowitz RA, Speer KP: The weighted abduction Grashey shoulder method, *Radiol Technol* 69:151–156, 1997.
3. Lawrence WS: A method of obtaining an accurate lateral roentgenogram of the shoulder joint, *AJR Am J Roentgenol* 5:193, 1918.
4. Lawrence WS: New position in radiographing the shoulder joint, *AJR Am J Roentgenol* 2:728, 1915.
5. Rafert JA, Long BW, Hernandez EM, et al: Axillary shoulder with exaggerated rotation: the Hill-Sachs defect, *Radiol Technol* 62:18–21, 1990.
6. Hill H, Sachs M: The grooved defect of the humeral head: a frequently unrecognized complication of dislocations of the shoulder joint, *Radiology* 35:690, 1940.
7. Rokous JR, Feagin JA, Abbott HG: Modified axillary roentgenogram, *Clin Orthop Relat Res* 82:84–86, 1972.
8. Rubin SA, Gray RL, Green WR: The scapular Y: a diagnostic aid in shoulder trauma, *Radiology* 110:725–726, 1974.
9. Neer CS, II: Supraspinatus outlet, *Orthop Trans* 11:234, 1987.
10. Neer CS, II: *Shoulder reconstruction*, Philadelphia, 1990, Saunders, pp 14–24.
11. Hall RH, Isaac F, Booth CR: Dislocations of the shoulder with special reference to accompanying small fractures, *J Bone Joint Surg Am* 41:489–494, 1959.
12. Garth WP, Jr, Slappey CE, Ochs CW: Roentgenographic demonstration of instability of the shoulder: the apical oblique projection, *J Bone Joint Surg Am* 66:1450–1453, 1984.
13. Fisk C: Adaptation of the technique for radiography of the bicipital groove, *Radiol Technol* 34:47–50, 1965.
14. Allman FL, Jr: Fractures and ligamentous injuries of the clavicle and its articulations, *J Bone Joint Surg Am* 49:774–784, 1967.
15. Rockwood CA, Green DP: *Fractures in adults*, ed 7, Philadelphia, 2009, Lippincott.
16. Alexander OM: Radiography of the acromioclavicular articulation, *Med Radiogr Photogr* 30:34–39, 1954.
17. Mazujian M: Lateral profile view of the scapula, *Xray Techn* 25:24–25, 1953.
18. Kwak DL, et al: Angled anteroposterior views of the shoulder, *Radiol Technol* 53:590, 1982.
19. Laquerrière Pierquin: De la nécessité d'employer une technique radiographique spéciale pour obtenir certains details squelettiques, *J Radiol Electr* 3:145, 1918.

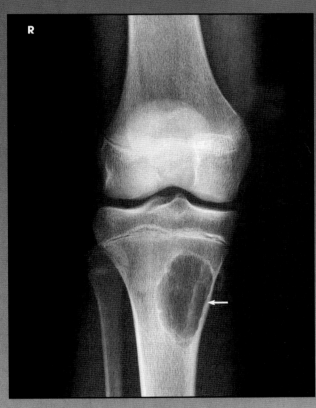
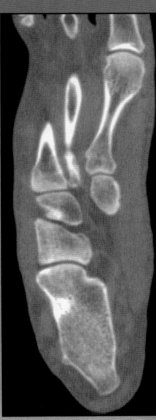

7

LOWER EXTREMITY

PROJECTIONS, POSITIONS, AND METHODS

Page	Essential	Anatomy	Projection	Position	Method
288	▲	Toes	AP or AP axial		
290		Toes	PA		
291	▲	Toes	AP oblique	Medial rotation	
292	▲	Toes	Lateral (mediolateral or lateromedial)		
296		Sesamoids	Tangential		LEWIS, HOLLY
298	▲	Foot	AP or AP axial		
302	▲	Foot	AP oblique	Medial rotation	
304		Foot	AP oblique	Lateral rotation	
306	▲	Foot	Lateral (mediolateral)		
308		Foot: *Longitudinal arch*	Lateral (lateromedial)	Standing	WEIGHT-BEARING
310		Feet	AP axial	Standing	WEIGHT-BEARING
311		Foot	AP axial	Standing	WEIGHT-BEARING COMPOSITE
313		Foot: *Congenital clubfoot*	AP		KITE
314		Foot: *Congenital clubfoot*	Lateral (mediolateral)		KITE
316		Foot: *Congenital clubfoot*	Axial (dorsoplantar)		KANDEL
317	▲	Calcaneus	Axial (plantodorsal)		
318		Calcaneus	Axial (dorsoplantar)		
319		Calcaneus	Axial (dorsoplantar)	Standing	WEIGHT-BEARING
320	▲	Calcaneus	Lateral (mediolateral)		
321		Calcaneus	Lateromedial oblique		WEIGHT-BEARING
322		Subtalar joint	Lateromedial oblique	Medial rotation foot	ISHERWOOD
323		Subtalar joint	AP axial oblique	Medial rotation ankle	ISHERWOOD
324		Subtalar joint	AP axial oblique	Lateral rotation ankle	ISHERWOOD
325	▲	Ankle	AP		
326	▲	Ankle	Lateral (mediolateral)		
328		Ankle	Lateral (lateromedial)		
329	▲	Ankle	AP oblique	Medial rotation	
330	▲	Ankle: *Mortise joint*	AP oblique	Medial rotation	
332		Ankle	AP oblique	Lateral rotation	
333	▲	Ankle	AP		STRESS
334		Ankles	AP	Standing	WEIGHT-BEARING
336	▲	Leg	AP		
338	▲	Leg	Lateral (mediolateral)		
340		Leg	AP oblique	Medial and lateral rotations	
342	▲	Knee	AP		
344		Knee	PA		

The icons in the Essential column indicate projections frequently performed in the United States and Canada. Students should become competent in these projections.
AP, Anteroposterior; *PA,* posteroanterior.

PROJECTIONS, POSITIONS, AND METHODS

Page	Essential	Anatomy	Projection	Position	Method
346	🌲	Knee	Lateral (mediolateral)		
348	🌲	Knees	AP	Standing	WEIGHT-BEARING
349		Knees	PA	Standing flexion	ROSENBERG, WEIGHT-BEARING
350	🌲	Knee	AP oblique	Lateral rotation	
351	🌲	Knee	AP oblique	Medial and lateral rotations	
352	🌲	Intercondylar fossa	PA axial		HOLMBLAD
354	🌲	Intercondylar fossa	PA axial		CAMP-COVENTRY
356		Intercondylar fossa	AP axial		BÉCLÈRE
357	🌲	Patella	PA		
358	🌲	Patella	Lateral (mediolateral)		
359		Patella and patellofemoral joint	Tangential		HUGHSTON
360		Patella and patellofemoral joint	Tangential		MERCHANT
362	🌲	Patella and patellofemoral joint	Tangential		SETTEGAST
364	🌲	Femur	AP		
366	🌲	Femur	Lateral (mediolateral)		
368		Lower Extremities: Long bone measurement	AP	Standing	WEIGHT-BEARING

The icons in the Essential column indicate projections frequently performed in the United States and Canada. Students should become competent in these projections.
AP, Anteroposterior; *PA,* posteroanterior.

The lower extremity and its girdle (considered in Chapter 8) are studied in four parts: (1) foot, (2) leg, (3) thigh, and (4) hip. The bones are composed, shaped, and placed so that they can carry the body in the upright position and transmit its weight to the ground with a minimal amount of stress to the individual parts.

Foot

The *foot* consists of 26 bones (Figs. 7.1 and 7.2):

- 14 phalanges (bones of the toes)
- 5 metatarsals (bones of the instep)
- 7 tarsals (bones of the ankle)

The bones of the foot are similar to the bones of the hand. Structural differences permit walking and support of the body's weight. For descriptive purposes, the foot is sometimes divided into the forefoot, midfoot, and hindfoot. The forefoot includes the metatarsals and toes. The midfoot includes five tarsals: cuneiforms, navicular, and cuboid bones. The hindfoot includes the talus and calcaneus. The bones of the foot are shaped and joined together to form a series of longitudinal and transverse arches. The longitudinal arch functions as a shock absorber to distribute the weight of the body in all directions, which permits smooth walking (see Fig. 7.2). The

transverse arch runs from side to side and assists in supporting the longitudinal arch. The superior surface of the foot is termed the *dorsum* or *dorsal surface,* and the inferior, or posterior, aspect of the foot is termed the *plantar surface.*

PHALANGES

Each foot has 14 *phalanges:* 2 in the great toe and 3 in each of the other toes. The phalanges of the great toe are termed *distal* and *proximal.* The phalanges of the other toes are termed *proximal, middle,* and *distal.* Each phalanx is composed of a body and two expanded articular ends: the proximal *base* and the distal *head.*

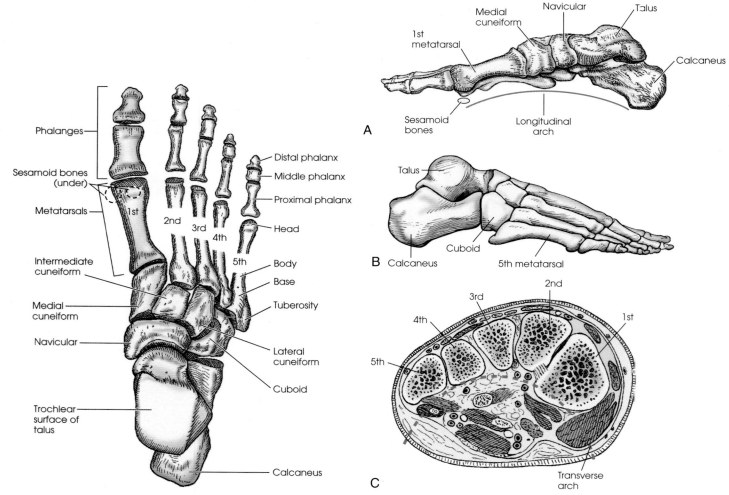

Fig. 7.1 Dorsal (superior) aspect of right foot.

Fig. 7.2 Right foot. (A) Medial aspect. (B) Lateral aspect. (C) Coronal section near base of metatarsals. Transverse arch shown.

METATARSALS

The five *metatarsals* are numbered one to five beginning at the medial or great toe side of the foot. The metatarsals consist of a *body* and two articular ends. The expanded proximal end is called the *base*, and the small, rounded distal end is termed the *head*. The five heads form the "ball" of the foot. The first metatarsal is the shortest and thickest. The second metatarsal is the longest. The base of the fifth metatarsal contains a prominent *tuberosity*, which is a common site of fractures.

TARSALS

The proximal foot contains seven *tarsals* (see Fig. 7.1):

- Calcaneus
- Talus
- Navicular
- Cuboid
- Medial cuneiform
- Intermediate cuneiform
- Lateral cuneiform

Beginning at the medial side of the foot, the cuneiforms are described as *medial, intermediate,* and *lateral.*

The *calcaneus* is the largest and strongest tarsal bone (Fig. 7.3). Some texts refer to it as the *os calcis.* It projects posteriorly and medially at the distal part of the foot. The long axis of the calcaneus is directed inferiorly and forms an angle of approximately 30 degrees. The posterior and inferior portions of the calcaneus contain the posterior *tuberosity* for attachment of the Achilles tendon. Superiorly, three articular facets join with the talus. They are called the *anterior, middle,* and *posterior facets*. Between the middle and posterior talar articular facets is a groove—the calcaneal sulcus—which corresponds to a similar groove on the inferior surface of the talus. Collectively, these sulci constitute the *sinus tarsi*. The interosseous ligament passes through this sulcus. The medial aspect of the calcaneus extends outward as a shelf-like overhang and is termed the *sustentaculum tali*. The lateral surface of the calcaneus contains the *trochlea*.

The *talus,* irregular in form and occupying the superior-most position of the foot, is the second largest tarsal bone (see Figs. 7.1 through 7.3). The talus articulates with four bones: tibia, fibula, calcaneus, and navicular bone. The superior surface, the *trochlear surface,* articulates with the tibia and connects the foot to the leg. The head of the talus is directed anteriorly and has articular surfaces that join the navicular bone and calcaneus. On the inferior surface is a groove, the *sulcus tali,* which forms the roof of the sinus tarsi. The inferior surface also contains three facets that align with the facets on the superior surface of the calcaneus.

The *cuboid* bone lies on the lateral side of the foot between the calcaneus and the fourth and fifth metatarsals (see Fig. 7.1). The *navicular* bone lies on the medial side of the foot between the talus and the three cuneiforms. The *cuneiforms* lie at the central and medial aspect of the foot between the navicular bone and the first, second, and third metatarsals. The *medial* cuneiform is the largest of the three cuneiform bones, and the *intermediate* cuneiform is the smallest.

The seven tarsals can be remembered using the following mnemonic:

Chubby	Calcaneus
Twisted	Talus
Never	Navicular
Could	Cuboid
Cha	Cuneiform—medial
Cha	Cuneiform—intermediate
Cha	Cuneiform—lateral

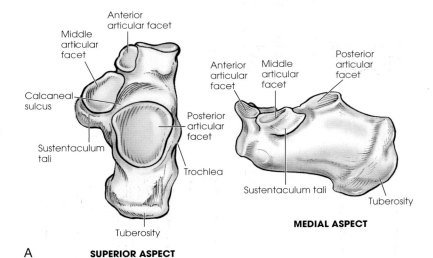

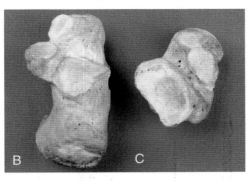

Fig. 7.3 (A) Articular surfaces of right calcaneus. (B) Photograph of superior aspect of right calcaneus. Note three articular facet surfaces. (C) Photograph of the inferior aspect of talus. Note three articular surfaces that articulate with the superior calcaneus.

SESAMOID BONES

Beneath the head of the first metatarsal are two small bones called *sesamoid bones.* They are detached from the foot and embedded within two tendons. These bones are seen on most adult foot radiographs. They are a common site of fractures and must be shown radiographically (see Fig. 7.2).

Leg

The leg has two bones: the *tibia* and the *fibula.* The tibia, the second largest bone in the body, is situated on the medial side of the leg and is a weight-bearing bone. Slightly posterior to the tibia on the lateral side of the leg is the fibula. The fibula does not bear any body weight.

TIBIA

The *tibia* (Fig. 7.4) is the larger of the two bones of the leg and consists of one body and two expanded extremities. The proximal end of the tibia has two prominent processes: the *medial* and *lateral condyles.* The superior surfaces of the condyles form smooth facets for articulation with the condyles of the femur. These two flatlike superior surfaces are called the *tibial plateaus,* and they slope posteriorly about 10 to 20 degrees. Between the two articular surfaces is a sharp projection, the *intercondylar eminence,* which terminates in two peaklike processes called the *medial* and *lateral intercondylar tubercles.* The lateral condyle has a facet at its distal posterior surface for articulation with the *head* of the fibula. On the anterior surface of the tibia, just below the condyles, is a prominent process called the *tibial tuberosity,* to which the ligamentum patellae attach. Extending along the anterior surface of the tibial body, beginning at the tuberosity, is a sharp ridge called the *anterior crest.*

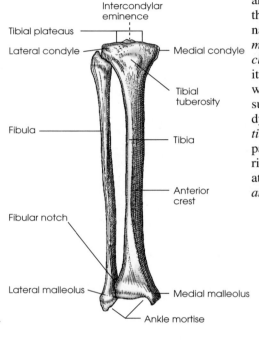

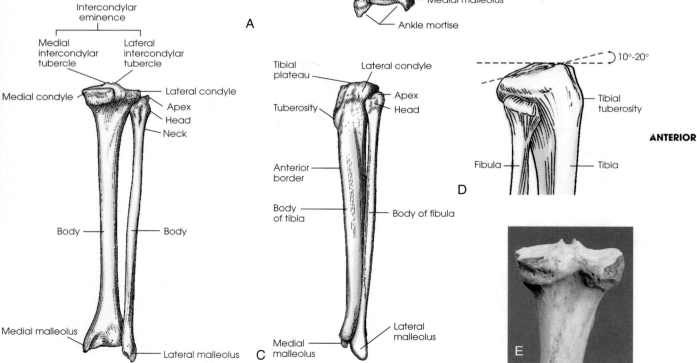

Fig. 7.4 Right tibia and fibula. (A) Anterior aspect. (B) Posterior aspect. (C) Lateral aspect. (D) Proximal end of tibia and fibula showing angle of the tibial plateau. (E) Photograph of superior and posterior aspects of the tibia.

The distal end of the tibia (Fig. 7.5) is broad, and its medial surface is prolonged into a large process called the *medial malleolus.* Its anterolateral surface contains the *anterior tubercle,* which overlays the fibula. The lateral surface is flattened and contains the triangular *fibular notch* for articulation with the fibula. The surface under the distal tibia is smooth and shaped for articulation with the talus.

FIBULA

The *fibula* is slender compared with its length and consists of one *body* and two articular extremities. The proximal end of the fibula is expanded into a *head,* which articulates with the lateral condyle of the tibia. At the lateroposterior aspect of the head is a conic projection called the *apex.*

The enlarged distal end of the fibula is the *lateral malleolus.* The lateral malleolus is pyramidal and is marked by several depressions at its inferior and posterior surfaces. Viewed axially, the lateral malleolus lies approximately 15 to 20 degrees more posterior than the medial malleolus (see Fig. 7.5C).

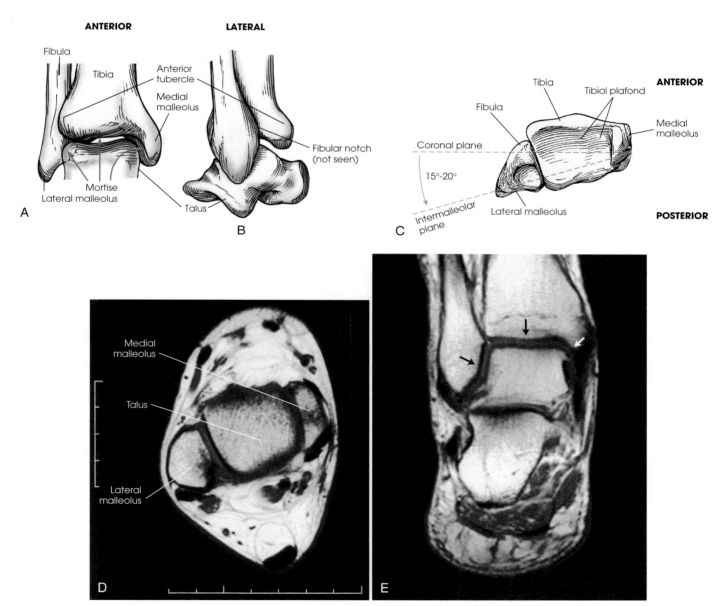

Fig. 7.5 (A) Right distal tibia and fibula in true anatomic position. Mortise joint and surrounding anatomy. Note slight overlap of anterior tubercle of tibia and superolateral talus over fibula. (B) Lateral aspect showing fibula positioned slightly posterior to tibia. (C) Inferior aspect. Note lateral malleolus lies more posterior than medial malleolus. (D) MRI axial plane of lateral and medial malleoli and talus. Lateral malleolus lies more posterior than medial malleolus. (E) MRI coronal plane of ankle clearly showing ankle mortise joint *(arrows).*

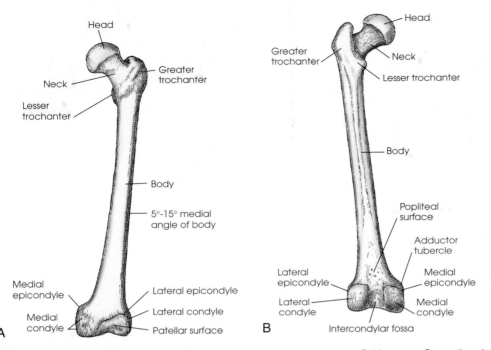

Femur

The *femur* is the longest, strongest, and heaviest bone in the body (Figs. 7.6 and 7.7). This bone consists of one body and two articular extremities. The *body* is cylindric and slightly convex anteriorly, and slants medially 5 to 15 degrees (see Fig. 7.6A). The extent of medial inclination depends on the breadth of the pelvic girdle. When the femur is vertical, the medial condyle is lower than the lateral condyle (see Fig. 7.6C). About a 5- to 7-degree difference exists between the two condyles. Because of this difference, on lateral radiographs of the knee the central ray is angled 5 to 7 degrees cephalad to "open" the joint space of the knee. The superior portion of the femur articulates with the acetabulum of the hip joint (considered with the pelvic girdle in Chapter 8).

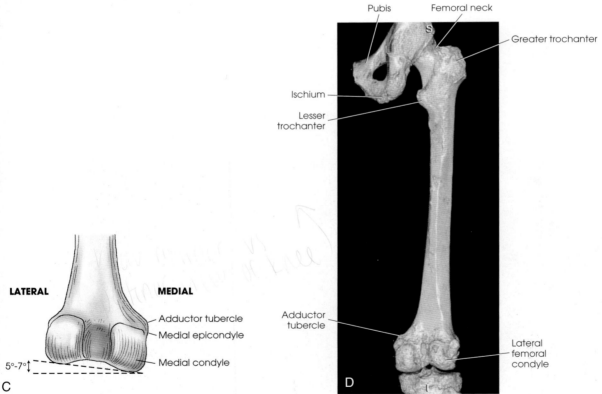

Fig. 7.6 (A) Anterior aspect of left femur. (B) Posterior aspect. (C) Distal end of posterior femur showing a 5- to 7-degree difference between medial and lateral condyle when the femur is vertical. (D) Three-dimensional CT scan showing posterior aspect and articulation with knee and hip.

The distal end of the femur is broadened and has two large eminences: the larger *medial condyle* and the smaller *lateral condyle*. Anteriorly, the condyles are separated by the *patellar surface*: a shallow, triangular depression. Posteriorly, the condyles are separated by a deep depression called the *intercondylar fossa*. A slight prominence above and within the curve of each condyle forms the *medial* and *lateral epicondyles*. The medial condyle contains the *adductor tubercle*, which is located on the posterolateral aspect. The tubercle is a raised bony area that receives the tendon of the adductor muscle. This tubercle is important to identify on lateral knee radiographs because it assists in identifying overrotation or underrotation. The triangular area superior to the intercondylar fossa on the posterior femur is the *trochlear groove*, over which the popliteal blood vessels and nerves pass.

The posterior area of the knee, between the condyles, contains a sesamoid bone in 3% to 5% of people. This sesamoid is called the *fabella* and is seen only on the lateral projection of the knee.

Patella

The *patella,* or knee cap (Fig. 7.8), is the largest and most constant sesamoid bone in the body (see Chapter 2). The patella is a flat, triangular bone situated at the distal anterior surface of the femur. The patella develops in the tendon of the quadriceps femoris muscle between 3 and 5 years of age. The *apex,* or tip, is directed inferiorly, lies ½ inch (1.3 cm) above the joint space of the knee, and is attached to the tuberosity of the tibia by the patellar ligament. The superior border of the patella is called the *base.*

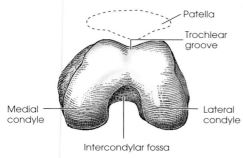

Fig. 7.7 Inferior aspect of left femur.

handwritten: condyles articulate w/ plateau's of tibia

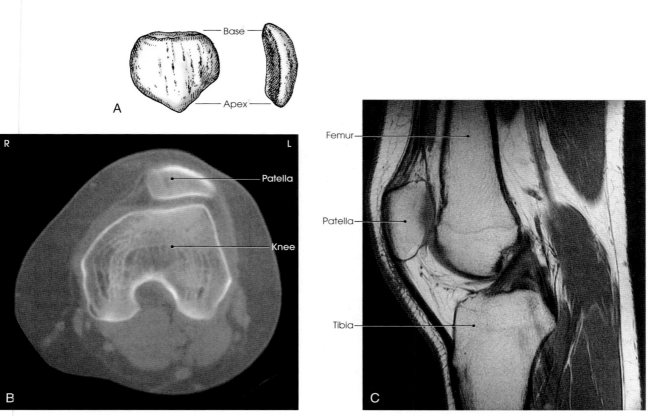

Fig. 7.8 (A) Anterior and lateral aspects of patella. (B) Axial CT scan of patella showing relationship to femur. (C) Sagittal MRI showing patellar relationship to femur and knee joint. The apex of the patella is ½ inch (1.2 cm) above the knee joint.

(B and C, Modified from Kelley LL, Petersen CM: *Sectional anatomy for imaging professionals,* ed 2, St Louis, 2007, Mosby.)

Knee Joint

The knee joint is one of the most complex joints in the human body. The femur, tibia, fibula, and patella are held together by a complex group of ligaments. These ligaments work together to provide stability for the knee joint. Although radiographers do not produce images of these ligaments, they need to have a basic understanding of their positions and interrelationships. Many patients with knee injuries do not have fractures, but they may have one or more torn ligaments, which can cause great pain and may alter the position of the bones. Fig. 7.9 shows the following important ligaments of the knee:

- Posterior cruciate ligament
- Anterior cruciate ligament
- Tibial collateral ligament
- Fibular collateral ligament

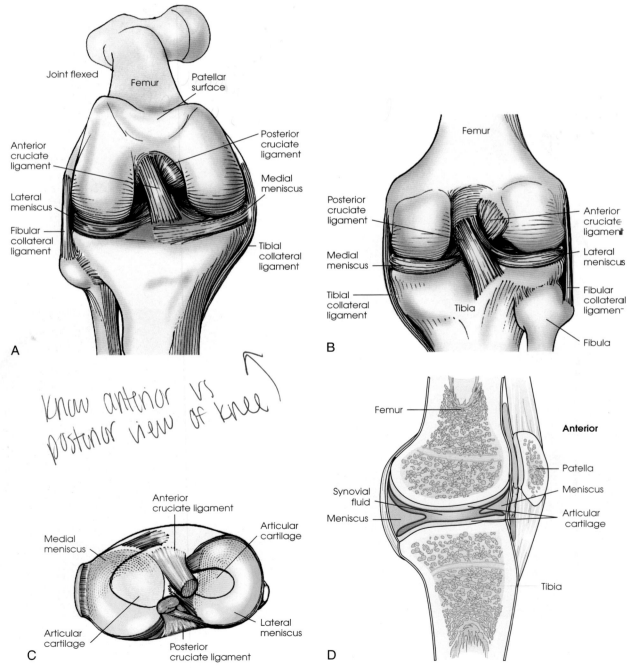

(handwritten note) Know anterior vs posterior view of knee

Fig. 7.9 Knee joint. (A) Anterior aspect with femur flexed. (B) Posterior aspect. (C) Superior surface of tibia. (D) Sagittal section.

The knee joint contains two fibrocartilage disks called the *lateral meniscus* and *medial meniscus* (Fig. 7.10; also see Fig. 7.9). The circular menisci lie on the tibial plateaus. They are thick at the outer margin of the joint and taper off toward the center of the tibial plateau. The center of the tibial plateau contains cartilage that articulates directly with the condyles of the knee. The menisci provide stability for the knee and act as a shock absorber. The menisci are commonly torn during injury. A knee arthrogram or a magnetic resonance imaging (MRI) scan must be performed to visualize a meniscus tear.

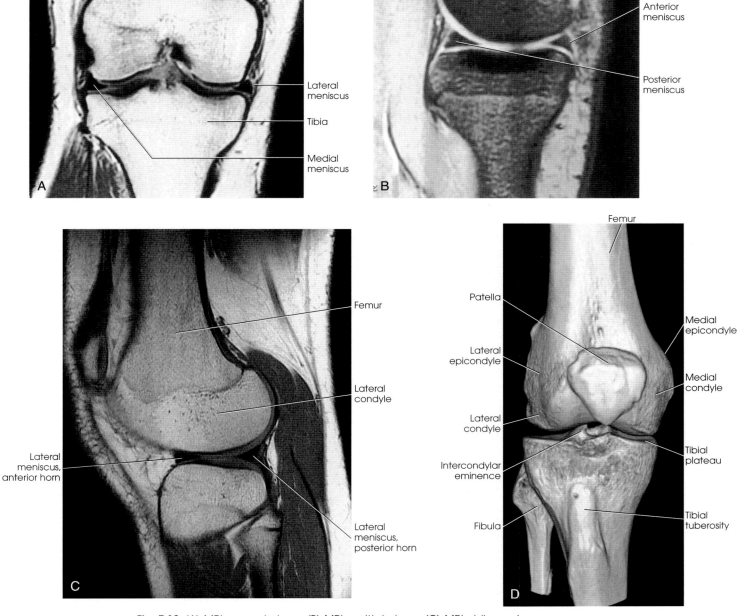

Fig. 7.10 (A) MRI coronal plane. (B) MRI sagittal plane. (C) MRI oblique plane. (D) Three-dimensional CT reformat of the knee joint.

Lower Extremity Articulations

The joints of the lower extremity are summarized in Table 7.1 and shown in Figs. 7.11 and 7.12. Beginning with the distal-most portion of the lower extremity, the articulations are as follows.

The *interphalangeal (IP) articulations,* between the phalanges, are *synovial hinges* that allow only flexion and extension. The joints between the distal and middle phalanges are the *distal interphalangeal (DIP) joints.* Articulations between the middle and proximal phalanges are the *proximal interphalangeal (PIP) joints.* With only two phalanges in the great toe, the joint is known simply as the *IP joint.*

TABLE 7.1
Joints of the lower extremity

| Joint | Structural classification | | Movement |
	Tissue	Type	
Interphalangeal	Synovial	Hinge	Freely movable
Metatarsophalangeal	Synovial	Ellipsoidal	Freely movable
Intermetatarsal	Synovial	Gliding	Freely movable
Tarsometatarsal	Synovial	Gliding	Freely movable
Calcaneocuboid	Synovial	Gliding	Freely movable
Cuneocuboid	Synovial	Gliding	Freely movable
Intercuneiform	Synovial	Gliding	Freely movable
Cuboidonavicular	Fibrous	Syndesmosis	Slightly movable
Naviculocuneiform	Synovial	Gliding	Freely movable
Subtalar			
Talocalcaneal	Synovial	Gliding	Freely movable
Talocalcaneonavicular	Synovial	Ball and socket	Freely movable
Ankle mortise			
Talofibular	Synovial	Hinge	Freely movable
Tibiotalar	Synovial	Hinge	Freely movable
Tibiofibular			
Proximal	Synovial	Gliding	Freely movable
Distal	Fibrous	Syndesmosis	Slightly movable
Knee			
Patellofemoral	Synovial	Gliding	Freely movable
Femorotibial	Synovial	Hinge modified	Freely movable

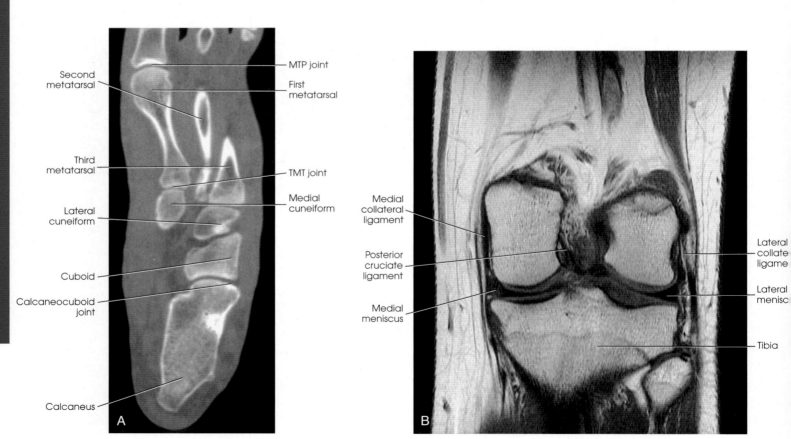

Fig. 7.11 (A) Axial CT scan of foot and calcaneus. (B) MRI coronal plane of the knee joint. Joint spaces are clearly shown.

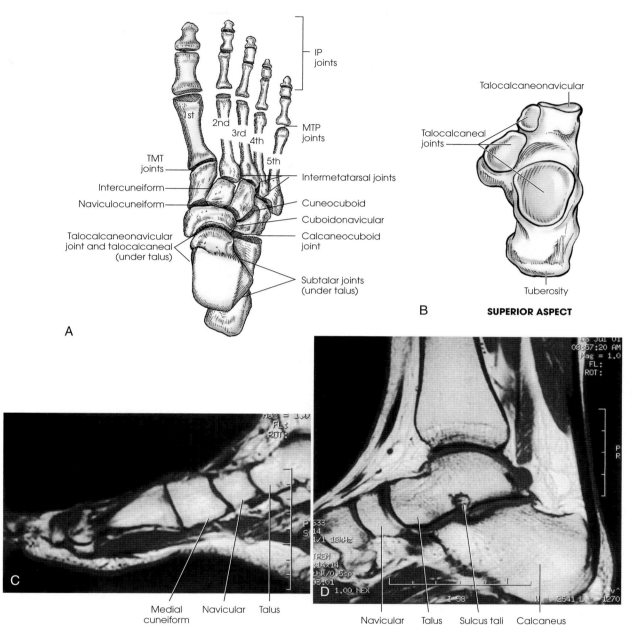

IP joints

MTP joints

TMT joints

Intercuneiform

Naviculocuneiform

Talocalcaneonavicular joint and talocalcaneal (under talus)

1st

2nd

3rd

4th

5th

Intermetatarsal joints

Cuneocuboid

Cuboidonavicular

Calcaneocuboid joint

Subtalar joints (under talus)

A

Talocalcaneonavicular

Talocalcaneal joints

Tuberosity

B   SUPERIOR ASPECT

C

Medial cuneiform   Navicular   Talus

D

Navicular   Talus   Sulcus tali   Calcaneus

Fig. 7.12 (A) and (B) Joints of the right foot. (C) MRI sagittal plane of the anterior foot. (D) MRI sagittal plane of the posterior foot and ankle. Joint spaces and articular surfaces are clearly shown.

The distal heads of the metatarsals articulate with the proximal ends of the phalanges at the *metatarsophalangeal* (MTP) articulations to form *synovial ellipsoidal* joints, which have movements of flexion, extension, and slight adduction and abduction. The proximal bases of the metatarsals articulate with one another (*intermetatarsal* articulations) and with the tarsals (*tarsometatarsal* [TMT] articulations) to form *synovial gliding* joints, which permit flexion, extension, adduction, and abduction movements.

The *intertarsal* articulations allow only slight gliding movements between the bones and are classified as *synovial gliding* or *synovial ball-and-socket* joints (see Table 7.1). The joint spaces are narrow and obliquely situated. When the joint surfaces of these bones are in question, it is necessary to angle the x-ray tube or adjust the foot to place the joint spaces parallel with the central ray.

The calcaneus supports the talus and articulates with it by an irregularly shaped, three-faceted joint surface, forming the *subtalar joint*. This joint is classified as a *synovial gliding* joint. Anteriorly, the calcaneus articulates with the cuboid at the calcaneocuboid joint. This joint is a synovial gliding joint. The talus rests on top of the calcaneus (see Fig. 7.12). It articulates with the navicular bone anteriorly, supports the tibia above, and articulates with the malleoli of the tibia and fibula at its sides.

Each of the three parts of the subtalar joint is formed by reciprocally shaped facets on the inferior surface of the talus and the superior surface of the calcaneus. Study of the superior and medial aspects of the calcaneus (see Fig. 7.3) helps the radiographer to understand better the problems involved in radiography of this joint.

The intertarsal articulations are:
- Calcaneocuboid
- Cuneocuboid
- Intercuneiform (two)
- Cuboidonavicular
- Naviculocuneiform
- Talocalcaneal
- Talocalcaneonavicular

The *ankle joint* is commonly called the *ankle mortise,* or *mortise joint.* It is formed by the articulations between the lateral malleolus of the fibula and the inferior surface and medial malleolus of the tibia (Fig. 7.13A). The mortise joint is often divided specifically into the *talofibular* and *tibiofibular* joints. These form a socket type of structure that articulates with the superior portion of the talus. The talus fits inside the mortise. The articulation is a synovial hinge type of joint. The primary action of the ankle joint consists of dorsiflexion (flexion) and plantar flexion (extension); however, in full plantar flexion, a small amount of rotation and abduction-adduction is permitted. The

mortise joint also allows inversion and eversion of the foot. Other movements at the ankle largely depend on the gliding movements of the intertarsal joints, particularly the one between the talus and the calcaneus.

The fibula articulates with the tibia at its distal and proximal ends. The *distal tibiofibular* joint is a *fibrous syndesmosis* joint allowing slight movement. The head of the fibula articulates with the posteroinferior surface of the lateral condyle of the tibia, which forms the *proximal tibiofibular* joint: a *synovial gliding* joint (see Fig. 7.13A).

The patella articulates with the patellar surface of the femur and protects the front of the knee joint. This articulation is called the *patellofemoral joint;* when the knee is extended and relaxed, the patella is freely movable over the patellar surface of the femur. When the knee is flexed as a *synovial gliding* joint, the patella is locked in position in front of the patellar surface. The knee joint, or *femorotibial* joint, is the largest joint in the body. It is called a *synovial modified-hinge joint.* In addition to flexion and extension, the knee joint allows slight medial and lateral rotation in the flexed position. The joint is enclosed in an articular capsule and is held together by numerous ligaments (see Figs. 7.9 and 7.13B).

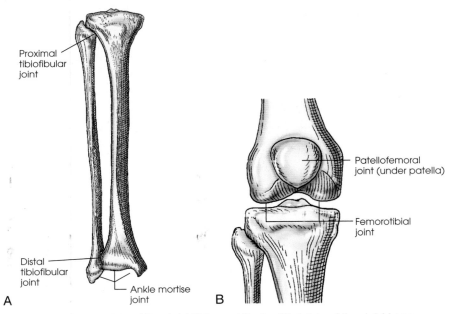

Proximal tibiofibular joint

Distal tibiofibular joint

Ankle mortise joint

A

Patellofemoral joint (under patella)

Femorotibial joint

B

Fig. 7.13 (A) Joints of the right tibia and fibula. (B) Joints of the right knee.

SUMMARY OF ANATOMY

Foot
Phalanges
Metatarsals
Tarsals
Dorsum (dorsal surface)
Plantar surface

Phalanges (14)
Proximal phalanx
Middle phalanx
Distal phalanx
Body
Base
Head

Metatarsals (5)
First metatarsal
Second metatarsal
Third metatarsal
Fourth metatarsal
Fifth metatarsal
Body
Base
Head
Tuberosity (fifth)

Tarsals (7)
Calcaneus
Tuberosity
Anterior facet
Middle facet

Posterior facet
Calcaneal sulcus
Sinus tarsi
Sustentaculum tali
Trochlea
Talus
Trochlear surface
Sulcus tali
Posterior articular surface
Cuboid
Navicular
Medial cuneiform
Intermediate cuneiform
Lateral cuneiform

Others
Sesamoid bones

Leg
Tibia
Fibula

Tibia
Body
Medial condyle
Lateral condyle
Tibial plateau
Intercondylar eminence
Medial intercondylar
Tubercle
Lateral intercondylar

Tubercle
Tibial tuberosity
Anterior crest
Medial malleolus
Anterior tubercle
Fibular notch

Fibula
Body
Head
Apex
Lateral malleolus

Thigh
Femur
Body
Medial condyle
Lateral condyle
Trochlear groove
Intercondylar fossa
Medial epicondyle
Lateral epicondyle
Adductor tubercle
Popliteal surface
Fabella

Patella
Apex
Base

Knee joint
Posterior cruciate ligament
Anterior cruciate ligament
Tibial collateral ligament
Fibular collateral ligament
Lateral meniscus
Medial meniscus

Articulations
Interphalangeal
Metatarsophalangeal
Intermetatarsal
Tarsometatarsal
Intertarsal
Subtalar
  Talocalcaneonavicular
  Talocalcaneal
Calcaneocuboid
Cuneocuboid
Intercuneiform
Cuboidonavicular
Naviculocuneiform
Ankle mortise
  Talofibular
  Tibiotalar
Tibiofibular
  Proximal
  Distal
Knee
  Patellofemoral
  Femorotibial

ABBREVIATIONS USED IN CHAPTER 7

ASIS	Anterior superior iliac spine
DIP[a]	Distal interphalangeal
IP[a]	Interphalangeal
PIP[a]	Proximal interphalangeal
MTP	Metatarsophalangeal
TMT	Tarsometatarsal

[a]The same abbreviations are used for joints in the hand.
See Addendum A for a summary of all abbreviations used in Volume 1.

SUMMARY OF PATHOLOGY

Condition	Definition
Bone cyst	Fluid-filled cyst with a wall of fibrous tissue
Congenital clubfoot	Abnormal twisting of the foot, usually inward and downward
Dislocation	Displacement of a bone from the joint space
Fracture	Disruption in the continuity of bone
Pott	Avulsion fracture of the medial malleolus with loss of the ankle mortise
Jones	Avulsion fracture of the base of the fifth metatarsal
Gout	Hereditary form of arthritis in which uric acid is deposited in joints
Metastases	Transfer of a cancerous lesion from one area to another
Osgood–Schlatter disease	Incomplete separation or avulsion of the tibial tuberosity
Osteoarthritis or degenerative joint disease	Form of arthritis marked by progressive cartilage deterioration in synovial joints and vertebrae
Osteomalacia or rickets	Softening of the bones due to vitamin D deficiency
Osteomyelitis	Inflammation of bone due to a pyogenic infection
Osteopetrosis	Increased density of atypically soft bone
Osteoporosis	Loss of bone density
Paget disease	Chronic metabolic disease of bone marked by weakened, deformed, and thickened bone that fractures easily
Tumor	New tissue growth where cell proliferation is uncontrolled
Chondrosarcoma	Malignant tumor arising from cartilage cells
Enchondroma	Benign tumor consisting of cartilage
Ewing sarcoma	Malignant tumor of bone arising in medullary tissue
Osteochondroma or exostosis	Benign bone tumor projection with a cartilaginous cap
Osteoclastoma or giant cell tumor	Lucent lesion in the metaphysis, usually at the distal femur
Osteoid osteoma	Benign lesion of cortical bone
Osteosarcoma	Malignant, primary tumor of bone with bone or cartilage formation

Eponymous (named) pathologies are listed in nonpossessive form to conform to the *AMA manual of style: a guide to authors and editors*, ed 10, Oxford, 2009, Oxford University Press.

SAMPLE EXPOSURE TECHNIQUE CHART ESSENTIAL PROJECTIONS

These techniques were accurate for the equipment used to produce each exposure. However, use caution when applying them in your department because "there is considerable variability in image receptor response owing to varying scatter sensitivity, the use of grids with different grid ratios, collimation, beam filtration, the choice of kilovoltage, source-to-image distance, and image receptor size."[1]

This chart was created in collaboration with Dennis Bowman, AS, RT(R), Clinical Instructor, Community Hospital of the Monterey Peninsula, Monterey, CA. http://digitalradiographysolutions.com/.

LOWER EXTREMITY

Part	cm	kVp[a]	SID[b]	Collimation	CR[c] mAs	CR[c] Dose (mGy)[e]	DR[d] mAs	DR[d] Dose (mGy)[e]
Toes—*all*[f]	1.5	63	40″	2″ × 6″ (5 × 15 cm)	2.0[g]	0.052	0.9[g]	0.023
Foot—*AP, oblique, lateral*[f]	5	70	40″	6″ × 11″ (15 × 28 cm)	2.5[g]	0.166	1.25[g]	0.082
Calcaneus—*axial*[f]	8	70	40″	4″ × 6″ (10 × 15 cm)	3.2[g]	0.201	1.8[g]	0.112
Calcaneus—*lateral*[f]	5	70	40″	4″ × 5″ (10 × 13 cm)	2.2[g]	0.130	1.1[g]	0.063
Ankle—*AP*[f]	11	70	40″	4″ × 9″ (10 × 23 cm)	3.2[g]	0.217	1.8[g]	0.121
Ankle—*lateral*[f]	7	70	40″	5″ × 9″ (13 × 23 cm)	2.2[g]	0.150	1.25[g]	0.084
Leg—*all*[h]	11	81	40″	6″ × 17″ (15 × 43 cm)	4.5[g]	0.468	2.0[g]	0.206
Leg—*all*[f]	12	70	40″	6″ × 17″ (15 × 43 cm)	3.6[g]	0.286	2.5[g]	0.199
Knee—*AP, oblique, lateral*[h]	12	85	40″	6″ × 11″ (15 × 28 cm)	5.0[g]	0.576	2.5[g]	0.283
Knee—*AP, oblique, lateral*[f]	13	70	40″	6″ × 11″ (15 × 28 cm)	5.0[g]	0.405	2.5[g]	0.202
Intercondylar fossa[f]	14	70	40″	6″ × 6″ (15 × 15 cm)	5.0[g]	0.398	2.5[g]	0.199
Patella—*PA*[h]	12	85	40″	6″ × 6″ (15 × 15 cm)	6.3[g]	0.698	3.2[g]	0.353
Patella—*lateral*[h]	12	85	40″	5″ × 5″ (13 × 13 cm)	2.8[g]	0.342	2.0[g]	0.190
Patella—*tangential*[f]	12	70	40″	5″ × 5″ (13 × 13 cm)	4.0[g]	0.259	2.0[g]	0.143
Femur—*AP, lateral*[h]	15	87.5	40″	8″ × 17″ (20 × 43 cm)	7.1[g]	0.949	3.6[g]	0.479
Femur—*proximal*[h]	19	87.5	40″	9″ × 17″ (23 × 43 cm)	14[g]	2.082	7.1[g]	1.052

[1]ACR-AAPM-SIMM Practice Parameter for Digital Radiography, revised 2017.
[a]kVp values are for a high-frequency generator.
[b]40-inch minimum; 44 to 48 inches recommended to improve spatial resolution (mAs increase needed, but no increase in patient dose will result).
[c]AGFA CR MD 4.0 General IP, central ray (CR) 75.0 reader, 400 speed class, with 6:1 (178LPI) grid when needed.
[d]GE Definium 8000, with 13:1 grid when needed.
[e]All doses are skin entrance for average adult (160- to 200-pound male, 150- to 190-pound female) at part thickness indicated.
[f]Tabletop, nongrid.
[g]Small focal spot.
[h]Bucky/Grid.

Radiation Protection

Protecting the patient from unnecessary radiation is a professional responsibility of the radiographer. In this chapter, the *Shield gonads* statement at the end of the *Position of part* sections indicates that the patient is to be protected from unnecessary radiation by using proper collimation and by placing lead shielding between the gonads and the radiation source, when necessary.

Toes

⚕ AP OR AP AXIAL PROJECTIONS

Because of the natural curve of the toes, the IP joint spaces are not best shown on the AP projection. When demonstration of these joint spaces is not critical, an AP projection may be performed (Figs. 7.14 and 7.15). An AP axial projection is recommended to open the joint spaces and reduce foreshortening (Figs. 7.16 and 7.17).

> **Image receptor:** Positioned by manufacturer or department protocol for proper anatomy display orientation; CR plate: 10 × 12 inches (24 × 30 cm) lengthwise.

Position of patient

- Have the patient seated or placed supine on the radiographic table.

Position of part

- With the patient in the supine or seated position, flex the knees, separate the feet about 6 inches (15 cm), and touch the knees together for immobilization.
- Center the toes directly over one half of the IR image receptor (IR) (see Figs. 7.14 and 7.16), or place a 15-degree foam wedge well under the foot and rest the toes near the elevated base of the wedge (Fig. 7.18).
- Adjust the IR half with its midline parallel to the long axis of the foot, and center it to the third MTP joint.
- *Shield gonads.*

NOTE: Some institutions may show the entire foot, whereas others radiograph only the toe or toes of interest.

Central ray

- Perpendicular through the third MTP joint (see Fig. 7.14) when it is not critical to demonstrate the joint spaces. To open the joint spaces, direct the central ray 15 degrees posteriorly through the third MTP joint (see Fig. 7.16), or elevate the foot on a 15-degree foam wedge (Fig. 7.19).

Collimation

- Adjust the radiation field to 1 inch (2.5 cm) on all sides of the toes, including 1 inch (2.5 cm) proximal to the MTP joint. Place side marker in the collimated exposure field.

Structures shown

The 14 phalanges of the toes; the distal portions of the metatarsals; and, on the axial projections, the IP joints.

EVALUATION CRITERIA

The following should be clearly seen:
- Evidence of proper collimation and the presence of a side marker placed clear of the anatomy of interest
- Entire toes, including distal ends of the metatarsals
- Toes separated from each other
- No rotation of phalanges; soft tissue width and midshaft concavity equal on both sides
- Open interphalangeal and metatarsophalangeal joint spaces on axial projections
- Bony trabecular detail and surrounding soft tissues

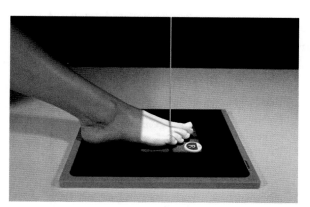

Fig. 7.14 AP toes, perpendicular CR.

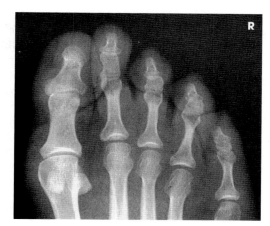

Fig. 7.15 AP toes, perpendicular CR.

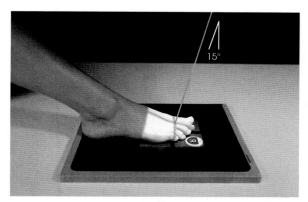

Fig. 7.16 AP axial toes, CR angulation of 15 degrees.

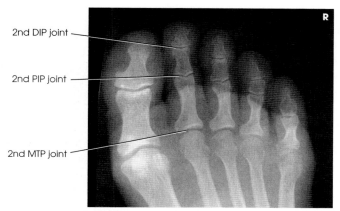

2nd DIP joint

2nd PIP joint

2nd MTP joint

Fig. 7.17 AP axial toes, CR angulation of 15 degrees.

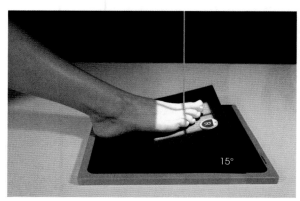

Fig. 7.18 AP axial, 15-degree foam wedge.

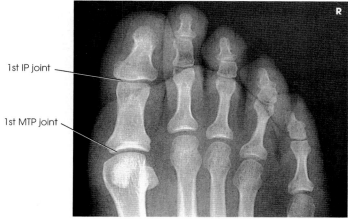

1st IP joint

1st MTP joint

Fig. 7.19 AP axial, toes on 15-degree wedge.

PA PROJECTION

Image receptor: Positioned by manufacturer or department protocol for proper anatomy display orientation; CR plate: 10 × 12 inches (24 × 30 cm) lengthwise.

Position of patient

- Have the patient lie prone on the radiographic table because this position naturally turns the foot over so that the dorsal aspect is in contact with the IR.

Position of part

- Place the toes in the appropriate position by elevating them on one or two small sandbags and adjusting the support to place the toes horizontally.

- Place the IR half under the toes with the midline of the side used parallel with the long axis of the foot, and center it to the third MTP joint (Fig. 7.20).

Central ray

- Perpendicular to the midpoint of the IR entering the third MTP joint (see Fig. 7.20). The IP joint spaces are shown well because the natural divergence of the x-ray beam coincides closely with the position of the toes (Fig. 7.21).

Collimation

- Adjust the radiation field to 1 inch (2.5 cm) on all sides of the toes, including 1 inch (2.5 cm) proximal to the MTP joint. Place side marker in the collimated exposure field.

Structures shown

The 14 phalanges of the toes, the IP joints, and the distal portions of the metatarsals.

EVALUATION CRITERIA

The following should be clearly seen:
- Evidence of proper collimation and the presence of a side marker placed clear of the anatomy of interest
- Entire toes, including distal ends of the metatarsals
- Toes separated from each other
- No rotation of phalanges; soft tissue width and midshaft concavity equal on both sides
- Open interphalangeal and metatarsophalangeal joint spaces
- Bony trabecular detail and surrounding soft tissues

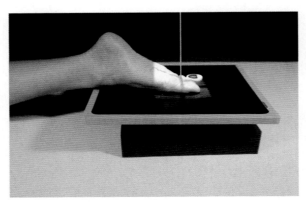

Fig. 7.20 PA toes.

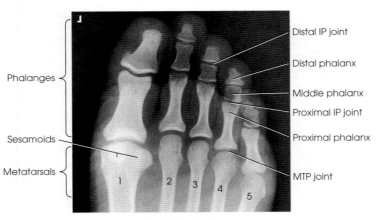

Fig. 7.21 PA toes.

♠ AP OBLIQUE PROJECTION
Medial rotation

Image receptor: Positioned by manufacturer or department protocol for proper anatomy display orientation; CR plate: 10 × 12 inches (24 ×30 cm) lengthwise.

Position of patient
- Place the patient in the supine or seated position on the radiographic table.
- Flex the knee of the affected side enough to have the sole of the foot resting firmly on the table.

Position of part
- Position the IR half under the toes.
- Medially rotate the lower leg and foot, and adjust the plantar surface of the foot to form a 30- to 45-degree angle from the plane of the IR (Fig. 7.22).
- Center the toes to the IR.
- *Shield gonads.*

Central ray
- Perpendicular and entering the third MTP joint.

Collimation
- Adjust the radiation field to 1 inch (2.5 cm) on all sides of the toes, including 1 inch (2.5 cm) proximal to the MTP joint. Place side marker in the collimated exposure field.

NOTE: Oblique projections of individual toes may be obtained by centering the affected toe to the portion of the IR being used and collimating closely. The foot may be placed in a medial oblique position for the first and second toes and in a lateral oblique position for the fourth and fifth toes. Either oblique position is adequate for the third (middle) toe.

Structures shown
An AP oblique projection of the phalanges shows the toes and the distal portion of the metatarsals rotated medially (Fig. 7.23).

EVALUATION CRITERIA
The following should be clearly seen:
- Evidence of proper collimation and the presence of a side marker placed clear of the anatomy of interest
- Entire toes, including distal ends of the metatarsals
- Toes separated from each other
- Proper rotation of toes, as demonstrated by more soft tissue width and more midshaft concavity on elevated side
- Open interphalangeal and second through fifth metatarsophalangeal joint spaces
- First MTP joint (not always opened)
- Bony trabecular detail and surrounding soft tissues

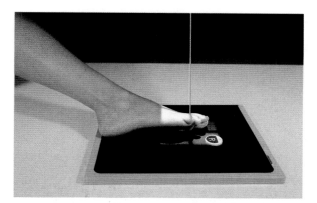

Fig. 7.22 AP oblique toes, medial rotation.

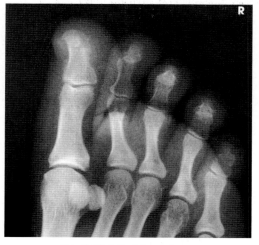

Fig. 7.23 AP oblique toes.

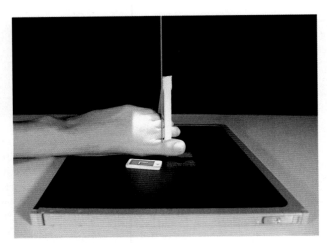

Fig. 7.24 Lateral great toe.

☀ LATERAL PROJECTIONS
Mediolateral or lateromedial

Image receptor: Positioned by manufacturer or department protocol for proper anatomy display orientation; CR plate: 10×12 inches (24×30 cm) lengthwise.

Position of patient

- Have the patient lie in the lateral recumbent position.
- Support the affected extremity on sandbags, and adjust it in a comfortable position.
- To prevent superimposition, tape the toes above the one being examined into a flexed position; a 4×4 inch gauze pad also may be used to separate the toes.

NOTE: Manipulate toes only if no deformity is apparent.

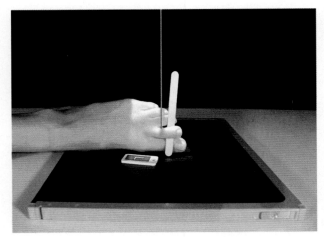

Fig. 7.25 Lateral second toe.

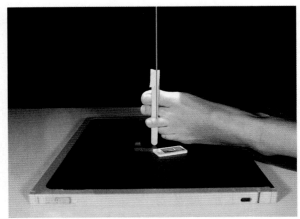

Fig. 7.26 Lateral third toe.

Position of part

Great toe, second toe

- Place the patient on the *unaffected* side for these two toes.
- Place an IR under the medial side of the foot and center it to the affected toe.
- Grasp the patient's extremity by the heel and knee, and adjust its position to place the toe in a true lateral position (plane through MTP joints will be perpendicular to IR).
- Adjust the long axis of the IR so that it is parallel with the long axis of the toe (Figs. 7.24 and 7.25).

Third, fourth, fifth toes

- Place the patient on the *affected* side for these three toes.
- Place an IR under the lateral side of the foot and center it to the toes.
- Grasp patient's extremity by heel and knee, and adjust its position to place the toes in a true lateral position (plane through MTP joints is perpendicular to IR).
- Adjust the long axis of the IR so that it is parallel with the long axis of the toe.
- Support the elevated heel on a sandbag or sponge for immobilization (Figs. 7.26–7.28).
- *Shield gonads.*

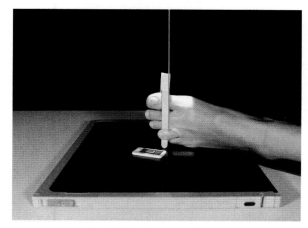

Fig. 7.27 Lateral fourth toe.

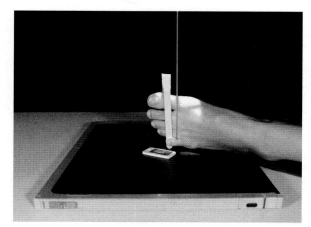

Fig. 7.28 Lateral fifth toe.

Central ray

- Perpendicular to the plane of the IR, entering the IP joint of the great toe or the proximal IP joint of the lesser toes.

Collimation

- Adjust the radiation field to 1 inch (2.5 cm) on all sides of the toes, including 1 inch (2.5 cm) proximal to the MTP joint. Place side marker in the collimated exposure field.

Structures shown

Lateral projection of the phalanges of the toe and the IP articulations projected free of the other toes (Figs. 7.29–7.33).

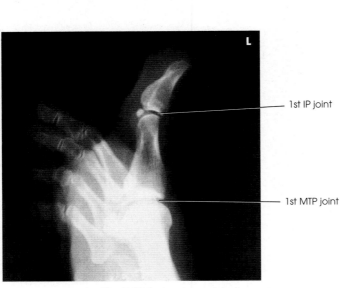

Fig. 7.29 Lateral great toe.

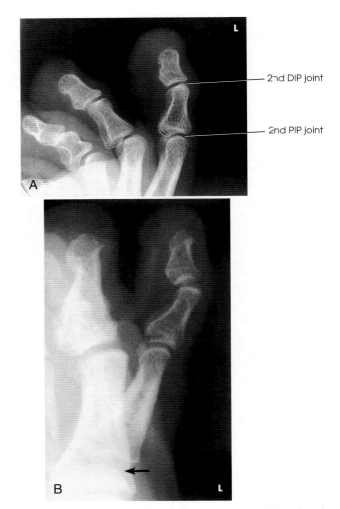

Fig. 7.30 (A) Lateral second toe. (B) Lateral second toe showing the MTP joint (arrow).

EVALUATION CRITERIA

The following should be clearly seen:

- Evidence of proper collimation and the presence of a side marker placed clear of the anatomy of interest
- Entire toe, without superimposition of adjacent toes; when superimposition cannot be avoided, the proximal phalanx must be shown
- Toe(s) in a true lateral position
  - Toenail in profile, if visualized and normal
  - Concave, plantar surfaces of the phalanges
  - No rotation of the phalanges
- Open interphalangeal joint spaces; the metatarsophalangeal joints are overlapped but may be seen in some patients
- Bony trabecular detail and surrounding soft tissues

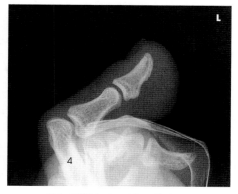

Fig. 7.32 Lateral fourth toe.

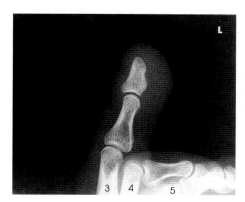

Fig. 7.31 Lateral third toe.

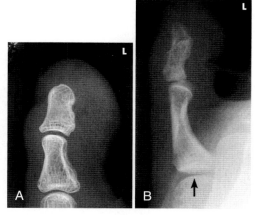

Fig. 7.33 (A) Lateral fifth toe. (B) Lateral fifth toe showing the MTP joint (arrow). Note that the distal IP joint is fused.

TANGENTIAL PROJECTION

LEWIS[1] AND HOLLY[2] METHODS

Image receptor: Positioned by manufacturer or department protocol for proper anatomy display orientation; CR plate: 10 × 12 inches (24 × 30 cm) lengthwise.

Position of patient

- Place the patient in the prone position for the Lewis method and in a sitting position for the Holly method.
- Elevate the ankle of the affected side on sandbags for stability, if needed. A folded towel may be placed under the knee for comfort.

Position of part

- Rest the great toe on the table in a position of dorsiflexion, and adjust it to place the ball of the foot perpendicular to the horizontal plane.
- Center the IR to the second metatarsal (Fig. 7.34).
- *Shield gonads.*

Central ray

- Perpendicular and tangential to the first MTP joint.

Collimation

- Adjust the radiation field to 3 × 3 inches (7.6 × 7.6 cm). Place side marker in the collimated exposure field.

Structures shown

Tangential projection of the metatarsal head in profile and the sesamoids (Fig. 7.35).

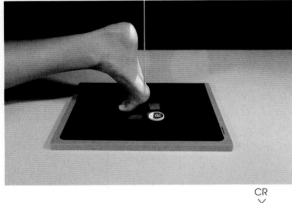

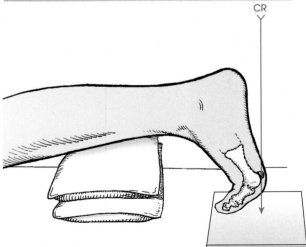

Fig. 7.34 Tangential sesamoids: Lewis method.

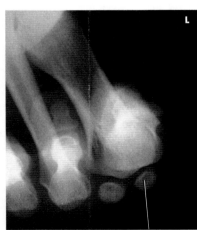

Sesamoid

Fig. 7.35 Tangential sesamoids: Lewis method with toes against the IR.

Sesamoids

EVALUATION CRITERIA

The following should be clearly seen:
- Evidence of proper collimation and the presence of a side marker placed clear of the anatomy of interest
- Sesamoids free of any portion of the first metatarsal
- Metatarsal heads
- Bony trabecular detail and surrounding soft tissues

NOTE: Holly[2] described a position that he believed was more comfortable for the patient. With the patient seated on the table, the foot is adjusted so that the medial border is vertical, and the plantar surface is at an angle of 75 degrees with the plane of the IR. The patient holds the toes in a flexed position with a strip of gauze bandage. The *central ray* is directed perpendicular to the head of the first metatarsal bone (Figs. 7.36–7.38).

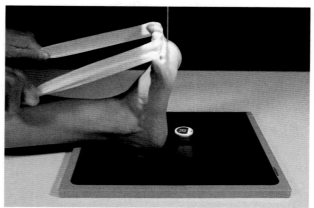

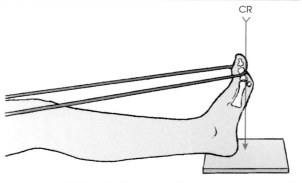

Fig. 7.36 Tangential sesamoids: Holly method.

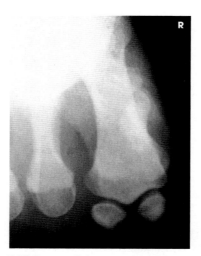

Fig. 7.37 Tangential sesamoids: Holly method with heel against the IR.

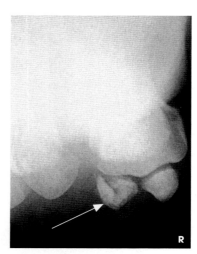

Fig. 7.38 Sesamoid with fracture *(arrow)*.

☀ AP OR AP AXIAL PROJECTION

Radiographs may be obtained by directing the central ray perpendicular to the plane of the IR or by angling the central ray 10 degrees posteriorly (toward the heel). When a 10-degree posterior angle is used, the central ray is perpendicular to the metatarsals, reducing foreshortening. The TMT joint spaces of the midfoot are also better shown (Figs. 7.39 and 7.40).

Image receptor: Positioned by manufacturer or department protocol for proper anatomy display orientation; CR plate: 10 × 12 inches (24 × 30 cm) lengthwise.

axial used to open joint spaces

Position of patient

- Place the patient in the supine or seated position.
- Flex the knee of the affected side enough to rest the sole of the foot firmly on the radiographic table.

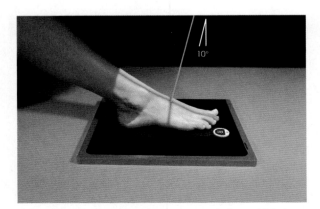

Fig. 7.39 AP axial foot with posterior angulation of 10 degrees.

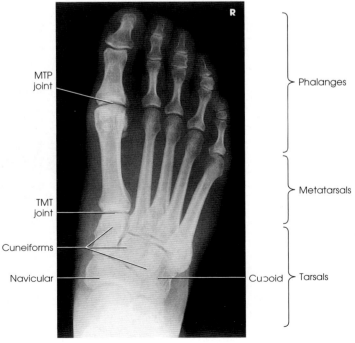

Fig. 7.40 AP axial foot with posterior angulation of 10 degrees.

Position of part

- Position the IR under the patient's foot, center it to the base of the third metatarsal, and adjust it so that its long axis is parallel with the long axis of the foot.
- Hold the leg in the vertical position by having the patient flex the opposite knee and lean it against the knee of the affected side.
- In this foot position, the entire plantar surface rests on the IR; it may be necessary to take precautions against the IR slipping by placing a sandbag on the table against the IR adjacent to the toes.
- Ensure that no rotation of the foot occurs.
- *Shield gonads.*

Central ray

- Directed one of two ways: (1) 10 degrees toward the heel entering the base of the third metatarsal (see Fig. 7.39), or (2) perpendicular to the IR and entering the base of the third metatarsal (Fig. 7.41). Palpating the prominent base of the fifth metatarsal assists in finding the third metatarsal. The third metatarsal base is in the midline, approximately 1 inch anterior (toward the toes) (Fig. 7.42).

Collimation

- Adjust the radiation field to 1 inch (2.5 cm) on the sides and 1 inch (2.5 cm) beyond the calcaneus and distal tip of the toes. Place side marker in the collimated exposure field.

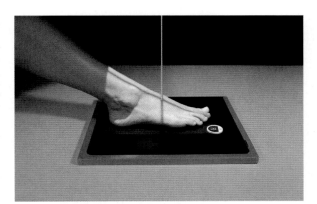

Fig. 7.41 AP foot with perpendicular CR.

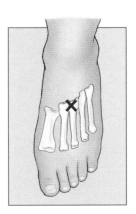

Fig. 7.42 Front view of foot in position showing CR entrance point.

◤ COMPENSATING FILTER

This projection can be improved with the use of a wedge-type compensating filter because of the difference in thickness between the toe area and the much thicker tarsal area (see Fig. 7.44).

Structures shown

AP (dorsoplantar) projection of the tarsals anterior to the talus, metatarsals, and phalanges (Figs. 7.43–7.45). This projection is used for localizing foreign bodies, determining the locations of fragments in fractures of the metatarsals and anterior tarsals, and performing general surveys of the bones of the foot.

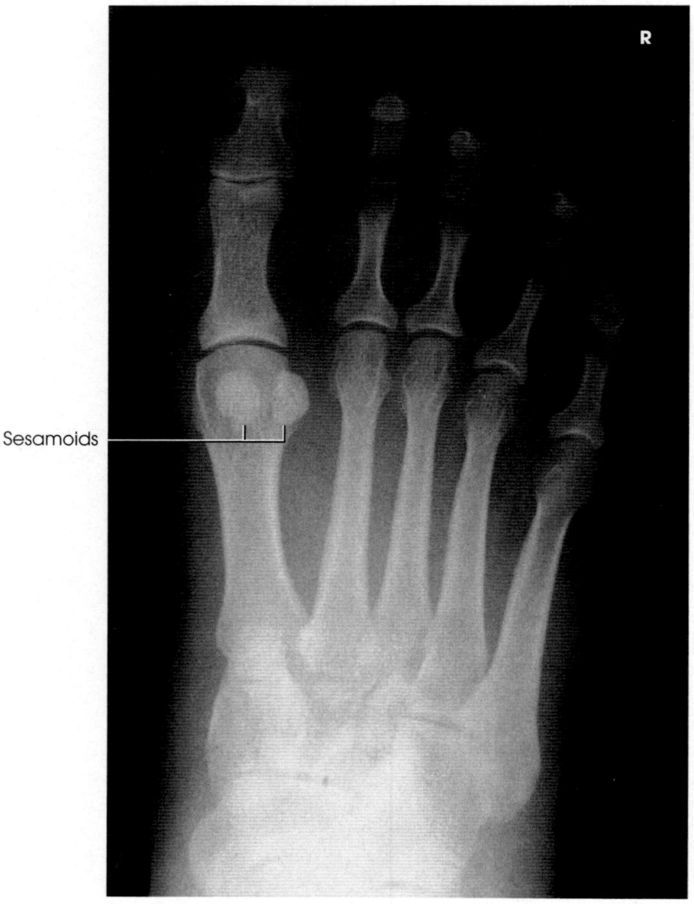

Sesamoids

Fig. 7.43 AP foot with perpendicular CR.

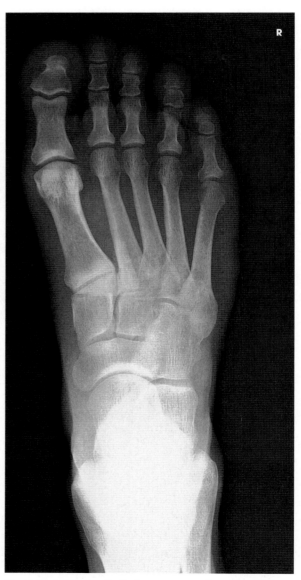

Fig. 7.44 AP foot with Ferlic compensating filter. Note how tarsal bones are better visualized.

EVALUATION CRITERIA

The following should be clearly seen:

- Evidence of proper collimation and the presence of a side marker placed clear of the anatomy of interest
- Anatomy from toes to tarsals; may include portions of talus and calcaneus
- No rotation of the foot, as demonstrated by equal amounts of space between the second through fourth metatarsals
- Overlap of the second through fifth metatarsal bases
- Axial projection resulting in improved demonstration of interphalangeal, meta-tarsophalangeal, and tarsometatarsal joint spaces
- Open joint space between medial and intermediate cuneiforms
- Bony trabecular detail and surrounding soft tissues

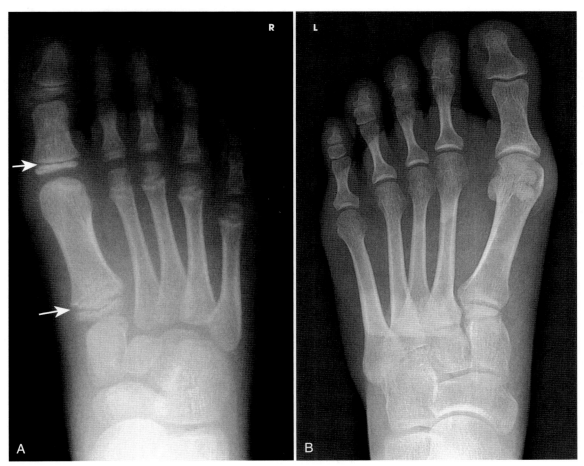

Fig. 7.45 (A) AP foot of a 6-year-old patient. Note epiphyseal lines *(arrows)*. (B) AP foot showing well-penetrated tarsal bones.

♠ AP OBLIQUE PROJECTION
Medial rotation

Image receptor: Positioned by manufacturer or department protocol for proper anatomy display orientation; CR plate: 10 × 12 inches (24 × 30 cm) lengthwise.

NOTE: The medial oblique is preferred over the lateral oblique because the plane through the metatarsals is more parallel to the IR, and it opens better the lateral side joints of the midfoot and hindfoot.

Position of patient
- Place the patient in the supine or seated position.
- Flex the knee of the affected side enough to have the plantar surface of the foot rest firmly on the radiographic table.

Position of part
- Place the IR under the patient's foot, parallel with its long axis, and center it to the midline of the foot at the level of the base of the third metatarsal.
- Rotate the patient's leg medially until the plantar surface of the foot forms an angle of 30 degrees to the plane of the IR (Fig. 7.46). If the angle of the foot is increased by more than 30 degrees, the lateral cuneiform tends to be thrown over the other cuneiforms.[3]
- *Shield gonads.*

Central ray
- Perpendicular to the base of the third metatarsal.

Collimation
- Adjust the radiation field to 1 inch (2.5 cm) on all sides and 1 inch (2.5 cm) beyond the calcaneus and distal tip of the toes. Place side marker in the collimated exposure field.

◥ COMPENSATING FILTER
This projection can be improved with the use of a wedge-type compensating filter because of the difference in thickness between the toe area and the much thicker tarsal area.

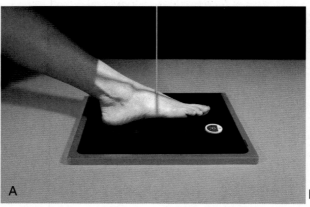
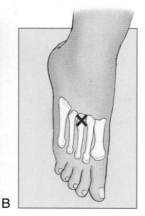

Fig. 7.46 (A) AP oblique foot, medial rotation. (B) Front view of oblique foot in position showing CR entrance point.

Structures shown

The joint spaces between the following: the cuboid and the calcaneus; the cuboid and the fourth and fifth metatarsals; the cuboid and the lateral cuneiform; and the talus and the navicular bone. The cuboid is shown in profile. The sinus tarsi is also well shown (Fig. 7.47A).

The following should be clearly seen:
- Evidence of proper collimation and the presence of a side marker placed clear of the anatomy of interest
- Entire foot, from toes to heel
- Proper rotation of foot
  - ☐ Third through fifth metatarsals free of superimposition
  - ☐ Bases of the first and second metatarsals superimposed on medial and intermediate cuneiforms
  - ☐ Navicular, lateral cuneiform, and cuboid with less superimposition than in the AP projection
- Tuberosity of the fifth metatarsal
- Lateral tarsometatarsal and intertarsal joints
- Sinus tarsi
- Bony trabecular detail and surrounding soft tissues

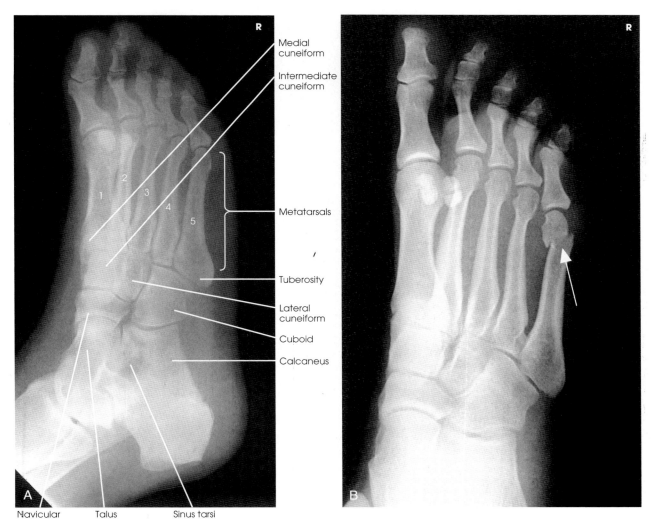

Medial cuneiform

Intermediate cuneiform

Metatarsals

Tuberosity

Lateral cuneiform

Cuboid

Calcaneus

Navicular   Talus   Sinus tarsi

Fig. 7.47 (A) AP oblique projection foot, medial rotation. (B) Fracture of distal aspect of fifth metatarsal (*arrow*). Calcaneus was not included, and technique was adjusted to visualize distal foot better.

AP OBLIQUE PROJECTION
Lateral rotation

Image receptor: Positioned by manufacturer or department protocol for proper anatomy display orientation; CR plate: 10 × 12 inch (24 × 30 cm) lengthwise.

Position of patient
- Place the patient in the supine position.
- Flex the knee of the affected side enough for the plantar surface of the foot to rest firmly on the radiographic table.

Position of part
- Place the IR under the patient's foot, parallel with its long axis, and center it to the midline of the foot at the level of the base of the third metatarsal.
- Rotate the leg laterally until the plantar surface of the foot forms an angle of 30 degrees to the IR.
- Support the elevated side of the foot on a 30-degree foam wedge to ensure consistent results (Fig. 7.48).
- *Shield gonads.*

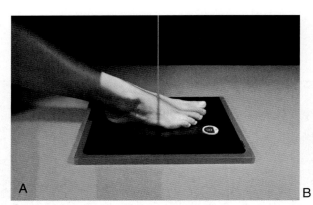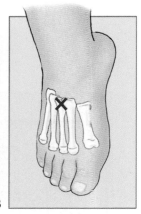

Fig. 7.48 (A) AP oblique foot, lateral rotation. (B) Front view of oblique foot in position showing CR entrance point.

Central ray

- Perpendicular to the base of the third metatarsal.

Collimation

- Adjust the radiation field to 1 inch (2.5 cm) on all sides and 1 inch (2.5 cm) beyond the calcaneus and distal tip of the toes. Place a side marker in the collimated exposure field.

Structures shown

The joint spaces between the first and second metatarsals and between the medial and intermediate cuneiforms (Fig. 7.49).

The following should be clearly seen:

- Evidence of proper collimation the presence of a side marker placed clear of the anatomy of interest
- Anatomy from toes to tarsals; may include portions of talus and calcaneus
- Proper rotation of foot
    - First and second metatarsal bases free of superimposition
    - Minimal superimposition between medial and intermediate cuneiforms
    - Navicular seen with less foreshortening than in the medial rotation AP oblique projection
- Bony trabecular detail and surrounding soft tissues

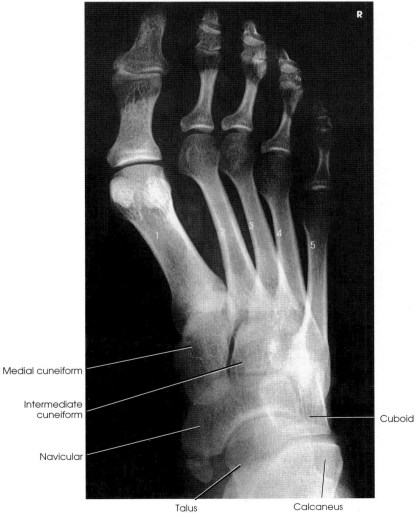
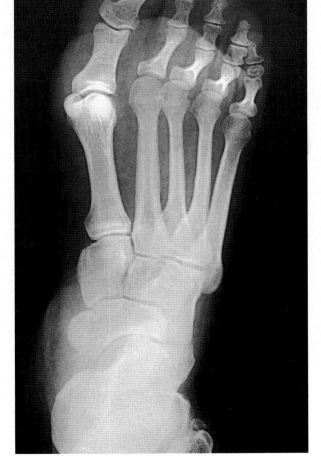

Fig. 7.49 AP oblique foot.

Medial cuneiform

Intermediate cuneiform

Navicular

Talus

Cuboid

Calcaneus

Foot

⚘ LATERAL PROJECTION
Mediolateral

The lateral (mediolateral) projection is routinely used in most radiology departments because it is the most comfortable position for the patient to assume.

Image receptor: Positioned by manufacturer or department protocol for proper anatomy display orientation; CR plate: 10 × 12 inches (24 × 30 cm) lengthwise.

Position of patient

- Have the patient lie on the radiographic table and turn toward the affected side until the leg and the foot are lateral.
- Place the opposite leg behind the affected leg.

Position of part

- Elevate the patient's knee enough to place the patella perpendicular to the horizontal plane, and adjust a sandbag support under the knee. The heel should not touch the IR, and the medial surface of the foot should be parallel with the plane of the IR.
- Adjust the foot to place the plantar surface of the forefoot perpendicular to the IR (Fig. 7.50).
- Center the IR to the midfoot, and adjust it so that its long axis is parallel with the long axis of the foot.
- Dorsiflex the foot to form a 90-degree angle with the lower leg.
- *Shield gonads.*

Central ray

- Perpendicular to the base of the third metatarsal.

Collimation

- Adjust the radiation field to 1 inch (2.5 cm) on all sides of the shadow of the foot and including the medial malleolus. Place a side marker in the collimated exposure field.

Structures shown

The entire foot in profile, the ankle joint, and the distal ends of the tibia and fibula (Figs. 7.51 and 7.52).

EVALUATION CRITERIA

The following should be clearly seen:
- Evidence of proper collimation and the presence of a side marker placed clear of the anatomy of interest
- Entire foot and distal leg
- Superimposed plantar surfaces of the metatarsal heads
- Fibula overlapping the posterior portion of the tibia
- Tibiotalar joint
- Bony trabecular detail and surrounding soft tissues

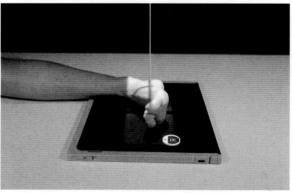

Fig. 7.50 Lateral foot.

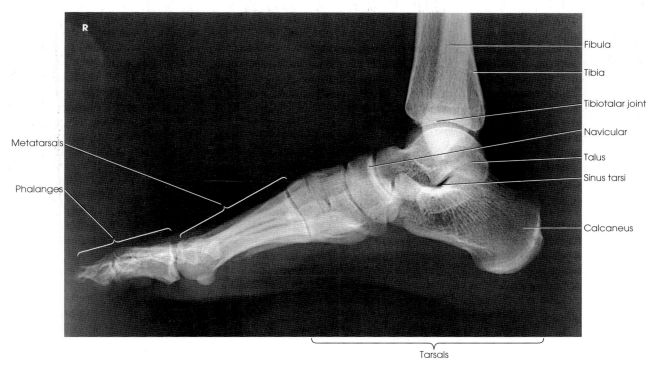

Fibula

Tibia

Tibiotalar joint

Navicular

Talus

Sinus tarsi

Calcaneus

Metatarsals

Phalanges

Tarsals

Fig. 7.51 Lateral (mediolateral) foot with anatomy identified.

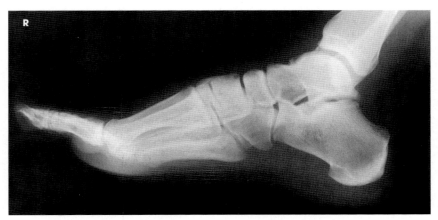

Fig. 7.52 Lateral (mediolateral foot) with foot not dorsiflexed completely.

Longitudinal Arch
LATERAL PROJECTION
Lateromedial
WEIGHT-BEARING METHOD
Standing

Image receptor: Positioned by manufacturer or department protocol for proper anatomy display orientation; CR plate: 10 × 12 inches (24 × 30 cm) lengthwise.

Position of patient

- Place the patient in the upright position, preferably on a low riser that has an IR groove. If such a riser is unavailable, use blocks to elevate the feet to the level of the x-ray tube (Figs. 7.53 and 7.54).
- If needed, use a mobile unit to allow the x-ray tube to reach the floor level.

Position of part

- Place the IR in the IR groove of the stool or between blocks.
- Have the patient stand in a natural position, one foot on each side IR, with the weight of the body equally distributed on the feet.
- Adjust the IR so that it is centered to the base of the third metatarsal, and place the medial surface of the foot against the IR.
- After the exposure, replace the IR and position the new one to image the opposite foot.
- *Shield gonads.*

Central ray

- Perpendicular to a point just above the base of the third metatarsal.

Collimation

- Adjust the radiation field to 1 inch (2.5 cm) on all sides of the shadow of the foot including 1 inch (2.5 cm) above the medial malleolus. Place a side marker in the collimated exposure field.

Structures shown

A lateromedial projection of the bones of the foot with weight-bearing. The projection is used to show the structural status of the longitudinal arch. The right and left sides are examined for comparison (Figs. 7.55 and 7.56).

EVALUATION CRITERIA

The following should be clearly seen:
- Evidence of proper collimation and the presence of a side marker placed clear of the anatomy of interest
- Entire foot and distal leg
- Superimposed plantar surfaces of the metatarsal heads
- Fibula overlapping the posterior portion of the tibia
- Tibiotalar joint
- Bony trabecular detail and surrounding soft tissues

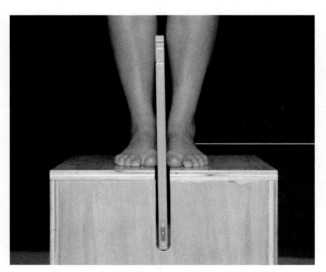

Fig. 7.53 Weight-bearing lateral foot.

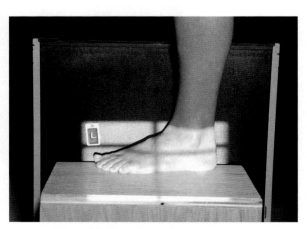

Fig. 7.54 Weight-bearing lateral foot.

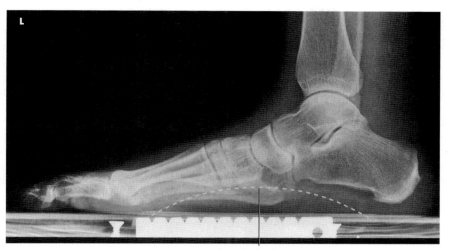

Longitudinal arch

Fig. 7.55 Weight-bearing lateral foot showing centimeter measuring scale built into standing platform.

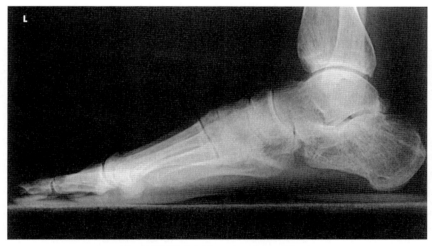

Fig. 7.56 Weight-bearing lateral foot.

AP AXIAL PROJECTION
WEIGHT-BEARING METHOD
Standing

Image receptor: Positioned by manufacturer or department protocol for proper anatomy display orientation; CR plate: 10 ×12 inches (24 × 30 cm) crosswise.

SID: 48 inches (122 cm). This SID is used to reduce magnification and improve spatial resolution in the image.

Position of patient
- Place the patient in the standing-upright position.

Position of part
- Place the IR on the floor, and have the patient stand on the IR with the feet centered on each side.

- Pull the patient's pant legs up to the knee level, if necessary.
- Ensure that right and left markers and an upright marker are placed on the IR.
- Ensure that the patient's weight is distributed equally on each foot (Fig. 7.57).
- The patient may hold the x-ray tube crane for stability.
- *Shield gonads.*

Central ray
- Angled 10 degrees toward the heel is optimal. A minimum of 15 degrees is usually necessary to have enough room to position the tube and allow the patient to stand. The central ray is positioned between the feet and at the level of the base of the third metatarsal.

Collimation
- Adjust the radiation field to 1 inch (2.5 cm) on all sides and 1 inch (2.5 cm) beyond the calcaneus and distal tip of the toes. Place a side marker in the collimated exposure field.

Structures shown
A weight-bearing AP axial projection of both feet, permitting accurate evaluation and comparison of the tarsals and metatarsals (Fig. 7.58).

The following should be clearly seen:
- Evidence of proper collimation and the presence of a side marker placed clear of the anatomy of interest
- Both feet centered on one image
- Anatomy from toes to tarsals; may include portions of talus and calcaneus
- Correct right and left marker placement and a weight-bearing marker
- Bony trabecular detail and surrounding soft tissues

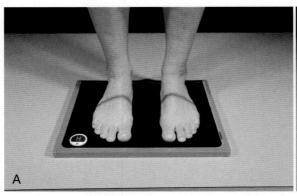
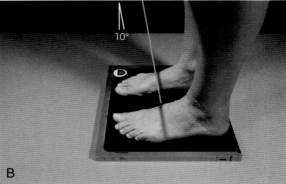

Fig. 7.57 Weight-bearing AP both feet, standing. (A) Correct position of both feet on the IR. (B) Lateral perspective of same projection shows position of feet on the IR and CR.

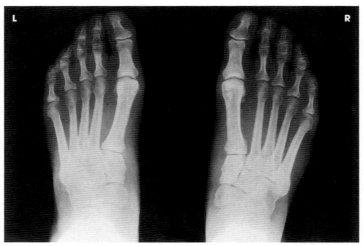

Fig. 7.58 Weight-bearing AP both feet, standing.

AP AXIAL PROJECTION
WEIGHT-BEARING COMPOSITE METHOD
Standing

Image receptor: Positioned by manufacturer or department protocol for proper anatomy display orientation; CR plate: 10 × 12 inches (24 × 30 cm) lengthwise.

Position of patient
- Place the patient in the standing-upright position. The patient should stand at a comfortable height on a low stool or on the floor.

Position of part
- With the patient standing upright, adjust the IR under the foot and center its midline to the long axis of the foot.
- To prevent superimposition of the leg shadow on that of the ankle joint, have the patient place the opposite foot one step backward for the exposure of the forefoot and one step forward for the exposure of the hindfoot or calcaneus.
- *Shield gonads.*

Central ray
- To use the masking effect of the leg, direct the central ray along the plane of alignment of the foot in both exposures.
- With the tube in front of the patient and adjusted for a posterior angulation of 15 degrees, center the central ray to the base of the third metatarsal for the first exposure (Figs. 7.59 and 7.60).

- Caution the patient to carefully maintain the position of the affected foot and to place the opposite foot one step forward in preparation for the second exposure.
- Move the tube behind the patient, adjust it for an anterior angulation of 25 degrees, and direct the central ray to the posterior surface of the ankle. The central ray emerges on the plantar surface at the level of the lateral malleolus (Figs. 7.61 and 7.62). An increase in technical factors is recommended for this exposure.

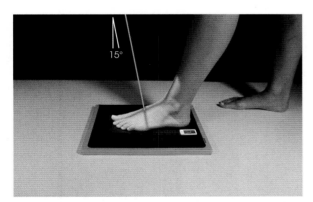

Fig. 7.59 Composite AP axial foot, posterior angulation of 15 degrees.

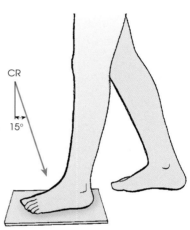

Fig. 7.60 Composite AP axial foot, posterior angulation of 15 degrees.

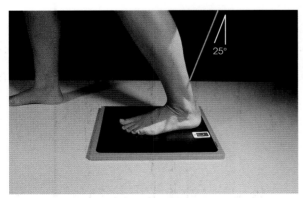

Fig. 7.61 Composite AP axial foot, anterior angulation of 25 degrees.

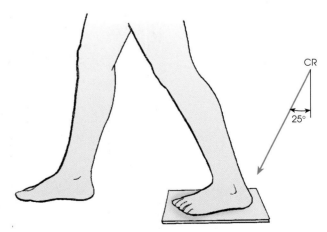

Fig. 7.62 Composite AP axial foot, anterior angulation of 25 degrees.

Collimation

• Adjust the radiation field to 1 inch (2.5 cm) on all sides and 1 inch (2.5 cm) beyond the calcaneus and distal tip of the toes. Place a side marker in the collimated exposure field.

Structures shown

A weight-bearing AP axial projection of all bones of the foot. The full outline of the foot is projected free of the leg (Fig. 7.63).

The following should be clearly seen:

■ Evidence of proper collimation and the presence of a side marker placed clear of the anatomy of interest
■ Entire foot, from toes to heel
■ Shadow of leg not overlapping the tarsals
■ Foot not rotated
■ Bony trabecular detail and surrounding soft tissues

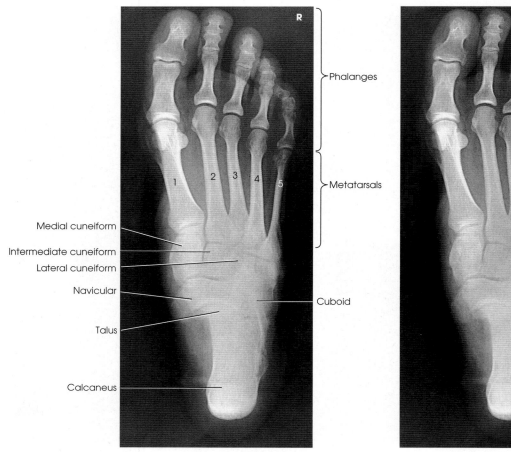

Fig. 7.63 Composite AP axial foot.

Congenital Clubfoot
AP PROJECTION
KITE METHOD

The typical clubfoot, or *talipes equinovarus,* shows three deviations from the normal alignment of the foot in relation to the weight-bearing axis of the leg. These deviations are plantar flexion and inversion of the calcaneus (equinus), medial displacement of the forefoot (adduction), and elevation of the medial border of the foot (supination). The typical clubfoot has numerous variations. Each of the typical abnormalities just described has varying degrees of deformity.

The classic Kite method[4,5]—exactly placed AP and lateral projections—for radiography of the clubfoot are used to show the anatomy of the foot and the bones or ossification centers of the tarsals and their relation to one another. *A primary objective makes it essential that no attempt be made to change the abnormal alignment of the foot when placing it on the IR.* Davis and Hatt[6] stated that even slight rotation of the foot can result in marked alteration in the radiographically projected relation of the ossification centers.

The AP projection shows the degree of adduction of the forefoot and the degree of inversion of the calcaneus.

Image receptor: Positioned by manufacturer or department protocol for proper anatomy display orientation; CR plate: 10×12 inches (24×30 cm) lengthwise.

Position of patient

- Place the infant in the supine position, with the hips and knees flexed to permit the foot to rest flat on the IR. Elevate the body on firm pillows to knee height to simplify gonad shielding and leg adjustment.

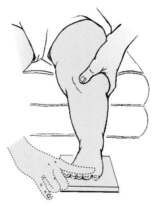

Fig. 7.64 AP foot to show clubfoot deformity.

Position of part

- Rest the feet flat on the IR with the ankles extended slightly to prevent superimposition of the leg shadow.
- Hold the infant's knees together or in such a way that the legs are exactly vertical (i.e., so that they do not lean medially or laterally).
- Using a lead glove, hold the infant's toes. When the adduction deformity is too great to permit correct placement of the legs and feet for bilateral images without overlap of the feet, each foot must be examined separately (Figs. 7.64 and 7.65).
- *Shield gonads.*

Central ray

- Perpendicular to the tarsals, midway between the tarsal areas for a bilateral projection.
- An approximately 15-degree posterior angle is generally required for the central ray to be perpendicular to the tarsals.
- Kite[4,5] stressed the importance of directing the central ray vertically for the purpose of projecting the true relationship of the bones and ossification centers.

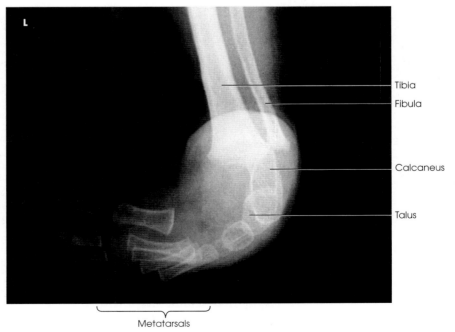

Tibia
Fibula

Calcaneus

Talus

Metatarsals

Fig. 7.65 AP projection showing nearly 90-degree adduction of forefoot.

Congenital Clubfoot
LATERAL PROJECTION
Mediolateral
KITE METHOD

The Kite method lateral radiograph shows the anterior talar subluxation and the degree of plantar flexion (equinus).

Position of patient

- Place the infant on his or her side in as near the lateral position as possible.
- Flex the uppermost extremity, draw it forward, and hold it in place.

Position of part

- After adjusting the IR under the foot, place a support that has the same thickness as the IR under the infant's knee to prevent angulation of the foot and to ensure a lateral foot position.
- Hold the infant's toes in position with tape or a protected hand (Figs. 7.66–7.70).
- *Shield gonads.*

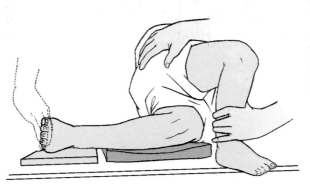

Fig. 7.66 Lateral foot.

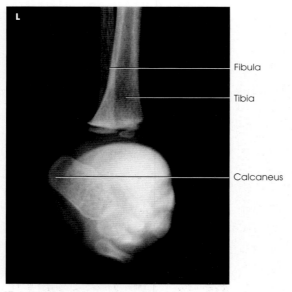

Fibula

Tibia

Calcaneus

Fig. 7.67 Lateral foot projection showing pitch of calcaneus. Other tarsals are obscured by adducted forefoot.

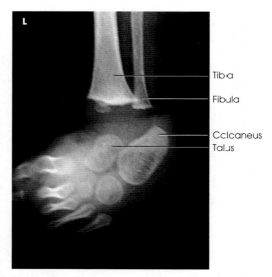

Tibia

Fibula

Calcaneus
Talus

Fig. 7.68 Nonroutine 45-degree medial rotation showing extent of talipes equinovarus.

Central ray

• Perpendicular to the midtarsal area.

EVALUATION CRITERIA

The following should be clearly seen:

■ Evidence of proper collimation and the presence of a side marker placed clear of the anatomy of interest
■ No medial or lateral angulation of the leg
■ Fibula in lateral projection overlapping the posterior half of the tibia
■ The need for a repeat examination if slight variations in rotation are seen in either image compared with previous radiographs

■ Talus, calcaneus, and metatarsals to allow assessment of alignment variations
■ Bony trabecular detail and surrounding soft tissues

NOTE: Freiberger et al.[7] recommended that dorsiflexion of an infant's foot could be obtained by pressing a small plywood board against the sole of the foot. An older child or adult is placed in the upright position for a horizontal projection. With the upright position, the patient leans the leg forward to dorsiflex the foot.

NOTE: Conway and Cowell[8] recommended tomography to show coalition at the middle facet and particularly the hidden coalition involving the anterior facet.

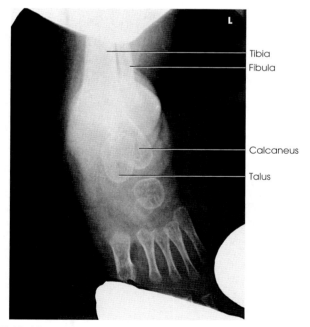

Fig. 7.69 AP projection after treatment (same patient as in Fig. 7.68).

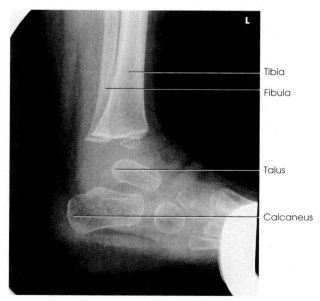

Fig. 7.70 Lateral projection after treatment (same patient as in Fig. 7.67).

Congenital Clubfoot
AXIAL PROJECTION
Dorsoplantar
KANDEL METHOD

Kandel[9] recommended the inclusion of a dorsoplantar axial projection in the examination of the patient with a clubfoot (Fig. 7.71).

For this method, the infant is held in a vertical or a bending-forward position. The plantar surface of the foot should rest on the IR, although a moderate elevation of the heel is acceptable when the equinus deformity is well marked. The central ray is directed 40 degrees anteriorly through the lower leg, as for the usual dorsoplantar projection of the calcaneus (Fig. 7.72).

Freiberger et al.[7] stated that sustentaculum talar joint fusion cannot be assumed on one projection because the central ray may not have been parallel with the articular surfaces. They recommended that three radiographs be obtained with varying central ray angulations (35, 45, and 55 degrees).

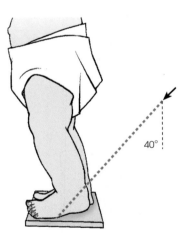

Fig. 7.71 Axial foot (dorsoplantar): Kandel method.

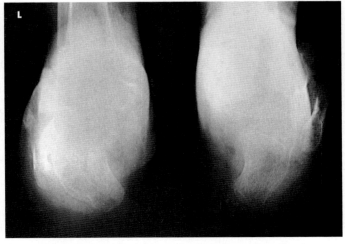

Fig. 7.72 Axial foot (dorsoplantar): Kandel method.

⚑ AXIAL PROJECTION
Plantodorsal

Image receptor: Positioned by manufacturer or department protocol for proper anatomy display orientation; CR plate: 10 ×12 inches (24 × 30 cm) lengthwise.

Position of patient
- Place the patient in the supine or seated position with the legs fully extended.

Position of part
- Place the IR under the patient's ankle, centered to the midline of the ankle (Figs. 7.73 and 7.74).
- Place a long strip of gauze around the ball of the foot. Have the patient grasp the gauze to hold the ankle in right-angle dorsiflexion.
- If the patient's ankles cannot be flexed enough to place the plantar surface of the foot perpendicular to the IR, elevate the leg on sandbags to obtain the correct position.
- *Shield gonads.*

Central ray
- Directed to the midpoint of the IR at a cephalic angle (entering the plantar surface and toward the heel) of 40 degrees to the long axis of the foot. The central ray enters near the base of the third metatarsal.

Collimation
- Adjust the radiation field to 1 inch (2.5 cm) on three sides of the shadow of the calcaneus and to include the fifth metatarsal base. Place side marker in the collimated exposure field.

◤ COMPENSATING FILTER
This projection can be improved significantly with the use of a compensating filter because of the increased density through the midportion of the foot.

Structures shown
An axial projection of the calcaneus (Fig. 7.75).

EVALUATION CRITERIA
The following should be clearly seen:
- Evidence of proper collimation and the presence of a side marker placed clear of the anatomy of interest
- Calcaneus and calcaneocuboid joint
- No rotation of the calcaneus—the first or fifth metatarsals not projected to the sides of the foot
- Bony trabecular detail and surrounding soft tissues

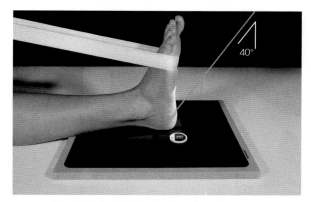

Fig. 7.73 Axial (plantodorsal) calcaneus.

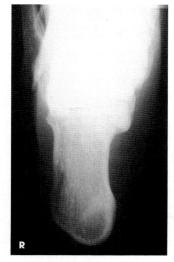

Fig. 7.74 Axial (plantodorsal) calcaneus. Note that anterior calcaneus is not penetrated.

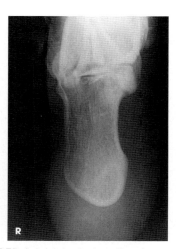

Fig. 7.75 Axial (plantodorsal) calcaneus. Image made using Ferlic swimmer's filter. Note penetration of anterior calcaneus and metatarsal joint spaces.

Calcaneus

AXIAL PROJECTION
Dorsoplantar

> **Image receptor:** Positioned by manufacturer or department protocol for proper anatomy display orientation; CR plate: 10 × 12 inches (24 × 30 cm) lengthwise.

Position of patient
- Place the patient in the prone position.

Position of part
- Elevate the patient's ankle on sandbags.
- Adjust the height and position of the sandbags under the ankle in such a way that the patient can dorsiflex the ankle enough to place the long axis of the foot perpendicular to the tabletop.

- Place the IR against the plantar surface of the foot, and support it in position with sandbags or a portable IR holder (Figs. 7.76 and 7.77).
- *Shield gonads.*

Central ray
- Directed to the midpoint of the IR at a caudal angle (enters posterior surface and toward the heel) of 40 degrees to the long axis of the foot. The central ray enters the dorsal surface of the ankle joint.

Collimation
- Adjust the radiation field to 1 inch (2.5 cm) on three sides of the shadow of the calcaneus and to include the fifth metatarsal base. Place side marker in the collimated exposure field.

▼ COMPENSATING FILTER

This projection can be improved significantly with the use of a compensating filter because of increased density through the midportion of the foot.

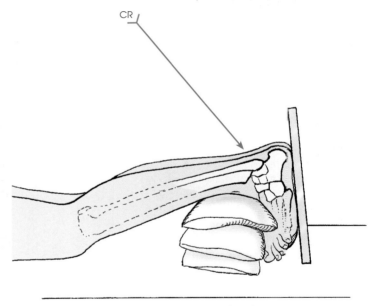

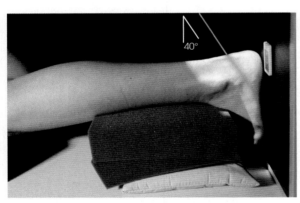

Fig. 7.76 Axial (dorsoplantar) calcaneus.

Fig. 7.77 Axial (dorsoplantar) calcaneus.

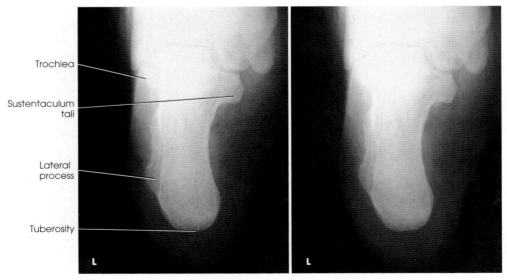

Trochlea

Sustentaculum tali

Lateral process

Tuberosity

Fig. 7.78 Axial (dorsoplantar) calcaneus.

Structures shown

An axial projection of the calcaneus and the calcaneocuboid joint (Fig. 7.78). Computed tomography (CT) is often used to show this bone (Fig. 7.79).

EVALUATION CRITERIA

The following should be clearly seen:
- Evidence of proper collimation and the presence of a side marker placed clear of the anatomy of interest
- Calcaneus and the calcaneocuboid joint
- Sustentaculum tali
- Calcaneus not rotated—the first or fifth metatarsals not projected to the sides of the foot
- Bony trabecular detail and surrounding soft tissues

WEIGHT-BEARING COALITION (HARRIS-BEATH) METHOD

This weight-bearing method, first described by Lilienfeld[10] (cit. Holzknecht), has come into use to show calcaneotalar coalition.[11–13] For this reason, it has been called the *coalition position*. It may also be called the Harris–Beath method.[11] It is more commonly used in Podiatry.

Position of patient

- Place the patient in the standing-upright position.

Position of part

- Center the IR to the long axis of the calcaneus, with the posterior surface of the heel at the edge of the IR.
- To prevent superimposition of the leg shadow, have the patient place the opposite foot one step forward (Fig. 7.80).

Central ray

- Angled 45 degrees anteriorly and directed through the posterior surface of the flexed ankle to a point on the plantar surface at the level of the base of the fifth metatarsal.

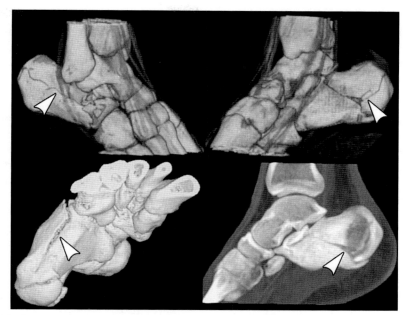

Fig. 7.79 CT images of calcaneal fracture with three-dimensional reconstruction. Conventional x-ray shows most fractures; however, complex regions, such as calcaneal-talar area, are best shown on CT. Note how bone *(arrows)* shows extent of fracture.

(From Jackson SA, Thomas RM: *Cross-sectional imaging made easy,* New York, 2004, Churchill Livingstone.)

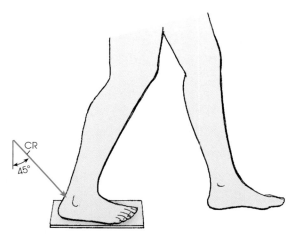

Fig. 7.80 Weight-bearing coalition method.

♠ LATERAL PROJECTION
Mediolateral

Image receptor: Positioned by manufacturer or department protocol for proper anatomy display orientation; CR plate: 10 × 12 inches (24 × 30 cm) lengthwise.

Position of patient
• Have the supine patient turn toward the affected side until the leg is approximately lateral. A support may be placed under the knee.

Position of part
• Adjust the calcaneus as for a lateral foot and to the center of the IR.
• Adjust the IR so that the long axis is parallel with the plantar surface of the heel (Fig. 7.81).
• *Shield gonads.*

Central ray
• Perpendicular to the calcaneus. Center about 1 inch (2.5 cm) distal to the medial malleolus. This places the central ray at the subtalar joint.

Collimation
• Adjust the radiation field to 1 inch (2.5 cm) beyond the posterior and inferior shadow of the heel. Include the medial malleolus and the base of the fifth metatarsal. Place side marker in the collimated exposure field.

Structures shown
The ankle joint and the calcaneus in lateral profile (Fig. 7.82).

EVALUATION CRITERIA
The following should be clearly seen:
■ Evidence of proper collimation and presence of side marker placed clear of anatomy of interest
■ Entire calcaneus, including ankle joint and adjacent tarsals
■ No rotation of the calcaneus
  □ Tuberosity in profile
  □ Sinus tarsi open
  □ Calcaneocuboid and talonavicular joints open
■ Bony trabecular detail and surrounding soft tissues

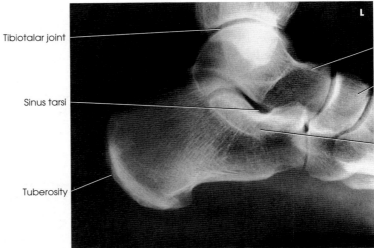
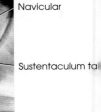

Tibiotalar joint
Sinus tarsi
Tuberosity
Talus
Navicular
Sustentaculum tali

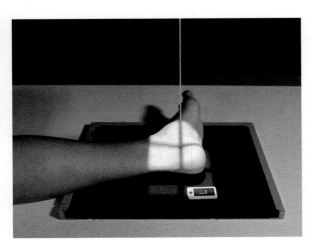

Fig. 7.81 Lateral calcaneus.

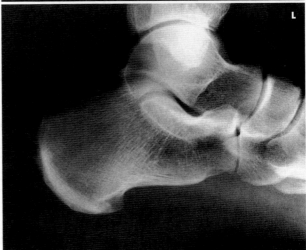

Fig. 7.82 Lateral calcaneus.

LATEROMEDIAL OBLIQUE PROJECTION
WEIGHT-BEARING METHOD

Image receptor: Positioned by manufacturer or department protocol for proper anatomy display orientation; CR plate: 10 × 12 inches (24 × 30 cm) lengthwise.

Position of patient

- Have the patient stand with the affected heel centered toward the lateral border of the IR (Fig. 7.83).
- A mobile radiographic unit may assist in this examination.

Position of part

- Adjust the patient's leg to ensure that it is exactly perpendicular.
- Center the calcaneus so that it is projected to the center of the IR.
- Center the lateral malleolus to the midline axis of the IR.
- *Shield gonads.*

Central ray

- Directed medially at a caudal angle of 45 degrees to enter the lateral malleolus.

Collimation

- Adjust the radiation field to 1 inch (2.5 cm) beyond the posterior and inferior shadow of the heel. Include the lateral malleolus and the metatarsal bases. Place a side marker in the collimated exposure field.

Structures shown

The calcaneal tuberosity and is useful in diagnosing stress fractures of the calcaneus or tuberosity (Fig. 7.84).

EVALUATION CRITERIA

The following should be clearly seen:
- Evidence of proper collimation and the presence of a side marker placed clear of the anatomy of interest
- Calcaneal tuberosity
- Sinus tarsi
- Cuboid, lateral cuneiform, and proximal metatarsals
- Bony trabecular detail and surrounding soft tissues

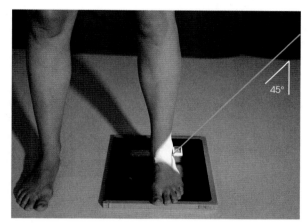

Fig. 7.83 Weight-bearing lateromedial oblique calcaneus.

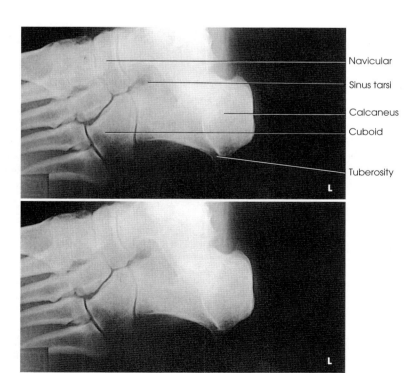

Navicular

Sinus tarsi

Calcaneus

Cuboid

Tuberosity

Fig. 7.84 Weight-bearing lateromedial oblique calcaneus.

LATEROMEDIAL OBLIQUE PROJECTION
ISHERWOOD METHOD
Medial rotation foot

Isherwood[14] devised a method for each of the three separate articulations of the subtalar joint: (1) a *medial rotation foot* position to show the anterior talar articulation, (2) a *medial rotation ankle* position to show the middle talar articulation, and (3) a *lateral rotation ankle* position to show the posterior talar articulation. Feist and Mankin[15] later described a similar position.

> **Image receptor:** Positioned by manufacturer or department protocol for proper anatomy display orientation; CR plate: 10 × 12 inches (24 × 30 cm) lengthwise.

Position of patient

- Place the patient in a semisupine or seated position, turned away from the side being examined.
- Ask the patient to flex the knee enough to place the ankle joint in nearly right-angle flexion and then to lean the leg and foot medially.

Position of part

- With the medial border of the foot resting on the IR, place a 45-degree foam wedge under the elevated leg.
- Adjust the leg so that its long axis is in the same plane as the central ray.
- Adjust the foot to be at a right angle.
- Place a support under the knee (Fig. 7.85).
- *Shield gonads.*

Central ray

- Perpendicular to a point 1 inch (2.5 cm) distal and 1 inch (2.5 cm) anterior to the lateral malleolus.

Collimation

- Adjust the radiation field to 1 inch (2.5 cm) beyond the posterior and inferior shadow of the heel. Include the lateral malleolus and the metatarsal bases. Place a side marker in the collimated exposure field.

Structures shown

The anterior subtalar articulation and an oblique projection of the tarsals (Fig. 7.86). The Feist-Mankin method produces a similar image representation.

The following should be clearly seen:
- Evidence of proper collimation and the presence of a side marker placed clear of the anatomy of interest
- Anterior talar articular surface
- Bony trabecular detail and surrounding soft tissues

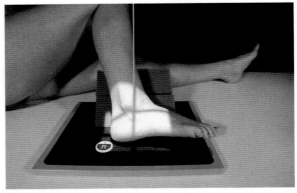

Fig. 7.85 Lateromedial oblique subtalar joint, medial rotation: Isherwood method.

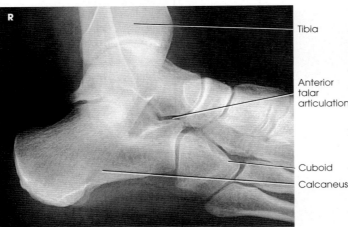

Tibia

Anterior talar articulation

Cuboid

Calcaneus

Fig. 7.86 Lateromedial oblique subtalar joint showing anterior articulation: Isherwood method.

Lower Extremity

AP AXIAL OBLIQUE PROJECTION

ISHERWOOD METHOD
Medial rotation ankle

Image receptor: Positioned by manufacturer or department protocol for proper anatomy display orientation; CR plate: 10 × 12 inches (24 × 30 cm) lengthwise.

Position of patient
- Have the patient assume a seated position on the radiographic table and turn with body weight resting on the flexed hip and thigh of the unaffected side.
- If a semilateral recumbent position is more comfortable, adjust the patient accordingly.

Position of part
- Ask the patient to rotate the leg and foot medially enough to rest the side of the foot and affected ankle on an optional 30-degree foam wedge (Fig. 7.87).
- Place a support under the knee. If the patient is recumbent, place another support under the greater trochanter.
- Dorsiflex the foot, then invert it, if possible, and have the patient maintain the position by pulling on a strip of 2- or 3-inch (5- to 7.6-cm) bandage looped around the ball of the foot.
- *Shield gonads.*

Central ray
- Directed to a point 1 inch (2.5 cm) distal and 1 inch (2.5 cm) anterior to the lateral malleolus at an angle of 10 degrees cephalad.

Collimation
- Adjust the radiation field to 1 inch (2.5 cm) beyond the posterior and inferior shadow of the heel. Include the lateral malleolus and the metatarsal bases. Place a side marker in the collimated exposure field.

Structures shown
The middle articulation of the subtalar joint and an "end-on" projection of the sinus tarsi (Fig. 7.88).

The following should be clearly seen:
- Evidence of proper collimation and the presence of a side marker placed clear of the anatomy of interest
- Middle (subtalar) articulation
- Open sinus tarsi
- Bony trabecular detail and surrounding soft tissues

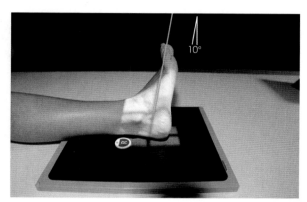

Fig. 7.87 AP axial oblique subtalar joint, medial rotation: Isherwood method.

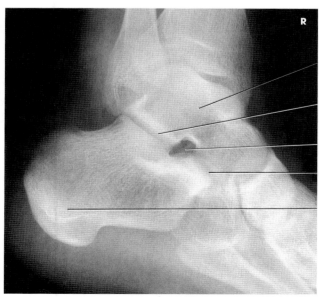
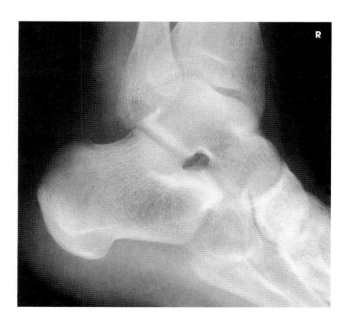

Talus

Posterior subtalar articulation

Sinus tarsi

Middle subtalar articulation

Calcaneus

Fig. 7.88 AP axial oblique subtalar joint: Isherwood method.

AP AXIAL OBLIQUE PROJECTION

ISHERWOOD METHOD
Lateral rotation ankle

Image receptor: Positioned by manufacturer or department protocol for proper anatomy display orientation; CR plate: 10 × 12 inches (24 × 30 cm) lengthwise.

Position of patient

- Place the patient in the supine or seated position.

Position of part

- Ask the patient to rotate the leg and foot laterally until the side of the foot and ankle rests against an optional 30-degree foam wedge.
- Dorsiflex the foot, evert it if possible, and have the patient maintain the position by pulling on a broad bandage looped around the ball of the foot (Fig. 7.89).
- *Shield gonads.*

Central ray

- Directed to a point 1 inch (2.5 cm) distal to the medial malleolus at an angle of 10 degrees cephalad.

Collimation

- Adjust the radiation field to 1 inch (2.5 cm) beyond the posterior and inferior shadow of the heel. Include the lateral malleolus and the metatarsal bases. Place a side marker in the collimated exposure field.

Structures shown

The posterior articulation of the subtalar joint in profile (Fig. 7.90).

The following should be clearly seen:

- Evidence of proper collimation and presence of side marker placed clear of anatomy of interest
- Posterior subtalar articulation
- Bony trabecular detail and surrounding soft tissues

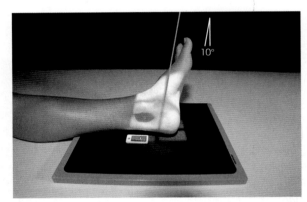

Fig. 7.89 AP axial oblique subtalar joint, lateral rotation: Isherwood method.

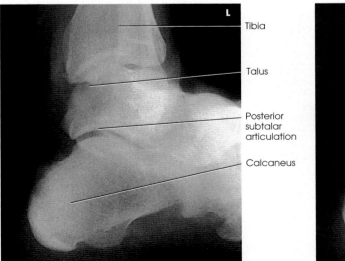
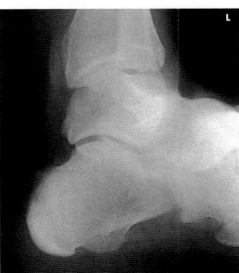

Tibia

Talus

Posterior subtalar articulation

Calcaneus

Fig. 7.90 AP oblique subtalar joint: Isherwood method.

♠ AP PROJECTION

Image receptor: Positioned by manufacturer or department protocol for proper anatomy display orientation; CR plate: 10 × 12 inches (24 × 30 cm) lengthwise.

Position of patient

- Place the patient in the supine or seated position with the affected extremity fully extended.

Position of part

- Adjust the ankle joint in the anatomic position (foot pointing straight up) to obtain a true AP projection. Flex the ankle and foot enough to place the long axis of the foot in the vertical position (Fig. 7.91).

- Ball and Egbert[16] stated that the appearance of the ankle mortise is not appreciably altered by moderate plantar flexion or dorsiflexion as long as the leg is not rotated either laterally or medially.
- *Shield gonads*.

Central ray

- Perpendicular through the ankle joint at a point midway between the malleoli.

Collimation

- Adjust the radiation field to 1 inch (2.5 cm) on the sides of the ankle and 8 inches (18 cm) lengthwise to include the heel. Place a side marker in the collimated exposure field.

Structures shown

AP projection of the ankle joint, the distal ends of the tibia and fibula, and the proximal portion of the talus.

NOTE: The inferior tibiofibular articulation and the talofibular articulation are not "open" or shown in profile in the true AP projection. This is a positive sign for the radiologist because it indicates that the patient has no ruptured ligaments or other types of separations. For this reason, it is important that the position of the ankle be anatomically "true" for the AP projection shown (Fig. 7.92).

EVALUATION CRITERIA

The following should be clearly seen:
- Evidence of proper collimation and the presence of a side marker placed clear of the anatomy of interest
- Ankle joint centered to exposure area
- Medial and lateral malleoli
- Talus
- No rotation of the ankle
  - Normal overlapping of the tibiofibular articulation with the anterior tubercle slightly superimposed over the fibula
  - Talus slightly overlapping the distal fibula
  - No overlapping of the medial talomalleolar articulation
- Tibiotalar joint space
- Bony trabecular detail and surrounding soft tissues

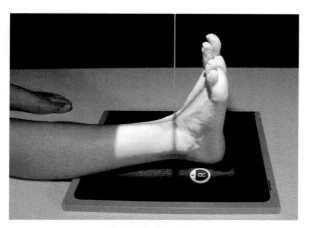

Fig. 7.91 AP ankle.

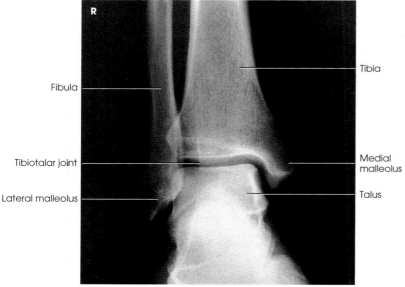
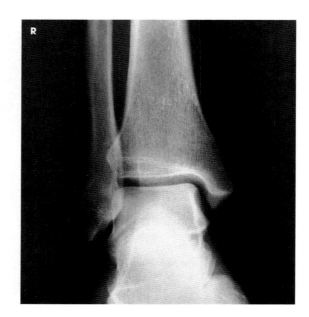

Fig. 7.92 AP ankle.

Fibula

Tibiotalar joint

Lateral malleolus

Tibia

Medial malleolus

Talus

▲ LATERAL PROJECTION
Mediolateral

Image receptor: Positioned by manufacturer or department protocol for proper anatomy display orientation; CR plate: 10 × 12 inches (24 × 30 cm) lengthwise.

Position of patient
- Have the supine patient turn toward the affected side until the ankle is lateral (Fig. 7.93).

Position of part
- Place the long axis of the IR parallel with the long axis of the patient's leg, and center it to the ankle joint.
- Ensure that the lateral surface of the foot is in contact with the IR.
- Dorsiflex the foot, and adjust it in the lateral position. Dorsiflexion is required to prevent lateral rotation of the ankle.
- *Shield gonads.*

Central ray
- Perpendicular to the ankle joint, entering the medial malleolus.

Collimation
- Adjust the radiation field to 1 inch (2.5 cm) on the sides of the ankle and 8 inches (18 cm) lengthwise. Include the heel and the fifth metatarsal base. Place a side marker in the collimated exposure field.

Structures shown
The resulting image shows a true lateral projection of the lower third of the tibia and fibula; the ankle joint; and the tarsals, including the base of the fifth metatarsal (Figs. 7.94 and 7.95).

EVALUATION CRITERIA
The following should be clearly seen:
- Evidence of proper collimation and the presence of a side marker placed clear of the anatomy of interest
- Ankle joint centered to exposure area
- Distal tibia and fibula, talus, calcaneus, and adjacent tarsals
- Ankle in true lateral position
  - ☐ Tibiotalar joint well visualized, with the medial and lateral talar domes superimposed
  - ☐ Fibula over the posterior half of the tibia
- Fifth metatarsal base and tuberosity should be seen to check for Jones fracture
- Bony trabecular detail and surrounding soft tissues

base of 5th metatarsal

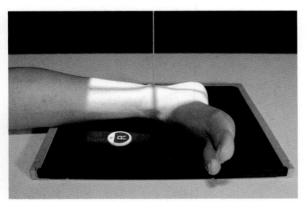

Fig. 7.93 Lateral ankle, mediolateral.

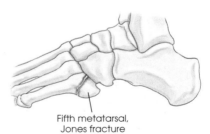

Fifth metatarsal, Jones fracture

Fig. 7.94 Bones shown on lateral ankle. Inclusion of base of fifth metatarsal on lateral ankle projection can reveal Jones fracture if present.

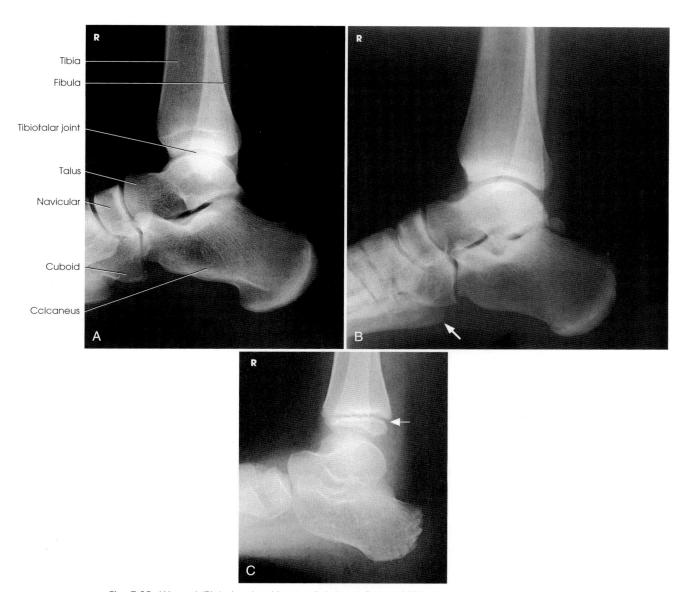

Tibia

Fibula

Tibiotalar joint

Talus

Navicular

Cuboid

Cclcaneus

Fig. 7.95 (A) and (B) Lateral ankle, mediolateral. Base of fifth metatarsal is seen *(arrow)*. (C) Lateral ankle of an 8-year-old child. Note tibial epiphysis *(arrow)*.

Lower Extremity

LATERAL PROJECTION

Lateromedial

The lateral projection of the ankle joint can be made with the medial side of the ankle in contact with the IR. Exact positioning of the ankle is more easily and more consistently obtained when the extremity is rested on its comparatively flat medial surface. However, this position is more difficult for patients than the more commonly performed mediolateral projection. For this reason, it is more commonly performed either upright or as a cross-table lateral.

> **Image receptor:** Positioned by manufacturer or department protocol for proper anatomy display orientation; CR plate: 10 × 12 inches (24 × 30 cm) lengthwise.

Position of patient

- Have the supine patient turn away from the affected side until the extended leg is placed laterally.

Position of part

- Center the IR to the ankle joint, and adjust the IR so that its long axis is parallel with the long axis of the leg.
- Adjust the foot in the lateral position.
- Have the patient turn anteriorly or posteriorly as required to place the patella perpendicular to the horizontal plane (Fig. 7.96A). This projection also can be performed as a cross table lateral with the patient supine (Fig. 7.96B).
- If necessary, place a support under the patient's knee.
- *Shield gonads.*

Central ray

- Perpendicular through the ankle joint, entering ½ inch (1.3 cm) superior to the lateral malleolus.

Collimation

- Adjust the radiation field to 1 inch (2.5 cm) on the sides of the ankle and 8 inches (18 cm) lengthwise. Include the heel and the fifth metatarsal base. Place a side marker in the collimated exposure field.

Structures shown

A lateral projection of the lower third of the tibia and fibula, the ankle joint, and the tarsals (Fig. 7.97).

EVALUATION CRITERIA

The following should be clearly seen:

- Evidence of proper collimation and presence of side marker placed clear of anatomy of interest
- Ankle joint centered to exposure area
- Distal tibia and fibula, talus, and adjacent tarsals
- Ankle in true lateral position
  - Tibiotalar joint well visualized, with the medial and lateral talar domes superimposed
  - Fibula over the posterior half of the tibia
- Bony trabecular detail and surrounding soft tissues

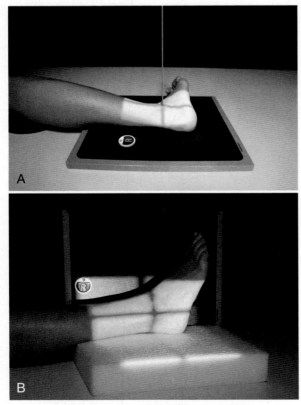

Fig. 7.96 Lateral ankle, lateromedial. (A) Positioned on tabletop. (B) Positioned as a cross-table lateral.

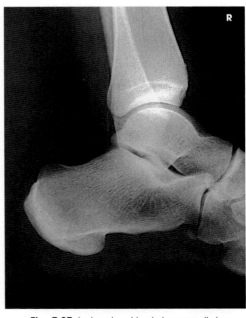

Fig. 7.97 Lateral ankle, lateromedial.

♠ AP OBLIQUE PROJECTION
Medial rotation

Image receptor: Positioned by manufacturer or department protocol for proper anatomy display orientation; CR plate: 10 × 12 inches (24 × 30 cm) lengthwise.

Position of patient

- Place the patient in the supine or seated position with the affected extremity fully extended.

Position of part

- Center the IR to the ankle joint midway between the malleoli, and adjust the IR so that its long axis is parallel with the long axis of the leg.
- Dorsiflex the foot enough to place the ankle at nearly right-angle flexion (Fig. 7.98). The ankle may be immobilized with sandbags placed against the sole of the foot or by having the patient hold the ends of a strip of bandage looped around the ball of the foot.
- Rotate the patient's entire *leg* for all oblique projections of the ankle by grasping the lower femur area with one hand and the foot with the other (see Fig. 7.98). Because the knee is a hinge joint, rotation of the leg can come only from the hip joint. Internally rotate the entire leg and foot together until the 45-degree oblique position is achieved (Fig. 7.99).

- The foot can be placed against a foam wedge for support.
- *Shield gonads.*

Central ray

- Perpendicular to the ankle joint, entering midway between the malleoli.

Collimation

- Adjust the radiation field to 1 inch (2.5 cm) on the sides of the ankle and 8 inches (18 cm) lengthwise to include the heel. Place a side marker in the collimated exposure field.

Structures shown

The 45-degree medial oblique projection shows the distal ends of the tibia and fibula, parts of which are often superimposed over the talus. The tibiofibular articulation also should be shown (Fig. 7.100).

The following should be clearly seen:

- ■ Evidence of proper collimation and the presence of a side marker placed clear of the anatomy of interest
- ■ Ankle joint centered to exposure area
- ■ Distal tibia, fibula, and talus
- ■ Proper 45-degree rotation of ankle
  - ☐ Tibiofibular articulation open
  - ☐ Distal tibia and fibula overlap some of the talus
- ■ Bony trabecular detail and surrounding soft tissues

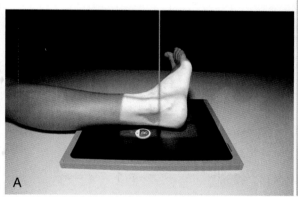
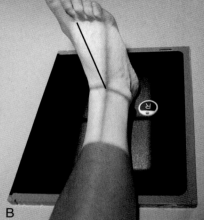

Fig. 7.99 (A) and (B) AP oblique ankle, 45-degree medial rotation.

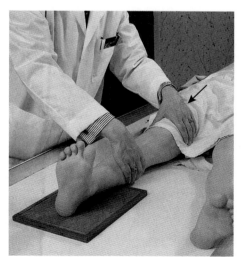

Fig. 7.98 Radiographer properly positioning the leg for an oblique projection of the ankle joint. Note the action of the left hand *(arrow)* in turning the leg medially. Proper positioning requires turning the leg but not the foot.

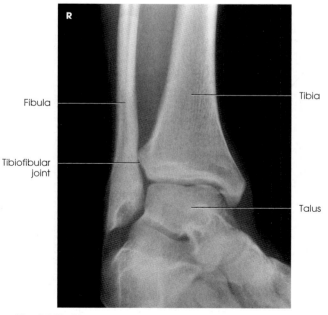

Fibula

Tibiofibular joint

Tibia

Talus

Fig. 7.100 AP oblique ankle, 45-degree medial rotation.

Mortise Joint[17]
▲ AP OBLIQUE
Medial rotation

Image receptor: Positioned by manufacturer or department protocol for proper anatomy display orientation; CR plate: 10 × 12 inches (24 × 30 cm) lengthwise.

Position of patient
- Place the patient in the supine or seated position.

Position of part
- Center the patient's ankle joint to the IR.
- Grasp the distal femur area with one hand and the foot with the other. Assist the patient by internally rotating the *entire leg* and *foot* together 15 to 20 degrees until the intermalleolar plane is parallel with the IR (Fig. 7.101).
- The plantar surface of the foot should be placed at a right angle to the leg.
- *Shield gonads.*

Central ray
- Perpendicular, entering the ankle joint midway between the malleoli.

Collimation
- Adjust the radiation field to 1 inch (2.5 cm) on the sides of the ankle and 8 inches (18 cm) lengthwise to include the heel. Place a side marker in the collimated exposure field.

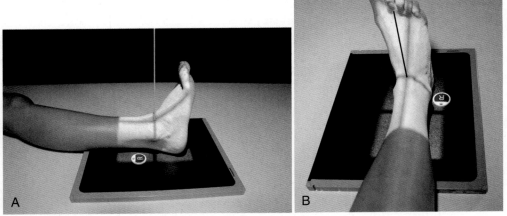

Fig. 7.101 (A) and (B) AP oblique ankle, 15- to 20-degree medial rotation to show ankle mortise joint.

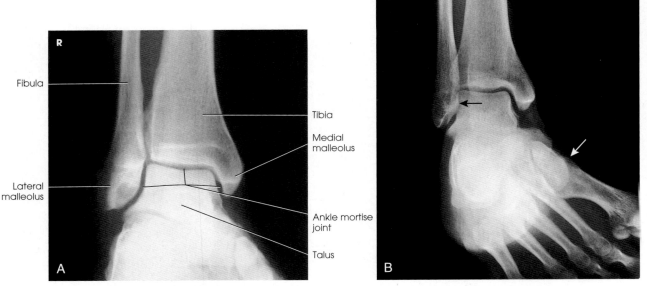

Fibula

Lateral malleolus

Tibia

Medial malleolus

Ankle mortise joint

Talus

Fig. 7.102 AP oblique ankle, 15- to 20-degree medial rotation to show ankle mortise joint. (A) Properly positioned leg to show mortise joint. (B) Poorly positioned leg; radiograph had to be repeated. The foot was turned medially *(white arrow)*, but the leg was not. Lateral mortise is closed *(black arrow)* because the "leg" was not medially rotated.

Structures shown

The entire ankle mortise joint in profile. The three sides of the mortise joint should be visualized (Figs. 7.102 and 7.103).

The following should be clearly seen:

- Evidence of proper collimation and the presence of a side marker placed clear of the anatomy of interest
- Entire ankle mortise joint centered to exposure area
- Distal tibia, fibula, and talus
- Proper 15- to 20-degree rotation of ankle
  - ☐ Talofibular articulation open
  - ☐ Tibiotalar articulation open
  - ☐ No overlap of the anterior tubercle of the tibia and the superolateral portion of the talus with the fibula
- Bony trabecular detail and surrounding soft tissues

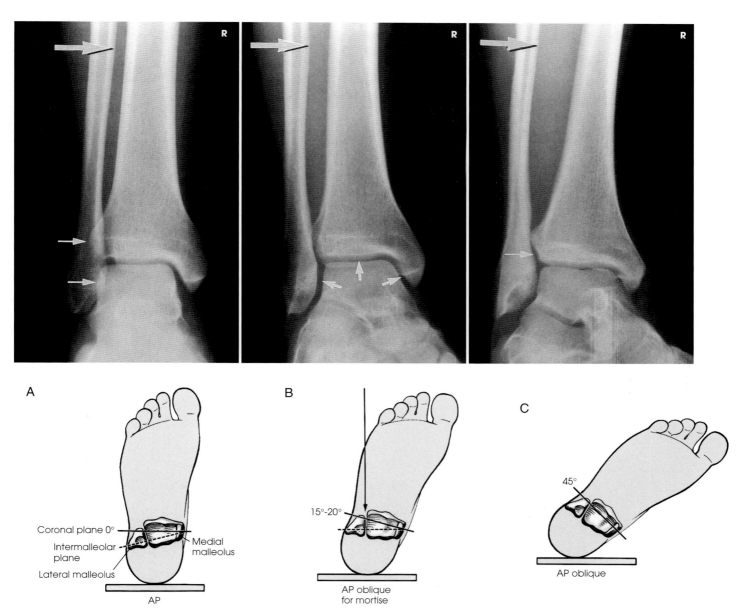

Fig. 7.103 Axial drawing of inferior surface of the tibia and fibula at the ankle joint along with matching radiographs. (A) AP ankle position with no rotation of the leg and foot. Drawing shows lateral malleolus positioned posteriorly when leg is in true anatomic position. Radiograph shows normal overlap of anterior tubercle and superolateral talus over fibula (arrows). (B) AP oblique ankle, 15- to 20-degree medial rotation to show ankle mortise. Drawing shows both malleoli parallel with IR. Radiograph clearly shows all three aspects of the mortise joint (arrows). (C) AP oblique ankle, 45-degree medial rotation. Radiograph shows the tibiofibular joint (arrow) and the entire distal fibula in profile. Larger upper arrow shows wider space created between tibia and fibula as the leg is turned medially for two AP oblique projections. This space should be observed when ankle radiographs are checked for proper positioning.

AP OBLIQUE PROJECTION
Lateral rotation

Image receptor: Positioned by manufacturer or department protocol for proper anatomy display orientation; CR plate: 10×12 inches (24×30 cm) lengthwise.

Position of patient

- Seat the patient on the radiographic table with the affected leg extended.

Position of part

- Place the plantar surface of the patient's foot in the vertical position, and laterally rotate the *leg* and *foot* 45 degrees.
- Rest the foot against a foam wedge for support, and center the ankle joint to the IR (Fig. 7.104).
- *Shield gonads.*

Central ray

- Perpendicular, entering the ankle joint midway between the malleoli.

Collimation

- Adjust the radiation field to 1 inch (2.5 cm) on the sides of the ankle and 8 inches (18 cm) lengthwise to include the heel. Place side marker in the collimated exposure field.

Structures shown

The lateral rotation oblique projection is useful in determining fractures and showing the superior aspect of the calcaneus (Fig. 7.105).

EVALUATION CRITERIA

The following should be clearly seen:
- Evidence of proper collimation and the presence of a side marker placed clear of the anatomy of interest
- Distal tibia, fibula, and talus
- Tibiotalar joint
- Calcaneal sulcus (superior portion of calcaneus)
- Bony trabecular detail and surrounding soft tissues

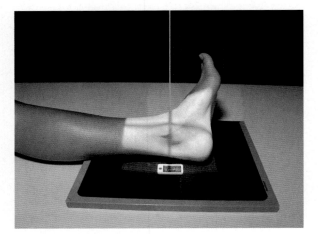

Fig. 7.104 AP oblique ankle, lateral rotation.

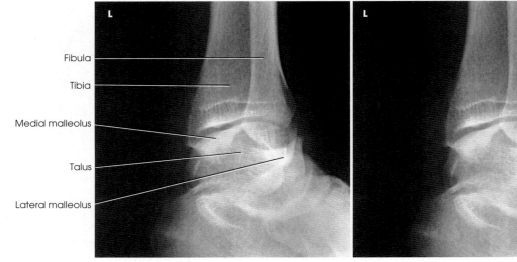

Fibula
Tibia
Medial malleolus
Talus
Lateral malleolus

Fig. 7.105 AP oblique ankle, lateral rotation.

▲ AP PROJECTION
STRESS METHOD

Stress studies of the ankle joint usually are obtained after an inversion or eversion injury to verify the presence of a ligamentous tear. Rupture of a ligament is shown by widening of the joint space on the side of the injury when, without moving or rotating the lower leg from the supine position, the foot is forcibly turned toward the opposite side.

When the injury is recent and the ankle is acutely sensitive to movement, the orthopedic surgeon may inject a local anesthetic into the sinus tarsi before performing the examination. The physician adjusts the foot when it must be turned into extreme stress and holds or straps it in position for the exposure. The patient usually can hold the foot in the stress position when the injury is not too painful or after he or she has received a local anesthetic by asymmetrically pulling on a strip of bandage looped around the ball of the foot (Figs. 7.106–7.108).

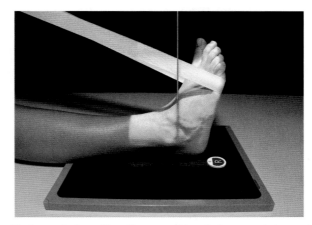

Fig. 7.106 AP ankle in neutral position. The use of lead glove and stress of the joint are required to obtain inversion and eversion radiographs (see Fig. 7.108).

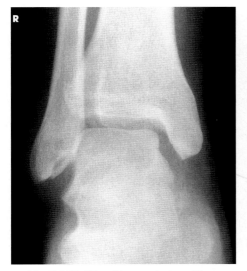

Fig. 7.107 AP ankle, neutral position.

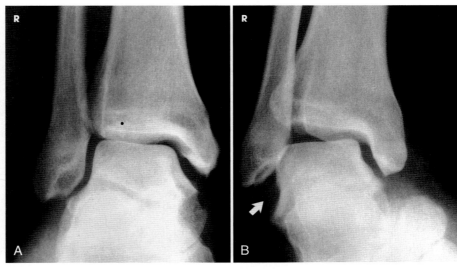

Fig. 7.108 (A) Eversion stress. No damage to medial ligament is indicated. (B) Inversion stress. Change in joint and rupture of lateral ligament (*arrow*) are seen.

AP PROJECTION
WEIGHT-BEARING METHOD
Standing
This projection is performed to identify ankle joint space narrowing with weight-bearing.

> **Image receptor:** Positioned by manufacturer or department protocol for proper anatomy display orientation; CR plate: 10 × 12 inches (24 × 30 cm) crosswise.

Position of patient
- Place the patient in the upright position, preferably on a low platform that has a cassette groove. If such a platform is unavailable, use blocks to elevate the feet to the level of the x-ray tube (Fig. 7.109).
- Ensure that the patient has proper support. Never stand the patient on the radiographic table.

Position of part
- Place the cassette in the cassette groove of the platform or between blocks.
- Have the patient stand with heels pushed back against the cassette and toes pointing straight ahead toward the x-ray tube.
- *Shield gonads.*

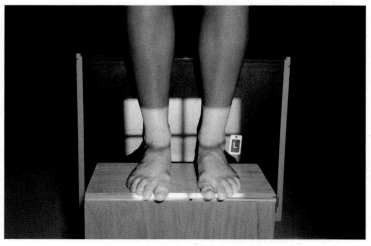

Fig. 7.109 AP weight-bearing ankles.

Central ray

- Perpendicular to the center of the cassette.

TECHNICAL NOTE: If needed, use a mobile unit to allow the x-ray tube to reach the floor level.

Collimation

- Adjust the radiation field to 1 inch (2.5 cm) outside the shadows of the feet but not beyond the IR borders, and 8 inches (18 cm) vertically to include the heel. Place a side marker in the collimated exposure field.

Structures shown

An AP projection of both ankle joints and the relationship of the distal tibia and fibula with weight-bearing. It also shows side-to-side comparison of the joint (Fig. 7.110).

EVALUATION CRITERIA

The following should be clearly seen:
- Evidence of proper collimation and the presence of a side marker placed clear of the anatomy of interest
- Both ankles centered on the image
- Medial mortise open
- Distal tibia and talus partially superimpose distal fibula
- Lateral mortise closed
- Bony trabecular detail and surrounding soft tissues

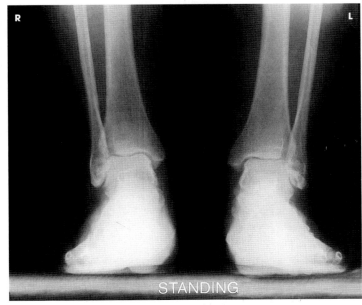

Fig. 7.110 AP weight-bearing ankles.

⚜ AP PROJECTION

For this projection and the lateral and oblique projections described in the following sections, the long axis of the IR is placed parallel with the long axis of the leg and centered to the midshaft. Unless the leg is unusually long, the IR extends beyond the knee and ankle joints enough to prevent their being projected off the IR by divergence of the x-ray beam. The IR must extend 1 to 1½ inches (2.5 to 3.8 cm) beyond the joints. When the leg is too long for these allowances, and the site of the lesion is unknown, two images should always be made. In these instances, the leg is imaged to include one joint, and a separate projection of the other joint is performed. Diagonal use of a 14 × 17 inch (35 × 43 cm) IR is

also an option if the leg is too long to fit lengthwise, and if such use is permitted by the facility. The use of a 48-inch (122-cm) SID reduces the divergence of the x-ray beam, and more of the body part is included.

> **Image receptor:** Positioned by manufacturer or department protocol for proper anatomy display orientation; CR plate: 14 × 17 inches (35 × 43 cm) lengthwise or diagonal.

Position of patient
- Place the patient in the supine position.

Position of part
- Adjust the patient's body so that the pelvis is not rotated.

- Adjust the leg so that the femoral condyles are parallel with the IR and the foot is vertical (Fig. 7.111).
- Flex the ankle until the foot is in the vertical position.
- If necessary, place a sandbag against the plantar surface of the foot to immobilize it in the correct position.
- *Shield gonads.*

Central ray
- Perpendicular to the center of the leg.

Collimation
- Adjust the radiation field to 1 inch (2.5 cm) on the sides and 1½ inches (4 cm) beyond the ankle and knee joints. Place a side marker in the collimated exposure field.

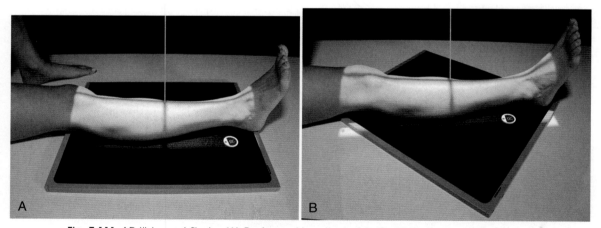

Fig. 7.111 AP tibia and fibula. (A) Performed lengthwise on IR. (B) Performed diagonal on the IR.

Structures shown

The tibia, fibula, and adjacent joints (Fig. 7.112).

EVALUATION CRITERIA

The following should be clearly seen:

- Evidence of proper collimation and the presence of a side marker placed clear of the anatomy of interest
- Ankle and knee joints on one or more images
- Entire leg without rotation
  - ☐ Proximal and distal articulations of the tibia and fibula moderately overlapped
  - ☐ Fibular midshaft free of tibial superimposition
- Bony trabecular detail and surrounding soft tissues

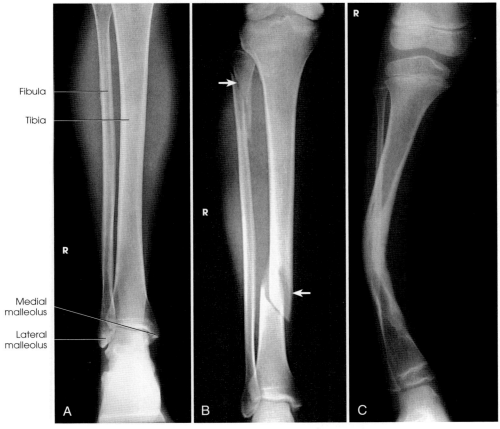

Fibula

Tibia

Medial malleolus

Lateral malleolus

Fig. 7.112 (A) AP tibia and fibula. Long leg length prevented showing entire leg. A separate knee projection had to be performed on this patient. (B) Short leg length allowed the entire leg to be shown. A spiral fracture of distal tibia with accompanying spiral fracture of proximal fibula (*arrows*) is seen. This radiograph shows the importance of including the entire length of a long bone in trauma cases. (C) AP tibia and fibula on a 4-year-old with neurofibromatosis.

♣ LATERAL PROJECTION
Mediolateral

Image receptor: Positioned by manufacturer or department protocol for proper anatomy display orientation; CR plate: 14 × 17 inches (35 × 43 cm) lengthwise or diagonal.

Position of patient
- Place the patient in the supine position.

Position of part
- Turn the patient toward the affected side with the leg on the IR.
- Adjust the rotation of the body to place the patella perpendicular to the IR, and ensure that a line drawn through the femoral condyles is also perpendicular (Fig. 7.113).
- Place sandbag supports where needed for the patient's comfort and to stabilize the body position (Fig. 7.113A).
- The knee may be flexed if necessary to ensure a true lateral position.
- The projection may be done with IR diagonal to include the ankle and knee joints or two projections are made, one of the leg to include a joint and one to include the other joint.

Alternative method
- When the patient cannot be turned from the supine position, the lateromedial lateral projection may be taken cross-table using a horizontal central ray.
- Lift the leg high enough for an assistant to slide a rigid support under the patient's leg.
- The IR may be placed between the legs, and the central ray may be directed from the lateral side.
- *Shield gonads.*

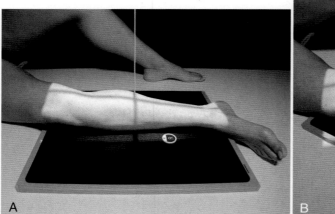
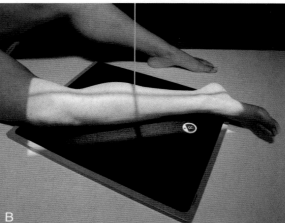

Fig. 7.113 Lateral tibia and fibula. (A) Performed lengthwise on the IR. (B) Performed diagonal on the IR.

Central ray

• Perpendicular to the midpoint of the leg.

Collimation

• Adjust the radiation field to 1 inch (2.5 cm) on the sides and 1½ inches (4 cm) beyond the ankle and knee joints. Place side marker in the collimated exposure field.

Structures shown

The tibia, fibula, and adjacent joints (Fig. 7.114).

The following should be clearly seen:

■ Evidence of proper collimation and the presence of a side marker placed clear of the anatomy of interest
■ Ankle and knee joints on one or more images
■ Entire leg in true lateral position
  □ Distal fibula superimposed by the posterior half of the tibia
  □ Slight overlap of the tibia on the proximal fibular head
  □ Moderate separation of the tibial and fibular bodies or shafts (except at their articular ends)
■ Possibly reduced superimposition of femoral condyles because of divergence of the beam
■ Bony trabecular detail and surrounding soft tissues

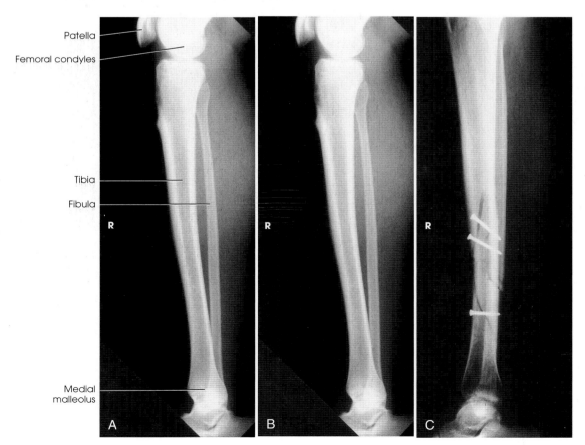

Fig. 7.114 (A) and (B) Lateral tibia and fibula. (C) Lateral postreduction tibia and fibula showing the fixation device. The leg was too long to fit on one image.

AP OBLIQUE PROJECTION
Medial and lateral rotations

Image receptor: Positioned by manufacturer or department protocol for proper anatomy display orientation; CR plate: 14 × 17 inches (35 × 43 cm) lengthwise or diagonal.

Position of patient

- Place the patient in the supine position on the radiographic table.

Position of part

- Perform oblique projections of the leg by alternately rotating the extremity 45 degrees medially (Fig. 7.115) or laterally (Fig. 7.116). For the medial rotation, ensure that the *leg* is turned inward, not just the foot.

- For the medial oblique projection, elevate the affected hip enough to rest the medial side of the foot and ankle against a 45-degree foam wedge, and place a support under the greater trochanter.
- *Shield gonads.*

Central ray

- Perpendicular to the midpoint of the IR.

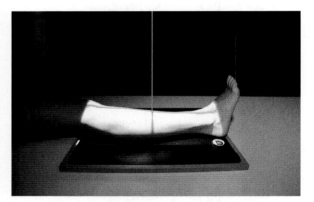

Fig. 7.115 AP oblique leg, medial rotation.

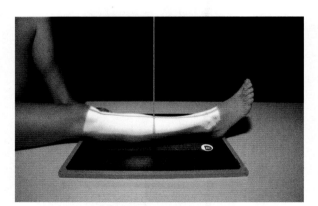

Fig. 7.116 AP oblique leg, lateral rotction.

Collimation

- Adjust the radiation field to 1 inch (2.5 cm) on the sides and 1½ inches (4 cm) beyond the ankle and knee joints. Place a side marker in the collimated exposure field.

Structures shown

A 45-degree oblique projection of the bones and soft tissues of the leg and one or both of the adjacent joints (Figs. 7.117 and 7.118).

The following should be clearly seen:
- Evidence of proper collimation and the presence of a side marker placed clear of the anatomy of interest
- Ankle and knee joints on one or more images
- Bony trabecular detail and surrounding soft tissues

Medial rotation

- Proper rotation of leg
  - Proximal and distal tibiofibular articulations
  - Maximum interosseous space between the tibia and fibula

Lateral rotation

- Proper rotation of leg
  - Fibula superimposed by lateral portion of tibia

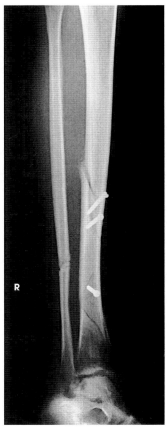

Fig. 7.117 AP oblique leg, medial rotation, showing the fixation device.

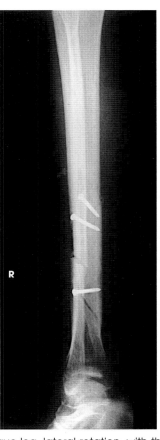

Fig. 7.118 AP oblique leg, lateral rotation, with the fixation device in place.

Lower Extremity

⚜ AP PROJECTION

Radiographs of the knee may be taken with or without the use of a grid, although a grid is most often used. Factors to consider in reaching a decision are the size of the patient's knee and the preference of the radiographer and physician.

Gonad shielding is needed during examinations of the lower extremities, when the path of the primary beam may be reasonably expected to be within 5 cm of the gonads. (Lead shielding is not shown on illustrations of the patient model because it would obstruct the demonstration of the body position.)

> **Image receptor + grid:** Positioned by manufacturer or department protocol for proper anatomy display orientation; CR plate: 10 × 12 inches (24 × 30 cm) lengthwise.

Position of patient

- Place the patient in the supine position, and adjust the body so that the pelvis is not rotated.

Position of part

- With the IR under the patient's knee, flex the joint slightly, locate the apex of the patella, and as the patient extends the knee, center the IR about ½ inch (1.3 cm) below the patellar apex. This centers the IR to the joint space.
- Adjust the patient's leg by placing the femoral epicondyles parallel with the IR for a true AP projection (Fig. 7.119). The patella lies slightly off center to the medial side. If the knee cannot be fully extended, a curved IR may be used.
- *Shield gonads.*

Central ray

- Directed to a point ½ inch (1.3 cm) inferior to the patellar apex.
- Variable, depending on the measurement between the anterior superior iliac spine (ASIS) and the tabletop (Fig. 7.120), as follows:[18]

<19 cm	3–5 degrees *caudad* (thin pelvis)
19–24 cm	0 degrees
>24 cm	3–5 degrees *cephalad* (large pelvis)

(handwritten: toward feet ↑ ; toward head ; important)

Collimation

- Adjust the radiation field to 8 × 10 inches (18 × 24 cm) on the collimator. Adjust to 1 inch (2.5 cm) beyond the sides. Place side marker in the collimated exposure field.

Structures shown

An AP projection of the knee structures (Fig. 7.121).

The following should be clearly seen:

- Evidence of proper collimation and the presence of a side marker placed clear of the anatomy of interest
- Knee fully extended if patient's condition permits
- Entire knee without rotation
  - ☐ Femoral condyles symmetric and tibia intercondylar eminence centered
  - ☐ Slight superimposition of the fibular head if the tibia is normal
  - ☐ Patella completely superimposed on the femur
  - ☐ Open femorotibial joint space, with interspaces of equal width on both sides if the knee is normal
  - ☐ Bony trabecular detail and surrounding soft tissues

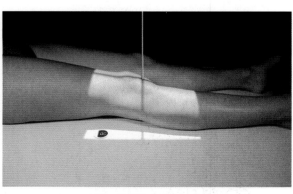

Fig. 7.119 AP knee.

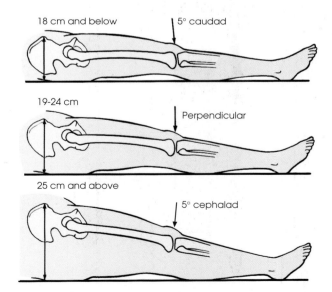

Fig. 7.120 Pelvic thickness and CR angles for AP knee radiographs.

(Modified from Martensen KM: Alternate AP knee method assures open joint space. Radiol Technol 64:19, 1992.)

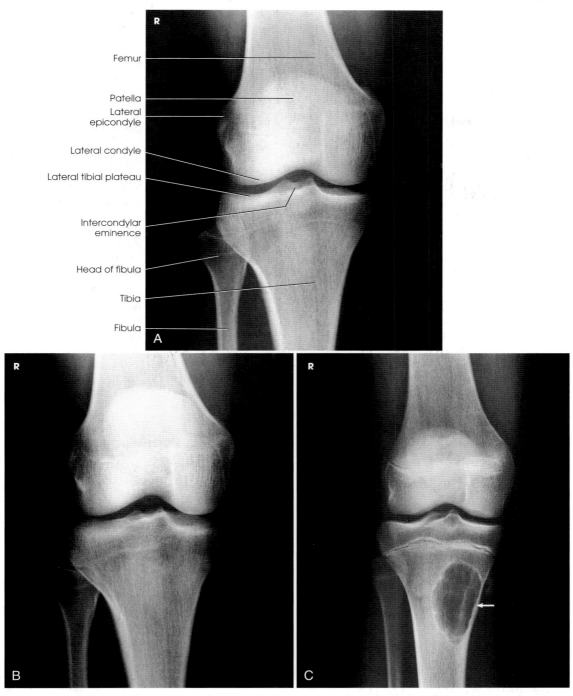

Femur

Patella

Lateral epicondyle

Lateral condyle

Lateral tibial plateau

Intercondylar eminence

Head of fibula

Tibia

Fibula

Fig. 7.121 (A) AP knee with CR angled 5 degrees cephalad. Patient's ASIS-to-tabletop distance was greater than 25 cm. (B) Same patient as in (A) with the CR perpendicular. Note that joint space is not opened as well. (C) AP knee on a 15-year-old. *Arrow* is pointing to a benign lesion in the tibia.

PA PROJECTION

Image receptor + grid: Positioned by manufacturer or department protocol for proper anatomy display orientation; CR plate: 10 × 12 inches (24 × 30 cm) lengthwise.

Position of patient

- Place the patient in the prone position with toes resting on the radiographic table, or place sandbags under the ankle for support.

Position of part

- Center a point ½ inch (1.3 cm) below the patellar apex to the center of the IR, and adjust the patient's leg so that the femoral epicondyles are parallel with the tabletop. Because the knee is balanced on the medial side of the obliquely located patella, care must be used in adjusting the knee (Fig. 7.122).
- *Shield gonads.*

Central ray

- Directed at an angle of 5 to 7 degrees caudad to exit a point ½ inch (1.3 cm) inferior to the patellar apex. Because the tibia and fibula are slightly inclined, the central ray is parallel with the tibial plateau. A perpendicular CR may be needed for patients with large thighs or when the foot is dorsiflexed.

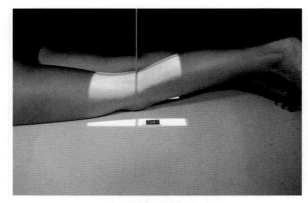

Fig. 7.122 PA knee.

Collimation

- Adjust the radiation field to 8 × 10 inches (18 × 24 cm) on the collimator. Adjust to 1 inch (2.5 cm) beyond the sides. Place side marker in the collimated exposure field.

Structures shown

A PA projection of the knee (Fig. 7.123).

The following should be clearly seen:
- Evidence of proper collimation and the presence of a side marker placed clear of the anatomy of interest
- Open the femorotibial joint space with interspaces of equal width on both sides if the knee is normal
- Knee fully extended if the patient's condition permits
- No rotation of the femur if the tibia is normal
- Slight superimposition of the fibular head with the tibia
- Bony trabecular detail and surrounding soft tissues

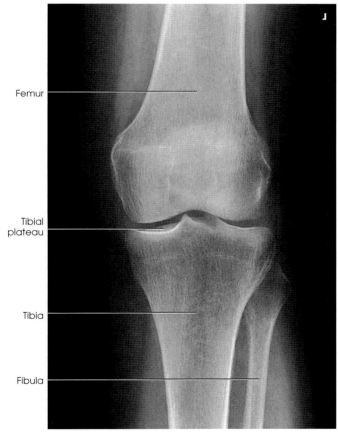

Femur

Tibial plateau

Tibia

Fibula

Fig. 7.123 PA knee.

LATERAL PROJECTION
Mediolateral

Image receptor + grid: Positioned by manufacturer or department protocol for proper anatomy display orientation; CR plate: 10 × 12 inches (24 × 30 cm) lengthwise.

Position of patient

- Ask the patient to turn onto the affected side. Ensure that the pelvis is not rotated.
- For a standard lateral projection, have the patient bring the affected knee forward and extend the other extremity behind it (Fig. 7.124). The other extremity may also be placed in front of the affected knee on a support block.

Position of part

- Flexion of 20 to 30 degrees is usually preferred because this position relaxes the muscles and shows the maximum volume of the joint cavity.[19]
- To prevent fragment separation in new or unhealed patellar fractures, the knee should not be flexed more than 10 degrees.
- Place a support under the ankle.
- Grasp the epicondyles and adjust them so that they are perpendicular to the IR (condyles superimposed). The patella is perpendicular to the plane of the IR (Fig. 7.125).
- *Shield gonads.*

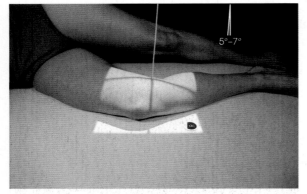

Fig. 7.124 Lateral knee showing a 5-degree cephalad angulation of CR.

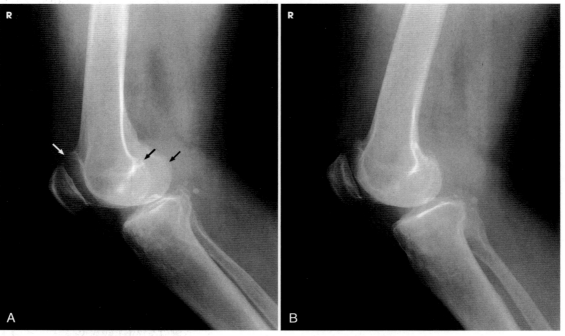

Fig. 7.125 (A) Improperly positioned lateral knee. Note that condyles are not superimposed *(black arrows)*, and the patella is a closed joint *(white arrow)*. (B) Same patient as in (A) after correct positioning. The condyles are superimposed, and the patellofemoral joint is open.

Central ray

- Directed to the knee joint 1 inch (2.5 cm) distal to the medial epicondyle at an angle of 5 to 7 degrees cephalad. This slight angulation of the central ray prevents the joint space from being obscured by the magnified image of the medial femoral condyle. In addition, in the lateral recumbent position, the medial condyle is slightly inferior to the lateral condyle.
- Center the IR to the central ray.

Collimation

- Adjust the radiation field to 8 × 10 inches (18 × 24 cm) on the collimator. Adjust to 1 inch (2.5 cm) anterior to the patella and 1 inch (2.5 cm) beyond the posterior shadow. Place side marker in the collimated exposure field.

Structures shown

A lateral image of the distal end of the femur, patella, knee joint, proximal ends of the tibia and fibula, and adjacent soft tissue (Fig. 7.126).

EVALUATION CRITERIA

The following should be clearly seen:
- Evidence of proper collimation and the presence of a side marker placed clear of the anatomy of interest
- Knee flexed 20 to 30 degrees in true lateral position as demonstrated by femoral condyles superimposed (locate the more magnified medial condyle)
  □ Anterior surface of medial condyle closer to patella results from over-rotation toward the image receptor (IR).
  □ Anterior surface of medial condyle farther from patella results from under-rotation away from the IR.
  □ Inferior surface of medial condyle caudal to lateral condyle results from insufficient cephalad central ray (CR) angle.
  □ Inferior surface of lateral condyle caudal to medial condyle results from too much cephalad CR angle.
- Fibular head and tibia slightly superimposed (overrotation causes less superimposition, and under-rotation causes more superimposition)
- Patella in a lateral profile
- Open patellofemoral joint space
- Open joint space between femoral condyles and tibia
- Bony trabecular detail and surrounding soft tissues

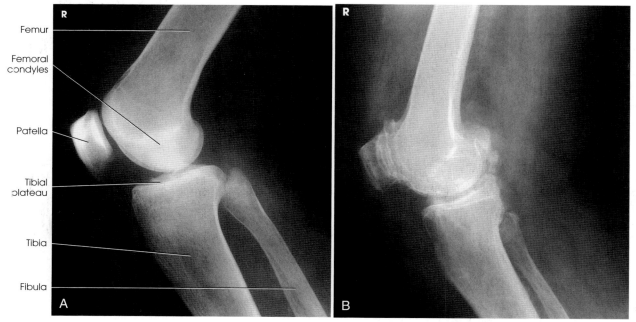

Femur

Femoral condyles

Patella

Tibial plateau

Tibia

Fibula

A

B

Fig. 7.126 (A) Lateral knee. (B) Lateral knee showing severe arthritis.

✿ AP PROJECTION
WEIGHT-BEARING METHOD
Standing

Leach et al.[20] recommended that a bilateral weight-bearing AP projection be routinely included in radiographic examination of arthritic knees. They found that a weight-bearing study often reveals narrowing of a joint space that appears normal on a non–weight-bearing study.

Image receptor + grid: Positioned by manufacturer or department protocol for proper anatomy display orientation; CR plate: 14 × 17 inches (35 × 43 cm) crosswise for bilateral image.

Position of patient

- Place the patient in the upright position with the back toward a vertical grid device.

Position of part

- Adjust the patient's position to center the knees to the IR.
- Place the toes straight ahead, with the feet separated enough for good balance.
- Ask the patient to stand straight with knees fully extended and weight equally distributed on the feet.
- Center the IR ½ inch (1.3 cm) below the apices of the patellae (Fig. 7.127).
- *Shield gonads.*

Central ray

- Horizontal and perpendicular to the center of the IR, entering at a point ½ inch (1.3 cm) below the apices of the patellae.

Collimation

- Adjust the radiation field to 14 × 17 inches (35 × 43 cm) on the collimator. Adjust to 1 inch (2.5 cm) beyond the sides. Place a side marker in the collimated exposure field.

Structures shown

The joint spaces of the knees. Varus and valgus deformities can also be evaluated with this procedure (Fig. 7.128).

The following should be clearly seen:
- Evidence of proper collimation and the presence of a side marker placed clear of the anatomy of interest
- Both knees without rotation
- Knee joint spaces centered to the exposure area
- Bony trabecular detail and surrounding soft tissues

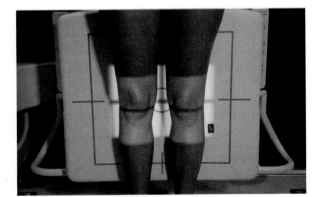

Fig. 7.127 AP bilateral weight-bearing knees.

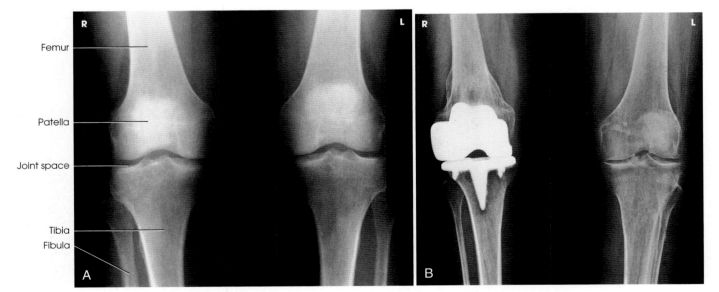

Femur

Patella

Joint space

Tibia
Fibula

A

B

Fig. 7.128 (A) AP bilateral weight-bearing knees. (B) Right knee has undergone total knee arthroplasty.

PA PROJECTION
ROSENBERG METHOD[21]
WEIGHT-BEARING
Standing flexion

> **Image receptor + grid:** Positioned by manufacturer or department protocol for proper anatomy display orientation; CR plate: 14 × 17 inches (35 × 43 cm) crosswise for bilateral knees.

Position of patient
- Place the patient in the standing position with the anterior aspect of the knees centered to the vertical grid device.

Position of part
- For a direct PA projection, have the patient stand upright with the knees in contact with the vertical grid device.
- Center the IR at a level ½ inch (1.3 cm) below the apices of the patellae.
- Have the patient grasp the edges of the grid device and flex the knees to place the femora at an angle of 45 degrees (Fig. 7.129).
- *Shield gonads.*

Central ray
- Horizontal and perpendicular to the center of the IR, entering at the midpopliteal area and exiting ½ inch (1.3 cm) below the patellar apex. The central ray is perpendicular to the tibia and fibula. A 10-degree caudal angle is sometimes used.

Collimation
- Adjust the radiation field to 14 × 17 inches (35 × 43 cm) on the collimator. Adjust to 1 inch (2.5 cm) beyond the sides. Place a side marker in the collimated exposure field.

Structures shown
The PA weight-bearing method is useful for evaluating joint space narrowing and showing articular cartilage disease on the posterior surface of the femoral condyles (Fig. 7.130). The image is similar to radiographs of the intercondylar fossa.

EVALUATION CRITERIA
The following should be clearly seen:
- Evidence of proper collimation and the presence of a side marker placed clear of the anatomy of interest
- Both knees without rotation
- Knee joints centered to exposure area
- Tibial plateaus in profile
- Intercondylar fossae visible
- Bony trabecular detail and surrounding soft tissues

NOTE: For a weight-bearing study of a single knee, the patient puts full weight on the affected side. The patient may balance with slight pressure on the toes of the unaffected side.

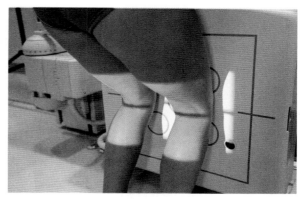

Fig. 7.129 PA projection with patient's knees flexed 45 degrees and using perpendicular CR.

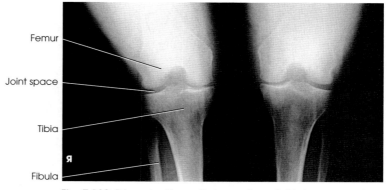

Femur

Joint space

Tibia

Fibula

Fig. 7.130 PA projection with knees flexed 45 degrees and CR directed 10 degrees caudad.

♠ AP OBLIQUE PROJECTION
Lateral rotation

Image receptor + grid: Positioned by manufacturer or department protocol for proper anatomy display orientation; CR plate: 10 × 12 inches (24 × 30 cm) lengthwise.

Position of patient
- Place the patient on the radiographic table in the supine position, and support the ankles.

Position of part
- If necessary, elevate the hip of the *unaffected* side enough to rotate the affected extremity.

- Support the elevated hip and knee of the unaffected side (Fig. 7.131).
- Center the IR ½ inch (1.3 cm) below the apex of the patella.
- Externally rotate the extremity 45 degrees.
- *Shield gonads.*

Central ray
- Directed ½ inch (1.3 cm) inferior to the patellar apex. The angle is variable, depending on the measurement between the ASIS and the tabletop, as follows:

<19 cm	3–5 degrees *caudad*
19–24 cm	0 degrees
>24 cm	3–5 degrees *cephalad*

Collimation
- Adjust the radiation field to 8 × 10 inches (18 × 24 cm) on the collimator. Adjust to 1 inch (2.5 cm) beyond the sides. Place a side marker in the collimated exposure field.

Structures shown
An AP oblique projection of the laterally rotated femoral condyles, patella, tibial condyles, and head of the fibula (Fig. 7.132).

EVALUATION CRITERIA
The following should be clearly seen:
- Evidence of proper collimation and the presence of a side marker placed clear of the anatomy of interest
- Medial femoral and tibial condyles
- Tibial plateaus
- Fibula superimposed over the lateral half of the tibia
- Margin of the patella projected slightly beyond the edge of the lateral femoral condyle
- Open knee joint
- Bony trabecular detail and surrounding soft tissues

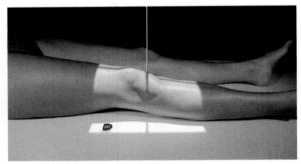

Fig. 7.131 AP oblique knee, lateral rotation.

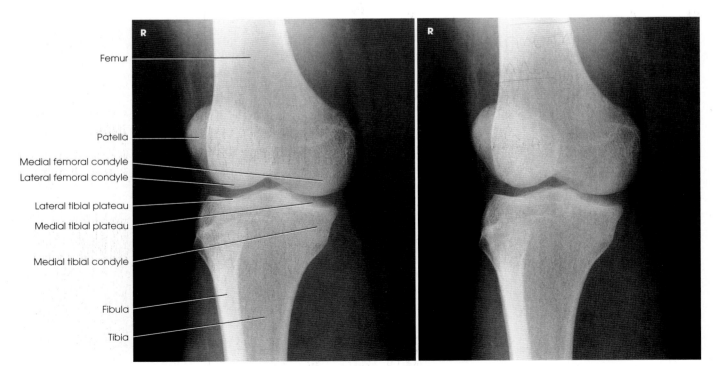

Fig. 7.132 AP oblique knee.

✦ AP OBLIQUE PROJECTION
Medial rotation

Image receptor + grid: Positioned by manufacturer or department protocol for proper anatomy display orientation; CR plate: 10 × 12 inches (24 × 30 cm) lengthwise.

Position of patient
- Place the patient on the table in the supine position, and support the ankles.

Position of part
- Medially rotate the extremity, and elevate the hip of the affected side enough to rotate the extremity 45 degrees.

- Place a support under the hip, if needed (Fig. 7.133).
- *Shield gonads.*

Central ray
- Directed ½ inch (1.3 cm) inferior to the patellar apex; the angle is variable, depending on the measurement between the ASIS and the tabletop, as follows:

<19 cm	3–5 degrees *caudad*
19–24 cm	0 degrees
>24 cm	3–5 degrees *cephalad*

Collimation
- Adjust the radiation field to 8 × 10 inches (18 × 24 cm) on the collimator. Adjust to 1 inch (2.5 cm) beyond the sides. Place a side marker in the collimated exposure field.

Structures shown
An AP oblique projection of the medially rotated femoral condyles, patella, tibial condyles, proximal tibiofibular joint, and head of the fibula (Fig. 7.134).

EVALUATION CRITERIA
The following should be clearly seen:
- ■ Evidence of proper collimation and the presence of a side marker placed clear of the anatomy of interest
- ■ Tibia and fibula separated at their proximal articulation
- ■ Posterior tibia
- ■ Lateral condyles of the femur and tibia
- ■ Both tibial plateaus
- ■ Margin of the patella projecting slightly beyond the medial side of the femoral condyle
- ■ Open knee joint
- ■ Bony trabecular detail and surrounding soft tissues

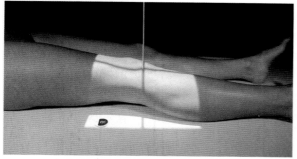

Fig. 7.133 AP oblique knee, medial rotation.

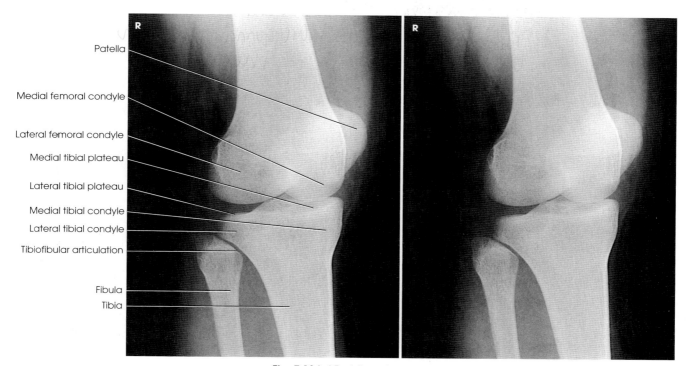

Patella
Medial femoral condyle
Lateral femoral condyle
Medial tibial plateau
Lateral tibial plateau
Medial tibial condyle
Lateral tibial condyle
Tibiofibular articulation
Fibula
Tibia

Fig. 7.134 AP oblique knee.

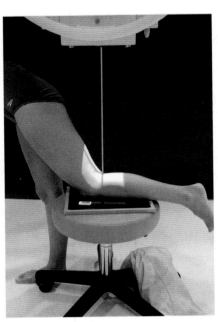

Fig. 7.135 PA axial intercondylar fossa, upright with the knee on a stool.

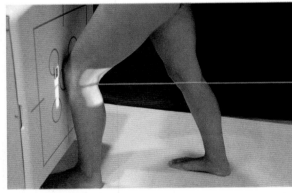

Fig. 7.136 PA axial intercondylar fossa, standing using the horizontal CR.

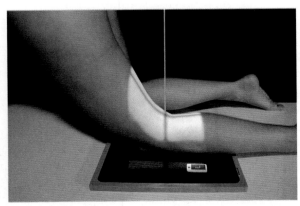

Fig. 7.137 PA axial intercondylar fossa, kneeling on a radiographic table: original Holmblad method.

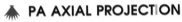

⚘ PA AXIAL PROJECTION
HOLMBLAD METHOD

The PA axial, or *tunnel,* projection, first described by Holmblad[22] in 1937, required that the patient assume a kneeling position on the radiographic table. In 1983, the Holmblad method[23] was modified so that if the patient's condition allowed, a standing position could be used.

> **Image receptor:** Positioned by manufacturer or department protocol for proper anatomy display orientation; CR plate: 10×12 inches (24×30 cm) lengthwise.

Position of patient

- After consideration of the patient's safety, place the patient in one of three positions: (1) standing with the knee of interest flexed and resting on a stool at the side of the radiographic table (Fig. 7.135); (2) standing at the side of the radiographic table with the affected knee flexed and placed in contact with the front of the IR (Fig. 7.136); or (3) kneeling on the radiographic table, as originally described by Holmblad, with the affected knee over the IR (Fig. 7.137). In all three approaches, the tibial portion of the knee is in contact with the IR, and the patient's upper body is stabilized with an appropriate support.

"me and my homie holmblad are gonna drive thru the tunnel"

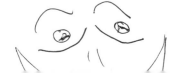

Position of part

- For all positions, place the IR against the anterior surface of the patient's knee, and center the IR to the apex of the patella. Flex the knee 70 degrees from full extension (20-degree difference from the central ray, as shown in Fig. 7.138).
- *Shield gonads.*

Central ray

- Perpendicular to the lower leg, entering the superior aspect of the popliteal fossa and exiting at the level of the patellar apex, for all three positions.

Collimation

- Adjust the radiation field to 8 × 10 inches (18 × 24 cm) on the collimator. Adjust to 1 inch (2.5 cm) beyond the sides. Place side marker in the collimated exposure field.

Structures shown

The intercondylar fossa and posteroinferior articular surfaces of the condyles of the femur, as well as the medial and lateral intercondylar tubercles of the intercondylar eminence and tibial plateaus in profile (Fig. 7.139). Holmblad[22] stated that the degree of flexion used in this position widens the joint space between the femur and tibia, and gives an improved image of the joint and the surfaces of the tibia and femur.

EVALUATION CRITERIA

The following should be clearly seen:
- Evidence of proper collimation and the presence of a side marker placed clear of the anatomy of interest
- Open intercondylar fossa
- Posteroinferior surface of the femoral condyles
- Knee joint space open, with one or both tibial plateaus in profile (superimposed anterior and posterior surfaces)
- Apex of the patella not superimposing the fossa
- No rotation, demonstrated by slight tibiofibular overlap and centered intercondylar eminence
- Bony trabecular detail and surrounding soft tissues

NOTE: The bilateral examination (Rosenberg method) is described on p. 349 (also see Fig. 7.130).

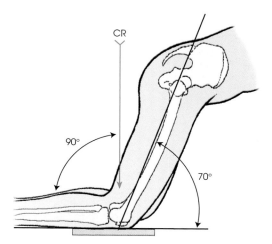

Fig. 7.138 Alignment relationship for any of three intercondylar fossa approaches: Holmblad method. CR is perpendicular to the tibia–fibula.

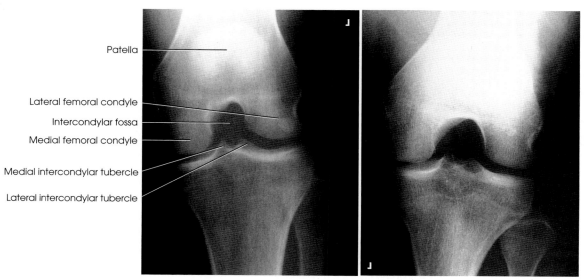

Patella
Lateral femoral condyle
Intercondylar fossa
Medial femoral condyle
Medial intercondylar tubercle
Lateral intercondylar tubercle

Fig. 7.139 PA axial (tunnel) intercondylar fossa: Holmblad method.

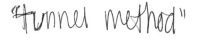

"Tunnel method"

PA AXIAL PROJECTION
CAMP-COVENTRY METHOD[24]

Image receptor: Positioned by manufacturer or department protocol for proper anatomy display orientation; CR plate: 10 × 12 inches (24 × 30 cm) lengthwise.

Position of patient
• Place the patient in the prone position, and adjust the body so that it is not rotated.

Position of part
• Flex the patient's knee to a 40- or 50-degree angle, place the femoral portion of the knee on the IR, and rest the foot on a suitable support.
• Center the upper half of the IR to the knee joint; the central ray angulation projects the joint to the center of the IR (Figs. 7.140 and 7.141).
• A protractor may be used beside the leg to determine the correct leg angle.
• Adjust the leg so that the knee has no medial or lateral rotation.
• *Shield gonads.*

Central ray
• Perpendicular to the long axis of the lower leg, entering the popliteal fossa and exiting at the patellar apex.
• Angled 40 degrees when the knee is flexed 40 degrees and 50 degrees when the knee is flexed 50 degrees.

Collimation
• Adjust the radiation field to 8 × 10 inches (18 × 24 cm) on the collimator. Adjust to 1 inch (2.5 cm) beyond the sides. Place a side marker in the collimated exposure field.

Structures shown
The intercondylar fossa and posteroinferior articular surfaces of the condyles of the femur, as well as the medial and lateral intercondylar tubercles of the intercondylar eminence and tibial plateaus in profile (Figs. 7.142 and 7.143).

The following should be clearly seen:
■ Evidence of proper collimation and the presence of a side marker placed clear of the anatomy of interest
■ Open intercondylar fossa
■ Posteroinferior surface of the femoral condyles
■ Knee joint space open, with one or both tibial plateaus in profile (superimposed anterior and posterior surfaces)
■ Apex of the patella not superimposing the fossa
■ No rotation, demonstrated by slight tibiofibular overlap and centered intercondylar eminence
■ Bony trabecular detail and surrounding soft tissues

NOTE: In examinations of the knee joint, an intercondylar fossa projection may be included to detect loose bodies ("joint mice"). This projection is also used in evaluating split and displaced cartilage in osteochondritis dissecans and flattening, or underdevelopment, of the lateral femoral condyle in congenital slipped patella.

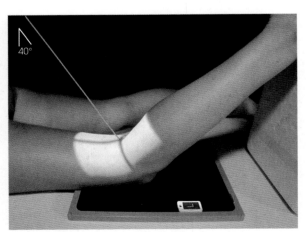

Fig. 7.140 PA axial (tunnel) intercondylar fossa: Camp-Coventry method.

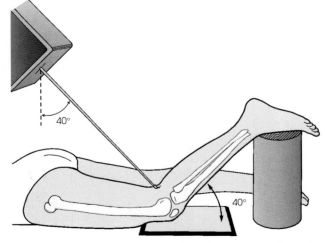

Fig. 7.141 PA axial (tunnel) intercondylar fossa: Camp-Coventry method.

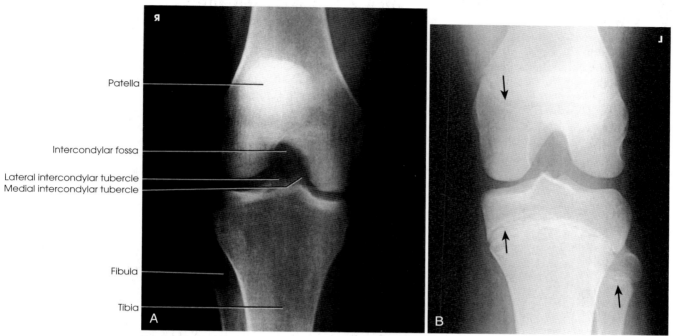

Patella

Intercondylar fossa

Lateral intercondylar tubercle
Medial intercondylar tubercle

Fibula

Tibia

Fig. 7.142 Camp-Coventry method. (A) Flexion of the knee at 40 degrees. (B) Flexion of the knee at 40 degrees in a 13-year-old patient. Note epiphyses *(arrows)*.

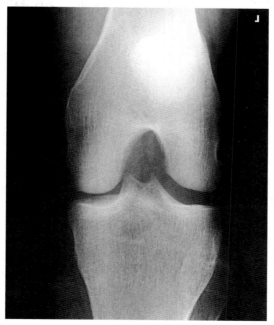

Fig. 7.143 Flexion of the knee at 50 degrees (same patient as in Fig. 7.142): Camp-Coventry method.

Intercondylar Fossa

AP AXIAL PROJECTION

BÉCLÈRE METHOD

Image receptor: Positioned by manufacturer or department protocol for proper anatomy display orientation; CR plate: 10 × 12 inches (24 × 30 cm) crosswise.

Position of patient

• Place the patient in the supine position, and adjust the body so that it is not rotated.

Position of part

• Flex the affected knee enough to place the long axis of the femur at an angle of 60 degrees to the long axis of the tibia.
• Support the knee on sandbags (Fig. 7.144).
• Place the IR under the knee, and position the IR so that the center point coincides with the central ray.

• Adjust the leg so that the femoral condyles are equidistant from the IR. Immobilize the foot with sandbags.
• *Shield gonads.*

Central ray

• Perpendicular to the long axis of the lower leg, entering the knee joint ½ inch (1.3 cm) below the patellar apex.

Collimation

• Adjust the radiation field to 8 × 10 inches (18 × 24 cm) on the collimator. Adjust to 1 inch (2.5 cm) beyond the sides. Place a side marker in the collimated exposure field.

Structures shown

The intercondylar fossa, intercondylar eminence, and knee joint (Fig. 7.145).

EVALUATION CRITERIA

The following should be clearly seen:
■ Evidence of proper collimation and the presence of a side marker placed clear of the anatomy of interest
■ Open intercondylar fossa
■ Posteroinferior surface of the femoral condyles
■ Intercondylar eminence and knee joint space
■ No superimposition of the fossa by the apex of the patella
■ No rotation, as demonstrated by slight tibiofibular overlap
■ Bony trabecular detail and surrounding soft tissues

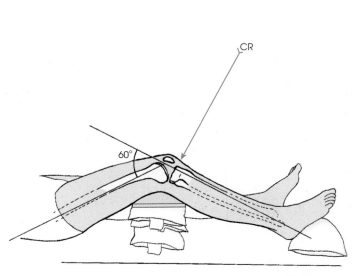

Fig. 7.144 AP axial intercondylar fossa with transverse IR: Béclère method.

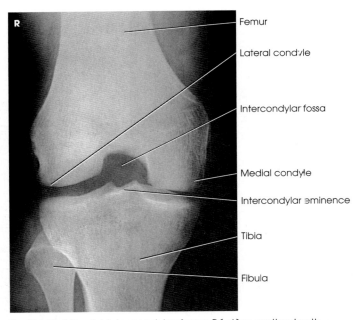

Fig. 7.145 AP axial intercondylar fossa: Béclère method with identified anatomy.

✦ PA PROJECTION

Image receptor + grid: Positioned by manufacturer or department protocol for proper anatomy display orientation; CR plate: 10 × 12 inches (24 × 30 cm) lengthwise.

Position of patient
- Place the patient in the prone position.
- If the knee is painful, place one sandbag under the thigh and another under the leg to relieve pressure on the patella.

Position of part
- Center the IR to the patella.
- Adjust the position of the leg to place the patella parallel with the plane of the IR. This usually requires that the heel be rotated 5 to 10 degrees laterally (Fig. 7.146).
- *Shield gonads.*

Central ray
- Perpendicular to the midpopliteal area exiting the patella.
- Collimate closely to the patellar area.

Collimation
- Adjust the radiation field to 6 × 6 inches (15 × 15 cm) on the collimator. Place a side marker in the collimated exposure field.

Structures shown
The PA projection of the patella provides improved spatial resolution over the AP projection because of a closer object-to-IR distance (OID) (Figs. 7.147 and 7.148).

EVALUATION CRITERIA

The following should be clearly seen:
- Evidence of proper collimation and the presence of a side marker placed clear of the anatomy of interest
- Patella completely superimposed by the femur
- No rotation
- Bony trabecular detail and surrounding soft tissues

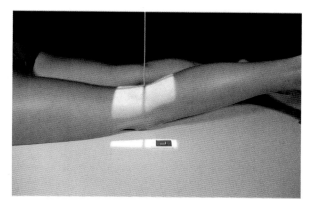

Fig. 7.146 PA patella.

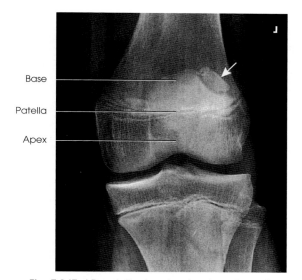

Fig. 7.147 AP patella showing fracture *(arrow)*.

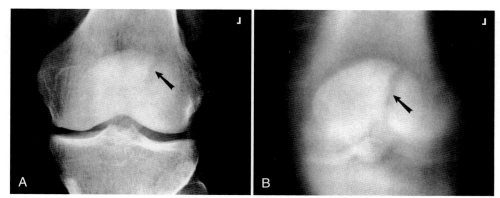

Fig. 7.148 (A) Conventional PA projection of patella shows vertical radiolucent line *(arrow)* passing through junction of lateral and middle third of patella. (B) On tomography, this defect extends from the superior to the inferior margin of patella. It is a bipartite patella, not a fracture.

⚑ LATERAL PROJECTION
Mediolateral

Image receptor + grid: Positioned by manufacturer or department protocol for proper anatomy display orientation; CR plate: 10 × 12 inches (24 × 30 cm) lengthwise.

Position of patient
- Place the patient in the lateral recumbent position.

Position of part
- Ask the patient to turn onto the affected hip. A sandbag may be placed under the ankle for support.
- Have the patient flex the unaffected knee and hip, and place the unaffected foot in front of the affected extremity for stability.
- Flex the affected knee approximately 5 to 10 degrees. Increasing the flexion reduces the patellofemoral joint space.
- Adjust the knee in the lateral position so that the femoral epicondyles are superimposed and the patella is perpendicular to the IR (Fig. 7.149).
- *Shield gonads.*
- Center the IR to the patella.

Central ray
- Perpendicular to the IR, entering the knee at the midpatellofemoral joint.

Collimation
- Adjust the radiation field to 4 × 4 inches (10 × 10 cm) on the collimator. Place a side marker in the collimated exposure field.

Structures shown
A lateral projection of the patella and patellofemoral joint space (Figs. 7.150 and 7.151).

EVALUATION CRITERIA

The following should be clearly seen:
- Evidence of proper collimation and the presence of a side marker placed clear of the anatomy of interest
- Knee flexed 5 to 10 degrees
- Patella in lateral profile
- Open patellofemoral joint space
- Bony trabecular detail and surrounding soft tissues

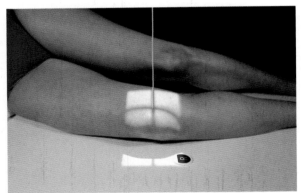

Fig. 7.149 Lateral patella, mediolateral.

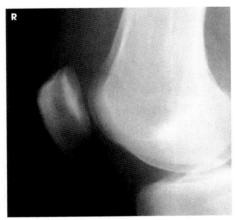

Fig. 7.150 Lateral patella, mediolateral.

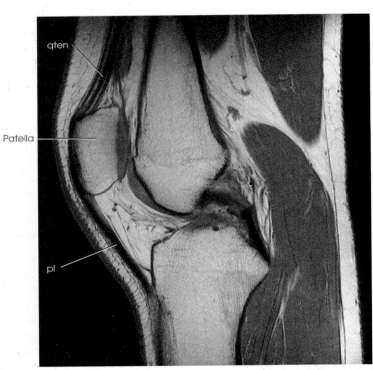

Fig. 7.151 Sagittal MRI shows patella, patellofemoral joint, and surrounding soft tissues. Quadriceps tendon (*qten*) and patellar ligament (*pl*) are shown on this image.

Lower Extremity

TANGENTIAL PROJECTION
HUGHSTON METHOD[25,26]

Radiography of the patella has been the topic of hundreds of articles. For a tangential radiograph, the patient may be placed in any of the following body positions: prone, supine, lying on the side, seated on the table, seated on the radiographic table with the leg hanging over the edge, or standing.

Various authors have described the degree of flexion of the knee joint as ranging from 20 to 120 degrees. Laurin[27] reported that patellar subluxation is easier to show when the knee is flexed 20 degrees and noted a limitation of using this small angle. Modern radiographic equipment often does not permit such small angles because of the large size of the collimator.

Fodor et al.[28] and Merchant et al.[29] recommended 45-degree flexion of the knee, and Hughston[25] recommended an approximately 55-degree angle with the central ray angled 45 degrees. In addition, Merchant et al.[29] stated that relaxation of the quadriceps muscles is required to show patellar subluxation.

> **Image receptor:** Positioned by manufacturer or department protocol for proper anatomy display orientation; CR plate: 10 × 12 inches (24 × 30 cm) lengthwise.

Position of patient
- Place the patient in a prone position with the foot resting on the radiographic table.
- Adjust the body so that it is not rotated.

Position of part
- Place the IR under the femoral portion of the knee, and slowly flex the affected knee so that the tibia and fibula form a 50- to 60-degree angle from the table.
- Rest the foot against the collimator, or support it in position (Fig. 7.152).
- Ensure that the collimator surface is not hot because this could burn the patient.
- Adjust the patient's leg so that it is not rotated medially or laterally from the vertical plane.
- *Shield gonads.*

Central ray
- Angled 45 degrees cephalad and directed through the patellofemoral joint.

Collimation
- Adjust the radiation field to 4 × 4 inches (10 × 10 cm) on the collimator. Place a side marker in the collimated exposure field.

Structures shown
The tangential image shows subluxation of the patella and patellar fractures and allows radiologic assessment of the femoral condyles (Fig. 7.153). Hughston recommended that both knees be examined for comparison.

EVALUATION CRITERIA
The following should be clearly seen:
- Evidence of proper collimation and the presence of a side marker placed clear of the anatomy of interest
- Patella in profile
- Femoral condyles and intercondylar sulcus
- Open patellofemoral articulation
- Bony trabecular detail and surrounding soft tissues

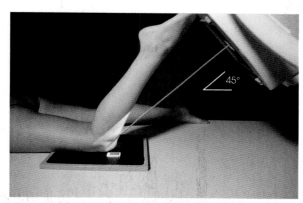

Fig. 7.152 Tangential patella and patellofemoral joint: Hughston method.

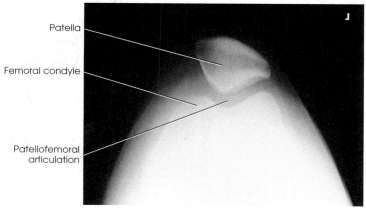

Fig. 7.153 Tangential patellofemoral joint: Hughston method.

Patella
Femoral condyle
Patellofemoral articulation

TANGENTIAL PROJECTION
MERCHANT METHOD[29]

Image receptor: Positioned by manufacturer or department protocol for proper anatomy display orientation; CR plate: 14 × 17 inches (35 × 43 cm) crosswise.

SID: A 6-foot (2-m) SID is recommended to reduce magnification.

Position of patient
- Place the patient supine with both knees at the end of the radiographic table.
- Support the knees and lower legs with an adjustable IR-holding device (Axial Viewer).[30]
- To increase comfort and relaxation of the quadriceps femoris, place pillows or a foam wedge under the patient's head and back.

Position of part
- Using the Axial Viewer device, elevate the patient's knees approximately 2 inches to place the femora parallel with the tabletop (Figs. 7.154 and 7.155).
- Adjust the angle of knee flexion to 40 degrees. (Merchant reported that the degree of angulation may be varied between 30 degrees and 90 degrees to show various patellofemoral disorders.)
- Strap both legs together at the calf level to control leg rotation and allow patient relaxation.
- Place the IR perpendicular to the central ray and resting on the patient's shins (a thin foam pad aids comfort) approximately 1 foot distal to the patellae.

- Ensure that the patient is able to relax. Relaxation of the quadriceps femoris is crucial for an accurate diagnosis. If these muscles are not relaxed, a subluxated patella may be pulled back into the intercondylar sulcus, showing a false normal appearance.
- Record the angle of knee flexion for reproducibility during follow-up examinations because the severity of patella subluxation commonly changes inversely with the angle of knee flexion.
- *Shield gonads.*

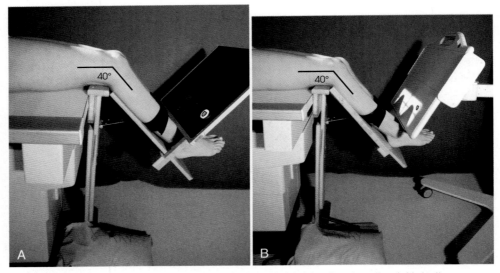

Fig. 7.154 Tangential patella and patellofemoral joint: Merchant method. Note the use of the Axial Viewer device. (A) Using a CR plate. (B) Using a DR detector in a rolling holder.

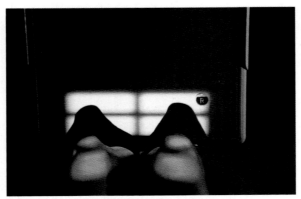

Fig. 7.155 DR detector in a rolling holder, from the patient's perspective. Note how the shadow of the knees is used to position the patella on the IR.

Central ray

- Perpendicular to the IR.
- With 40-degree knee flexion, angle the central ray 30 degrees caudad from the horizontal plane (60 degrees from vertical) to achieve a 30-degree central ray-to-femur angle. The central ray enters midway between the patellae at the level of the patellofemoral joint (superior aspect of patella).

Collimation

- Adjust the radiation field to 2 inches (5 cm) above the patellar shadow and 1 inch on the sides. Place a side marker in the collimated exposure field.

Structures shown

The bilateral tangential image shows an axial projection of the patellae and patellofemoral joints (Fig. 7.156). Because of the right-angle alignment of the IR and central ray, the patellae are seen as nondistorted, albeit slightly magnified, images.

The following should be clearly seen:

- Evidence of proper collimation and the presence of a side marker placed clear of the anatomy of interest
- Patellae in profile
- Femoral condyles and intercondylar sulcus
- Open patellofemoral articulation
- Bony trabecular detail and surrounding soft tissues

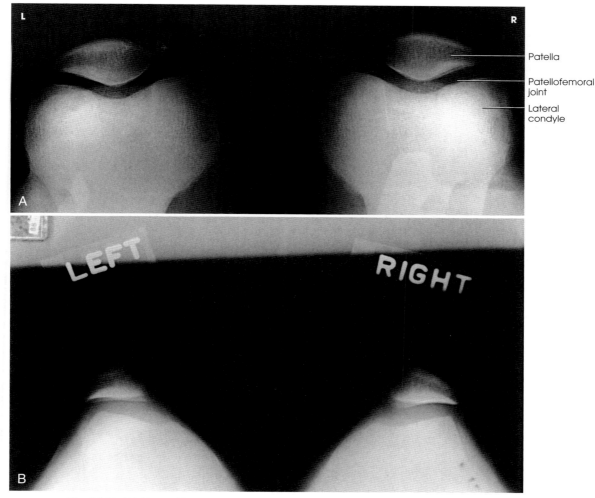

Patella

Patellofemoral joint

Lateral condyle

Fig. 7.156 (A) Normal tangential radiograph of congruent patellofemoral joints, showing patellae to be well centered with normal trabecular pattern. (B) Abnormal tangential radiograph showing abnormally shallow intercondylar sulci, misshapen and laterally subluxated patellae, and incongruent patellofemoral joints (left worse than right).

(Courtesy Alan J. Merchant.)

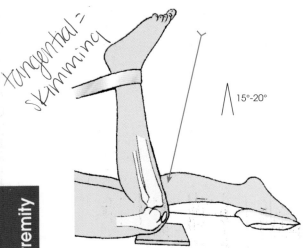

tangential = skimming

Fig. 7.157 Tangential patella and patellofemoral joint: Settegast method.

15°-20°

♠ TANGENTIAL PROJECTION
SETTEGAST METHOD

Because of the danger of fragment displacement by the acute knee flexion required for this procedure, this projection should not be attempted until a transverse fracture of the patella has been ruled out with a lateral image, or if the patient is in pain.

> **Image receptor:** Positioned by manufacturer or department protocol for proper anatomy display orientation; CR plate: 10 × 12 inches (24 × 30 cm) lengthwise.

Position of patient

- Place the patient in the supine or prone position. The latter is preferable because the knee can usually be flexed to a greater degree, and immobilization is easier (Figs. 7.157 and 7.158).

- If the patient is seated on the radiographic table, hold the IR securely in place (Fig. 7.159). Alternative positions are shown in Figs. 7.160 and 7.161.

Position of part

- Flex the patient's knee slowly as much as possible or until the patella is perpendicular to the IR if the patient's condition permits. With *slow, even flexion,* the patient should be able to tolerate the position, whereas quick, uneven flexion may cause too much pain.

- If desired, loop a long strip of bandage around the patient's ankle or foot. Have the patient grasp the ends over the shoulder to hold the leg in position. Gently adjust the leg so that its long axis is vertical.

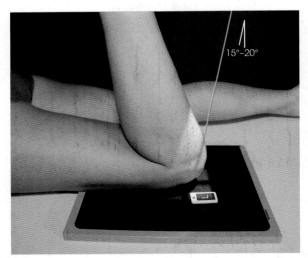

15°-20°

Fig. 7.158 Tangential patella and patellofemoral joint: Settegast method.

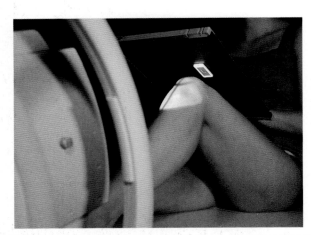

Fig. 7.159 Tangential patella and patellofemoral joint: Settegast method.

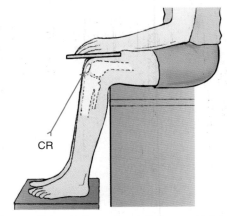

CR

Fig. 7.160 Tangential patella and patellofemoral joint: patient seated.

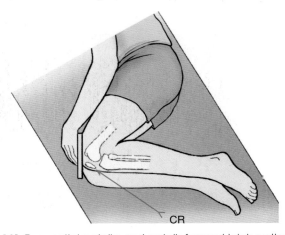

CR

Fig. 7.161 Tangential patella and patellofemoral joint: patient lateral.

- Place the IR transversely under the knee, and center it to the joint space between the patella and the femoral condyles.
- *Shield gonads.*
- By maintaining the same OID and SID relationships, this position can be obtained with the patient in a lateral or seated position (Figs. 7.160 and 7.161).

NOTE: When the central ray is directed toward the patient's upper body (Figs. 7.159 and 7.160), the thorax and thyroid should be shielded. *Gonad shielding* (not shown) should be used in all patients.

Central ray

- Perpendicular to the joint space between the patella and the femoral condyles when the joint is perpendicular. When the joint is not perpendicular, the degree of central ray angulation depends on the degree of flexion of the knee. The angulation typically is 15 to 20 degrees.
- Close collimation is recommended.

Collimation

Cephallic

- Adjust the radiation field to 4 × 4 inches (10 × 10 cm) on the collimator. Place a side marker in the collimated exposure field.

Structures shown

The articulating surfaces of the patellofemoral joint. Vertical fractures of the patella will be shown (Figs. 7.162 and 7.163).

EVALUATION CRITERIA

The following should be clearly seen:
- Evidence of proper collimation and the presence of a side marker placed clear of the anatomy of interest
- Patella in profile
- Femoral condyles and intercondylar sulcus
- Open patellofemoral articulation
- Bony trabecular detail and surrounding soft tissues

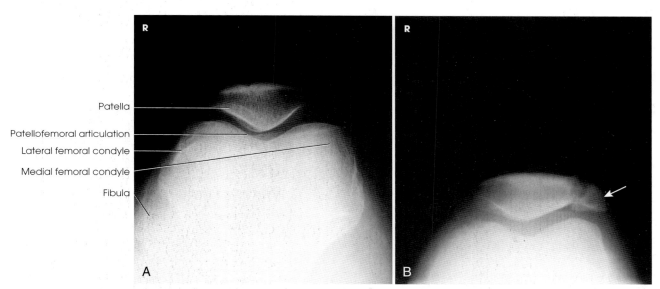

Patella
Patellofemoral articulation
Lateral femoral condyle
Medial femoral condyle
Fibula

Fig. 7.162 (A) Tangential patella and patellofemoral joint: Settegast method. (B) Fracture *(arrow)*.

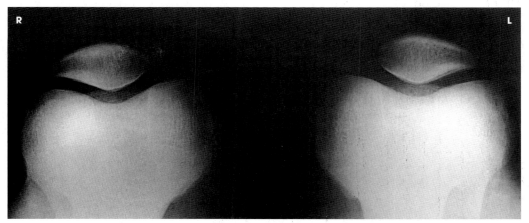

Fig. 7.163 Bilateral patella examination. For this examination, the legs should be strapped together at the level of the calf, using appropriate binding to control femoral rotation.

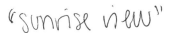

"sunrise view"

♠ AP PROJECTION

If the femoral heads are separated by an unusually broad pelvis, the bodies (shafts) are more strongly angled toward the midline.

Image receptor + grid: Positioned by manufacturer or department protocol for proper anatomy display orientation; CR plate: 14 ×17 inches (35 × 43 cm) lengthwise.

Position of patient
- Place the patient in the supine position.
- Check the pelvis to ensure it is not rotated.

Position of part
- Center the affected thigh to the midline of the IR. When the patient is too tall to include the entire femur, include on a single image the joint closest to the area of interest.

With the knee included
- For projection of the *distal* femur, rotate the patient's extremity internally to place it in true anatomic position. The extremity is naturally turned externally when the patient is lying on the table. Ensure that the epicondyles are parallel with the IR.
- Place the bottom of the IR 2 inches (5 cm) below the knee joint (Fig. 7.164).

With the hip included
- For projection of the *proximal* femur, which must include the hip joint, place the top of the IR at the level of the ASIS (Fig. 7.165).
- Rotate the extremity internally 10 to 15 degrees to place the femoral neck in profile.
- *Shield gonads.*

Central ray
- Perpendicular to the midfemur and the center of the IR.

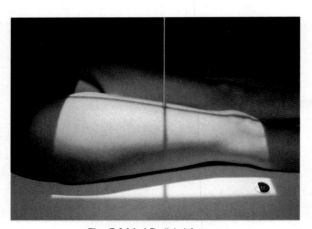

Fig. 7.164 AP distal femur.

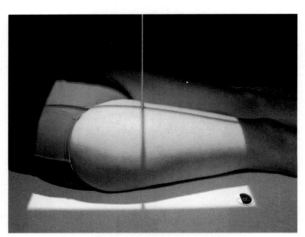

Fig. 7.165 AP right proximal femur.

Collimation

- Adjust the radiation field to 1 inch (2.5 cm) on the sides of the shadow of the thigh and 17 inches (43 cm) in length. Place a side marker in the collimated exposure field.

Structures shown

An AP projection of the femur, including the knee joint or hip or both (Figs. 7.166 and 7.167).

EVALUATION CRITERIA

The following should be clearly seen:
- Evidence of proper collimation and the presence of a side marker placed clear of the anatomy of interest
- Most of the femur and the joint nearest to the pathologic condition or site of injury (a second projection of the other joint is recommended)
- Femoral neck not foreshortened on the proximal femur
- Lesser trochanter not seen beyond the medial border of the femur or only a very small portion seen on the proximal femur
- No knee rotation on the distal femur
- Gonad shielding when indicated, but without the shield covering the proximal femur
- Any orthopedic appliance in its entirety
- Bony trabecular detail and surrounding soft tissues

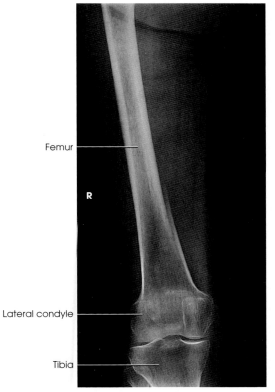

Fig. 7.166 AP right distal femur.

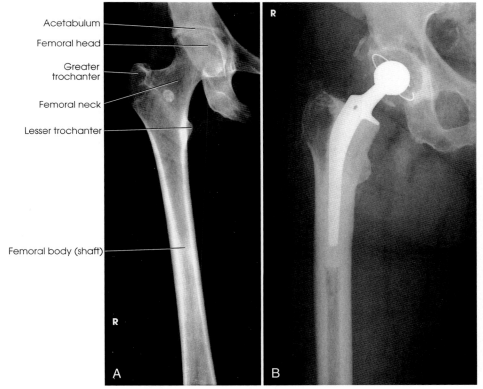

Fig. 7.167 (A) AP proximal femur. (B) AP proximal femur showing "total hip" arthroplasty procedure.

🔥 LATERAL PROJECTION
Mediolateral

Image receptor + grid: Positioned by manufacturer or department protocol for proper anatomy display orientation; CR plate: 14 × 17 inches (35 × 43 cm) lengthwise.

Position of patient

- Ask the patient to turn onto the affected side.
- Adjust the body position, and center the affected thigh to the midline of the grid.

Position of part
With the knee included

- For projection of the *distal* femur, draw the patient's uppermost extremity posterior and support it (Fig. 7.168). This position can also be accomplished by drawing the upper extremity forward and supporting it at hip level (Fig. 7.169).
- Adjust the pelvis in a true lateral position.
- Flex the affected knee about 45 degrees, place a sandbag under the ankle, and adjust the body rotation to place the epicondyles perpendicular to the tabletop.
- Adjust the position of the Bucky tray so that the IR projects approximately 2 inches (5 cm) beyond the knee to be included.

With the hip included

- For projection of the *proximal* femur, place the top of the IR at the level of the ASIS.
- Draw the upper most extremity posteriorly, and support it.
- Adjust the pelvis so that it is rolled posteriorly just enough to prevent superimposition; 10 to 15 degrees from the lateral position is sufficient (Fig. 7.170).
- *Shield gonads.*

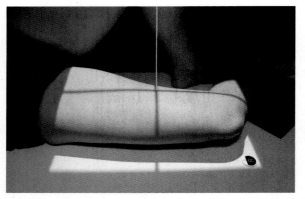

Fig. 7.168 Lateral distal femur, unaffected extremity positioned posterior.

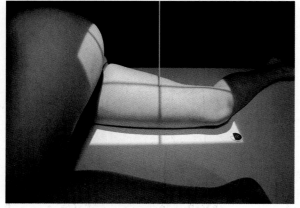

Fig. 7.169 Lateral distal femur, unaffected extremity positioned anterior.

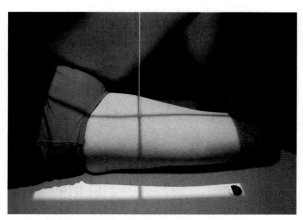

Fig. 7.170 Lateral proximal femur.

Central ray
- Perpendicular to the midfemur and the center of the IR.

Collimation
- Adjust the radiation field to 1 inch (2.5 cm) on the sides of the shadow of the thigh and 17 inches (43 cm) in length. Place a side marker in the collimated exposure field.

Structures shown
A lateral projection of about three-quarters of the femur and the adjacent joint. If needed, use two IRs to show the entire length of the adult femur (Figs. 7.171 and 7.172).

EVALUATION CRITERIA
The following should be clearly seen:
- Evidence of proper collimation and the presence of a side marker placed clear of the anatomy of interest
- Most of the femur and the joint nearest to the pathologic condition or site of injury (a second radiograph of the other end of the femur is recommended)
- Any orthopedic appliance in its entirety
- Bony trabecular detail and surrounding soft tissues

With the knee included
- Superimposed anterior surface of the femoral condyles
- Patella in profile
- Open patellofemoral space
- Inferior surface of the femoral condyles not superimposed because of divergent rays

With the hip included
- Opposite thigh not over proximal femur and hip joint
- Greater trochanter superimposed over distal femoral neck
- Lesser trochanter visible on medial aspect of proximal femur

NOTE: Because of the danger of fragment displacement, the aforementioned position is not recommended for patients with fracture or patients who may have destructive disease. Patients with these conditions should be examined in the supine position by placing the IR vertically along the medial or lateral aspect of the thigh and knee and then directing the central ray horizontally. A wafer grid or a grid-front IR should be used to minimize scattered radiation.

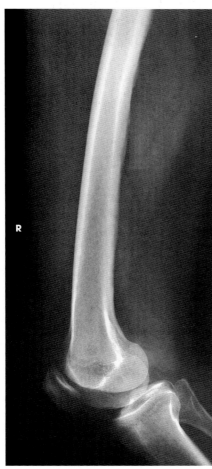

Fig. 7.171 Lateral distal femur.

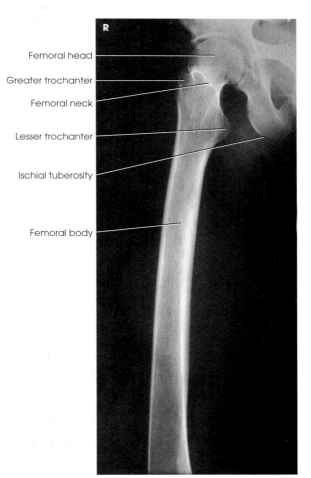

Femoral head
Greater trochanter
Femoral neck
Lesser trochanter
Ischial tuberosity
Femoral body

Fig. 7.172 Lateral proximal femur.

Long Bone Measurement

Long bone measurement to evaluate for length discrepancy may be accomplished by radiography, microdose digital radiography, ultrasonography (US), computed tomography (CT), and MRI.[31] Traditional radiographic methods included orthoroentgenography, scanography, and teleoroentgenography. Both the orthoroentgenogram and the scanogram required three precisely centered exposures at the hip, knee, and ankle joints, and include the use of a radiopaque ruler taped to the table between the extremities. The IR size is the primary difference, with the orthoroentgenogram using a single IR that remained stationary while the table and the x-ray tube moved to an unexposed section. The scanogram technique uses three separate IRs. The teleoroentgenogram was a single upright AP exposure of both extremities on a special long IR at an SID of at least 6 ft (180 cm). Digital imaging, using either DR or CR, usually employs a hybrid of these traditional techniques by obtaining the three exposures centered at the hip, knee, and ankle joints with the patient standing upright. Digital postprocessing "stitches" the three images together, creating an image similar to the orthoroentgenogram and the teleoroentgenogram, for equally accurate measurements of the entire lower extremities with a lower radiation dose than that used in the traditional methods.[31,32] A scanogram procedure also can be accomplished using digital imaging. Other variations are also performed including full lower extremity length cassettes that contain multiple CR IPs creating images similar to those accomplished with the teloroentgenographic procedure. Although long bone measurement procedures are occasionally performed for the upper extremities, the procedure is most frequently applied to the lower extremities. This section will focus on long bone measurement imaging of the lower extremities.

Radiation Protection

Differences in extremity length are common in children and may occur in association with various disorders. Patients with unequal bone growth may require yearly imaging evaluations. More frequent examinations may be necessary in patients who have undergone surgical procedures to equalize extremity length. For these reasons, radiation protection is a primary consideration in imaging for long bone measurement. Gonad shielding is recommended, as are careful patient positioning, secure immobilization, and accurate centering of a closely collimated beam of radiation to prevent unnecessary repeat exposures. Microdose digital radiography yields the lowest dose but requires specialized equipment, which can be cost-prohibitive. MRI and US have promise as means to safely image for long bone measurement, with recent research demonstrating 99% accuracy and reliability for MRI measurements.[31,33]

Long Bone Measurement Procedure

Modern radiographic procedures for long bone measurements of the lower extremities are accomplished with digital imaging technology. For this reason, the section will present the procedural details used with DR or CR. Both upright "stitched" entire leg procedures and supine scanogram procedures will be discussed in detail. Procedures with long cassettes are being phased out, so they will not be included.

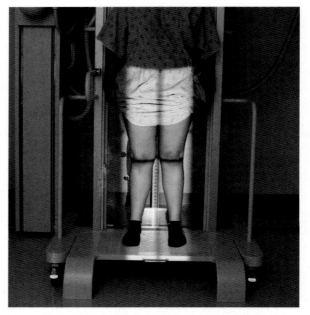

Fig. 7.173 Patient in position for radiograph of lower extremities: hips, knees, and ankles. The patient is placed in the anatomic position. The patient is standing on a raised platform so that the ankles are included.

UPRIGHT LEG MEASUREMENT PROCEDURE

Image receptor + grid: Positioned by manufacturer or department protocol for proper anatomy display orientation; CR plate: 14 × 17 inches (35 × 43 cm).

Position of patient

- Stand the patient upright with the back against the vertical imaging stand.

Position of part

- Adjust and immobilize the extremities for an AP projection.
- If the two lower extremities are examined simultaneously, separate the ankles 5 to 6 inches (13 to 15 cm) and place the specialized ruler between the patient and the IR, with the top at the level of the pelvis and extending down between the legs (Fig. 7.173).
- If the extremities are examined separately, position the patient with the special ruler behind each extremity.

Localization of joints

- Localize each joint and mark the central ray centering point. If a significant discrepancy in length is suspected it may be necessary to mark the joints of each side independently.
- Locate the *hip joint* by placing a mark 1 to $1\frac{1}{4}$ inches (2.5 to 3.2 cm) (depending on the size of the patient) laterodistally and at a right angle to the midpoint of an imaginary line extending from the ASIS to the pubic symphysis.
- Locate the *knee joint* just below the apex of the patella at the level of the depression between the femoral and tibial condyles.
- Locate the *ankle joint* directly below the depression midway between the malleoli.

Procedure

The three-exposure sequence may be made manually, with the radiographer moving the tube and IR for each exposure, or automatically, with the equipment programmed by the radiographer adjusting the field to include the ASIS at the top of the field and the ankles at the bottom (Fig. 7.174). For the automated procedure, the radiographer activates the sequence, and the tube and DR detector move first to the hip joint level, then to the knee joint level, and finally to the ankle joint level.

For both the manual and automated procedures, exposures are made as follows:

- The exposure field is centered to the patient's hip, and the first IR is exposed (see Fig. 7.174A).
- The exposure field is centered to the patient's knee joint, and the second IR is exposed (see Fig. 7.174B).
- The exposure field is centered to the patient's ankle joint, and the third IR is exposed (see Fig. 7.174C).

When a significant discrepancy in length of the two extremities exists, it will not be possible to place the CR at the level of both joints for a bilateral procedure. In these cases, the radiography must use professional judgment to place the CR as close as possible to the center of both joints.

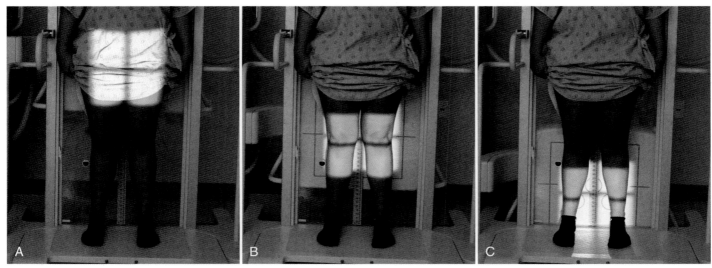

Fig. 7.174 Upright leg measurement procedure. Three radiographs are taken. (A) The first includes the hips; (B) the second includes the knees; (C) the third includes the ankles.

Central ray

- Perpendicular to the center of the IR for the manual procedure. For the automated procedure, there may be a small cephalad angle for the hip exposure and a small caudad angle for the ankle exposure.

Collimation

- Adjust the radiation field to approximately 14 × 17 inches (35 × 43 cm) on the collimator. For smaller patients, collimate to within 1 inch (2.5 cm) of shadow of the lateral thighs.

Structures shown

A composite of the three exposures digitally stitched into one image, which includes all anatomy from the hip joints to the ankle joints (Fig. 7.175).

The following should be clearly seen:

- Evidence of proper collimation and the presence of a side marker placed clear of the anatomy of interest
- Image of the special ruler
- All lower extremity anatomy, including the hip joint, the knee joint, and the ankle joint
- Bony trabecular detail and surrounding soft tissues

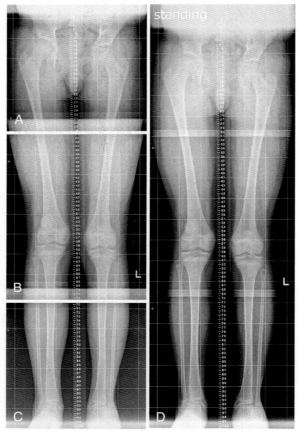

Fig. 7.175 The three images that include the (A) hips, (B) knees, and (C) ankles are digitally "stitched" together to create a composite image (D) of the entire lower extremity.

SUPINE SCANOGRAM PROCEDURE

Image receptor + grid: Positioned by manufacturer or department protocol for proper anatomy display orientation; CR plate: 14 × 17 inches (35 × 43 cm).

Position of patient

- Place the patient in the supine position.

Position of part

- Adjust and immobilize the extremities for an AP projection.
- If the two lower extremities are examined simultaneously, separate the ankles 5 to 6 inches (13 to 15 cm) and place the specialized ruler between the patient and the IR, with the top at the level of the pelvis and extending down between the legs.
- If the extremities are examined separately, position the patient with the special ruler behind each extremity.

Localization of joints

- Localize each joint and mark the central ray centering point. If a significant discrepancy in length is suspected it may be necessary to mark the joints of each side independently.
- Locate the *hip joint* by placing a mark 1 to 1¼ inches (2.5 to 3.2 cm) (depending on the size of the patient) laterodistally and at a right angle to the midpoint of an imaginary line extending from the ASIS to the pubic symphysis.
- Locate the *knee joint* just below the apex of the patella at the level of the depression between the femoral and tibial condyles.
- Locate the *ankle joint* directly below the depression midway between the malleoli.

Procedure

Three exposures are made, with the radiographer moving the tube and IR for each exposure.

Exposures are made as follows:

- The exposure field is centered to the patient's hip, and the first IR is exposed (Fig. 7.176A).
- The exposure field is centered to the patient's knee joint, and the second IR is exposed (see Fig. 7.176B).
- The exposure field is centered to the patient's ankle joint, and the third IR is exposed (see Fig. 7.176C).

When a significant discrepancy in length of the two extremities exists, it will not be possible to place the CR at the level of both joints for a bilateral procedure. In these cases, the radiography must use professional judgment to place the CR as close as possible to the center of both joints.

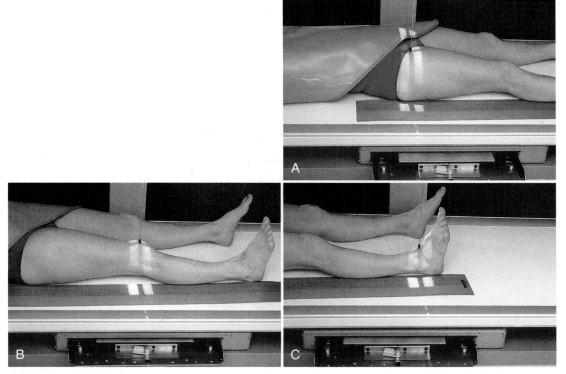

Fig. 7.176 Supine scanogram procedure. Three radiographs are taken. (A) The first is at the level of the hip joints; (B) the second is at the level of the knee joints; and (C) the third is at the level of the ankle joints.

Central ray

- Perpendicular to the center of the IR at the level of the joints for a bilateral procedure and through each joint space for a unilateral procedure.

Collimation

- Adjust the radiation field to 6 inches (15 cm) in length and to 1 inch (2.5 cm) beyond the lateral shadow of the hip, knee, or ankle.

Structures shown

Three images that include the special ruler, one of the hip joint(s), one of the knee joint(s), and one of the ankle joint(s) (Fig. 7.177).

The following should be clearly seen:

- Evidence of proper collimation and the presence of a side marker placed clear of the anatomy of interest
- Image of the special ruler
- Pertinent lower extremity anatomy on each image, including the hip joint, the knee joint, or the ankle joint
- Bony trabecular detail and surrounding soft tissues

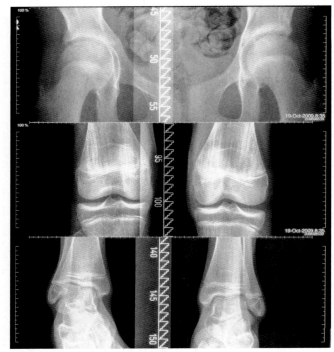

Fig. 7.177 Scanogram images. The three images include both joints at each level and the special ruler.

Lower Extremity

Other Long Bone Measurement Techniques

Although lower extremity long bone measurement procedures are commonly performed using DR or CR, large children's hospitals may perform these procedures using low-dose/microdose systems. An example of this type of equipment is seen in Fig. 7.178. This particular system uses two slit-beam x-ray sources and dual digital IRs to capture both PA/AP and lateral images simultaneously by scanning the selected portion of the body. Since these patients require multiple imaging procedures, the initial procedure can be done with a low dose exposure. Subsequent procedures are usually done with microdose exposures since detailed images are not required. The resulting image (Fig. 7.179) has only preliminary measurement lines because the image data set is registered in space, so the accompanying software allows the surgeon to create very precise measurements needed for surgical planning or follow-up.

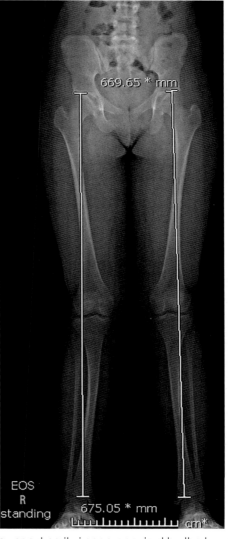

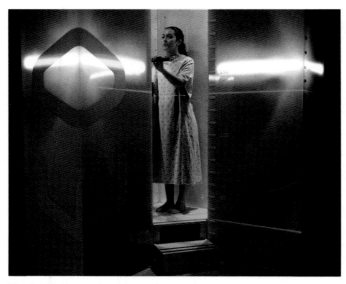

Fig. 7.178 The patient is positioned for a lower extremity long bone measurement procedure using a low-dose slit-scanning system. AP and lateral images are acquired simultaneously. The green laser lines define the area to be scanned.

Fig. 7.179 Lower extremity image acquired by the low-dose system from Fig. 7.178.

Helms and McCarthy[34] reported a method for using CT to measure discrepancies in leg length. Temme et al.[35] compared conventional orthoroentgenograms with CT scans for long bone measurements. Both sets of investigators concluded that the CT scanogram is more consistently reproduced and that it causes less radiation exposure to the patient than the conventional radiographic approach (Figs. 7.180 and 7.181).

The accuracy of the CT examination depends on proper placement of the cursor. Helms and McCarthy[34] found that accuracy improved when the cursors were placed three times and the values obtained were averaged. These authors also reported that CT examinations used radiation doses that were 50 to 200 times less than those used with conventional radiography, while Sabharwal and Kumar[31] reported the CT dose as 80% less than

that of orthoroentgenograms. CT examination requires about the same amount of time as conventional radiography, and the costs are comparable.[31]

Although uncommon, long bone measurement imaging is also performed on the upper extremities (Figs. 7.182 and 7.183).

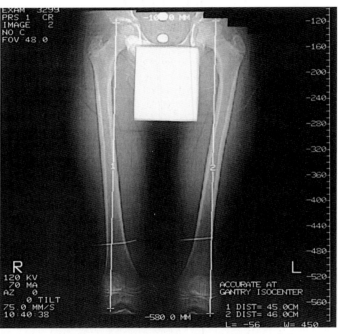

Fig. 7.180 CT measurement of femurs. The right femur is 1 cm shorter than the left femur.

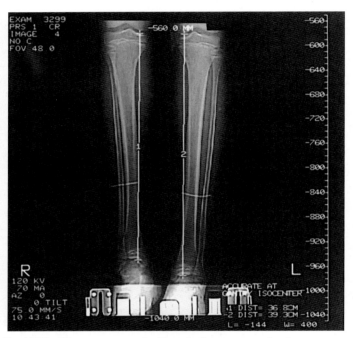

Fig. 7.181 CT measurement of legs in the same patient as Fig. 7.180.

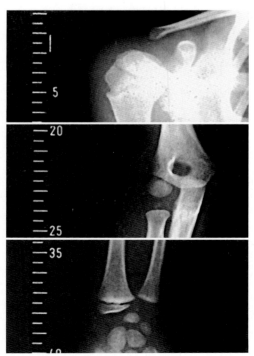

Fig. 7.182 Scanogram images of an upper extremity.

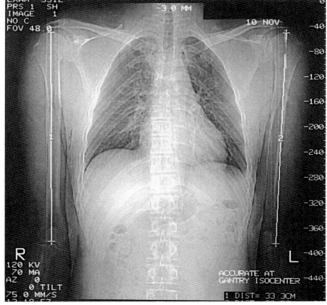

Fig. 7.183 CT measurement of arms.

References

1. Lewis RW: Nonroutine views in roentgen examination of the extremities, *Surg Gynecol Obstet* 67:38, 1938.
2. Holly EW: Radiography of the tarsal sesamoid bones, *Med Radiogr Photogr* 31:73, 1955.
3. Doub HP: A useful position for examining the foot, *Radiology* 16:764, 1931.
4. Kite JH: Principles involved in the treatment of congenital clubfoot, *J Bone Joint Surg* 21:595, 1939.
5. Kite JH: *The clubfoot*, New York, 1964, Grune & Stratton.
6. Davis LA, Hatt WS: Congenital abnormalities of the feet, *Radiology* 64:818, 1955.
7. Freiberger RH, et al: Roentgen examination of the deformed foot, *Semin Roentgenol* 5:341, 1970.
8. Conway JJ, Cowell HR: Tarsal coalition: clinical significance and roentgenographic demonstration, *Radiology* 92:799–811, 1969.
9. Kandel B: The suroplantar projection in the congenital clubfoot of the infant, *Acta Orthop Scand* 22:161–173, 1952.
10. Lilienfeld L: *Anordnung der normalisierten Röntgenaufnahmen des menschlichen Körpers*, ed 4, Berlin, 1927, Urban & Schwarzenberg.
11. Harris RI, Beath T: Etiology of peroneal spastic flat foot, *J Bone Joint Surg Br* 30:624–634, 1948.
12. Coventry MB: Flatfoot with special consideration of tarsal coalition, *Minn Med* 33:1091–1097, 1950.
13. Vaughan WH, Segal G: Tarsal coalition, with special reference to roentgenographic interpretation, *Radiology* 60:855–863, 1953.
14. Isherwood I: A radiological approach to the subtalar joint, *J Bone Joint Surg Br* 43:566, 1961.
15. Feist JH, Mankin HJ: The tarsus: basic relationships and motions in the adult and definition of optimal recumbent oblique projection, *Radiology* 79:250–263, 1962.
16. Ball RP, Egbert EW: Ruptured ligaments of the ankle, *AJR Am J Roentgenol* 50:770, 1943.
17. Frank ED, Kravetz NA, O'Neill DE, et al: Radiography of the ankle mortise, *Radiol Technol* 62:354–359, 1991.
18. Martensen KM: Alternate AP knee method assures open joint space, *Radiol Technol* 64:19–23, 1992.
19. Sheller S: Roentgenographic studies on epiphyseal growth and ossification in the knee, *Acta Radiol* 195:1–303, 1960.
20. Leach RE, Gregg T, Siber FJ: Weight-bearing radiography in osteoarthritis of the knee, *Radiology* 97:265–268, 1970.
21. Rosenberg TD, Paulos LE, Parker RD, et al: The forty-five degree posteroanterior flexion weight-bearing radiograph of the knee, *J Bone Joint Surg Am* 70:1479–1483, 1988.
22. Holmblad EC: Postero-anterior x-ray view of the knee in flexion, *JAMA* 109:1196, 1937.
23. Turner GW, Burns CB, Previtte RG, Jr: Erect positions for "tunnel" views of the knee, *Radiol Technol* 55:640–642, 1983.
24. Camp JD, Coventry MB: Use of special views in roentgenography of the knee joint, *US Naval Med Bull* 42:56, 1944.
25. Hughston JC: Subluxation of the patella, *J Bone Joint Surg Am* 50:1003–1026, 1968.
26. Kimberlin GE: Radiological assessment of the patellofemoral articulation and subluxation of the patella, *Radiol Technol* 45:129–137, 1973.
27. Laurin CA, Lévesque HP, Dussault R, et al: The abnormal lateral patellofemoral angle: a diagnostic roentgenographic sign of recurrent patellar subluxation, *J Bone Joint Surg Am* 60:55–60, 1968.
28. Fodor J, et al: Accurate radiography of the patellofemoral joint, *Radiol Technol* 53:570, 1982.
29. Merchant AC, Mercer RL, Jacobsen RH, et al: Roentgenographic analysis of patellofemoral congruence, *J Bone Joint Surg Am* 56:1391–1396, 1974.
30. Merchant AC: The Axial Viewer, Orthopedic Products, 2500 Hospital Dr., Bldg. 7, Mountain View, CA 94040.
31. Sabharwal S, Kumar A: Methods for assessing leg length discrepancy, *Clin Orthop Relat Res* 466:2910–2922, 2008.
32. Khakharia S, Bigman D, Fragomen AT, et al: Comparison of PACS and hard-copy 51-inch radiographs for measuring leg length and deformity, *Clin Orthop Relat Res* 469:244–250, 2011.
33. Doyle AJ, Winsor S: Magnetic resonance imaging (MRI) lower limb length measurement, *J Med Imaging Radiat Oncol* 55:191–194, 2011.
34. Helms CA, McCarthy S: CT scanograms for measuring leg length discrepancy, *Radiology* 151:802, 1984.
35. Temme JB, Chu WK, Anderson JC: CT scanograms compared with conventional orthoroentgenograms in long bone measurement, *Radiol Technol* 59:65–68, 1987.

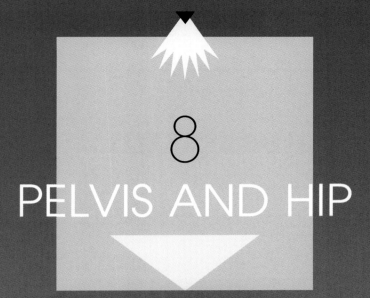

8

PELVIS AND HIP

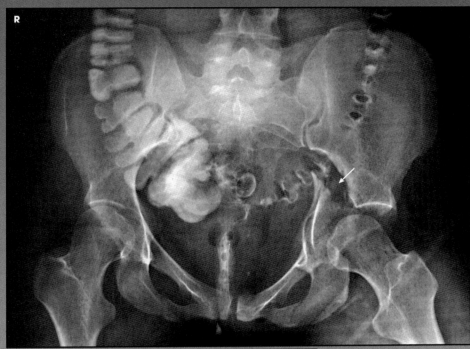

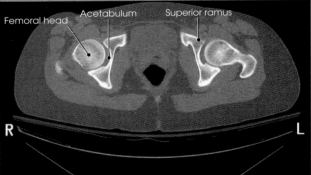

Femoral head · Acetabulum · Superior ramus

R · L

PROJECTIONS, POSITIONS, AND METHODS

Page	Essential	Anatomy	Projection	Position	Method
389	⚚	Pelvis and proximal femora	AP		
392		Pelvis and proximal femora	Lateral	R or L	
394	⚚	Femoral necks	AP oblique		MODIFIED CLEAVES
396		Femoral necks	Axiolateral		ORIGINAL CLEAVES
398	⚚	Hip	AP		
400	⚚	Hip	Lateral (mediolateral)		LAUENSTEIN, HICKEY
402	⚚	Hip	Axiolateral		DANELIUS-MILLER
404		Hip	Modified axiolateral		CLEMENTS-NAKAYAMA
406		Acetabulum	PA axial oblique	RAO or LAO	TEUFEL
408	⚚	Acetabulum	AP oblique	RPO or LPO	JUDET, MODIFIED JUDET
410		Anterior pelvic bones	AP axial (outlet)		TAYLOR
412		Anterior pelvic bones	Superoinferior axial (inlet)		BRIDGEMAN
413		Ilium	AP and PA oblique	RPO and LPO, RAO and LAO	

The icons in the Essential column indicate projections frequently performed in the United States and Canada. Students should become competent in these projections.
AP, Anteroposterior; *L*, left; *LAO*, left anterior oblique; *LPO*, left posterior oblique; *PA*, posteroanterior; *R*, right; *RAO*, right anterior oblique; *RPO*, right posterior oblique.

The *pelvis* serves as a base for the trunk and a girdle for the attachment of the lower limbs. The pelvis consists of four bones: two *hip bones,* the *sacrum,* and the *coccyx.* The *pelvic girdle* is composed of only the two hip bones.

Hip Bone

The *hip bone* is often referred to as the *os coxae,* and some textbooks continue to refer to it as the *innominate bone.* The most widely used term is *hip bone* (Figs. 8.1 and 8.2).

The hip bone consists of the *ilium, pubis,* and *ischium* (Fig. 8.3A). These three bones join together to form the *acetabulum,* the cup-shaped socket that receives the head of the femur. The ilium, pubis, and ischium are separated by cartilage in children but become fused into one bone in adults.

The hip bone is divided further into two distinct areas: the *iliopubic column* and the *ilioischial column* (see Fig. 8.3B). These columns are used to identify fractures around the acetabulum.

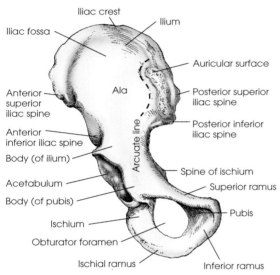

Fig. 8.1 Anterior aspect of right hip bone.

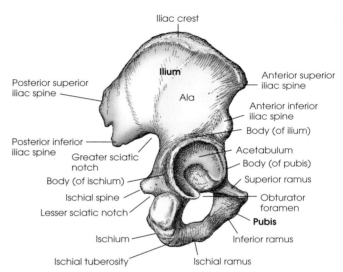

Fig. 8.2 Lateral aspect of right hip bone.

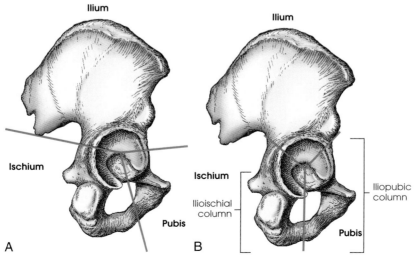

Fig. 8.3 (A) Lateral aspect of right hip bone showing its three parts. (B) Lateral aspect of hip bone showing ilioischial and iliopubic columns.

ILIUM

The *ilium* consists of a *body* and a broad, curved portion called the *ala*. The body of the ilium forms approximately two-fifths of the acetabulum superiorly (see Figs. 8.1 and 8.2). The ala projects superiorly from the body to form the prominence of the hip. The ala has three borders: anterior, posterior, and superior. The anterior and posterior borders present four prominent projections:

- Anterior superior iliac spine (ASIS)
- Anterior inferior iliac spine
- Posterior superior iliac spine
- Posterior inferior iliac spine

The *ASIS* is an important and frequently used radiographic positioning reference point. The superior margin extending from the ASIS to the posterior superior iliac spine is called the *iliac crest*. The medial surface of the wing contains the *iliac fossa* and is separated from the body of the bone by a smooth, arc-shaped ridge—the *arcuate line*—which forms part of the circumference of the pelvic brim. The arcuate line passes obliquely, inferiorly, and medially to its junction with the pubis. The inferior and posterior portions of the wing present a large, rough surface—the *auricular surface*—for articulation with the sacrum. This articular surface and the articular surface of the adjacent sacrum have irregular elevations and depressions that cause a partial interlock of the two bones. The ilium curves inward below this surface, forming the *greater sciatic notch*.

PUBIS

The *pubis* consists of a *body,* the *superior ramus,* and the *inferior ramus*. The body of the pubis forms approximately one-fifth of the acetabulum anteriorly (see Figs. 8.1 and 8.2). The superior ramus projects inferiorly and medially from the acetabulum to the midline of the body. There the bone curves inferiorly and then posteriorly and laterally to join the ischium. The lower prong is termed the *inferior ramus*.

ISCHIUM

The *ischium* consists of a *body* and the *ischial ramus*. The body of the ischium forms approximately two-fifths of the acetabulum posteriorly (see Figs. 8.1 and 8.2). It projects posteriorly and inferiorly from the acetabulum to form an expanded portion called the *ischial tuberosity*. When the body is in a seated or upright position, its weight rests on the two ischial tuberosities. The ischial ramus projects anteriorly and medially from the tuberosity to its junction with the inferior ramus of the pubis. By this posterior union, the rami of the pubis and ischium enclose the *obturator foramen*. At the superoposterior border of the body is a prominent projection called the *ischial spine*. An indentation, the *lesser sciatic notch,* is just below the ischial spine.

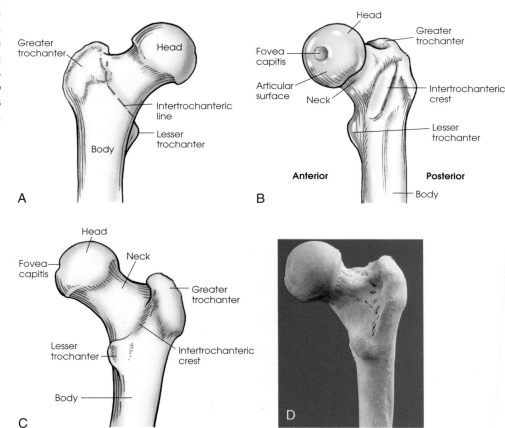

Fig. 8.4 Proximal right femur. (A) Anterior aspect. (B) Medial aspect. The body is positioned 15 to 20 degrees posterior from the head. (C) Posterior aspect. (D) Posterior aspect of right proximal human femur. Note anatomic details and compare with C.

Proximal Femur

The *femur* is the longest, strongest, and heaviest bone in the body. The proximal end of the femur consists of a *head,* a *neck,* and two large processes—the *greater* and *lesser trochanters* (Fig. 8.4). The smooth, rounded head is connected to the femoral body by a pyramid-shaped neck and is received into the acetabular cavity of the hip bone. A small depression at the center of the head, the *fovea capitis,* attaches to the ligamentum capitis femoris (Fig. 8.5; also see Fig. 8.4). The neck is constricted near the head but expands to a broad base at the *body* of the bone. The neck projects medially, superiorly, and anteriorly from the body. The trochanters are situated at the junction of the body and the base of the neck. The greater trochanter is at the superolateral part of the femoral body, and the lesser trochanter is at the posteromedial part. The prominent ridge extending between the trochanters at the base of the neck on the posterior surface of the body is called the *intertrochanteric crest.* The less prominent ridge connecting the trochanters anteriorly is called the *intertrochanteric line.* The femoral neck and the intertrochanteric crest are two common sites of fracture in elderly adults. The superior portion of the greater trochanter projects above the neck and curves slightly posteriorly and medially.

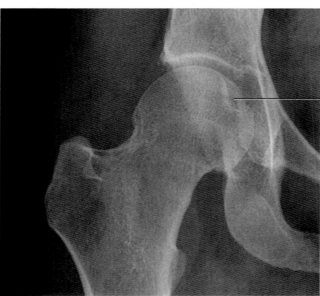

Fovea capitis

Fig. 8.5 Hip joint. AP hip demonstrating the fovea capitis.

The angulation of the neck of the femur varies considerably with age, sex, and stature. In the average adult, the neck projects anteriorly from the body at an angle of approximately 15 to 20 degrees and superiorly at an angle of approximately 120 to 130 degrees to the long axis of the femoral body (Fig. 8.6). The longitudinal plane of the femur is angled about 10 degrees from vertical. In children, the latter angle is wider—that is, the neck is more vertical in position. In wide pelves, the angle is narrower, placing the neck in a more horizontal position.

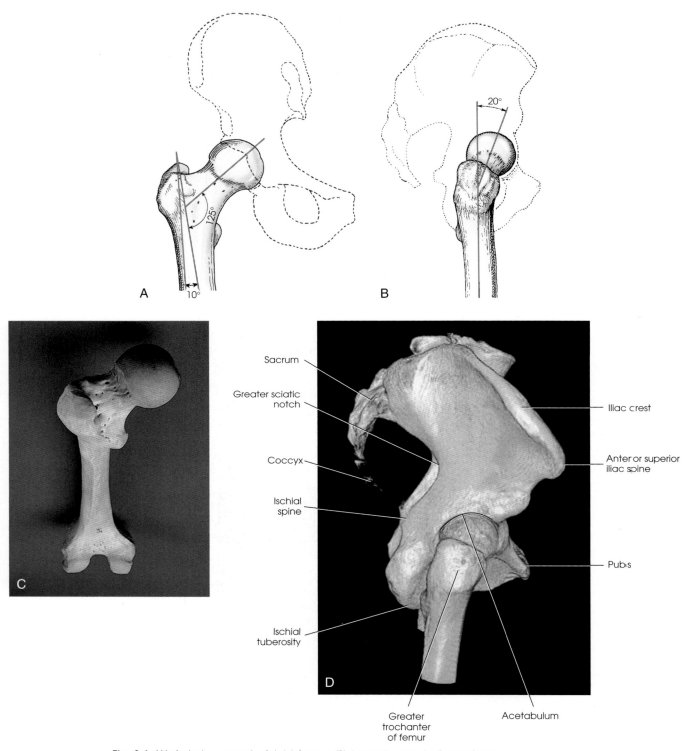

Fig. 8.6 (A) Anterior aspect of right femur. (B) Lateral aspect of right femur. (C) Superoinferior view of posterior aspect of a human femur showing 15- to 20-degree anterior angle of femoral neck. (D) Three-dimensional CT scan of lateral hip bone and proximal femur.

Articulations of the Pelvis

Table 8.1 and Fig. 8.7 provide a summary of the three joints of the pelvis and upper femora. The articulation between the acetabulum and the head of the femur (the hip joint) is a *synovial ball-and-socket* joint that permits free movement in all directions. The knee and ankle joints are hinge joints; the wide range of motion of the lower limb depends on the ball-and-socket joint of the hip. Because the knee and ankle joints are hinge joints, medial and lateral rotations of the foot cause rotation of the entire limb, which is centered at the hip joint.

The pubes of the hip bones articulate with each other at the anterior midline of the body, forming a joint called the *pubic symphysis*. The pubic symphysis is a *cartilaginous symphysis* joint.

The right and left ilia articulate with the sacrum posteriorly at the *sacroiliac* (SI) joints. These two joints angle 25 to 30 degrees relative to the midsagittal plane (MSP) (see Fig. 8.7B). The SI articulations are *synovial irregular gliding* joints. Because the bones of the SI joints interlock, movement is limited or nonexistent.

TABLE 8.1

Joints of the pelvis and upper femora

| Joint | Structural classification | | Movement |
	Tissue	Type	
Hip joint	Synovial	Ball and socket	Freely movable
Pubic symphysis	Cartilaginous	Symphysis	Slightly movable
Sacroiliac	Synovial	Irregular gliding[a]	Slightly movable

[a]Some anatomists term this a synovial fibrous joint.

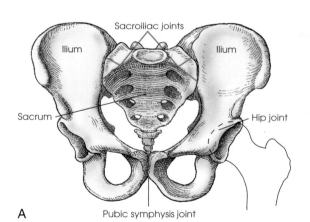

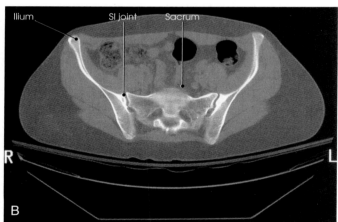

Fig. 8.7 (A) Joints of pelvis and upper femora. (B) Axial CT image of pelvis showing SI joints. Note 25- to 30-degree angulation of joint.

(B, Modified from Kelley L, Petersen CM: *Sectional anatomy for imaging professionals*, ed 2, St Louis, 2007, Mosby.)

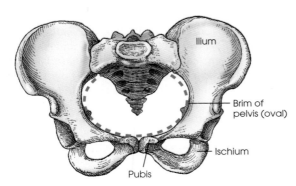

Ilium

Brim of
pelvis (oval)

Ischium

Pubis

Fig. 8.8 Female pelvis.

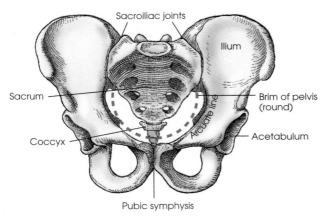

Sacroiliac joints

Ilium

Sacrum

Brim of pelvis
(round)

Arcuate line

Coccyx

Acetabulum

Pubic symphysis

Fig. 8.9 Male pelvis.

Pelvis

The female pelvis (Fig. 8.8) is lighter in structure than the male pelvis (Fig. 8.9). It is wider and shallower, and the inlet is larger and more oval in shape. The sacrum is wider; it curves more sharply posteriorly and the sacral promontory is flatter. The width and depth of the pelvis vary with stature and gender (Table 8.2). The female pelvis is shaped for childbearing and delivery.

The pelvis is divided into two portions by an oblique plane that extends from the upper anterior margin of the sacrum to the upper margin of the pubic symphysis. The boundary line of this plane is called the *brim of the pelvis* (see Figs. 8.8 and 8.9). The region above the brim is called the *false* or *greater pelvis,* and the region below the brim is called the *true* or *lesser pelvis.*

The brim forms the *superior aperture,* or *inlet,* of the true pelvis. The *inferior aperture,* or *outlet,* of the true pelvis is measured from the tip of the coccyx to the inferior margin of the pubic symphysis in the AP direction and between the ischial tuberosities in the horizontal direction. The region between the inlet and the outlet is called the *pelvic cavity* (Fig. 8.10).

When the body is in the upright or seated position, the brim of the pelvis forms an angle of approximately 60 degrees to the horizontal plane. This angle varies with other body positions; the degree and direction of the variation depend on the lumbar and sacral curves.

TABLE 8.2
Female and male pelvis characteristics

Feature	Female	Male
Shape	Wide, shallow	Narrow, deep
Bony structure	Light	Heavy
Superior aperture (inlet)	Oval	Round
Inferior aperture (outlet)	Wide	Narrow

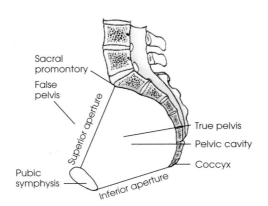

Sacral
promontory

False
pelvis

Superior aperture

True pelvis

Pelvic cavity

Coccyx

Pubic
symphysis

Inferior aperture

Fig. 8.10 Midsagittal section showing inlet and outlet of true pelvis.

Localizing Anatomic Structures

The bony landmarks used in radiography of the pelvis and hips are as follows:
- Iliac crest
- ASIS
- Pubic symphysis
- Greater trochanter of the femur
- Ischial tuberosity
- Tip of the coccyx

Most of these points are palpable, even in hypersthenic patients (Fig. 8.11). The highest point of the iliac crest, located on the posterior aspect of the ilium, may be more difficult to locate in heavily muscled patients. To avoid positioning errors, this structure may be more easily palpated while the patient breathes out because the abdominal muscles will then be relaxed.

The highest point of the greater trochanter, which can be palpated immediately below the depression in the soft tissues of the lateral surface of the hip, is in approximately the same horizontal plane as the midpoint of the hip joint and the coccyx. The most prominent point of the greater trochanter is in the same horizontal plane as the pubic symphysis (see Fig. 8.11).

The greater trochanter is most prominent laterally and more easily palpated when the lower leg is medially rotated. When properly used, medial rotation assists in localization of hip and pelvis centering points and avoids foreshortening of the femoral neck during radiography. Improper rotation of the lower

leg can rotate the pelvis. Consequently, positioning of the lower leg is important in radiographing the hip and pelvis. Traumatic injuries or pathologic conditions of the pelvis or lower limb may rule out the possibility of medial rotation.

The pubic symphysis can be palpated on the midsagittal plane and on the same horizontal plane as the greater trochanters. By placing the fingertips at this location and performing a brief downward palpation with the hand flat, palm down, and fingers together, the radiographer can locate the superior margin of the pubic symphysis. *To avoid possible embarrassment or misunderstanding, the radiographer should advise the patient in advance that this and other palpations of pelvic landmarks are part of normal procedure and necessary for an accurate examination.* When performed in an efficient and professional manner with respect for the patient's condition, such palpations are generally well tolerated.

The hip joint can be located by palpating the ASIS and the superior margin of the pubic symphysis (Fig. 8.12). The midpoint of a line drawn between these two points is directly above the center of the dome of the acetabular cavity. A line drawn at right angles to the midpoint of the first line lies parallel to the long axis of the femoral neck of an average adult in the anatomic position. The femoral head lies 1.5 inches (3.8 cm) distal, and the femoral neck is 2.5 inches (6.3 cm) distal to this midpoint.

For accurate localization of the femoral neck in atypical patients or in patients in whom the limb is not in the anatomic position, a line is drawn between the ASIS and the superior margin of the pubic symphysis; a second line is then drawn from a point 1 inch (2.5 cm) inferior to the greater trochanter to the midpoint of the previously marked line. The femoral head and neck lie along this line (see Fig. 8.12A).

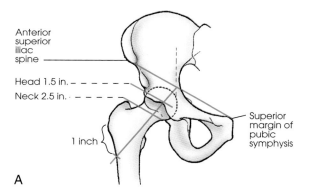

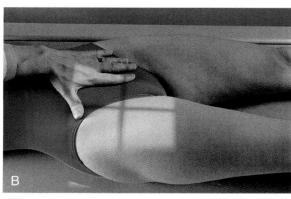

Anterior superior iliac spine

Head 1.5 in.

Neck 2.5 in.

1 inch

Superior margin of pubic symphysis

A

B

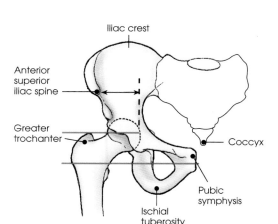

Iliac crest

Anterior superior iliac spine

Greater trochanter

Ischial tuberosity

Pubic symphysis

Coccyx

Fig. 8.11 Bony landmarks and localization planes of pelvis.

Fig. 8.12 (A) Method of localizing right hip joint and long axis of femoral neck. (B) Suggested method of localizing right hip. Left thumb is on the ASIS, and second finger is on superior margin of the pubic symphysis. Central ray is positioned 1.5 inches distal to center of line drawn between the ASIS and pubic symphysis.

ALTERNATIVE POSITIONING LANDMARK

In many radiology departments, it is no longer considered appropriate practice for a radiographer to palpate the pubic bone as a landmark for location of anatomy during radiographic positioning. Bello[1] described an alternative positioning landmark for the pelvis and hip—which can be generalized for radiography of any body part—recommending use of the pubic symphysis as a positioning landmark. His research determined that the distance from the ASIS to the superior aspect of the pubic symphysis ranges from 2.5 to 3.5 inches (6.3 to 8.8 cm), with an average of 3.0 inches (7.5 cm). He also found the same distance from the superior margin of the iliac crest to the ASIS—average 3.0 inches (7.5 cm). However, this article was not published through the peer-review process and the sample size was small, so the *Atlas* authors cannot advocate use of these measurements without support of more formal research and peer-reviewed publication.

SUMMARY OF ANATOMY			
Pelvis	Anterior superior iliac spine (ASIS)	**Ischium**	Intertrochanteric crest
Hip bones (two)	Anterior inferior iliac spine	Body	Intertrochanteric line
Sacrum	Posterior superior iliac spine	Ischial ramus	
Coccyx	Posterior inferior iliac spine	Ischial tuberosity	**Articulations**
Pelvic girdle	Iliac crest	Obturator foramen	Hip
	Iliac fossa	Ischial spine	Pubic symphysis
Hip bone	Arcuate line	Lesser sciatic notch	Sacroiliac joints
Ilium	Auricular surface	Ilioischial column	
Pubis	Greater sciatic notch		**Pelvis**
Ischium		**Femur (proximal aspect)**	Brim of the pelvis
Acetabulum	**Pubis**	Head	Greater or false pelvis
	Body	Neck	Lesser or true pelvis
Ilium	Superior ramus	Body	Superior aperture or inlet
Body	Inferior ramus	Fovea capitis	Inferior aperture or outlet
Ala	Iliopubic column	Greater trochanter	Pelvic cavity
Superior spine		Lesser trochanter	Intertrochanteric crest
Inferior spine			Intertrochanteric line

ABBREVIATIONS USED IN CHAPTER 8	
ASIS	Anterior superior iliac spine
MCP	Midcoronal plane
MSP	Midsagittal plane
SI	Sacroiliac

See Addendum A for a summary of all abbreviations used in Volume 1.

SUMMARY OF PATHOLOGY

Condition	Definition
Ankylosing spondylitis	Rheumatoid arthritis variant involving the SI joints and spine
Congenital hip dysplasia	Malformation of the acetabulum causing displacement of the femoral head
Dislocation	Displacement of a bone from the joint space
Fracture	Disruption in the continuity of bone
Legg-Calvé-Perthes disease	Flattening of the femoral head due to vascular interruption
Metastasis	Transfer of a cancerous lesion from one area to another
Osteoarthritis or degenerative joint disease	Form of arthritis marked by progressive cartilage deterioration in synovial joints and vertebrae
Osteopetrosis	Increased density of atypically soft bone
Osteoporosis	Loss of bone density
Paget disease	Thick, soft bone marked by bowing and fractures
Slipped epiphysis	Proximal portion of femur dislocated from distal portion at the proximal epiphysis
Tumor	New tissue growth where cell proliferation is uncontrolled
Chondrosarcoma	Malignant tumor arising from cartilage cells
Multiple myeloma	Malignant neoplasm of plasma cells involving the bone marrow and causing destruction of the bone

Eponymous (named) pathologies are listed in nonpossessive form to conform to the AMA manual of style: a guide for authors and editors, ed 10, Oxford, 2009, Oxford University Press.

SAMPLE EXPOSURE TECHNIQUE CHART ESSENTIAL PROJECTIONS

These techniques were accurate for the equipment used to produce each exposure. However, use caution in applying them in your department because "there is considerable variability in image receptor response owing to varying scatter sensitivity, the use of grids with different grid ratios, collimation, beam filtration, the choice of kilovoltage, source-to-image distance, and image receptor size." Generator output characteristics and IR energy sensitivities vary widely.[1]

This chart was created in collaboration with Dennis Bowman, AS, RT(R), Clinical Instructor, Community Hospital of the Monterey Peninsula, Monterey, CA. http://digitalradiographysolutions.com/.

PELVIS AND PROXIMAL FEMORA

Part	cm	kVp[a]	SID[b]	Collimation	CR[c] mAs	CR[c] Dose (mGy)[e]	DR[d] mAs	DR[d] Dose (mGy)[e]
Pelvis and proximal femora—AP[f]	19	85	40″	17″ × 14″ (43 × 35 cm)	25[g]	3.620	12.5[g]	1.805
Femoral necks—AP oblique[f]	19	85	40″	17″ × 10″ (43 × 25 cm)	28[g]	3.960	14[g]	1.977
Hip—AP[f]	18	85	40″	8″ × 12″ (20 × 30 cm)	20[g]	2.740	10[g]	1.367
Hip—lateral (Lauenstein-Hickey)[f]	18	85	40″	10″ × 8″ (25 × 20 cm)	18[g]	2.430	9[g]	1.206
Hip—axiolateral (Danelius-Miller)[f]	24	90	40″	12″ × 8″ (30 × 20 cm)	71[g]	12.48	32[g]	5.600

[1]ACR-AAPM-SIMM Practice Parameter for Digital Radiography, Revised 2017.
[a]kVp values are for a high-frequency generator.
[b]40- inch minimum; 44 to 48 inches recommended to improve spatial resolution (mAs increase needed, but no increase in patient dose will result).
[c]AGFA CR MD 4.0 General IP, CR 75.0 reader, 400 speed class, with 6:1 (178LPI) grid when needed.
[d]GE Definium 8000, with 13:1 grid when needed.
[e]All doses are skin entrance for average adult (160- to 200-lb male, 150- to 190-lb female) at part thickness indicated.
[f]Bucky/Grid.
[g]Large focal spot.

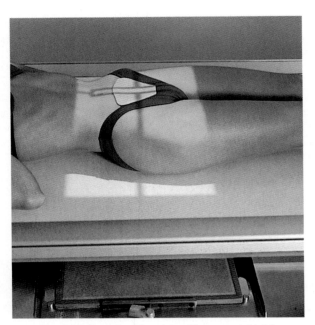

Fig. 8.13 Female AP pelvis with gonad shield.

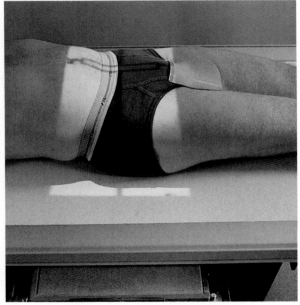

Fig. 8.14 Male AP pelvis with gonad shield.

Radiation Protection

Protection of the patient from unnecessary radiation is a professional responsibility of the radiographer (see Chapter 1 for specific guidelines). In this chapter, the *Shield gonads* statement at the end of the *Position of part* section indicates that the patient is to be protected from unnecessary radiation by restricting the radiation beam through the use of proper collimation. In addition, placing lead shielding between the gonads and the radiation source is appropriate when the clinical objectives of the examination are not compromised (Figs. 8.13 and 8.14).[2]

♣ AP PROJECTION

Image receptor + grid: Positioned by manufacturer or department protocol for proper anatomy display orientation; CR plate 14 × 17 inches (35 × 43 cm) crosswise.

Position of patient
- Place the patient on the table in the supine position.

Position of part
- Center the MSP of the body to the midline of the grid and adjust it in a true supine position.
- Unless contraindicated because of trauma or pathologic factors, medially rotate the feet and lower limbs about 15 to 20 degrees to place the femoral necks parallel with the plane of the image receptor (IR) (Figs. 8.15 and 8.16).

Medial rotation is easier for the patient to maintain if the knees are supported. The heels should be placed about 8 to 10 inches (20 to 24 cm) apart.
- Immobilize the legs with a sandbag across the ankles if necessary.
- Check the distance from the ASIS to the tabletop on each side to ensure that the pelvis is not rotated.

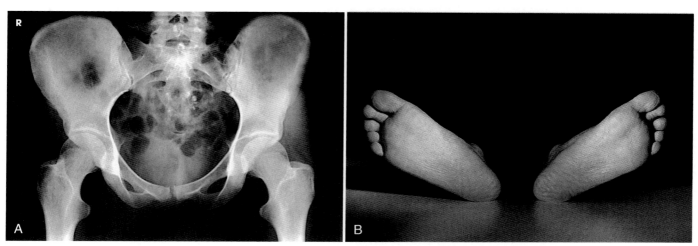

Fig. 8.15 (A) AP pelvis with femoral necks and trochanters poorly positioned because of lateral rotation of limbs. (B) Feet and lower limbs in natural, laterally rotated tabletop position, causing poor profile of proximal femora in A.

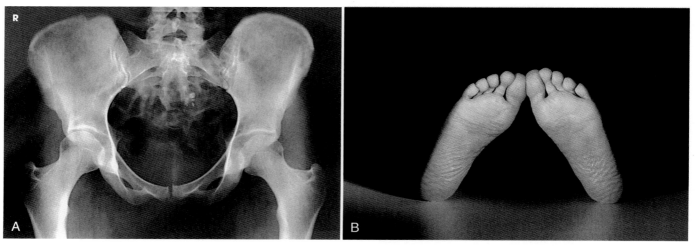

Fig. 8.16 (A) AP pelvis with femoral necks and trochanters in correct position. (B) Feet and lower limbs medially rotated 15 to 20 degrees, correctly placed with upper femora in correct profile in (A).

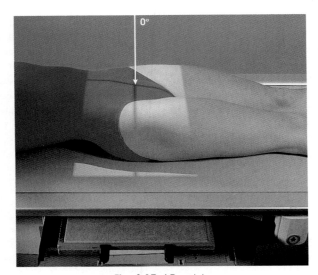

Fig. 8.17 AP pelvis.

- Center the IR at the level of the soft tissue depression just above the palpable prominence of the greater trochanter (approximately 1.5 inches [3.8 cm]), which is also midway between the ASIS and the pubic symphysis. In average-sized patients, the center of the IR is about 2 inches (5 cm) inferior to the ASIS and 2 inches (5 cm) superior to the pubic symphysis (Fig. 8.17).
- If the pelvis is deep, palpate for the iliac crest and adjust the position of the IR so that its upper border projects 1 to 1 1/2 inches (2.5 to 3.8 cm) above the crest.
- *Shield gonads.*
- *Respiration:* Suspend.

Central ray

- Perpendicular to the midpoint of the IR.

Collimation

- Adjust radiation field to 14 × 17 inches (35 × 43 cm) on the collimator. For smaller patients, collimate 1 inch (2.5 cm) beyond the skin shadow on the sides. Place side marker in the collimated exposure field.

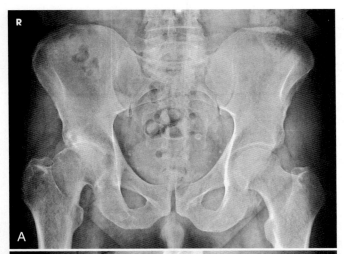

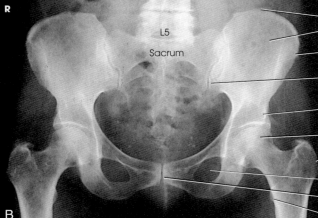

Iliac crest
Ala
L5
Anterior superior iliac spine
Sacrum
Sacroiliac joint
Anterior inferior iliac spine
Femoral head
Greater trochanter
Obturator foramen
Pubic symphysis
Lesser trochanter

Fig. 8.18 (A) Male AP pelvis. (B) Female AP pelvis.

Structures shown

An AP projection of the pelvis and of the head, neck, trochanters, and proximal one-third or one-fourth of the shaft of the femora (Fig. 8.18).

EVALUATION CRITERIA

The following should be clearly seen:

- Evidence of proper collimation and presence of side marker placed clear of anatomy of interest
- Entire pelvis and proximal femora
- Both ilia and greater trochanters equidistant from the edge of the radiograph
- Lower vertebral column centered to the middle of the radiograph
- No rotation of pelvis
  - Symmetric ilia
  - Symmetric obturator foramina
  - Ischial spines equally seen
  - Sacrum and coccyx aligned with the pubic symphysis
- Proper rotation of proximal femora
  - Femoral necks in their full extent without superimposition
  - Greater trochanters in profile
  - Lesser trochanters, if seen, visible on the medial border of the femora
- Bony trabecular detail and surrounding soft tissues

Congenital dislocation of the hip

Martz and Taylor[3] recommended two AP projections of the pelvis to show the relationship of the femoral head to the acetabulum in patients with congenital dislocation of the hip. The first projection is obtained with the central ray directed perpendicular to the pubic symphysis to detect any lateral or superior displacement of the femoral head. The second projection is obtained with the central ray directed to the pubic symphysis at a cephalic angulation of 45 degrees (Fig. 8.19). This angulation casts the shadow of an anteriorly displaced femoral head above that of the acetabulum and the shadow of a posteriorly displaced head below that of the acetabulum.

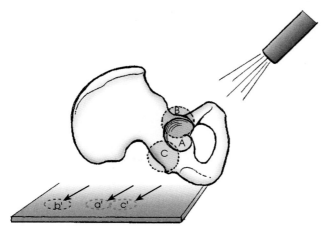

Fig. 8.19 Special projection taken for congenital dislocation of hip.

LATERAL PROJECTION
Right or left position

Image receptor + grid: Positioned by manufacturer or department protocol for proper anatomy display orientation; CR plate 14 × 17 inches (35 × 43 cm) lengthwise.

Position of patient
- Place the patient in the lateral recumbent, dorsal decubitus, or upright position.

Position of part
Recumbent position
- When the patient can be placed in the lateral position, center the midcoronal plane (MCP) of the body to the midline of the grid.
- Extend the thighs enough to prevent the femora from obscuring the pubic arch.
- Place a support under the lumbar spine and adjust it to place the vertebral column parallel with the tabletop (Fig. 8.20). If the vertebral column is allowed to sag, it tilts the pelvis in the longitudinal plane.
- Adjust the pelvis in a true lateral position, with the ASIS lying in the same vertical plane.
- Place one knee directly over the other knee. A pillow or other support between the knees promotes stabilization and patient comfort.
- Berkebile et al.[4] recommended a dorsal decubitus lateral projection of the pelvis to show the "gull wing" sign in cases of fracture-dislocation of the acetabular rim and posterior dislocation of the femoral head.

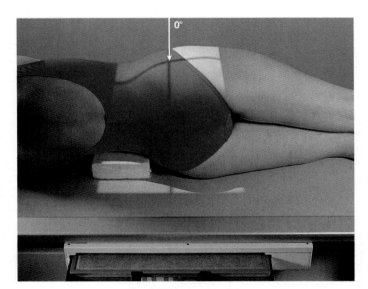

Fig. 8.20 Lateral pelvis.

Upright position

- Place the patient in the lateral position in front of a vertical grid device, and center the MCP of the body to the midline of the grid.
- Have the patient stand straight, with the weight of the body equally distributed on the feet, so that the MSP is parallel with the plane of the IR.
- If the limbs are of unequal length, place a support of suitable height under the foot of the shorter side.
- Have the patient grasp the side of the stand for support.
- *Shield gonads.*
- *Respiration:* Suspend.

Central ray

- Perpendicular to a point centered at the level of the soft tissue depression just above the palpable prominence of the greater trochanter (approximately 2 inches [5 cm]) and to the midpoint of the IR.
- Center the IR to the central ray.

Collimation

- Adjust radiation field to 14 × 17 inches (35 × 43 cm). Place side marker in the collimated exposure field.

Structures shown

A lateral radiograph of the lumbosacral junction, sacrum, coccyx, and superimposed hip bones and upper femora (Fig. 8.21).

The following should be clearly seen:

- Evidence of proper collimation and presence of side marker placed clear of anatomy of interest
- Entire pelvis and the proximal femora
- Sacrum and coccyx
- Pelvis in true lateral position without rotation
  - ☐ Superimposed posterior margins of the ischium and ilium
  - ☐ Superimposed femora
  - ☐ Superimposed acetabular shadows (The larger circle of the fossa [farther from the IR] is equidistant from the smaller circle of the fossa nearer the IR throughout their circumference.)
- Pubic arch unobscured by the femora
- Bony trabecular detail and surrounding soft tissues

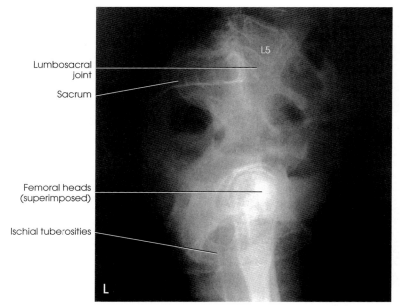

Lumbosacral joint

Sacrum

Femoral heads (superimposed)

Ischial tuberosities

L5

L

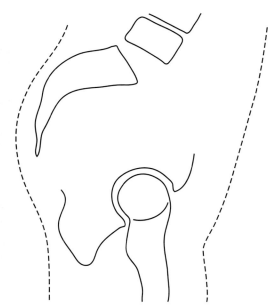

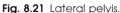

Fig. 8.21 Lateral pelvis.

♠ AP OBLIQUE PROJECTION
MODIFIED CLEAVES METHOD

Image receptor + grid: Positioned by manufacturer or department protocol for proper anatomy display orientation; CR plate: 14 × 17 inches (35 × 43 cm) crosswise.

This projection is often called the bilateral *frog-leg* position.

NOTE: This examination is contraindicated for a patient suspected to have a fracture or other pathologic disease.

Position of patient
• Place the patient in the supine position.

Position of part
• Center the MSP of the body to the midline of the grid.
• Flex the patient's elbows, and rest the hands on the upper chest.
• Adjust the patient so that the pelvis is not rotated. This position can be achieved by placing the two ASISs equidistant from the radiographic table.
• Place a compression band across the patient well above the hip joints for stability if necessary.

Bilateral projection
Step 1
• Have the patient flex the hips and knees and draw the feet up as much as possible (i.e., enough to place the femora in a nearly vertical position if the affected side permits).
• Instruct the patient to hold this position, which is relatively comfortable, while the x-ray tube and IR are adjusted.

Step 2
• Center the IR 1 inch (2.5 cm) superior to the pubic symphysis.

Step 3
• Abduct the thighs as much as possible and have the patient turn the feet inward to brace the soles against each other for support. According to Cleaves, the angle may vary between 25 and 45 degrees, depending on how vertically the femora can be placed.
• Center the feet to the midline of the grid (Fig. 8.22).
• If possible, abduct the thighs approximately 45 degrees from the vertical plane to place the long axes of the femoral necks parallel with the plane of the IR.
• Check the position of the thighs, being careful to abduct them to the same degree.

Unilateral projection
• Adjust the body position to center the ASIS of the affected side to the midline of the grid.
• Have the patient flex the hip and knee of the affected side and draw the foot up to the opposite knee as much as possible.
• After adjusting the perpendicular central ray and positioning the IR tray, have the patient brace the sole of the foot against the opposite knee and abduct the thigh laterally approximately 45 degrees (Fig. 8.23). The pelvis may rotate slightly.
• *Shield gonads.*
• *Respiration:* Suspend.

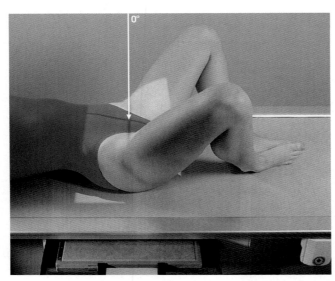

Fig. 8.22 AP oblique femoral necks with perpendicular central ray: modified Cleaves method.

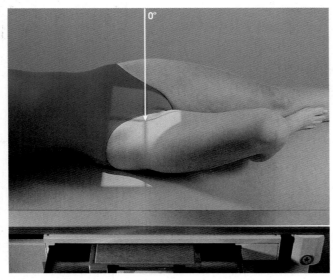

Fig. 8.23 Unilateral AP oblique femoral neck: modified Cleaves method.

Central ray

- Perpendicular to enter the patient's MSP at the level 1 inch (2.5 cm) superior to the pubic symphysis. May center lower to include more of the femur. For the unilateral position, direct the central ray to the femoral neck (see Fig. 8.12).

Collimation

Adjust radiation field to 14 × 17 inches (35 × 43 cm) on the collimator. For smaller patients, collimate 1 inch (2.5 cm) beyond the skin shadow on the sides. Place side marker in the collimated exposure field.

Structures shown

The bilateral image shows an AP oblique projection of the femoral heads, necks, and trochanteric areas onto one radiograph for comparison (Figs. 8.24 through 8.26).

EVALUATION CRITERIA

The following should be clearly seen:

- Evidence of proper collimation and presence of side marker placed clear of anatomy of interest
- No rotation of the pelvis, as demonstrated by a symmetric appearance
- Acetabulum, femoral head, and femoral neck
- Lesser trochanter on the medial side of the femur
- Femoral neck without superimposition by the greater trochanter; excess abduction causes the greater trochanter to obstruct the neck
- Femoral axes extended from the hip bones at equal angles
- Bony trabecular detail and surrounding soft tissues

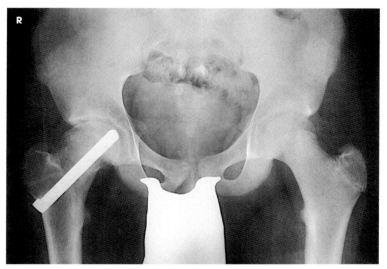

Fig. 8.24 AP femoral necks. Note fixation device in right hip and male gonad shield.

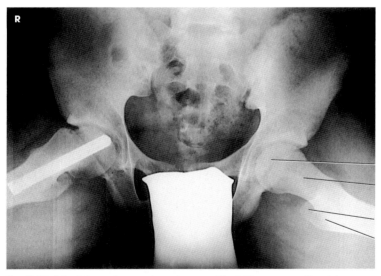

Femoral head
Femoral neck
Greater trochanter
Lesser trochanter

Fig. 8.25 AP oblique femoral necks: modified Cleaves method (same patient as in Fig. 8.24).

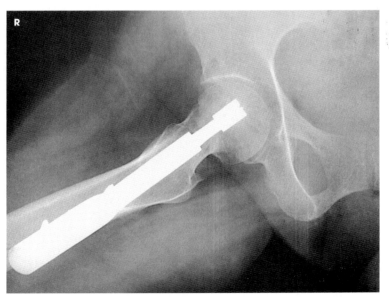

Fig. 8.26 AP oblique femoral neck: modified Cleaves method.

AXIOLATERAL PROJECTION
ORIGINAL CLEAVES METHOD[5]

NOTE: This examination is contraindicated for patients with suspected fracture or pathologic condition.

Image receptor + grid: Positioned by manufacturer or department protocol for proper anatomy display orientation; CR plate: 14 × 17 inches (35 × 43 cm) crosswise.

Position of patient
• Place the patient in the supine position.

Position of part

NOTE: This is the same part position as the modified Cleaves method previously described. The projection can be performed unilaterally or bilaterally.

• Before having the patient abduct the thighs (described in step 3 on p. 394), direct the x-ray tube parallel to the long axes of the femoral shafts (Fig. 8.27).
• Adjust the IR so that the midpoint coincides with the central ray.
• *Shield gonads.*
• *Respiration:* Suspend.

Central ray
• Parallel with the femoral shafts. According to Cleaves,[5] the angle may vary between 25 and 45 degrees, depending on how vertically the femora can be placed.

Collimation
• Adjust radiation field to 14 × 17 inches (35 × 43 cm) on the collimator. For smaller patients, collimate 1 inch (2.5 cm) beyond the skin shadow on the sides. Place side marker in the collimated exposure field.

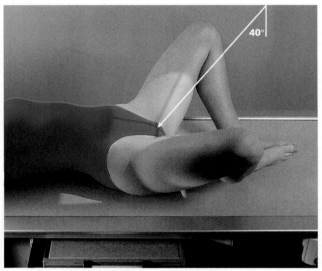

Fig. 8.27 Axiolateral femoral necks: Cleaves method.

Structures shown

An axiolateral projection of the femoral heads, necks, and trochanteric areas (Fig. 8.28).

EVALUATION CRITERIA

The following should be clearly seen:

- Evidence of proper collimation and presence of side marker placed clear of anatomy of interest
- No rotation of the pelvis, as demonstrated by a symmetric appearance
- Axiolateral projections of the femoral necks
- Femoral necks without overlap from the greater trochanters
- Small parts of the lesser trochanters on the posterior surfaces of the femora
- Small parts of the greater trochanters on the posterior and anterior surfaces of the femora
- Both sides equidistant from the edge of the radiograph
- Greater amount of the proximal femur on a unilateral examination
- Femoral neck angles approximately 15 to 20 degrees superior to the femoral bodies
- Bony trabecular detail and surrounding soft tissues

Congenital dislocation of the hip

The diagnosis of congenital dislocation of the hip in newborns has been discussed in numerous articles. Andren and von Rosén[6] described a method that is based on certain theoretic considerations. Their method requires accurate and judicious application of the positioning technique to make an accurate diagnosis. The Andren–von Rosén approach involves taking a bilateral hip projection with both legs forcibly abducted to at least 45 degrees with appreciable inward rotation of the femora. Knake and Kuhns[7] described the construction of a device that controlled the degree of abduction and rotation of both limbs. They reported that the device essentially eliminated and greatly simplified positioning difficulties, reducing the number of repeat examinations.

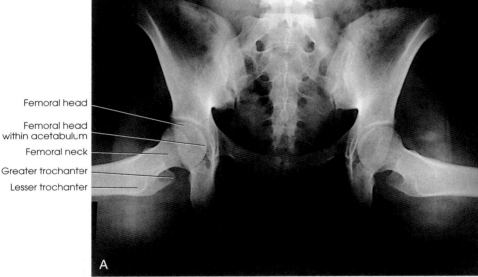

Femoral head
Femoral head within acetabulum
Femoral neck
Greater trochanter
Lesser trochanter

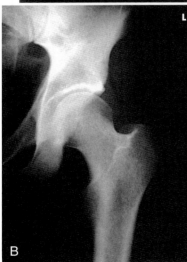
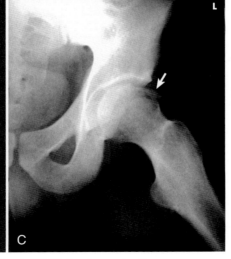

Fig. 8.28 Axiolateral femoral necks: Cleaves method. (A) Bilateral examination. (B) and (C) Unilateral hip examination of a patient who fell. No fractures were seen on initial AP hip radiograph (B), and a second projection using the Cleaves method was performed. Chip fracture of femoral head *(arrow)* was seen (C). At least two projections are required in trauma diagnoses.

♠ AP PROJECTION

Image receptor + grid: Positioned by manufacturer or department protocol for proper anatomy display orientation; CR plate: 10 × 12 inches (24 × 30 cm) lengthwise.

Position of patient
- Place the patient in the supine position.

Position of part
- Adjust the patient's pelvis so that it is not rotated. This is accomplished by placing the ASIS equidistant from the table (Figs. 8.29 and 8.30).
- Place the patient's arms in a comfortable position.
- Medially rotate the lower limb and foot approximately 15 to 20 degrees to place the femoral neck parallel with the plane of the IR unless this maneuver is contraindicated or other instructions are given.
- Place a support under the knee and a sandbag across the ankle. This makes it easier for the patient to maintain this position.
- *Shield gonads.*
- *Respiration:* Suspend.

Central ray
- Perpendicular to the femoral neck; using the localizing technique previously described (see Fig. 8.12), place the central ray approximately 2.5 inches (6.4 cm) distal on a line drawn perpendicular to the midpoint of a line between the ASIS and the pubic symphysis (see Fig. 8.30B).
- Center the IR to the central ray.
- Make any necessary adjustments in the IR size and central ray point when an entire orthopedic device is to be shown on one image.

Collimation
- Adjust radiation field to 10 × 12 inches (24 × 30 cm) on the collimator. Place side marker in the collimated exposure field.

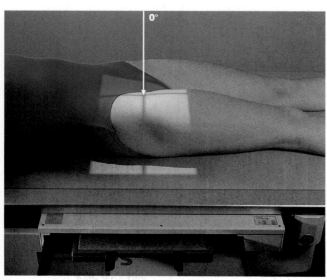

Fig. 8.29 AP hip.

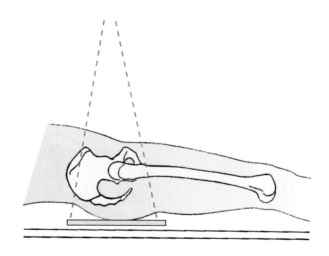

A

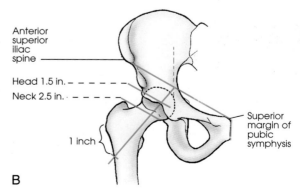

B

Fig. 8.30 (A) AP hip. (B) Localization planes of pelvis.

Anterior superior iliac spine

Head 1.5 in.
Neck 2.5 in.

1 inch

Superior margin of pubic symphysis

Structures shown

The head, neck, trochanters, and proximal one-third of the body of the femur (Fig. 8.31). In the initial examination of a hip lesion, whether traumatic or pathologic in origin, the AP projection is often obtained using an IR large enough to include the entire pelvic girdle and upper femora. Progress studies may be restricted to the affected side.

EVALUATION CRITERIA

The following should be clearly seen:

- Evidence of proper collimation and presence of side marker placed clear of anatomy of interest
- Regions of the ilium and pubic bones adjoining the pubic symphysis
- Hip joint
- Proximal one-third of the femur
- Femoral head, penetrated and seen through the acetabulum
- Entire long axis of the femoral neck not foreshortened
- Greater trochanter in profile
- Lesser trochanter usually not projected beyond the medial border of the femur or only a very small amount of the trochanter visible
- Any orthopedic appliance in its entirety
- Bony trabecular detail and surrounding soft tissues

NOTE: Trauma patients who have sustained severe injury usually are not transferred to the radiographic table but are radiographed on the stretcher or bed. After the localization point has been established and marked, one assistant should be on each side of the stretcher to grasp the sheet and lift the pelvis just enough for placement of the IR, while a third person supports the injured limb. Any necessary manipulation of the limb must be made by a physician.

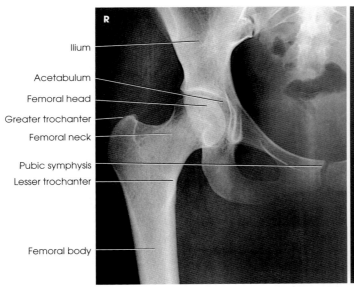
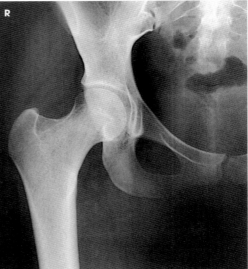

Ilium
Acetabulum
Femoral head
Greater trochanter
Femoral neck
Pubic symphysis
Lesser trochanter
Femoral body

Fig. 8.31 AP hip.

♠ LATERAL PROJECTION
Mediolateral
LAUENSTEIN AND HICKEY METHODS

NOTE: This examination is contraindicated for patients with a suspected fracture or pathologic condition.

The Lauenstein and Hickey methods are used to show the hip joint and the relationship of the femoral head to the acetabulum. This position is similar to the previously described modified Cleaves method.

> **Image receptor + grid:** Positioned by manufacturer or department protocol for proper anatomy display orientation; CR plate: 10 × 12 inches (24 × 30 cm) crosswise.

Position of patient
- From the supine position, rotate the patient slightly toward the affected side to an oblique position. The degree of obliquity depends on how much the patient can abduct the leg.

Position of part
- Adjust the patient's body, and center the affected hip to the midline of the grid.
- Ask the patient to flex the affected knee and draw the thigh up to a position at nearly a right angle to the hip bone.
- Keep the body of the affected femur parallel to the table.
- Extend the opposite limb and support it at hip level and under the knee.
- Rotate the pelvis no more than necessary to accommodate flexion of the thigh and avoid superimposition of the affected side (Fig. 8.32).
- *Shield gonads.*
- *Respiration:* Suspend.

Central ray
- Perpendicular through the hip joint, which is located midway between the ASIS and the pubic symphysis for the Lauenstein method (Fig. 8.33) and at a cephalic angle of 20 to 25 degrees and an additional 1 inch (2.5 cm) more inferior for the Hickey method (Fig. 8.34).
- Center the IR to the central ray.

Collimation
- Adjust radiation field to 10 × 12 inches (24 × 30 cm) on the collimator. Place side marker in the collimated exposure field.

Structures shown
A lateral projection of the hip, including the acetabulum, the proximal end of the femur, and the relationship of the femoral head to the acetabulum (see Figs. 8.33 and 8.34).

EVALUATION CRITERIA
The following should be clearly seen:
- Evidence of proper collimation and presence of side marker placed clear of anatomy of interest
- Hip joint centered to the radiograph
- Hip joint, acetabulum, and femoral head
- Femoral neck overlapped by the greater trochanter in the Lauenstein method
- With cephalic angulation in the Hickey method, the femoral neck free of superimposition
- Bony trabecular detail and surrounding soft tissues

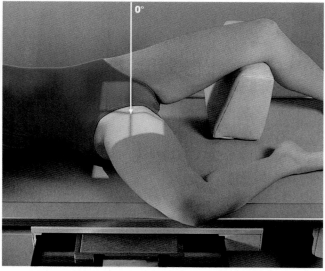

Fig. 8.32 Mediolateral hip: Lauenstein method.

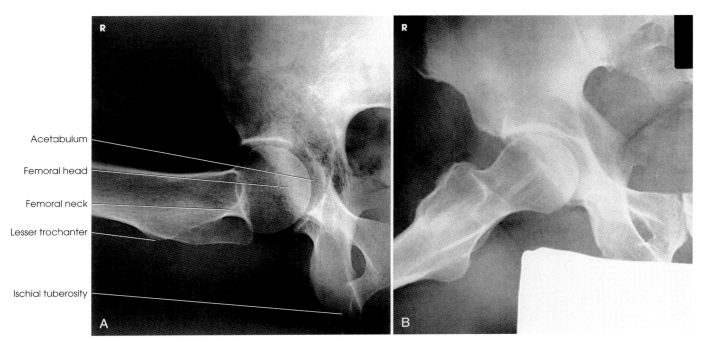

Acetabulum

Femoral head

Femoral neck

Lesser trochanter

Ischial tuberosity

Fig. 8.33 (A) Mediolateral hip with perpendicular central ray: Lauenstein method.
(B) Mediolateral hip with perpendicular central ray using male gonad (contact) shield.

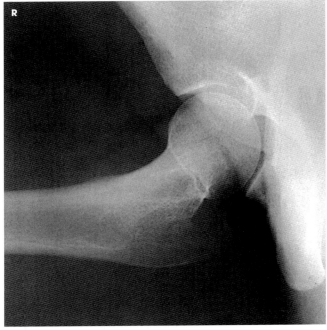

Fig. 8.34 Mediolateral hip with 20-degree cephalad angulation: Hickey method.

♠ AXIOLATERAL PROJECTION
DANELIUS-MILLER METHOD

This projection is often called the *cross-table* or *surgical-lateral* projection.

> **Image receptor + grid:** Positioned by manufacturer or department protocol for proper anatomy display orientation; CR plate: 10 × 12 inches (24 × 30 cm) lengthwise.

Position of patient
- Place the patient in the supine position.

Position of part
- When examining a patient who is thin or lying on a soft bed, elevate the pelvis on a firm pillow or folded sheets sufficiently to center the most prominent point of the greater trochanter to the midline of the IR. The support must not extend beyond the lateral surface of the body; otherwise it would interfere with placement of the IR.
- When the pelvis is elevated, support the affected limb at hip level on sandbags or firm pillows.

- Flex the knee and hip of the unaffected side to elevate the thigh in a vertical position.
- Rest the unaffected leg on a suitable support that does not interfere with the central ray. Special support devices are available. *Do not rest the foot on the x-ray tube or collimator.*
- Adjust the pelvis so that it is not rotated (Figs. 8.35 and 8.36).
- Unless contraindicated, grasp the heel and medially rotate the foot and lower limb of the affected side about 15 or 20 degrees. A sandbag may be used to hold the leg and foot in this position, and a small support can be placed under the knee. Manipulation of patients with unhealed fractures should be performed by a physician.

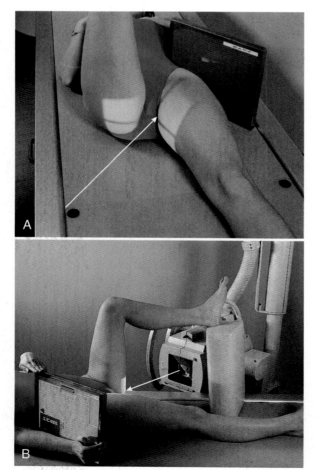

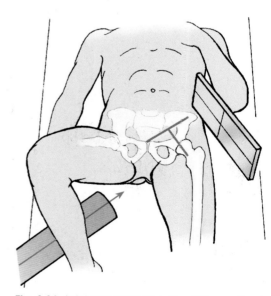

Fig. 8.35 (A) Axiolateral hip: Danelius-Miller method, IR supported with sandbags. (B) Same projection, patient holding IR. Foot is on a footrest.

Fig. 8.36 Axiolateral hip: Danelius-Miller method.

Position of IR

- Place the IR in the vertical position with its upper border in the soft tissue crease above the iliac crest.
- Angle the IR away from the body until it is exactly parallel with the long axis of the femoral neck.
- Support the IR in this position with sandbags or a vertical IR holder. These are the preferred methods. Alternatively, the patient may support the IR with a hand.
- Be careful to position the grid vertically but with the lead strips oriented horizontally.
- *Shield gonads.*
- *Respiration:* Suspend.

Central ray

- Perpendicular to the long axis of the femoral neck. The central ray enters the groin area at a point midway between the anterior and posterior surfaces of the upper thigh and passes through the femoral neck, which is about 2.5 inches (6.4 cm) below the point of intersection of the localization lines described previously (see Fig. 8.12).

Collimation

- Adjust radiation field to 10 × 12 inches (24 × 30 cm) on the collimator. Place side marker in the collimated exposure field.

▼ COMPENSATING FILTER

This projection is improved dramatically and can be performed with one exposure with the use of a specially designed compensating filter.

Structures shown

The acetabulum, head, neck, and trochanters of the femur (Fig. 8.37).

The following should be clearly seen:

- Evidence of proper collimation and presence of side marker placed clear of anatomy of interest
- Hip joint with the acetabulum
- Femoral neck without overlap from the greater trochanter
- Small amount of the lesser trochanter on the posterior surface of the femur
- Small amount of the greater trochanter on the anterior and posterior surfaces of the proximal femur when the femur is properly inverted
- Ischial tuberosity below the femoral head and neck
- Soft tissue shadow of the unaffected thigh not overlapping the hip joint or proximal femur
- Any orthopedic appliance in its entirety
- Bony trabecular detail and surrounding soft tissues

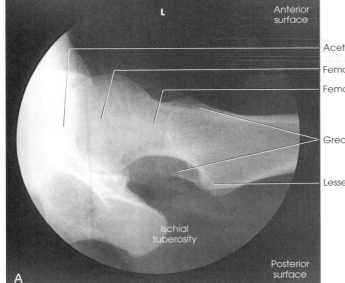
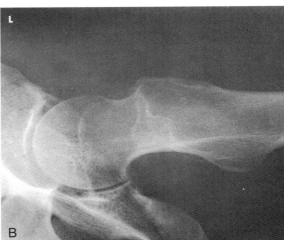

Fig. 8.37 (A) Axiolateral hip: Danelius-Miller method. (B) Same projection with use of compensating filter. Note excellent detail of acetabular area and femur.

MODIFIED AXIOLATERAL PROJECTION

CLEMENTS-NAKAYAMA MODIFICATION

When the patient has bilateral hip fractures, bilateral hip arthroplasty (plastic surgery of the hip joints), or limitation of movement of the unaffected leg, the Danelius-Miller method cannot be used. Clements and Nakayama[8] described a modification using a 15-degree posterior angulation of the central ray (Fig. 8.38).

Image receptor + grid: Positioned by manufacturer or department protocol for proper anatomy display orientation; CR plate: 10 × 12 inches (24 × 30 cm) lengthwise.

Position of patient

- Position the patient supine on the radiographic table with the affected side near the edge of the table.

Position of part

- For this position, do not rotate the lower limb internally. Instead, the limb remains in a neutral or slightly externally rotated position.
- Support a grid IR on the Bucky tray so that its lower margin is below the patient. Position the grid so that the lines run parallel with the floor.
- Adjust the grid parallel to the axis of the femoral neck, and tilt its top back 15 degrees.
- *Shield gonads.*
- *Respiration:* Suspend.

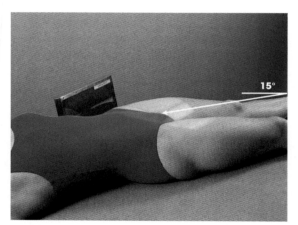

Fig. 8.38 Axiolateral hip: Clements-Nakayama method.

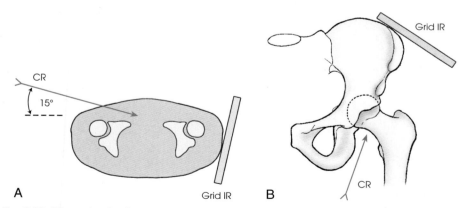

Fig. 8.39 CR angles for Clements-Nakayama method. (A) 15 degrees posteriorly. Note grid IR tilted 15 degrees. (B) Perpendicular to femoral neck and grid IR.

Central ray

- Directed 15 degrees posteriorly and aligned perpendicular to the femoral neck and the grid IR (Fig. 8.39).

Collimation

- Adjust radiation field to 10 × 12 inches (24 × 30 cm) on the collimator. Place side marker in the collimated exposure field.

Structures shown

The acetabulum and proximal femur—including the head, neck, and trochanters—in lateral profile. The Clements-Nakayama modification (Fig. 8.40) can be compared with the Danelius-Miller approach described previously (Fig. 8.41).

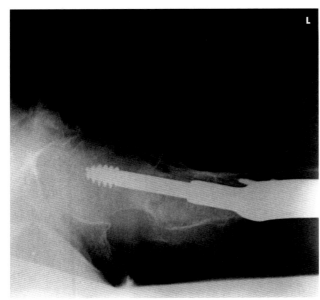

Fig. 8.40 Clements-Nakayama method with 15-degree central ray angulation in same patient as in Fig. 8.41.

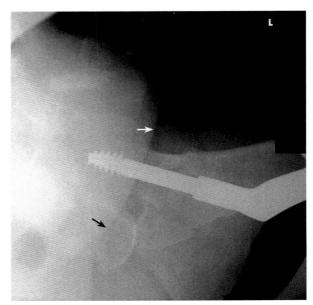

Fig. 8.41 Postoperative Danelius-Miller method used for a patient who was unable to flex unaffected hip. Contralateral thigh (*arrows*) is obscuring femoral head and acetabular area.

PA AXIAL OBLIQUE PROJECTION
TEUFEL METHOD
RAO or LAO position

Image receptor + grid: Positioned by manufacturer or department protocol for proper anatomy display orientation; CR plate: 10 × 12 inches (24 × 30 cm) lengthwise.

Position of patient
- Have the patient lie recumbent in an anterior oblique position on the affected side.

Position of part
- Align the body and center the hip being examined to the midline of the grid.
- Elevate the unaffected side so that the anterior surface of the body forms a 38-degree angle from the table (Fig. 8.42).

- Have the patient support the body on the forearm and flexed knee of the elevated side.
- With the IR in the Bucky tray, adjust the position of the IR so that its midpoint coincides with the central ray.
- *Shield gonads.*
- *Respiration:* Suspend.

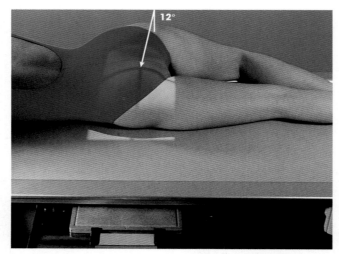

Fig. 8.42 PA axial oblique acetabulum: Teufel method.

Central ray

- Directed through the acetabulum at an angle of 12 degrees cephalad. The central ray enters the body at the inferior level of the coccyx and approximately 2 inches (5 cm) lateral to the MSP toward the side being examined.

Collimation

- Adjust radiation field to 10 × 12 inches (24 × 30 cm) on the collimator. Place side marker in the collimated exposure field.

Structures shown

The fovea capitis and the superoposterior wall of the acetabulum (Fig. 8.43).

The following should be clearly seen:

- Evidence of proper collimation and presence of side marker placed clear of anatomy of interest
- Hip joint and acetabulum near the center of the radiograph
- Femoral head in profile to show the concave area of the fovea capitis
- Superoposterior wall of the acetabulum
- Bony trabecular detail and surrounding soft tissues

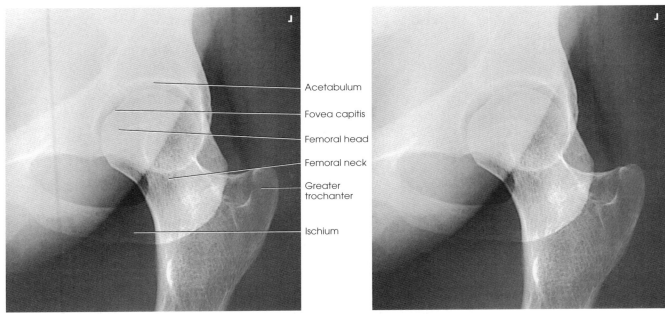

Acetabulum

Fovea capitis

Femoral head

Femoral neck

Greater trochanter

Ischium

Fig. 8.43 PA axial oblique acetabulum: Teufel method.

♠ AP OBLIQUE PROJECTION

JUDET METHOD[9]
MODIFIED JUDET METHOD[10]

RPO and LPO positions

Judet et al.[9] described *two* 45-degree posterior oblique positions that are useful in diagnosing fractures of the acetabulum: the internal oblique position (affected side up) and the external oblique position (affected side down). Both positions must be performed to demonstrate the entire acetabulum, as well as the iliopubic and ilioischial columns of the affected side.

Image receptor + grid: Positioned by manufacturer or department protocol for proper anatomy display orientation; CR plate: 10 × 12 inches (24 × 30 cm) lengthwise.

Internal oblique

The internal oblique position is used for a patient with a suspected fracture of the *iliopubic column* (anterior) and the posterior rim of the acetabulum.

NOTE: The *iliopubic column* (anterior), composed of a short segment of the ilium and the pubis, extends up as far as the anterior spine of the ilium and from the symphysis pubis and obturator foramen through the acetabulum to the ASIS.

Position of patient

- Place the patient in a posterior oblique position with the affected hip *up*.

Position of part

- Align the body and center the hip being examined to the middle of the IR.
- Elevate the affected side so that the MCP of the body forms a 45-degree angle from the table (Fig. 8.44A).
- *Shield gonads.*
- *Respiration:* Suspend.

Central ray

- Perpendicular to the IR and entering 2 inches (5 cm) inferior to the ASIS of the affected side

External oblique

The external oblique is used for a patient with a suspected fracture of the *ilioischial column* (posterior) and the anterior rim of the acetabulum.

Position of patient

- Place the patient in a posterior oblique position with the affected hip *down*.

Position of part

- Align the body and center the hip being examined to the middle of the IR.
- Elevate the unaffected side so that the MCP of the body forms a 45-degree angle from the table (Fig. 8.44B).
- *Shield gonads.*
- *Respiration:* Suspend.

Central ray

- Perpendicular to the IR and entering at the pubic symphysis

Collimation

- Adjust radiation field to 10 × 12 inches (24 × 30 cm) on the collimator. Place side marker in the collimated exposure field.

Structures shown

The acetabular rim (Fig. 8.45).

NOTE: The *ilioischial column* (posterior), composed of the vertical portion of the ischium and the portion of the ilium immediately above the ischium, extends from the obturator foramen through the posterior aspect of the acetabulum.

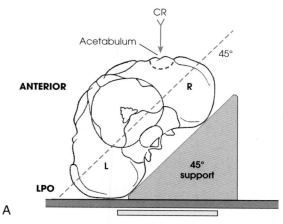
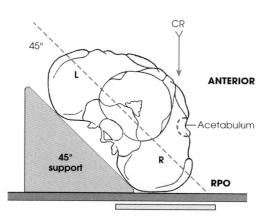

Fig. 8.44 AP oblique projection, Judet method for right hip. (A) LPO places right hip in *internal* oblique position. (B) RPO places right hip in *external* oblique position.

EVALUATION CRITERIA

The following should be clearly seen:
- Evidence of proper collimation and presence of side marker placed clear of anatomy of interest
- Acetabulum centered to the IR
- The iliopubic column and the posterior rim of the affected acetabulum on the internal oblique

- The ilioischial column and the anterior rim of the acetabulum on the external oblique
- Bony trabecular detail and surrounding soft tissues

NOTE: Rafert and Long[10] described a modification of the Judet method on trauma patients. The patient is not required to lie on the affected side for the external oblique (Fig. 8.46).

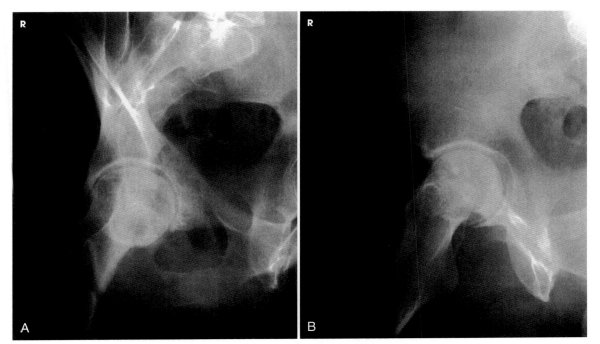

Fig. 8.45 AP oblique projection, Judet method, right hip. (A) LPO. (B) RPO.

(From Long BW, Rafert JA: *Orthopedic radiography*, Philadelphia, 1995, Saunders.)

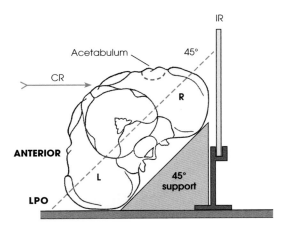

Fig. 8.46 AP oblique projection, *modified Judet method* for right hip on a trauma patient. *External* oblique projection is obtained using cross-table CR and grid IR. *Internal oblique* is obtained on a trauma patient in same position using vertical CR (same as Fig. 8.44A).

AP AXIAL OUTLET PROJECTION

TAYLOR METHOD[11]

Image receptor + grid: Positioned by manufacturer or department protocol for proper anatomy display orientation; CR plate: 14 × 17 inches (35 × 43 cm) crosswise.

Position of patient

- Place the patient in the supine position.

Position of part

- Center the MSP of the patient's body to the midline of the grid and adjust the pelvis so that it is not rotated. The ASIS should be equidistant from the table (Fig. 8.47).
- Flex the knees slightly with a support underneath if the patient is uncomfortable.
- With the IR in the Bucky tray, adjust the tray's position so that the midpoint of the IR coincides with the central ray.
- *Shield gonads.*
- *Respiration:* Suspend.

Central ray

Men

- Directed 20 to 35 degrees cephalad and entering the midline at a point 2 inches (5 cm) inferior to the superior border of the pubic symphysis

Women

- Directed 30 to 45 degrees cephalad and entering the midline at a point 2 inches (5 cm) inferior to the superior border of the pubic symphysis

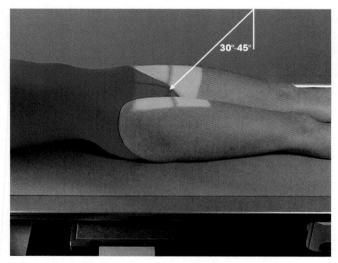

Fig. 8.47 AP axial pelvic bones: Taylor method.

Collimation

- Adjust radiation field to 14 × 17 inches (35 × 43 cm) on the collimator. For smaller patients, collimate 1 inch (2.5 cm) beyond the skin shadow on the sides. Place side marker in the collimated exposure field.

Structures shown

The superior and inferior rami without the foreshortening seen in a PA or AP projection because the central ray is more perpendicular to the rami (Figs. 8.48 and 8.49).

The following should be clearly seen:

- Evidence of proper collimation and presence of side marker placed clear of anatomy of interest
- Pubic and ischial bones magnified with pubic bones superimposed over the sacrum and coccyx
- Symmetric obturator foramina
- Pubic and ischial rami near the center of the radiograph
- Hip joints
- Bony trabecular detail and surrounding soft tissues

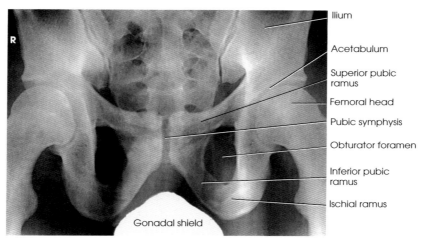

Ilium

Acetabulum

Superior pubic ramus

Femoral head

Pubic symphysis

Obturator foramen

Inferior pubic ramus

Ischial ramus

Gonadal shield

Fig. 8.48 Male AP axial pelvic bones: Taylor method.

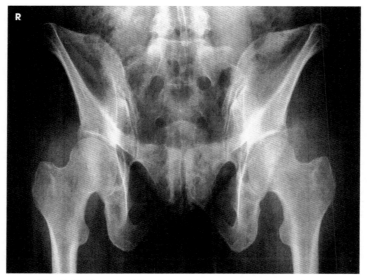

Fig. 8.49 Female AP axial pelvic bones: Taylor method.

SUPEROINFERIOR AXIAL INLET PROJECTION

BRIDGEMAN METHOD[12]

Image receptor + grid: Positioned by manufacturer or department protocol for proper anatomy display orientation; CR plate: 14 × 17 inches (35 × 43 cm) crosswise.

Position of patient

- Place the patient on the radiographic table in the supine position.

Position of part

- Center the MSP of the patient's body to the midline of the grid.
- Flex the knees slightly and support them to relieve strain.

- Adjust the pelvis so that the ASISs are equidistant from the table.
- With the IR in the Bucky tray, center it at the level of the greater trochanters (Fig. 8.50).
- *Shield gonads.*
- *Respiration:* Suspend.

Central ray

- Directed 40 degrees caudad, entering the midline at the level of ASIS

Collimation

- Adjust radiation field to 14 × 17 inches (35 × 43 cm) on the collimator. For smaller patients, collimate 1 inch (2.5 cm) beyond the skin shadow on the sides. Place side marker in the collimated exposure field.

Structures shown

An axial projection of the pelvic ring, or inlet, in its entirety (Fig. 8.51).

EVALUATION CRITERIA

The following should be clearly seen:

- Evidence of proper collimation and presence of side marker placed clear of anatomy of interest
- Medially superimposed superior and inferior rami of the pubic bones
- Nearly superimposed lateral two-thirds of the pubic and ischial bones
- Symmetric pubes and ischial spines
- Hip joints
- Anterior pelvic bones
- Bony trabecular detail and surrounding soft tissues

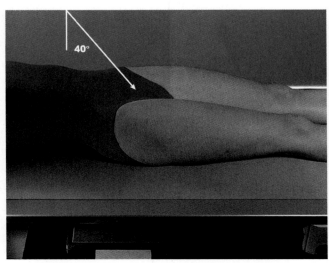

Fig. 8.50 AP axial pelvic bones: Bridgeman method.

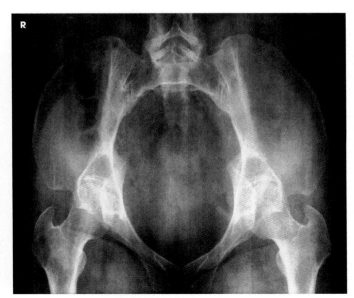

Fig. 8.51 AP axial inlet projection.

AP AND PA OBLIQUE PROJECTIONS

Image receptor + grid: Positioned by manufacturer or department protocol for proper anatomy display orientation; CR plate: 10 × 12 inches (24 × 30 cm) lengthwise.

RPO and LPO positions
Position of patient
- Place the patient in the supine position.

Position of part
- Center the sagittal plane passing through the hip joint of the affected side to the midline of the grid.
- Elevate the unaffected side approximately 40 degrees to place the broad surface of the wing of the affected ilium parallel with the plane of the IR.
- Support the elevated shoulder, hip, and knee on sandbags.
- Adjust the position of the uppermost limb to place the ASIS in the same transverse plane (Fig. 8.52).
- Center the IR at the level of the ASIS.
- *Shield gonads.*
- *Respiration:* Suspend.

RAO and LAO positions
Position of patient
- Place the patient in the prone position.

Position of part
- Center the sagittal plane passing through the hip joint of the affected side to the midline of the grid.
- Elevate the unaffected side about 40 degrees to place the affected ilium perpendicular to the plane of the IR.
- Have the patient rest on the forearm and flexed knee of the elevated side.
- Adjust the position of the uppermost thigh to place the iliac crests in the same horizontal plane.
- Center the IR at the level of the ASIS (Fig. 8.53).
- *Shield gonads.*
- *Respiration:* Suspend.

Central ray
- Perpendicular to the midpoint of the IR

Collimation
- Adjust radiation field to 10 × 12 inches (24 × 30 cm) on the collimator. Place side marker in the collimated exposure field.

Structures shown
AP oblique image shows an unobstructed projection of the ala and sciatic notches and a profile image of the acetabulum (Fig. 8.54). PA oblique image shows the ilium in profile and the femoral head within the acetabulum (Fig. 8.55).

EVALUATION CRITERIA
The following should be clearly seen:
- Evidence of proper collimation and presence of side marker placed clear of anatomy of interest
- Entire ilium
- Hip joint, proximal femur, and SI joint
- Bony trabecular detail and surrounding soft tissues

AP Oblique Projection
- Broad surface of the iliac wing without rotation

PA Oblique Projection
- Ilium in profile

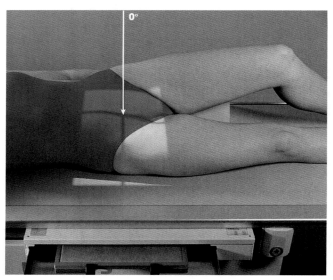

Fig. 8.52 AP oblique ilium, RPO.

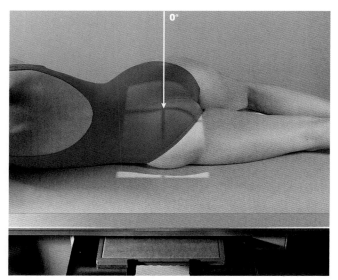

Fig. 8.53 PA oblique ilium, LAO.

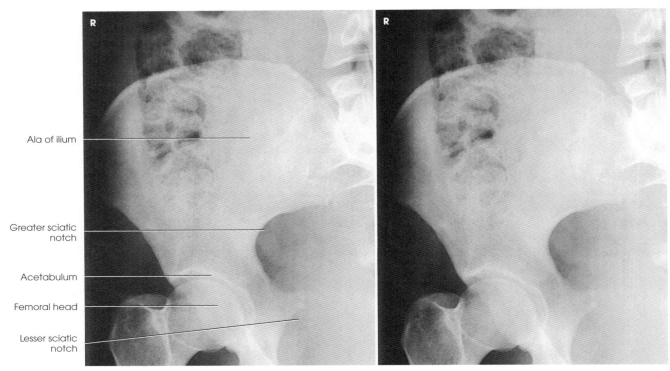

Ala of ilium

Greater sciatic notch

Acetabulum

Femoral head

Lesser sciatic notch

Fig. 8.54 AP oblique ilium, RPO.

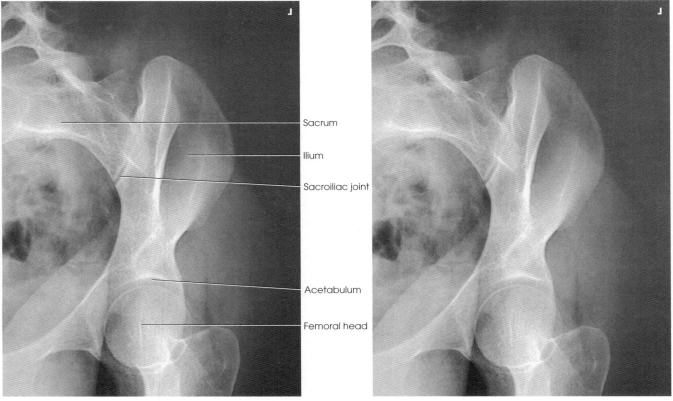

Sacrum

Ilium

Sacroiliac joint

Acetabulum

Femoral head

Fig. 8.55 PA oblique ilium, LAO.

References

1. Bello A, Jr: An alternative positioning landmark, *Radiol Technol* 5:477–478, 1999.
2. Fauber TL: Gonadal shielding in radiography: a best practice?, *Radiol Technol* 88:127–134, 2016.
3. Martz CD, Taylor CC: The 45-degree angle roentgenographic study of the pelvis in congenital dislocation of the hip, *J Bone Joint Surg Am* 36:528–532, 1954.
4. Berkebile RD, Fischer DL, Albrecht LF: The gull-wing sign: value of the lateral view of the pelvis in fracture dislocation of the acetabular rim and posterior dislocation of the femoral head, *Radiology* 84:937–939, 1965.
5. Cleaves EN: Observations on lateral views of the hip, *AJR Am J Roentgenol* 34:964, 1938.
6. Andren L, von Rosén S: The diagnosis of dislocation of the hip in newborns and the primary results of immediate treatment, *Acta Radiol* 49:89–95, 1958.
7. Knake JE, Kuhns LR: A device to aid in positioning for the Andren-von Rosén hip view, *Radiology* 117:735–736, 1975.
8. Clements RS, Nakayama HK: Radiographic methods in total hip arthroplasty, *Radiol Technol* 51:589–600, 1980.
9. Judet R, Judet J, Letournel E: Fractures of the acetabulum: classification and surgical approaches for open reduction, *J Bone Joint Surg Am* 46:1615–1646, 1964.
10. Rafert JA, Long BW: Showing acetabular trauma with more clarity, less pain, *Radiol Technol* 63:92–97, 1991.
11. Taylor R: Modified anteroposterior projection of the anterior bones of the pelvis, *Radiog Clin Photog* 17:67, 1941.
12. Bridgeman CF: Radiography of the hip bone, *Med Radiog Photog* 28:38–46, 1952.

References

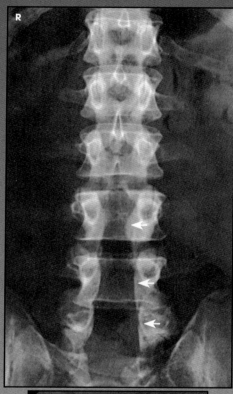

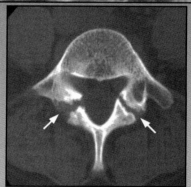

9

VERTEBRAL COLUMN

SUMMARY OF PROJECTIONS

PROJECTIONS, POSITIONS, AND METHODS

Page	Essential	Anatomy	Projection	Position	Method
437	✦	Dens	AP		FUCHS
438	✦	Atlas and axis	AP	Open mouth	
440		Atlas and axis	Lateral	R or L	
441	✦	Cervical vertebrae	AP axial		
443	✦	Cervical vertebrae	Lateral	R or L	GRANDY
445	✦	Cervical vertebrae	Lateral	R or L flexion and extension	
447	✦	Cervical intervertebral foramina	AP axial oblique	RPO and LPO	
448		Cervical intervertebral foramina	AP oblique	Flexion and extension	
449	✦	Cervical intervertebral foramina	PA axial oblique	RAO and LAO	
451		Cervical vertebrae	AP		OTTONELLO
453		Cervical and upper thoracic vertebrae: *vertebral arch (pillars)*	AP axial		
455		Cervical and upper thoracic vertebrae: *vertebral arch (pillars)*	AP axial oblique	R and L head rotations	
456	✦	Cervicothoracic region	Lateral	R or L	SWIMMER'S TECHNIQUE
458	✦	Thoracic vertebrae	AP		
461	✦	Thoracic vertebrae	Lateral	R or L	
464		Thoracic zygapophyseal joints	AP, PA oblique	RAO and LAO, RPO and LPO	

PROJECTIONS, POSITIONS, AND METHODS

Page	Essential	Anatomy	Projection	Position	Method
467	⚜	Lumbar-lumbosacral vertebrae	AP		
467		Lumbar-lumbosacral vertebrae	PA		
471	⚜	Lumbar-lumbosacral vertebrae	Lateral	R or L	
473	⚜	L5–S1 lumbosacral junction	Lateral	R or L	
475	⚜	Lumbar zygapophyseal joints	AP oblique	RPO and LPO	
477	⚜	Lumbar zygapophyseal joints	PA oblique	RAO and LAO	
479	⚜	Lumbosacral junction and sacroiliac joints	AP, PA axial		FERGUSON
481	⚜	Sacroiliac joints	AP oblique	RPO and LPO	
483	⚜	Sacroiliac joints	PA oblique	RAO and LAO	
485	⚜	Sacrum and coccyx	AP, PA axial		
487	⚜	Sacrum and coccyx	Lateral	R or L	
489		Lumbar intervertebral disks	PA	R and L bending	WEIGHT-BEARING
491	⚜	Thoracolumbar spine: scoliosis	PA, lateral		FRANK ET AL.
495	⚜	Thoracolumbar spine: scoliosis	PA		FERGUSON
497	⚜	Lumbar spine: spinal fusion	AP	R and L bending	
499	⚜	Lumbar spine: spinal fusion	Lateral	R or L flexion and extension	

Icons in the Essential column indicate projections that are frequently performed in the United States and Canada. Students should be competent in these projections.

AP, Anteroposterior; *L*, left; *LAO*, left anterior oblique; *LPO*, left posterior oblique; *PA*, posteroanterior; *R*, right; *RAO*, right anterior oblique; *RPO*, right posterior oblique.

Vertebral Column

The *vertebral column,* or *spine,* forms the central axis of the skeleton and is centered in the midsagittal plane of the posterior part of the trunk. The vertebral column has many functions: It encloses and protects the spinal cord, acts as a support for the trunk, supports the skull superiorly, and provides for attachment for the deep muscles of the back and the ribs laterally. The upper limbs are supported indirectly via the ribs, which articulate with the sternum. The sternum articulates with the shoulder girdle. The vertebral column articulates with each hip bone at the sacroiliac joints. This articulation supports the vertebral column and transmits the weight of the trunk through the hip joints to the lower limbs.

The vertebral column is composed of small segments of bone called *vertebrae.* Disks of fibrocartilage are interposed between the vertebrae and act as cushions. The vertebral column is held together by ligaments, and it is jointed and curved so that it has considerable flexibility and resilience.

In early life, the vertebral column usually consists of 33 small, irregularly shaped bones. These bones are divided into five groups and are named according to the region they occupy (Fig. 9.1). The seven superior-most vertebrae occupy the region of the neck and are termed *cervical vertebrae.* The succeeding 12 bones lie in the dorsal, or posterior, portion of the thorax and are called the *thoracic vertebrae.* The five vertebrae occupying the region of the loin are termed *lumbar vertebrae.* The next five vertebrae, located in the pelvic region, are termed *sacral vertebrae.* The terminal vertebrae, also in the pelvic region, vary from three to five in number in adults and are termed the *coccygeal vertebrae.*

The 24 vertebral segments in the upper three regions remain distinct throughout life and are termed the *true* or movable vertebrae. The pelvic segments in the two lower regions are called *false* or fixed vertebrae because of the change they undergo in adults. The sacral segments usually fuse into one bone called the *sacrum,* and the coccygeal segments, referred to as the *coccyx,* also fuse into one bone.

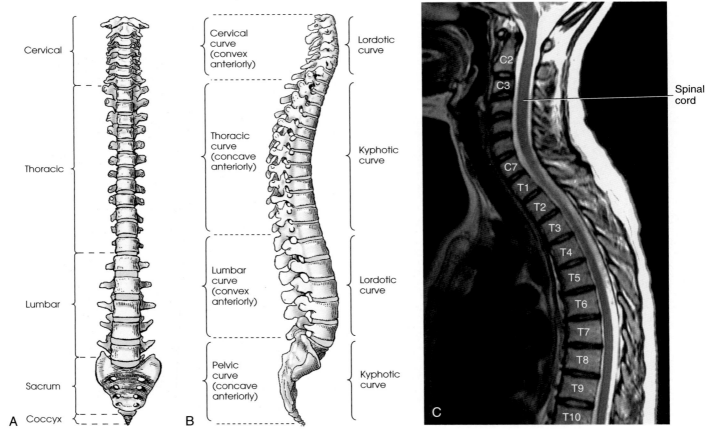

Fig. 9.1 (A) Anterior aspect of vertebral column. (B) Lateral aspect of vertebral column, showing regions and curvatures. (C) Midsagittal MRI scan of cervical and thoracic spine. Note curves and spinal cord protected by vertebrae.

Vertebral Curvature

Viewed from the side, the vertebral column has four curves that arch anteriorly and posteriorly from the midcoronal plane of the body. The *cervical, thoracic, lumbar,* and *pelvic* curves are named for the regions they occupy.

In this text, the vertebral curves are discussed in reference to the *anatomic position* and are referred to as "convex anteriorly" or "concave anteriorly." Because physicians and surgeons evaluate the spine from the posterior aspect of the body, *convex* and *concave* terminology can be the exact opposites. When viewed posteriorly, the normal lumbar curve can correctly be referred to as "concave posteriorly." Whether the curve is described as "convex anteriorly" or "concave posteriorly," the curvature of the patient's spine is the same. The cervical and lumbar curves, which are convex anteriorly, are called *lordotic* curves. The thoracic and pelvic curves are concave anteriorly and are called *kyphotic* curves (see Fig. 9.1B).

The cervical and thoracic curves merge smoothly.

The lumbar and pelvic curves join at an obtuse angle termed the *lumbosacral angle.* The acuity of the angle in the junction of these curves varies among patients. The thoracic and pelvic curves are called *primary curves* because they are present at birth. The cervical and lumbar curves are called *secondary* or *compensatory curves* because they develop after birth. The cervical curve, which is the least pronounced of the curves, develops when an infant begins to hold the head up at about 3 or 4 months of age and begins to sit alone at about 8 or 9 months of age. The lumbar curve develops when the child begins to walk at about 1 to 1½ years of age. The lumbar and pelvic curves are more pronounced in females, who have a more acute angle at the lumbosacral junction.

Any abnormal increase in the anterior concavity (or posterior convexity) of the thoracic curve is termed *kyphosis* (Fig. 9.2B). Any abnormal increase in the anterior convexity (or posterior concavity) of the lumbar or cervical curve is termed *lordosis.*

In frontal view, the vertebral column varies in width in several regions (see Fig. 9.1). In general, the width of the spine gradually increases from the second cervical vertebra to the superior part of the sacrum and then decreases sharply. A *slight* lateral curvature is sometimes present in the upper thoracic region. The curve is to the right in right-handed persons and to the left in left-handed persons. For this reason, the lateral curvature of the vertebral column is believed to be the result of muscle action and to be influenced by occupation. An abnormal lateral curvature of the spine is called *scoliosis.* This condition also causes the vertebrae to rotate toward the concavity. The vertebral column develops a second or compensatory curve in the opposite direction to keep the head centered over the feet (see Fig. 9.2A).

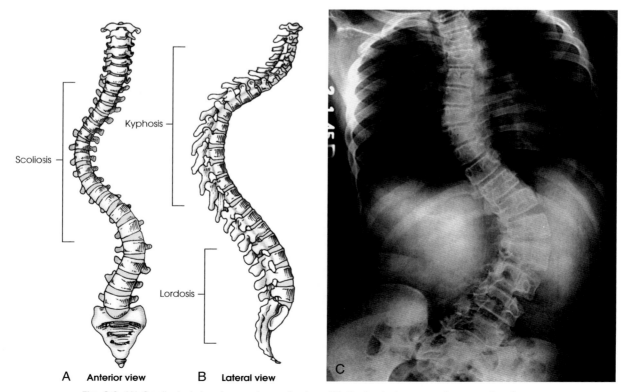

Fig. 9.2 (A) Scoliosis, lateral curvature of spine. (B) Kyphosis, increased convexity of thoracic spine, and lordosis, increased concavity of lumbar spine. (C) PA thoracic and lumbar spine showing severe scoliosis.

Typical Vertebra

A typical vertebra is composed of two main parts—an anterior mass of bone called the *body* and a posterior ringlike portion called the *vertebral arch* (Figs. 9.3 and 9.4). The vertebral body and arch enclose a space called the *vertebral foramen*. In the articulated column, the vertebral foramina form the *vertebral canal*.

The body of the vertebra is approximately cylindric in shape and is largely composed of cancellous bony tissue covered by a layer of compact tissue. From the superior aspect, the posterior surface is flattened, and from the lateral aspect, the anterior and lateral surfaces are concave. The superior and inferior surfaces of the bodies are flattened and are covered by a thin plate of *articular cartilage.*

In the articulated spine, the vertebral bodies are separated by *intervertebral disks,* forming the cartilaginous intervertebral joints. These disks account for approximately one-fourth of the length of the vertebral column. Each disk has a central mass of soft, pulpy, semigelatinous material called the *nucleus pulposus,* which is surrounded by an outer fibrocartilaginous disk called the *annulus fibrosus.* It is common for the pulpy nucleus to rupture or protrude into the vertebral canal, impinging on a spinal nerve. This condition is called *herniated nucleus pulposus* (HNP) or, more commonly, *slipped disk.* HNP most often occurs in the lumbar region as a result of improper body mechanics, and it can cause considerable discomfort and pain. HNP also occurs in the cervical spine as a result of trauma (i.e., whiplash injuries) or degeneration.

The vertebral arch (see Figs. 9.3 and 9.4) is formed by two *pedicles* and two *laminae* that support four articular processes, two transverse processes, and one spinous process. The pedicles are short, thick processes that project posteriorly, one from each side, from the superior and lateral parts of the posterior surface of the vertebral body. The superior and inferior surfaces of the pedicles, or roots, are concave. These concavities are called *vertebral notches.* By articulation with the vertebrae above and below, the notches form *intervertebral foramina* for the transmission of spinal nerves and blood vessels. The broad, flat *laminae* are directed posteriorly and medially from the pedicles.

The *transverse processes* project laterally and slightly posteriorly from the junction of the pedicles and laminae. The *spinous process* projects posteriorly and inferiorly from the junction of the laminae in the posterior midline. A congenital defect of the vertebral column in which the laminae fail to unite posteriorly at the midline is called *spina bifida.* In serious cases of spina bifida, the spinal cord may protrude from the affected individual's body.

Four articular processes—two superior and two inferior—arise from the junction of the pedicles and laminae to articulate with the vertebrae above and below (see Fig. 9.4). The articulating surfaces of the four articular processes are covered with fibrocartilage and are called *facets.* In a typical vertebra, each *superior articular process* has an articular facet on its posterior surface, and each *inferior articular process* has an articular facet on its anterior surface. The planes of the facets vary in direction in the different regions of the vertebral column and often vary within the same vertebra. The articulations between the articular processes of the vertebral arches are the synovial intervertebral joints, referred to as *zygapophyseal joints.* Some texts refer to these joints as *interarticular facet joints.*

The movable vertebrae, with the exception of the first and second cervical vertebrae, are similar in general structure. Each group has certain distinguishing characteristics, however, that must be considered in radiography of the vertebral column.

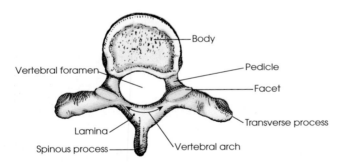

Fig. 9.3 Superior aspect of thoracic vertebra, showing structures common to all vertebral regions.

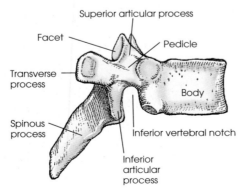

Fig. 9.4 Lateral aspect of thoracic vertebra, showing structures common to all vertebral regions.

Cervical Vertebrae

The first two cervical vertebrae are atypical in that they are structurally modified to join the skull. The seventh vertebra is also atypical and is slightly modified to join the thoracic spine. Atypical and typical vertebrae are described in the following sections.

ATLAS

The *atlas,* the first cervical vertebra (C1), is a ringlike structure with no body and a very short spinous process (Fig. 9.5). The atlas consists of an *anterior arch,* a *posterior arch,* two *lateral masses,* and two *transverse processes.* The anterior and posterior arches extend between the lateral masses. The ring formed by the arches is divided into anterior and posterior portions by a ligament called the *transverse atlantal ligament.* The anterior portion of the ring receives the dens (odontoid process) of the axis, and the posterior portion transmits the proximal spinal cord.

The transverse processes of the atlas are longer than those of the other cervical vertebrae, and they project laterally and slightly inferiorly from the lateral masses. Each lateral mass bears a superior and an inferior articular process. The superior processes lie in a horizontal plane, are large and deeply concave, and are shaped to articulate with the occipital condyles of the occipital bone of the cranium.

AXIS

The *axis,* the second cervical vertebra (C2; Figs. 9.6 and 9.7), has a strong conical process arising from the upper surface of its body. This process, called the *dens* or *odontoid process,* is received into the anterior portion of the atlantal ring to act as the pivot or body for the atlas. At each side of the dens on the superior surface of the vertebral body are the superior articular processes, which are adapted to join with the inferior articular processes of the atlas. These joints, which differ in position and direction from the other cervical zygapophyseal joints, are clearly visualized in an AP projection if the patient is properly positioned. The inferior articular processes of the axis have the same direction as the processes of the succeeding cervical vertebrae. The laminae of the axis are broad and thick. The spinous process is horizontal in position. Fig. 9.8 shows the relationship of C1 and C2 with the occipital condyles.

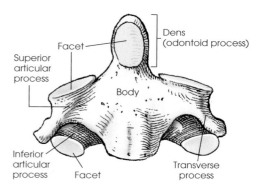

Fig. 9.6 Anterior aspect of axis (C2).

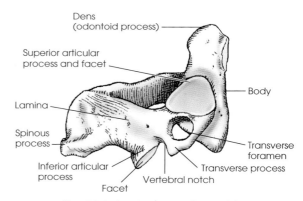

Fig. 9.7 Lateral aspect of axis (C2).

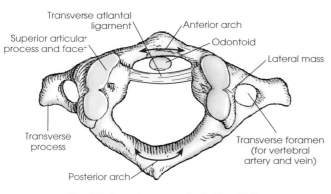

Fig. 9.5 Superior aspect of atlas (C1).

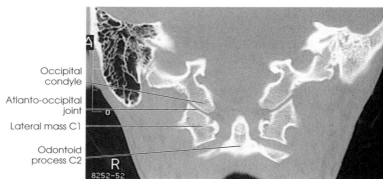

Fig. 9.8 Coronal MRI shows atlas, axis, and occipital bone of skull and their relationship.

(Courtesy Siemens Medical Systems, Iselin, NJ.)

SEVENTH VERTEBRA

The seventh cervical vertebra (C7), termed the *vertebra prominens,* has a long, prominent spinous process that projects almost horizontally to the posterior. The spinous process of this vertebra is easily palpable at the posterior base of the neck. It is convenient to use this process as a guide in localizing other vertebrae.

TYPICAL CERVICAL VERTEBRA

The *typical cervical vertebrae* (C3–C6) have a small, transversely located, oblong body with slightly elongated anteroinferior borders (Fig. 9.9). The result is AP overlapping of the bodies in the articulated column. The transverse processes of

the typical cervical vertebra arise partly from the sides of the body and partly from the vertebral arch. These processes are short and wide, are perforated by the *transverse foramina* for transmission of the vertebral artery and vein, and present a deep concavity on their upper surfaces for passage of the spinal nerves. All cervical vertebrae contain three foramina: the right and left transverse foramina and the vertebral foramen.

The pedicles of the typical cervical vertebra project laterally and posteriorly from the body, and their superior and inferior vertebral notches are nearly equal in depth. The laminae are narrow and thin. The spinous processes are short,

have double-pointed (bifid) tips, and are directed posteriorly and slightly inferiorly. Their palpable tips lie at the level of the interspace below the body of the vertebra from which they arise.

The superior and inferior articular processes are located posterior to the transverse processes at the point where the pedicles and laminae unite. Together the processes form short, thick columns of bone called *articular pillars.* The fibrocartilaginous articulating surfaces of the articular pillars contain facets. The zygapophyseal facet joints of the second through seventh cervical vertebrae lie at right angles to the midsagittal plane and are clearly shown in a lateral projection (Fig. 9.10A).

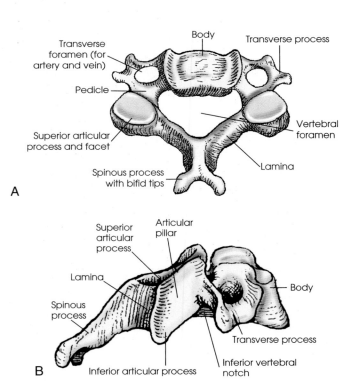

Fig. 9.9 (A) Superior aspect of typical cervical vertebra. (B) Lateral aspect of typical cervical vertebra.

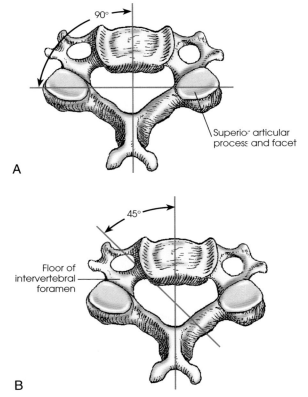

Fig. 9.10 (A) Direction of cervical zygapophyseal joints. (B) Direction of cervical intervertebral foramina.

The intervertebral foramina of the cervical region are directed anteriorly at a 45-degree angle from the midsagittal plane of the body (Fig. 9.11; also see Fig. 9.10B). The foramina are also directed at a 15-degree inferior angle to the horizontal plane of the body. Accurate radiographic demonstration of these foramina requires a 15-degree longitudinal angulation of the central ray and a 45-degree medial rotation of the patient (or a 45-degree medial angulation of the central ray). A lateral projection is necessary to show the cervical zygapophyseal joints. The positioning rotations required for showing the intervertebral foramina and zygapophyseal joints of the cervical spine are summarized in Table 9.1. A full view of the cervical spine along with surrounding tissues is shown in Fig. 9.12.

TABLE 9.1

Positioning rotations needed to show intervertebral foramina and zygapophyseal joints

Area of spine	Intervertebral foramina	Zygapophyseal joint
Cervical spine	45 degrees[a] oblique AP side up PA side down	Lateral
Thoracic spine	Lateral	70 degrees[a] oblique AP side up PA side down
Lumbar spine	Lateral	30–60 degrees[a] oblique AP side down PA side up

[a]From the anatomic position.

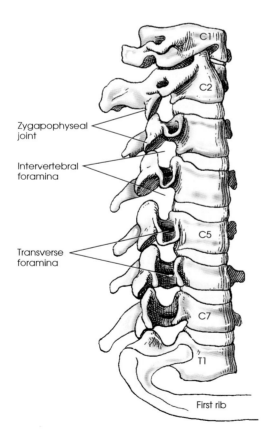

Fig. 9.11 Anterior oblique of cervical vertebrae, showing intervertebral transverse foramina and zygapophyseal joints.

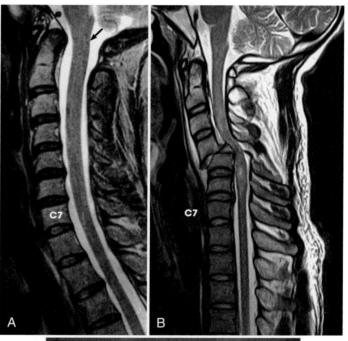

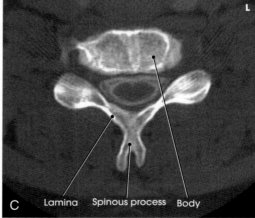

Fig. 9.12 (A) MRI sagittal plane of cervical spine. Note position of spinal cord (*arrow*) in relation to vertebral bodies. (B) MRI sagittal plane showing anterior displacement of C4 on C5. Narrowed spinal canal compresses spinal cord causing paralysis. (C) Axial CT of typical cervical vertebra.

(B, Modified from Jackson SA, Thomas RM: *Cross-sectional imaging made easy,* New York, 2004, Churchill Livingstone. C, Modified from Kelley LL, Petersen CM: *Sectional anatomy for imaging professionals,* ed 2, St. Louis, 2007, Mosby.)

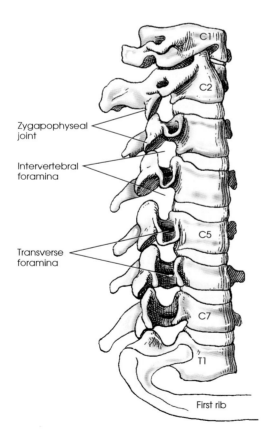

Thoracic Vertebrae

The bodies of the thoracic vertebrae increase in size from the first to the twelfth vertebrae. They also vary in form, with the superior thoracic bodies resembling cervical bodies and the inferior thoracic bodies resembling lumbar bodies. The bodies of the typical (third through ninth) thoracic vertebrae are approximately triangular in form (Figs. 9.13 and 9.14). These vertebral bodies are deeper posteriorly than anteriorly, and their posterior surface is concave from side to side.

The posterolateral margins of each thoracic body have *costal facets* for articulation with the heads of the ribs (Fig. 9.15). The body of the first thoracic vertebra presents a whole costal facet near its superior border for articulation with the head of the first rib and presents a *demifacet* (half-facet) on its inferior border for articulation with the head of the second rib. The bodies of the second through eighth thoracic vertebrae contain demifacets superiorly and inferiorly. The ninth thoracic vertebra has only a superior demifacet. Finally, the tenth, eleventh, and twelfth thoracic vertebral bodies have a single whole facet at the superior margin for articulation with the eleventh and twelfth ribs (Table 9.2).

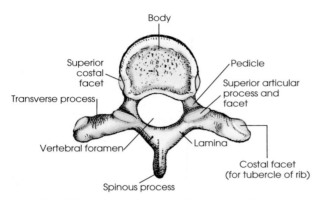

Fig. 9.13 Superior aspect of thoracic vertebra.

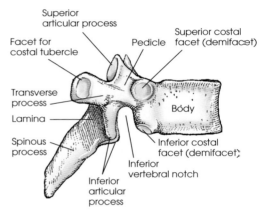

Fig. 9.14 Lateral aspect of thoracic vertebra.

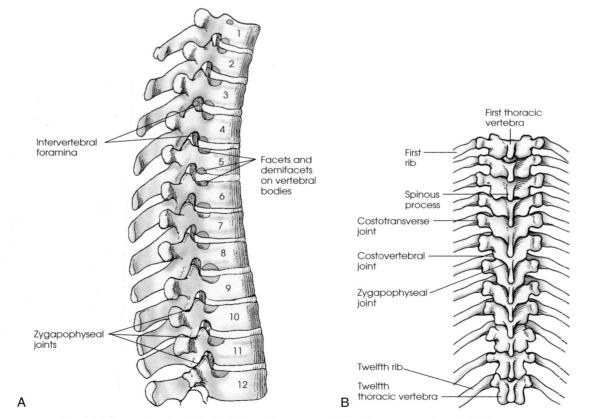

Fig. 9.15 Thoracic spine. (A) Posterior oblique aspect showing zygapophyseal joints, intervertebral foramina, and facets and demifacets (see Table 9.2). (B) Posterior aspect showing attachment of ribs and joints.

The transverse processes of the thoracic vertebrae project obliquely, laterally, and posteriorly. With the exception of the eleventh and twelfth pairs, each process has on the anterior surface of its extremity a small concave facet for articulation with the tubercle of a rib. The laminae are broad and thick, and they overlap the subjacent lamina. The spinous processes are long. From the fifth to the ninth vertebrae, the spinous processes project sharply inferiorly and overlap each other, but they are less vertical above and below this region. The palpable tip of each spinous process of the fifth to ninth thoracic vertebrae corresponds in position to the interspace *below* the vertebra from which it projects.

The zygapophyseal joints of the thoracic region (except the inferior articular processes of the twelfth vertebra) angle anteriorly approximately 15 to 20 degrees to form an angle of 70 to 75 degrees (open anteriorly) to the midsagittal plane of the body (Fig. 9.16A; also see Fig. 9.15). To show the zygapophyseal joints of the thoracic region radiographically, the patient's body must be rotated 70 to 75 degrees from the anatomic position or 15 to 20 degrees from the lateral position.

The intervertebral foramina of the thoracic region are perpendicular to the midsagittal plane of the body (see Figs. 9.15 and 9.16B). These foramina are clearly shown radiographically with the patient in a true lateral position (see Table 9.1). During inspiration, the ribs are elevated. The arms must also be raised enough to elevate the ribs, which otherwise cross the intervertebral foramina. A full view of the thoracic vertebrae along with surrounding tissues is seen in Fig. 9.17.

TABLE 9.2
Costal facets and demifacets

Vertebrae	Vertebral border	Facet/demifacet[a]
T1	Superior	Whole facet
	Inferior	Demifacet
T2–T8	Superior	Demifacet
	Inferior	Demifacet
T9	Superior	Demifacet
	Inferior	None
T10–T12	Superior	Whole facet
	Inferior	None

[a]On *each side* of a vertebral body.

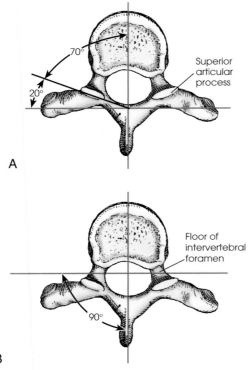

A

B

Fig. 9.16 (A) Direction of thoracic zygapophyseal joints. (B) Direction of thoracic intervertebral foramina.

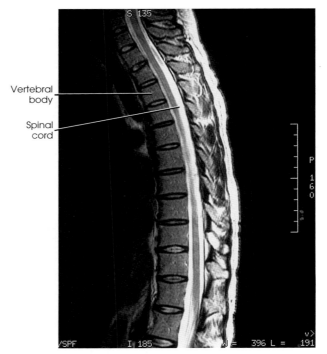

Fig. 9.17 MRI sagittal plane of thoracic vertebrae region showing vertebral bodies and relationship to spinal cord.

Lumbar Vertebrae

The lumbar vertebrae have large, bean-shaped bodies that increase in size from the first to the fifth vertebra in this region. The lumbar bodies are deeper anteriorly than posteriorly, and their superior and inferior surfaces are flattened or slightly concave (Fig. 9.18A). At their posterior surface, these vertebrae are flattened anteriorly to posteriorly, and they are transversely concave. The anterior and lateral surfaces are concave from the top to the bottom (see Fig. 9.18B).

The transverse processes of lumbar vertebrae are smaller than those of thoracic vertebrae. The superior three pairs are directed almost exactly laterally, whereas the inferior two pairs are inclined slightly superiorly. The lumbar pedicles are strong and are directed posteriorly; the laminae are thick. The spinous processes are large, thick, and blunt, and they have an almost horizontal projection posteriorly. The palpable tip of each spinous process corresponds in position with the interspace below the vertebra from which it projects. The *mammillary process* is a smoothly rounded projection on the back of each superior articular process. The *accessory process* is at the back of the root of the transverse process.

The body of the fifth lumbar segment is considerably deeper in front than behind, which gives it a wedge shape that adapts it for articulation with the sacrum. The intervertebral disk of this joint is also more wedge-shaped than the disks in the interspaces above the lumbar region. The spinous process of the fifth lumbar vertebra is smaller and shorter, and the transverse processes are much thicker than those of the upper lumbar vertebrae.

The laminae lie posterior to the pedicles and transverse processes. The part of the lamina between the superior and inferior articular processes is called the *pars interarticularis* (Fig. 9.19).

The zygapophyseal joints of the lumbar region (Figs. 9.20 and 9.21A) are inclined posteriorly from the coronal plane, forming an average angle (open posteriorly) of 30 to 60 degrees to the midsagittal plane of the body.

The average angle increases from cephalad to caudad with L1–L2 at 15 degrees, L2–L3 at 30 degrees, and L3–L4 through L5–S1 at 45 degrees. Table 9.3 shows that these joint angles may vary widely at each level. Numerous upper joints have no angle, and many lower joints have an angle of 60 degrees or more. Although the customary 45-degree oblique body position shows most clinically significant lumbar zygapophyseal joints (L3 through S1), 25% of L1–L2 and L2–L3 joints are shown on an AP projection, and a small percentage of L4–L5 and L5–S1 joints are seen on a lateral projection.

The intervertebral foramina of the lumbar region are situated at right angles to the midsagittal plane of the body, except for the fifth, which turns slightly anteriorly (Fig. 9.21B). The superior four pairs of foramina are shown radiographically with the patient in a true lateral position; the last pair requires slight obliquity of the body (see Table 9.1).

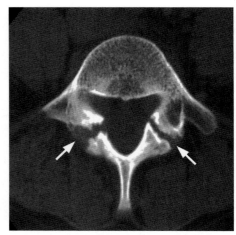

Fig. 9.19 Axial CT image of L5 showing fractures of right and left pars interarticularis (arrows).

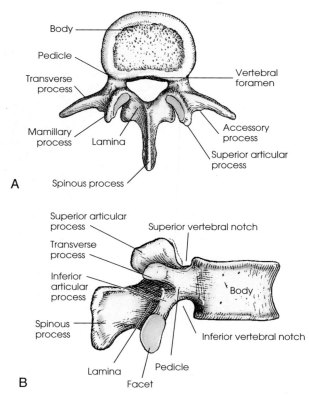

Fig. 9.18 (A) Superior aspect of lumbar vertebra. (B) Lateral aspect of lumbar vertebra.

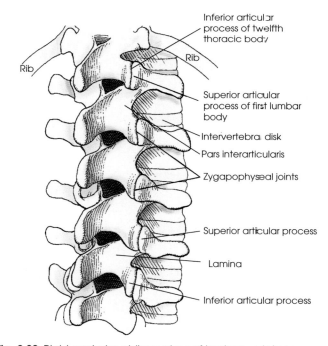

Fig. 9.20 Right posterior oblique view of lumbar vertebrae, showing zygapophyseal joints and pars interarticularis.

Spondylolysis is an acquired bony defect occurring in the pars interarticularis—the area of the lamina between the two articular processes. The defect may occur on one or both sides of the vertebra, resulting in a condition termed *spondylolisthesis*. This condition is characterized by the anterior displacement of one vertebra over another, generally the fifth lumbar over the sacrum. Spondylolisthesis almost exclusively involves the lumbar spine (Fig. 9.22).

Spondylolisthesis is of radiologic importance because oblique-position radiographs show the "neck" area of the "Scottie dog" (i.e., the pars interarticularis). (Oblique positions involving the lumbar spine, including the Scottie dog, are presented later in this chapter, starting with Fig. 9.95.) A full view of the lumbar vertebrae along with surrounding tissues is seen in Fig. 9.23.

TABLE 9.3

Lumbar zygapophyseal joint angle[a]

Joint	Average angle (degrees)	Average range (degrees)	% at 0 degrees[b]	% at 90 degrees[c]
L1–L2	15	0–30	25	0
L2–L3	30	0–30	25	0
L3–L4	45	15–45	10	0
L4–L5	45	45–60	3	2
L5–S1	45	45–60	5	7

[a]In relation to the sagittal plane.
[b]Joint space oriented parallel to sagittal plane.
[c]Joint space perpendicular to sagittal plane.
From Bogduk N, Twomey L: *Clinical anatomy of the lumbar spine,* ed 3, London, 1997, Churchill Livingstone.

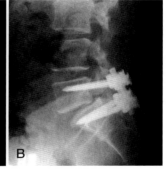

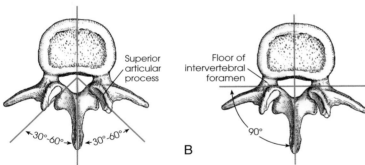

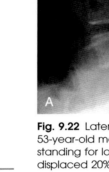

Fig. 9.21 (A) Direction of lumbar zygapophyseal joints. (B) Superior aspect showing orientation of lumbar intervertebral foramina. (C) Axial CT image of lumbar spine showing angles of zygapophyseal joints *(arrows)*.

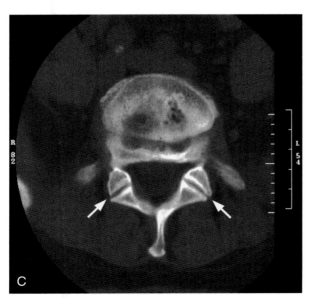

Fig. 9.22 Lateral lumbar spine showing spondylolisthesis. (A) A 53-year-old man presenting with pain in the legs and difficulty standing for longer than 5 minutes without pain. L4 is anteriorly displaced 20% over L5. (B) Surgery performed to stabilize spondylolisthesis. The patient recovered fully from pain.

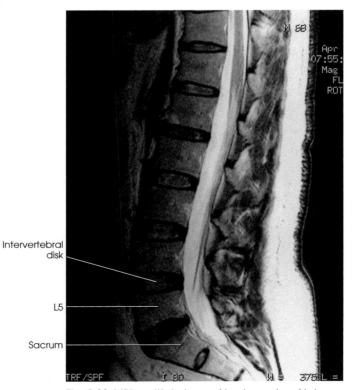

Fig. 9.23 MRI sagittal plane of lumbar spine. Note intervertebral disks between vertebral bodies.

Sacrum

The *sacrum* is formed by fusion of the five sacral vertebral segments into a curved, triangular bone (Figs. 9.24 and 9.25). The sacrum is wedged between the iliac bones of the pelvis, with its broad base directed obliquely, superiorly, and anteriorly, and its apex directed posteriorly and inferiorly. Although the size and degree of curvature of the sacrum vary considerably in different patients, the bone is normally longer, narrower, more evenly curved, and more vertical in position in males than in females. The female sacrum is more acutely curved, with its greatest curvature in the lower half of the bone; it also lies in a more oblique plane, which results in a sharper angle at the junction of the lumbar and pelvic curves.

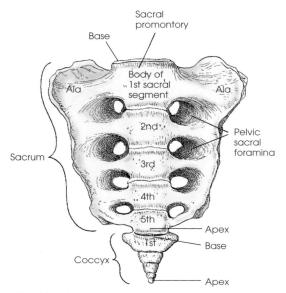

Fig. 9.24 Anterior aspect of sacrum and coccyx.

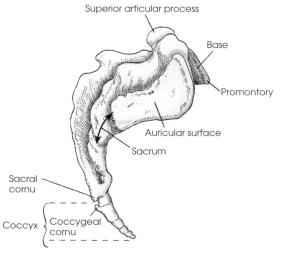

Fig. 9.25 Lateral aspect of sacrum and coccyx.

The superior portion of the first sacral segment remains distinct and resembles the vertebrae of the lumbar region (Fig. 9.26). The superior surface of the *base* of the sacrum corresponds in size and shape to the inferior surface of the last lumbar segment, with which it articulates to form the lumbosacral junction. The concavities on the upper surface of the pedicles of the first sacral segment and the corresponding concavities on the lower surface of the pedicles of the last lumbar segment form the last pair of intervertebral foramina. The *superior articular processes* of the first sacral segment articulate with the inferior articular processes of the last lumbar vertebra to form the last pair of zygapophyseal joints.

At its superior anterior margin, the base of the sacrum has a prominent ridge termed the *sacral promontory*. Directly behind the bodies of the sacral segments is the *sacral canal*, which is the continuation of the vertebral canal. The sacral canal is contained within the bone and transmits the sacral nerves (Fig. 9.27). Each of the anterior and posterior walls of the sacral canal is perforated by four pairs of *pelvic sacral foramina* for passage of the sacral nerves and blood vessels.

On each side of the sacral base is a large, winglike lateral mass called the *ala*. At the superoanterior part of the lateral surface of each ala is the *auricular surface*—a large articular process for articulation with similarly shaped processes on the iliac bones of the pelvis.

The inferior surface of the *apex* of the sacrum has an oval facet for articulation with the coccyx and the *sacral cornua*—two processes that project inferiorly from the posterolateral aspect of the last sacral segment to join the *coccygeal cornua*.

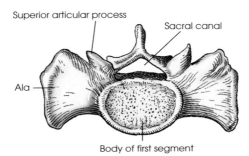

Fig. 9.26 Superior aspect of sacrum.

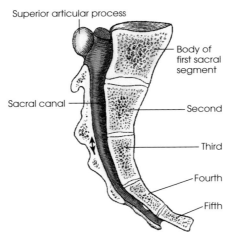

Fig. 9.27 Sagittal section of sacrum.

Coccyx

The *coccyx* is composed of three to five (usually four) rudimentary *vertebrae* that have a tendency to fuse into one bone in the adult (see Figs. 9.24 and 9.25). The coccyx diminishes in size from its *base* inferiorly to its *apex*. From its articulation with the sacrum, it curves inferiorly and anteriorly, often deviating from the midline of the body. The *coccygeal cornua* project superiorly from the posterolateral aspect of the first coccygeal segment to join the sacral cornua.

Vertebral Articulations

The joints of the vertebral column are shown in Fig. 9.28 and are summarized in Table 9.4. A detailed description follows.

The vertebral articulations consist of two types of joints: (1) *intervertebral* joints, which are between the two vertebral bodies and are *cartilaginous symphysis* joints that permit only slight movement of individual vertebrae but considerable motility for the column as a whole, and (2) *zygapophyseal* joints, which are between the articulation processes of the vertebral arches and are *synovial gliding* joints that permit free movement (see Fig. 9.20). Movements permitted in the vertebral column by the combined action of the joints are flexion, extension, lateral flexion, and rotation.

The articulations between the atlas and the occipital bone are *synovial ellipsoidal* joints and are called the *atlantooccipital articulations* (see Fig. 9.8). The anterior arch of the atlas rotates around the dens of the axis to form the *atlantoaxial* joint, which is a synovial gliding articulation and a *synovial pivot* articulation (see Table 9.4).

In the thoracic region, the heads of the ribs articulate with the bodies of the vertebrae to form the *costovertebral* joints, which are synovial gliding articulations. The tubercles of the ribs and the transverse processes of the thoracic vertebrae articulate to form *costotransverse* joints, which are also synovial gliding articulations (see Fig. 9.15).

The articulations between the sacrum and the two ilia—the sacroiliac joints—are discussed in Chapter 8.

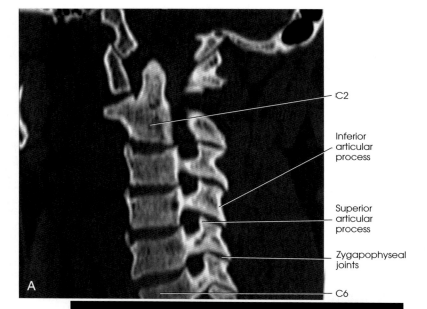

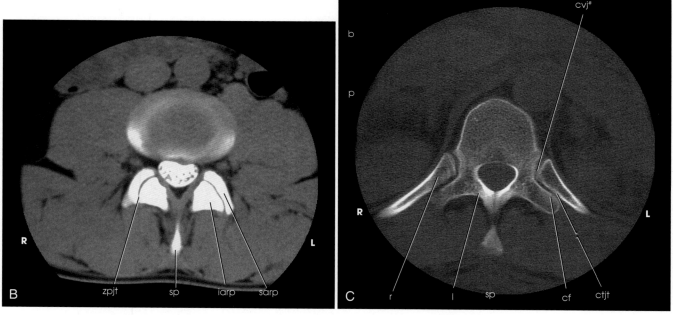

Fig. 9.28 Vertebral articulations. (A) CT reformat of cervical spine showing zygapophyseal joints. (B) CT scan of lumbar spine showing zygapophyseal joints. *iarp,* Inferior articulating process; *sarp,* superior articulating process; *zpjt,* zygapophyseal joint. (C) CT scan of thoracic vertebra. *cf,* Costal facet; *ctjt,* costotransverse joint; *cvjt,* costovertebral joint; *l,* lamina; *r,* rib.

SUMMARY OF ANATOMY

Vertebral column (spine)
Vertebrae (24)
  Cervical (7)
  Thoracic (12)
  Lumbar (5)
  Sacral
  Coccygeal
True vertebrae
False vertebrae
Sacrum
Coccyx

Vertebral curvature
Curves
  Cervical
  Thoracic
  Lumbar
  Pelvic
Lordotic curve
Kyphotic curve
Lumbosacral angle
Primary curves
Secondary or
  compensatory curves

Typical vertebra
Body
Vertebral arch
Vertebral foramen
Vertebral canal
Articular cartilage plate
Intervertebral disks
  Nucleus pulposus
  Annulus fibrosus
Pedicles
Vertebral notches
Intervertebral foramina
Laminae
Transverse processes
Spinous process
Facets
Superior articular processes
Inferior articular processes

Cervical vertebrae
Atlas (first)
  Anterior arch
  Posterior arch
  Lateral masses
  Transverse atlantal
    ligament
Axis (second)
  Dens (odontoid process)
Cervical (seventh)
  Vertebra prominens
Typical cervical vertebra
  Transverse foramina
  Articular pillars

Thoracic vertebrae
Costal facets
Demifacets

Lumbar vertebrae
Mammillary process
Accessory process
Pars interarticularis

Sacrum
Base
Superior articular processes
Sacral promontory
Sacral canal
Pelvic sacral foramina
Ala
Auricular surface
Apex
Sacral cornua

Coccyx
Base
Apex
Coccygeal cornua

Vertebral articulations
Atlantooccipital
Atlantoaxial
  Lateral (2)
  Medial (1—dens)
Costovertebral
Costotransverse
Intervertebral
Zygapophyseal (facet)

ABBREVIATIONS USED IN CHAPTER 9

EAM	External acoustic meatus
HNP	Herniated nucleus pulposus
IOML	Infraorbitomeatal line
MSP	Midsagittal plane

See Addendum A for a summary of all abbreviations used in Volume 1.

TABLE 9.4
Joints of the vertebral column

| | Structural classification | | |
Joint	Tissue	Type	Movement
Atlantooccipital	Synovial	Ellipsoidal	Freely movable
Atlantoaxial			
Lateral (2)	Synovial	Gliding	Freely movable
Medial (1—dens)	Synovial	Pivot	Freely movable
Intervertebral	Cartilaginous	Symphysis	Slightly movable
Zygapophyseal	Synovial	Gliding	Freely movable
Costovertebral	Synovial	Gliding	Freely movable
Costotransverse	Synovial	Gliding	Freely movable

SUMMARY OF PATHOLOGY

Condition	Definition
Ankylosing spondylitis	Rheumatoid arthritis variant involving the sacroiliac joints and spine
Fracture	Disruption in the continuity of bone
Clay shoveler's	Avulsion fracture of the spinous process in the lower cervical and upper thoracic region
Compression	Fracture that causes compaction of bone and a decrease in length or width
Hangman's	Fracture of the anterior arch of C2 owing to hyperextension
Jefferson	Comminuted fracture of the ring of C1
Herniated nucleus pulposus	Rupture or prolapse of the nucleus pulposus into the spinal canal
Kyphosis	Abnormally increased anterior concavity (posterior convexity) in the thoracic curvature
Lordosis	Abnormally increased anterior convexity (posterior concavity) of the cervical and lumbar spine
Metastasis	Transfer of a cancerous lesion from one area to another
Osteoarthritis or degenerative joint disease and vertebrae	Form of arthritis marked by progressive cartilage deterioration in synovial joints
Osteopetrosis	Increased density of atypically soft bone
Osteoporosis	Loss of bone density
Paget disease	Thick, soft bone marked by bowing and fractures
Scheuermann disease or adolescent kyphosis	Kyphosis with onset in adolescence
Scoliosis	Lateral deviation of the spine with possible vertebral rotation
Spina bifida	Failure of the posterior encasement of the spinal cord to close
Spondylolisthesis	Forward displacement of a vertebra over a lower vertebra, usually L5–S1
Spondylolysis	Breaking down of the vertebra
Subluxation	Incomplete or partial dislocation
Tumor	New tissue growth where cell proliferation is uncontrolled
Multiple myeloma	Malignant neoplasm of plasma cells involving the bone marrow and causing destruction of bone

Eponymous (named) pathologies are listed in nonpossessive form to conform to the *AMA manual of style: a guide to authors and editors*, ed 10, Oxford, 2009, Oxford University Press.

These techniques were accurate for the equipment used to produce each exposure. However, use caution when applying them in your department because "there is considerable variability in image receptor response owing to varying scatter sensitivity, the use of grids with different grid ratios, collimation, beam filtration, the choice of kilovoltage, source-to-image distance, and image receptor size."[1]

This chart was created in collaboration with Dennis Bowman, AS, RT(R), Clinical Instructor, Community Hospital of the Monterey Peninsula, Monterey, CA. http://digitalradiographysolutions.com/.

VERTEBRAL COLUMN

Part	cm	kVp[a]	SID[b]	Collimation	CR[c] mAs	CR[c] Dose (mGy)[e]	DR[d] mAs	DR[d] Dose (mGy)[e]
Atlas and axis—AP[f]	11	85	40"	6" × 4" (15 × 10 cm)	8[g]	0.776	3.6[g]	0.346
Dens—AP (Fuchs)[f]	14	85	40"	5" × 5" (13 × 13 cm)	12.5[g]	1.380	7.1[g]	0.782
Cervical vertebrae—AP axial[f]	11	85	40"	5" × 10" (13 × 25 cm)	6.3[g]	0.697	3.2[g]	0.351
Cervical vertebrae—lateral (Grandy)[f]	11	85	72"	7" × 10" (18 × 25 cm)	16[g]	1.848	8[g]	0.921
Cervical vertebrae—hyperflexion and hyperextension[f]	11	85	72"	8" × 10" (20 × 25 cm)	18[g]	2.092	7.1[g]	0.821
Cervical intervertebral foramina—AP and PA axial oblique[f]	11	85	72"	6" × 10" (15 × 25 cm)	22[g]	2.530	10[g]	1.144
Cervicothoracic region—lateral (swimmer's)[f]	24	96	40"	7" × 12" (18 × 30 cm)	65[h]	14.23	28[h]	6.110
Thoracic vertebrae—AP[f]	21	90	40"	5" × 17" (13 × 43 cm)	20[h]	3.270	8[h]	1.296
Thoracic vertebrae—lateral[f]	33	90	40"	8" × 17" (20 × 43 cm)	50[h]	12.87	25[h]	6.410
Lumbar vertebrae—AP[f]	21	90	40"	9" × 14" (23 × 35 cm)	20[h]	3.650	10[h]	1.826
Lumbar vertebrae—lateral[f]	27	96	40"	8" × 14" (20 × 35 cm)	56[h]	13.66	28[h]	6.790
Lumbar L5–S1—lateral[f]	31	96	40"	5" × 5" (13 × 13 cm)	100[h]	18.01	45[h]	8.060
Zygapophyseal joints—AP oblique[f]	23	90	40"	8" × 14" (20 × 35 cm)	36[h]	7.010	18[h]	3.480
Lumbosacral junction and sacroiliac joints—AP axial[f]	17	90	40"	10" × 8" (25 × 20 cm)	28[h]	4.560	14[h]	2.270
Sacroiliac joints—AP oblique[f]	17	90	40"	10" × 7" (25 × 18 cm)	36[h]	5.820	16[h]	2.580
Sacrum—AP axial[f]	17	90	40"	8" × 7" (20 × 18 cm)	28[h]	4.480	14[h]	2.233
Sacrum—lateral[f]	31	96	40"	8" × 5" (20 × 13 cm)	100[h]	19.95	45[h]	10.07
Coccyx—AP axial[f]	17	85	40"	4" × 5" (10 × 13 cm)	32[h]	3.480	14[h]	1.519
Coccyx—lateral[f]	31	85	40"	4" × 5" (10 × 13 cm)	90[h]	10.98	40[h]	4.580
Thoracolumbar spine-scoliosis—PA (Frank and Ferguson)[f]	23	90	40"	8" × 17" (20 × 43 cm)	28[h]	5.530	12.5[h]	2.460

[1]ACR-AAPM-SIMM Practice Parameter for Digital Radiography, revised 2017.
[a]kVp values are for a high-frequency generator.
[b]40 inches minimum; 44–48 inches recommended to improve spatial resolution (mAs increase needed, but no increase in patient dose will result).
[c]AGFA CR MD 4.0 General IP, CR 75.0 reader, 400 speed class, with 6:1 (178LPI) grid when needed.
[d]GE Definium 8000, with 13:1 grid when needed.
[e]All doses are skin entrance for average adult (160 to 200 pound male, 150 to 190 pound female) at part thickness indicated.
[f]Bucky/Grid.
[g]Small focal spot.
[h]Large focal spot.

SUMMARY OF OBLIQUE PROJECTIONS

Projection	Position—degrees	Structures shown	CR (degrees)
Cervical obliques			
AP obliques	LPO—45	R: IFs (side up)	15–20
	RPO—45	L: IFs (side up)	15–20
PA obliques	LAO—45	L: IFs (side down)	15–20
	RAO—45	R: IFs (side down)	15–20
Thoracic obliques			
AP obliques	LPO—70	R: Z joints (joints up)	0
	RPO—70	L: Z joints (joints up)	0
PA obliques	LAO—70	L: Z joints (joints down)	0
	RAO—70	R: Z joints (joints down)	0
Lumbar obliques			
AP obliques	LPO—45	L: Z joints (joints down)	0
	RPO—45	R: Z joints (joints down)	0
PA obliques	LAO—45	R: Z joints (joints up)	0
	RAO—45	L: Z joints (joints up)	0
Sacroiliac obliques			
AP obliques	LPO—25–30	R: SI joint (joint up)	0
	RPO—25–30	L: SI joint (joint up)	0
PA obliques	LAO—25–30	L: SI joint (joint down)	0
	RAO—25–30	R: SI joint (joint down)	0

▲ AP PROJECTION
FUCHS METHOD

Fuchs[1] recommended the AP projection to show the dens when its upper half is not clearly shown in the open-mouth position. This patient position must not be attempted if fracture or degenerative disease of the upper cervical region is suspected.

> **Image receptor +grid:** Positioned by manufacturer or department protocol for proper anatomy display orientation; CR plate: 10 × 12 inches (24 × 30 cm) crosswise.

Position of patient
- Place the patient in the supine position.
- Center the midsagittal plane (MSP) of the body to the midline of the grid.
- Place the arms along the sides of the body.
- Place a support under the patient's knees for comfort.

Position of part
- Place the IR in the Bucky tray, and center the IR to the level of the tips of the mastoid processes.
- Extend the chin until the tip of the chin and the tip of the mastoid process are vertical (Fig. 9.29).
- Adjust the head so that the MSP is perpendicular to the plane of the grid.
- *Shield gonads.*
- *Respiration:* Suspend.

Central ray
- Perpendicular to the midpoint of the IR; enters the neck on the MSP just distal to the tip of the chin

Collimation
- Adjust radiation field to 5 × 5 inches (13 × 13 cm) on the collimator. Place the side marker in the collimated exposure field.

Structures shown
An AP projection of the dens lying within the circular foramen magnum (Fig. 9.30).

EVALUATION CRITERIA
The following should be clearly seen:
- Evidence of proper collimation and presence of the side marker placed clear of anatomy of interest
- Entire dens within the foramen magnum
- No rotation of the head or neck, demonstrated by symmetry of the mandible, cranium, and vertebrae
- Bony trabecular detail and surrounding soft tissues

PA PROJECTION
JUDD METHOD

Because of the difficulty in positioning the patient, especially a patient who has a potential fracture, this projection is no longer described in full. In addition, computed tomography (CT) is now used to evaluate the upper cervical area. This method is described in the tenth and previous editions.

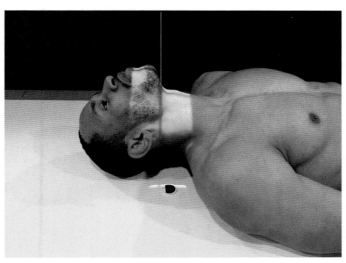

Fig. 9.29 AP dens: Fuchs method.

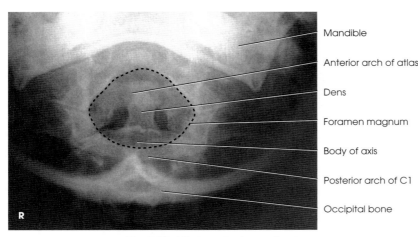

Mandible

Anterior arch of atlas

Dens

Foramen magnum

Body of axis

Posterior arch of C1

Occipital bone

Fig. 9.30 AP dens: Fuchs method.

▲ AP PROJECTION
Open-mouth

The open-mouth technique was described by Albers-Schönberg[2] in 1910 and by George[3] in 1919.

> **Image receptor + grid:** Positioned by manufacturer or department protocol for proper anatomy display orientation; CR plate: 10 × 12 inches (24 × 30 cm).

> **SID:** A 30-inch (76-cm) SID may be used for this projection to increase the field of view of the odontoid area. See Chapter 1 for use of a 30-inch (76-cm) SID.

Position of patient
- Place the patient in the supine position.
- Center the MSP of the body to the midline of the grid.

- Place the patient's arms along the sides of the body, and adjust the shoulders to lie in the same horizontal plane.
- Place a support under the patient's knees for comfort.

Position of part
- Place the IR in the Bucky tray, and center the IR at the level of the axis.
- Adjust the patient's head so that the MSP is perpendicular to the plane of the table (Figs. 9.31 and 9.32).
- Select the exposure factors, and move the x-ray tube into position so that any minor change can be made quickly after the final adjustment of the patient's head. Although this position is not easy to hold, the patient is usually able to cooperate fully unless he or she is kept in the final, strained position too long.
- Have the patient open the mouth as wide as possible, and then adjust the head so that a line from the lower edge of the upper incisors to the tip of the mastoid process (occlusal plane) is perpendicular to the IR. A small support under the back of the head may be needed to facilitate opening of the mouth while proper alignment of the upper incisors and mastoid tips is maintained.
- *Shield gonads.*
- *Respiration:* Instruct the patient to keep the mouth wide open and to phonate "ah" softly during the exposure. This places the tongue in the floor of the mouth so that it is not projected on the atlas and axis and prevents movement of the mandible.

Central ray
- Perpendicular to the center of the IR and entering the midpoint of the open mouth

Collimation
- Adjust radiation field to 5 × 5 inches (13 × 13 cm) on the collimator. Place the side marker in the collimated exposure field.

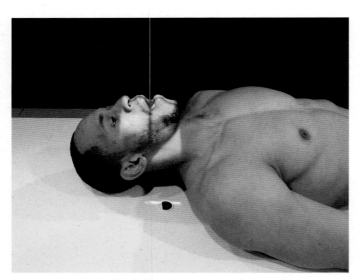

Fig. 9.31 AP atlas and axis.

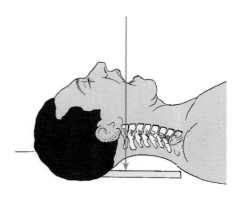

Fig. 9.32 Open-mouth spine alignment.

Structures shown

An AP projection of the atlas and axis through the open mouth (Figs. 9.33 and 9.34). If the patient has a deep head or a long mandible, the entire atlas is not shown. When the exactly superimposed shadows of the occlusal surface of the upper central incisors and the base of the skull are in line with those of the tips of the mastoid processes, the position cannot be improved. If the patient cannot open the mouth, tomography may be required (Fig. 9.35).

EVALUATION CRITERIA

The following should be clearly seen:

- Evidence of proper collimation and presence of the side marker placed clear of anatomy of interest
- Dens, atlas, axis, and articulations between the first and second cervical vertebrae
- Entire articular surfaces of the atlas and axis (to check for lateral displacement)
- Mouth open wide
- Superimposed occlusal plane of the upper central incisors and the base of the skull, demonstrating proper neck flexion
  - □ If the upper incisors are projected over the dens, the neck is flexed too much toward the chest.
  - □ If the base of the skull is projected over the dens, the neck is extended too much.
- Shadow of the tongue not projected over the atlas and axis
- Mandibular rami equidistant from dens, demonstrating proper head rotation
- Bony trabecular detail and surrounding soft tissues

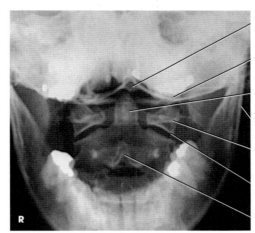

Occipital base

Occlusal surface of teeth

Dens (odontoid process)

Mandibular ramus

Lateral mass of atlas

Inferior articular process of atlas

Spinous process of axis

Fig. 9.33 Open-mouth atlas and axis.

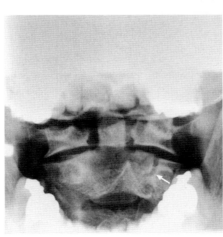

Fig. 9.34 Open-mouth atlas and axis, showing fracture of left lateral mass of axis (*arrow*), performed at a 30-inch SID.

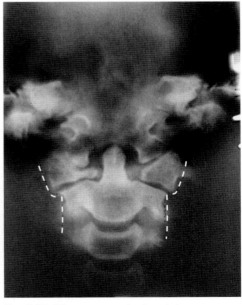

Fig. 9.35 AP upper cervical vertebrae tomogram of a patient who fell and landed on his head. A bursting-type Jefferson fracture caused outward displacement of both lateral masses of atlas. A tomogram is often necessary to show upper cervical area in trauma patients who cannot move their heads or open their mouths.

LATERAL PROJECTION
Right or left position

> **Image receptor + grid:** Positioned by manufacturer or department protocol for proper anatomy display orientation; CR plate: 10 × 12 inches (24 × 30 cm).

Position of patient
- Place the patient in the supine position.
- Place the arms along the sides of the body, and adjust the shoulders to lie in the same horizontal plane.
- Place a sponge or pad under the patient's head unless traumatic injury has been sustained, in which case the neck should not be moved.

Position of part
- With the IR in the vertical position and in contact with the upper neck, center it at the level of the atlantoaxial articulation (1 inch [2.5 cm] distal to the tip of the mastoid process).

- Adjust the IR so that it is parallel with the MSP of the neck, and then support the IR in position (Figs. 9.36 and 9.37).
- Extend the neck slightly so that the shadow of the mandibular rami does not overlap that of the spine.
- Adjust the head so that the MSP is perpendicular to the table.
- *Shield gonads.*
- *Respiration:* Suspend.

Central ray
- Perpendicular to a point 1 inch (2.5 cm) distal to the adjacent mastoid tip

Collimation
- Adjust radiation field to 5 × 5 inches (13 × 13 cm) on the collimator. Place the side marker in the collimated exposure field.

Structures shown
A lateral projection of the atlas and axis. The atlantooccipital articulations are also shown (Fig. 9.38).

EVALUATION CRITERIA
The following should be clearly seen:
- Evidence of proper collimation and presence of the side marker placed clear of anatomy of interest
- Upper cervical vertebrae
- MSP of head and neck parallel to plane of IR, without tilt or rotation
    - Superimposed laminae of the axis and superimposed posterior arches of the atlas
    - Nearly superimposed rami of the mandible
- Neck extended so that the mandibular rami does not overlap the axis or atlas
- Bony trabecular detail and surrounding soft tissues

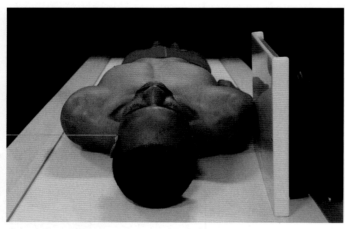

Fig. 9.36 Position for lateral atlas and axis.

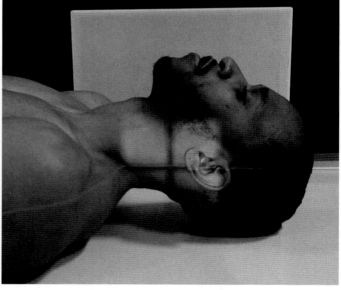

Fig. 9.37 Side view as seen for centering CR.

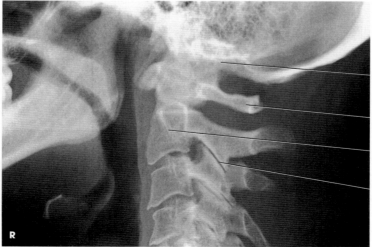

Atlantooccipital articulation

Posterior arch atlas

Body of axis

C2-C3 Zygapophyseal joint

Fig. 9.38 Lateral atlas and axis.

Vertebral Column

⚘ AP AXIAL PROJECTION

Image receptor + grid: Positioned by manufacturer or department protocol for proper anatomy display orientation; CR plate: 10 × 12 inches (24 × 30 cm) lengthwise.

Position of patient

- Place the patient in the supine or upright position with the back against the IR holder.
- Adjust the patient's shoulders to lie in the same horizontal plane to prevent rotation.

Position of part

- Center the MSP of the patient's body to the midline of the table or vertical grid device.
- Extend the chin enough so that the occlusal plane is perpendicular to the tabletop. This prevents superimposition of the mandible and midcervical vertebrae (Figs. 9.39 and 9.40).
- Center the IR at the level of C4.
- Adjust the head so that the MSP is in straight alignment and perpendicular to the IR.

- Provide support for the head of any patient who has a pronounced lordotic curvature. This support helps compensate for the curvature and reduces image distortion.
- *Shield gonads.*
- *Respiration:* Suspend.

Central ray

- Directed through C4 at an angle of 15 to 20 degrees cephalad. The central ray enters at or slightly inferior to the most prominent point of the thyroid cartilage, commonly called the "Adam's apple."

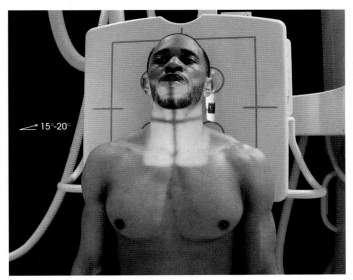

Fig. 9.39 AP axial cervical vertebrae: upright.

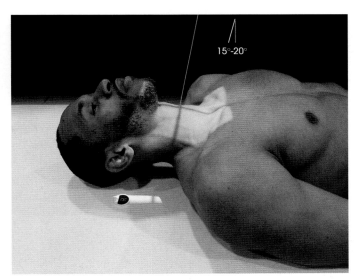

Fig. 9.40 AP axial cervical vertebrae: recumbent.

Cervical Vertebrae

Collimation

• Adjust radiation field to 10 inches (25 cm) lengthwise and 1 inch (2.5 cm) beyond the skin shadow on the sides. Place the side marker in the collimated exposure field.

Structures shown

The lower five cervical bodies and the upper two or three thoracic bodies, the interpediculate spaces, the superimposed transverse and articular processes, and the intervertebral disk spaces (Fig. 9.41). This projection is also used to show the presence or absence of cervical ribs.

EVALUATION CRITERIA

The following should be clearly seen:

■ Evidence of proper collimation and presence of the side marker placed clear of anatomy of interest

■ Area from superior portion of C3 to T2 and surrounding soft tissue

■ Shadows of the mandible and occiput superimposed over the atlas and most of the axis

■ Open intervertebral disk spaces

■ MSP of head and neck perpendicular to plane of IR, without tilt or rotation

    □ Spinous processes equidistant to the pedicles and aligned with the midline of the cervical bodies

    □ Mandibular angles and mastoid processes equidistant to the vertebrae

■ Bony trabecular detail and surrounding soft tissues

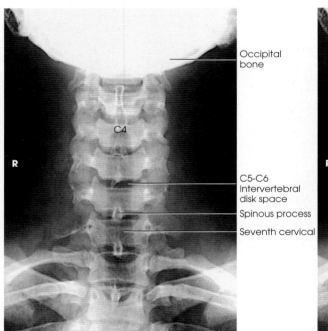
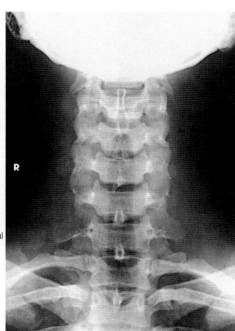

Fig. 9.41 AP axial cervical vertebrae.

Occipital bone

C4

C5-C6 Intervertebral disk space

Spinous process

Seventh cervical

R

R

Vertebral Column

✦ LATERAL PROJECTION
GRANDY METHOD[4]
Right or left position

Image receptor + grid: Positioned by manufacturer or department protocol for proper anatomy display orientation; CR plate: 10 × 12 inches (24 × 30 cm) lengthwise.

SID: A 60- to 72-inch (152- to 183-cm) SID is recommended to compensate for the increased OID. A longer distance helps show C7.

Position of patient
- Place the patient in a true lateral position, either seated or standing, before a vertical grid device. The long axis of the cervical vertebrae should be parallel to the plane of the IR.
- Have the patient sit or stand straight, and adjust the height of the IR so that it is centered at the level of C4. The top of the IR is about 1 inch (2.5 cm) above the external acoustic meatus (EAM).

Position of part
- Center the coronal plane that passes through the mastoid tips to the midline of the IR.
- Move the patient close enough to the vertical grid device to permit the adjacent shoulder to rest against the device for support (Fig. 9.42). (This projection may be performed without the use of a grid.)
- Rotate the shoulders anteriorly or posteriorly according to the natural kyphosis of the back: If the patient is round shouldered, rotate the shoulders anteriorly; otherwise, rotate them posteriorly.
- Adjust the shoulders to lie in the same horizontal plane, depress them as much as possible, and immobilize them by attaching one small sandbag to each *wrist*. The sandbags should be of equal weight.

- Be careful to ensure that the patient does not elevate the shoulder.
- Elevate the chin slightly, or have the patient protrude the mandible to prevent superimposition of the mandibular rami and the spine. At the same time and with the MSP of the head vertical, ask the patient to look steadily at one spot on the wall; this helps maintain the position of the head.
- *Shield gonads.*
- *Respiration:* Suspend respiration at the end of full expiration to obtain maximum depression of the shoulders.

NOTE: If cervical spine trauma is suspected, this projection must be performed **first** and "cleared" by the radiologist before additional images are performed. Refer to Chapter 12 in Volume 2 for details related to performing this projection on patients with suspected cervical spine trauma.

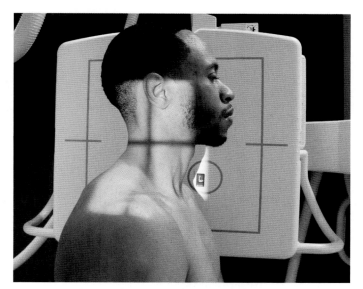

Fig. 9.42 Lateral cervical vertebrae: Grandy method.

Central ray

- Horizontal and perpendicular to C4. With such centering, the magnified outline of the shoulder *farthest* from the IR is projected below the lower cervical vertebrae.

Collimation

- Adjust radiation field to 10 × 12 inches (24 × 30 cm) on the collimator. Place the side marker in the collimated exposure field.

Structures shown

The cervical bodies and their intervertebral disk spaces, the articular pillars, the lower five zygapophyseal joints, and the spinous processes (Figs. 9.43 and 9.44). Depending on how well the shoulders can be depressed, a good lateral projection must include C7; sometimes T1 and T2 can also be seen.

EVALUATION CRITERIA

The following should be clearly seen:

- Evidence of proper collimation and presence of the side marker placed clear of anatomy of interest
- All seven cervical vertebrae and at least one-third of the T1 (otherwise a separate radiograph of the cervicothoracic region is recommended)
- C4 in the center of the radiograph
- Neck extended so that mandibular rami are not overlapping the atlas or axis
- No rotation or tilt of the cervical spine
  - ☐ Superimposed zygapophyseal joints and open intervertebral disk spaces
  - ☐ Superimposed or nearly superimposed rami of the mandible
  - ☐ Spinous processes shown in profile
- Bony trabecular detail and surrounding soft tissues

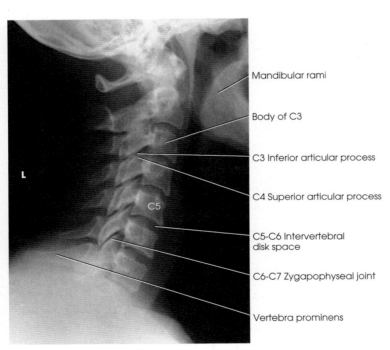

Mandibular rami

Body of C3

C3 Inferior articular process

C4 Superior articular process

C5-C6 Intervertebral disk space

C6-C7 Zygapophyseal joint

Vertebra prominens

Fig. 9.43 Lateral cervical vertebrae: Grandy method.

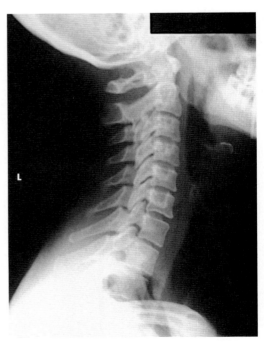

Fig. 9.44 Same projection as in Fig. 9.43 provides excellent visualization of all seven cervical vertebrae and T1.

♠ LATERAL PROJECTION
Right or left position
Flexion and extension

NOTE: This procedure must not be attempted until cervical spine pathology or fracture has been ruled out.

Functional studies of the cervical vertebrae in the lateral position are performed to show normal intersegmental movement or changes in intersegmental alignment resulting from trauma or disease. The spinous processes are elevated and widely separated in the flexion position and are depressed in close approximation in the extension position.

Image receptor + grid: Positioned by manufacturer or department protocol for proper anatomy display orientation; CR plate: 10 × 12 inches (24 × 30 cm) lengthwise.

SID: A 60- to 72-inch (152- to 183-cm) SID is recommended to compensate for the increased OID. A longer distance helps show C7.

Position of patient
- Place the patient in a true lateral position, either seated or standing, before a vertical grid device.
- Have the patient sit or stand straight, and adjust the height of the IR so that it is centered at the level of C4. The top of the IR is about 2 inches (5 cm) above the EAM.

Position of part
- Move the patient close enough to the vertical grid device to permit the adjacent shoulder to rest against the grid for support.
- Keep the MSP of the patient's head and neck parallel with the plane of the IR.
- Alternatively, perform the projection without using a grid.

Flexion
- Ask the patient to drop the head forward and then draw the chin as close as possible to the chest, so that the cervical vertebrae are placed in a position of maximum flexion for the first exposure (Fig. 9.45).

Extension
- Ask the patient to elevate the chin as much as possible, so that the cervical vertebrae are placed in a position of maximum extension for the second exposure (Fig. 9.46).
- *Shield gonads.*
- *Respiration:* Suspend.

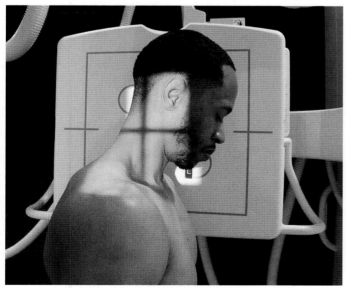

Fig. 9.45 Lateral cervical vertebrae: hyperflexion.

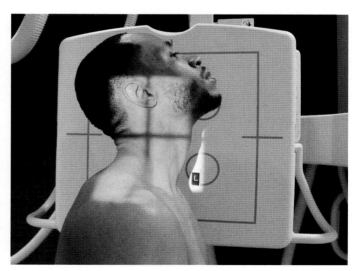

Fig. 9.46 Lateral cervical vertebrae: hyperextension.

Central ray

- Horizontal and perpendicular to C4

Collimation

- Adjust radiation field to 10 × 12 inches (24 × 30 cm) on the collimator. For flexion, light should extend from EAC anteriorly to C7 spinous process posteriorly. For extension, light should extend from midmandible anteriorly to C7 spinous process posteriorly. Place the side marker in the collimated exposure field.

Structures shown

Intersegmental alignment of the cervical spine when flexed (Fig. 9.47) and extended (Fig. 9.48). The intervertebral disks and the zygapophyseal joints are also shown.

NOTE: The radiologist evaluates the posterior aspect of vertebral bodies for intersegmental alignment.

The following should be clearly seen:

- Evidence of proper collimation and presence of the side marker placed clear of anatomy of interest
- All seven cervical vertebrae in true lateral position
- No rotation or tilt of the cervical spine
  - □ Superimposed zygapophyseal joints and open intervertebral disk spaces
  - □ Superimposed or nearly superimposed rami of the mandible
  - □ Spinous processes shown in profile
- Bony trabecular detail and surrounding soft tissues

Flexion

- Body of the mandible almost vertical in a normal patient
- All seven spinous processes in profile, elevated and widely separated

Extension

- Body of the mandible almost horizontal in a normal patient
- All seven spinous processes in profile, depressed and closely spaced

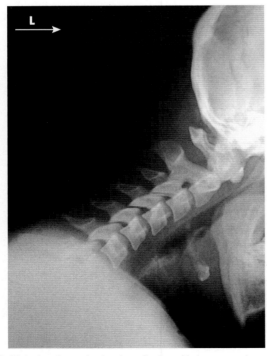

Fig. 9.47 Lateral cervical spine: flexion. Note correct marking.

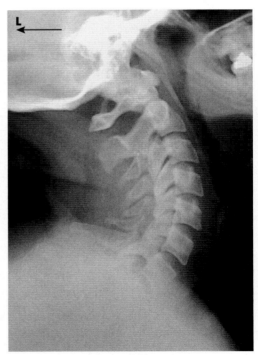

Fig. 9.48 Lateral cervical spine: extension. Note correct marking.

☀ AP AXIAL OBLIQUE PROJECTION

RPO and LPO positions

Oblique projections for showing the cervical intervertebral foramina were first described by Barsóny and Koppenstein.[5,6] Both sides are examined for comparison.

Image receptor + grid: Positioned by manufacturer or department protocol for proper anatomy display orientation; CR plate: 10 × 12 inches (24 × 30 cm) lengthwise.

SID: A 60- to 72-inch (152- to 183-cm) SID is recommended to compensate for the increased OID.

Position of patient

• Place the patient in a supine or upright position facing the x-ray tube. The upright position (standing or seated) is preferable for the patient's comfort and makes it easier to position the patient.

Position of part

• Adjust the body (including the head) at a 45-degree angle, and center the cervical spine to the midline of the IR.
• Center the IR to the third cervical body (1 inch [2.5 cm] superior to the most prominent point of the thyroid cartilage) to compensate for the cephalic angulation of the central ray.

Upright posterior oblique position

• Ask the patient to sit or stand straight without strain and to rest the adjacent shoulder firmly against the vertical grid device for support.
• Ensure that the degree of body rotation is 45 degrees.
• While the patient looks straight ahead, elevate and, if needed, protrude the chin so that the mandible does not overlap the spine (Fig. 9.49). Turning the chin to the side causes slight rotation of the superior vertebrae and should be avoided.

Recumbent posterior oblique position

• Rotate the patient's head and body approximately 45 degrees.
• Center the cervical spine to the midline of the grid.
• Place suitable supports under the lower thorax and the elevated hip.
• Place a support under the patient's head, and adjust it so that the cervical column is horizontal.
• Check and adjust the 45-degree body rotation.
• Elevate the patient's chin and protrude the jaw as for the upright study (Fig. 9.50). Turning the chin to the side causes slight rotation of the superior vertebrae and should be avoided.
• *Shield gonads.*
• *Respiration:* Suspend.

NOTE: See p. 436 for the Summary of Oblique Projections.

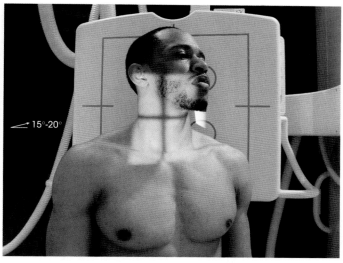

Fig. 9.49 Upright AP axial oblique right intervertebral foramina: LPO position.

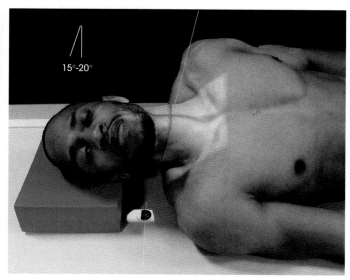

Fig. 9.50 Recumbent AP axial oblique left intervertebral foramina: RPO position.

Central ray

- Directed to C4 at a cephalad angle of 15 to 20 degrees so that the central ray coincides with the orientation of the foramina

Collimation

- Adjust radiation field to 10 × 12 inches (24 × 30 cm) on the collimator. Place the side marker in the collimated exposure field.

Structures shown

The intervertebral foramina and pedicles *farthest* from the IR and an oblique projection of the bodies and other parts of the cervical vertebrae (Fig. 9.51). (See the Summary of Oblique Projections, p. 436.)

The following should be clearly seen:

- Evidence of proper collimation and presence of the side marker placed clear of anatomy of interest
- All seven cervical and the first thoracic vertebrae
- Appropriate 45-degree rotation of body and neck
  - Open intervertebral foramina *farthest* from the IR, from C2–C3 to C7–T1
  - Uniform size and contour of the foramina
- Appropriately elevated chin
  - Mandible not overlapping the atlas and axis
  - Occipital bone not overlapping the atlas and axis
- Open intervertebral disk spaces
- Bony trabecular detail and surrounding soft tissues

AP OBLIQUE PROJECTION
Flexion and extension

Boylston[7] suggested using functional studies of the cervical vertebrae in the oblique to show fractures of the articular processes and obscure dislocations and subluxations. When acute injury has been sustained, manipulation of the patient's head must be performed by a physician.

The patient is placed in a direct frontal body position facing the x-ray tube, with the shoulders held firmly against the grid device. The head is carefully rotated maximally to one side and is kept in that position while the neck is fully flexed for the first exposure and fully extended for the second exposure. Both sides are examined for comparison.

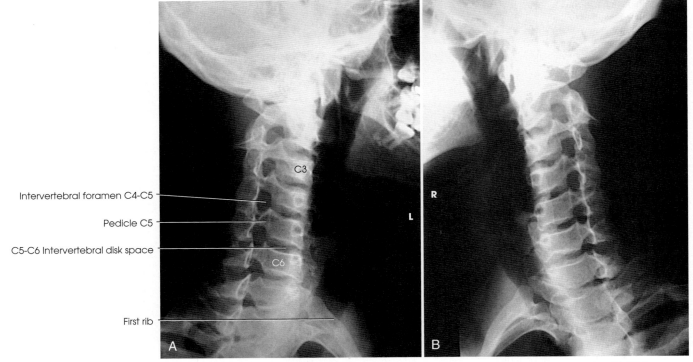

Intervertebral foramen C4-C5

Pedicle C5

C5-C6 Intervertebral disk space

First rib

Fig. 9.51 AP axial oblique intervertebral foramina. (A) LPO position showing right side. (B) RPO position showing left side.

⚜ PA AXIAL OBLIQUE PROJECTION
RAO and LAO positions

Image receptor + grid: Positioned by manufacturer or department protocol for proper anatomy display orientation; CR plate: 10 × 12 inches (24 × 30 cm) lengthwise.

SID: A 60- to 72-inch (152- to 183-cm) SID is recommended to compensate for the increased OID.

Position of patient
- Place the patient prone or upright with the back toward the x-ray tube. For the patient's comfort and accurate adjustment of the part, the standing or seated-upright position is preferred.

Position of part
- *Upright anterior oblique position:* Ask the patient to sit or stand straight with the arms by the side and rest the shoulder against the grid device. Rotate the patient's entire body to a 45-degree angle. Center the cervical spine to the midline of the grid device (Fig. 9.52).

- *Recumbent anterior oblique position:* Place the patient's body at an angle of 45 degrees and the cervical spine centered to the midline of the grid. Have the patient use the forearm and flexed knee of the elevated side to support the body and maintain the position (Figs. 9.53 and 9.54). Place a suitable support under the patient's head to position the long axis of the cervical column parallel with the IR.
- To allow for the caudal angulation of the central ray, center the IR at the level of C5 (1 inch [2.5 cm] caudal to the most prominent point of the thyroid cartilage).
- Adjust the position of the patient's head so that the MSP is aligned with the plane of the spine.
- Elevate and protrude the patient's chin just enough to prevent superimposition of the mandible with the upper cervical vertebrae. Turning the chin to the side causes rotation of the superior vertebrae and should be avoided. (The chin has to be turned slightly for the recumbent anterior oblique position.)
- *Shield gonads.*
- *Respiration:* Suspend.

Central ray
- Directed to C4 at an angle of 15 to 20 degrees caudad so that it coincides with the orientation of the foramina.

Collimation
- Adjust radiation field to 10 × 12 inches (24 × 30 cm) in the collimator. Place the side marker in the collimated exposure field.

Structures shown
The intervertebral foramina and pedicles *closest* to the IR and an oblique projection of the bodies and other parts of the cervical column (Fig. 9.55). (See the Summary of Oblique Projections, p. 436.)

EVALUATION CRITERIA
The following should be clearly seen:
- Evidence of proper collimation and presence of the side marker placed clear of anatomy of interest
- All seven cervical and the first thoracic vertebrae
- Appropriate 45-degree rotation of body and neck
  - ☐ Open intervertebral foramina *closest* to the IR, from C2–C3 to C7–T1
  - ☐ Uniform size and contour of the foramina
- Appropriately elevated chin
  - ☐ Mandible not overlapping the atlas and axis
  - ☐ Occipital bone not overlapping the atlas and axis
- Open intervertebral disk spaces
- Bony trabecular detail and surrounding soft tissues

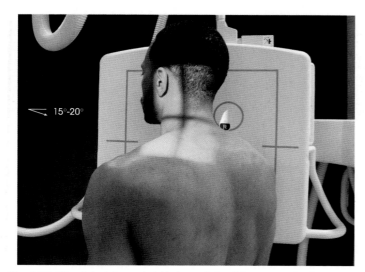

Fig. 9.52 PA axial oblique right intervertebral foramina: RAO position.

15°–20°

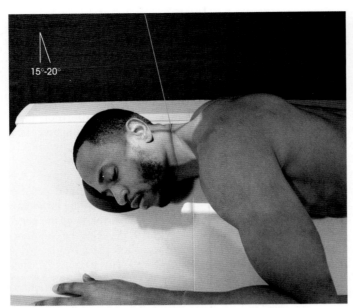

Fig. 9.53 PA axial oblique right intervertebral foramina: RAO position.

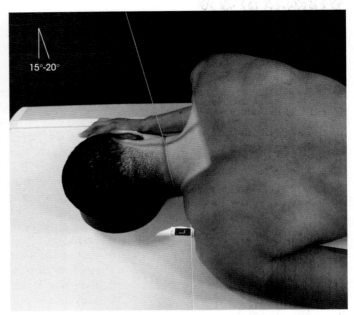

Fig. 9.54 PA axial oblique left intervertebral foramina: LAO position.

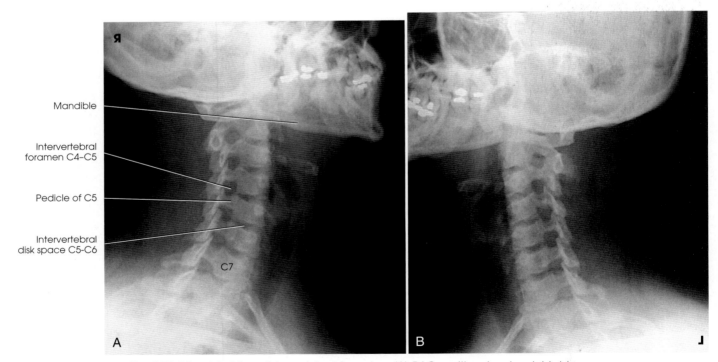

Mandible

Intervertebral foramen C4–C5

Pedicle of C5

Intervertebral disk space C5-C6

C7

A

B

Fig. 9.55 PA axial oblique intervertebral foramina. (A) RAO position showing right side. (B) LAO position showing left side.

AP PROJECTION
OTTONELLO METHOD

With the Ottonello method, the mandibular shadow is blurred or obliterated by having the patient perform an even chewing motion of the mandible during the exposure. The patient's head must be rigidly immobilized to prevent movement of the vertebrae. The exposure time must be long enough to cover several complete excursions of the mandible. This projection is also referred to as the "wagging jaw."

> **Image receptor + grid:** Positioned by manufacturer or department protocol for proper anatomy display orientation; CR plate: 10 × 12 inches (24 × 30 cm) lengthwise.

Position of patient
- Place the patient in the supine position.
- Center the MSP of the body to the midline of the grid.
- Place the patient's arms along the sides of the body, and adjust the shoulders to lie in the same horizontal plane.
- Place a support under the knees for the patient's comfort.

Position of part
- Adjust the patient's head so that the MSP is aligned with the lower body and is perpendicular to the table.
- Elevate the patient's chin enough to place the occlusal surface of the upper incisors and the mastoid tips in the same vertical plane.

- Immobilize the head, and have the patient practice opening and closing the mouth until the mandible can be moved smoothly without striking the teeth together (Fig. 9.56).
- Place the IR in a Bucky tray, and center the IR at the level of C4.
- To blur the mandible, use an exposure technique with low milliamperage (mA) and long exposure time (minimum of 1 second).
- *Shield gonads.*
- *Respiration:* Suspend.

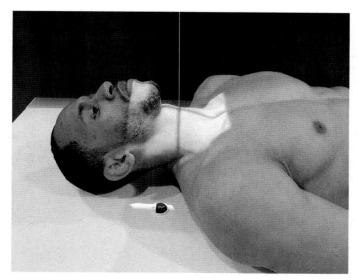

Fig. 9.56 AP cervical vertebrae: Ottonello method.

Central ray

- Perpendicular to C4; the central ray enters at the most prominent point of the thyroid cartilage.

Collimation

- Adjust radiation field to 10 × 12 inches (24 × 30 cm) on the collimator. Place the side marker in the collimated exposure field.

Structures shown

The entire cervical spine, with the mandible blurred or obliterated (Figs. 9.57 and 9.58).

The following should be clearly seen:
- Evidence of proper collimation and presence of the side marker placed clear of anatomy of interest
- All seven cervical vertebrae
- Blurred mandible with resultant visualization of the underlying atlas and axis
- Bony trabecular detail and surrounding soft tissues

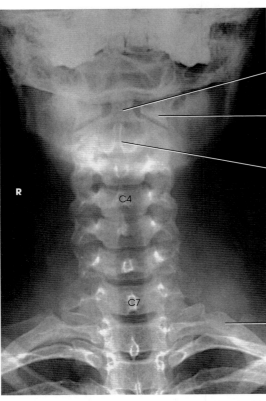

Dens

C1 lateral mass

Spinous process of C2

R

C4

C7

First rib

Fig. 9.57 AP cervical spine: Ottonello method with chewing motion of mandible and use of perpendicular central ray.

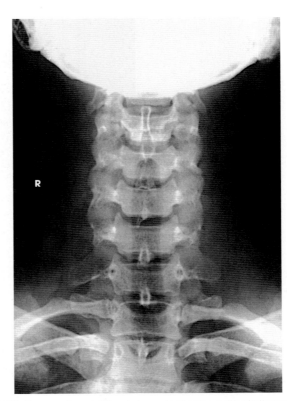

R

Fig. 9.58 Conventional AP axial cervical spine with stationary mandible and 15- to 20-degree cephalad angulation of central ray.

Vertebral Arch (Pillars)
AP AXIAL PROJECTION[8]

NOTE: The procedure must not be attempted until cervical spine pathology or fracture has been ruled out.

The vertebral arch projections, sometimes referred to as *pillar* or *lateral mass* projections, are used to show the posterior elements of the cervical vertebrae, the upper three or four thoracic vertebrae, the articular processes and their facets, the laminae, and the spinous processes. The central ray angulations that are employed project the vertebral arch elements free of the anteriorly situated vertebral bodies and transverse processes. When the central ray angulation is correct, the resultant image resembles a hemisection of the vertebrae. In addition to frontal plane delineation of the articular pillars and facets, vertebral arch projections are especially useful for showing the cervicothoracic spinous processes in patients with whiplash injury.[9]

Image receptor + grid: Positioned by manufacturer or department protocol for proper anatomy display orientation; CR plate: 10 × 12 inches (24 × 30 cm).

Position of patient
- Adjust the patient in the supine position with the MSP of the body centered to the midline of the grid.
- Depress the patient's shoulders, and adjust them to lie in the same horizontal plane.

Position of part
- With the MSP of the head perpendicular to the table, fully *extend* the patient's neck (Figs. 9.59 and 9.60).
- If the patient cannot tolerate full extension without undue discomfort, the oblique projection described in the next section is recommended.
- *Shield gonads.*
- *Respiration:* Suspend.

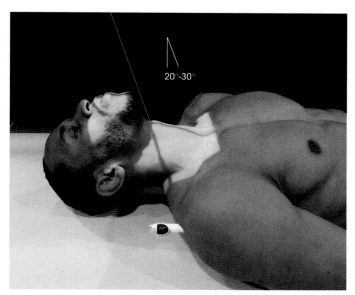

Fig. 9.59 AP axial vertebral arch.

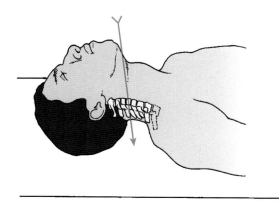

Fig. 9.60 AP axial vertebral arch.

Central ray

- Directed to C7 at an average angle of 25 degrees caudad (range, 20 to 30 degrees). The central ray enters the neck in the region of the thyroid cartilage.
- The degree of the central ray angulation is determined by the cervical lordosis. The goal is to have the central ray coincide with the plane of the articular facets so that a greater angle is required when the cervical curve is accentuated, and a lesser angle is required when the curve is diminished.
- To reduce an accentuated cervical curve and place C3–C7 in the same plane as T1–T4, the originators[8] of this technique have suggested that a radiolucent wedge be placed under the patient's neck and shoulders, with the head extended over the edge of the wedge.

Collimation

- Adjust radiation field to 10×12 inches (24×30 cm) on the collimator. Place the side marker in the collimated exposure field.

Structures shown

The posterior portion of the cervical and upper thoracic vertebrae, including the articular and spinous processes (Fig. 9.61).

EVALUATION CRITERIA

The following should be clearly seen:
- Evidence of proper collimation and presence of the side marker placed clear of anatomy of interest
- Vertebral arch structures, especially the superior and inferior articulating processes (pillars), without overlapping of the vertebral bodies and transverse processes
- Articular processes
- Open zygapophyseal joints between the articular processes
- Bony trabecular detail and surrounding soft tissues

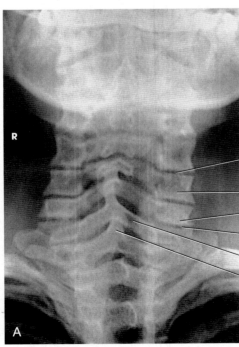
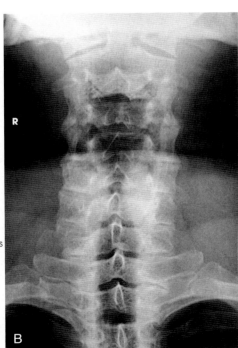

Zygapophyseal joint
Pillar or lateral mass
Inferior articular process
Superior articular process
Lamina
Spinous process

Fig. 9.61 AP axial. (A) Central ray parallel with plateau of articular processes. (B) Head fully extended but inadequate central ray angulation; central ray not parallel with zygapophyseal joints.

Vertebral Arch (Pillars)
AP AXIAL OBLIQUE PROJECTION
Right and left head rotations[10]

These radiographic projections are used to show the vertebral arches or pillars when the patient cannot fully extend the head for the AP axial projection. Both sides are examined for comparison.

> **Image receptor + grid:** Positioned by manufacturer or department protocol for proper anatomy display orientation; CR plate: 10 × 12 inches (24 × 30 cm).

Position of patient
• Place the patient in the supine position.

Position of part
• Rotate the patient's head 45 to 50 degrees, turning the jaw away from the side of interest. A 45- to 50-degree rotation of the head usually shows the articular processes of C2–C7 and T1. A rotation of 60 to 70 degrees is sometimes required to show the processes of C6 and T1–T4 (Fig. 9.62).
• Position the IR so that the top edge is at the level of the mastoid tip.
• *Shield gonads.*
• *Respiration:* Suspend.

Central ray
• Directed to exit the spinous process of C7 at an average angle of 35 degrees caudad (range, 30 to 40 degrees).

Collimation
• Adjust radiation field to 10 × 12 inches (24 × 30 cm) on the collimator. Place the side marker in the collimated exposure field.

Structures shown
The posterior arch and pillars of the cervical and upper thoracic vertebrae with open zygapophyseal joints (Fig. 9.63).

The following should be clearly seen:
■ Evidence of proper collimation and presence of the side marker placed clear of anatomy of interest
■ Vertebral arch structures, especially the superior and inferior articulating processes (pillars), without overlapping of the vertebral bodies and transverse processes
■ Articular processes on the side of interest
■ Open zygapophyseal joints between the articular processes
■ Bony trabecular detail and surrounding soft tissues

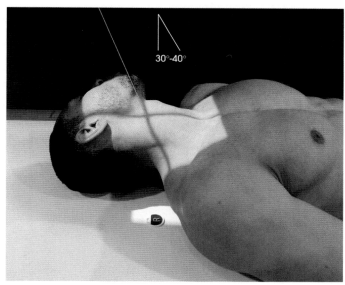

Fig. 9.62 AP axial oblique showing right vertebral arches.

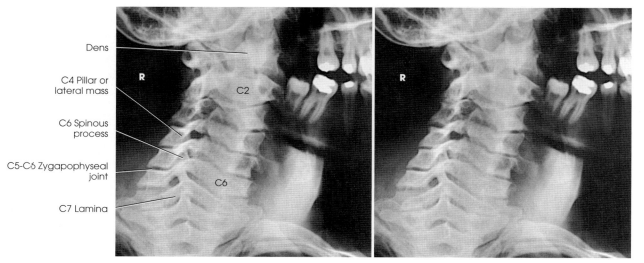

Dens

C4 Pillar or lateral mass

C6 Spinous process

C5-C6 Zygapophyseal joint

C7 Lamina

Fig. 9.63 AP axial oblique showing right vertebral arches.

Cervical and Upper Thoracic Vertebrae

♠ LATERAL PROJECTION
SWIMMER'S TECHNIQUE
Right or left position

The *swimmer's technique* is performed when shoulder superimposition obscures C7 on a lateral cervical spine projection or when a lateral projection of the upper thoracic vertebra is needed. After reviewing the original publications of Twining[11] and Pawlow[12] and other pertinent publications,[13-15] the authors determined that the current technique descriptions are a combination of their recommendations. The following description identifies the historical origins and provides the authors' recommendations for the optimal positioning technique.

Image receptor + grid: Positioned by manufacturer or department protocol for proper anatomy display orientation; CR plate: 10 × 12 inches (24 × 30 cm) lengthwise.

Position of patient
- *Recumbent:* Place the patient in a lateral recumbent position with the head elevated on the patient's arm or other firm support (Fig. 9.64).
- *Upright:* Place the patient in a lateral position, either seated or standing, against a vertical grid device (Fig. 9.65).

Position of part
- Center the midcoronal plane of the body to the midline of the grid.
- Extend the arm closest to the IR above the head. If the patient is upright, flex the elbow and rest the forearm on the patient's head[11] (see Fig. 9.65). In addition, the humeral head can be moved anteriorly[12] (recommended) or posteriorly.[13]
- Position the arm away from the IR down along the patient's side, and depress the shoulder as much as possible.[11] In addition, the humeral head can be moved in the opposite direction to that of the other shoulder[12,13] (posterior recommended).

- Adjust the head and body in a true lateral position, with the MSP parallel to the plane of the IR. If the patient is recumbent, a support may be placed under the lower thorax.
- Center the IR at the level of the C7–T1 intervertebral disk space, which is located 2 inches (5 cm) above the jugular notch.
- *Shield gonads.*
- *Respiration:* Suspend; or if patient can cooperate and can be immobilized, a breathing technique can be used to blur the lung anatomy.

Central ray
- Directed to the C7–T1 intervertebral disk space: perpendicular[12] if the shoulder away from the IR is well depressed or at a caudal angle of 3 to 5 degrees[14] when the shoulder is immobile and cannot be depressed sufficiently.
- Monda[15] recommended angling 5 to 15 degrees cephalad to show better the intervertebral disk spaces when the spine is tilted because of broad shoulders or a nonelevated lower spine. The proper angle results in a central ray perpendicular to the long axis of the tilted spine.

NOTE: See Chapter 12 in Volume 2 for a description of positioning used for patients with suspected cervical spine trauma.

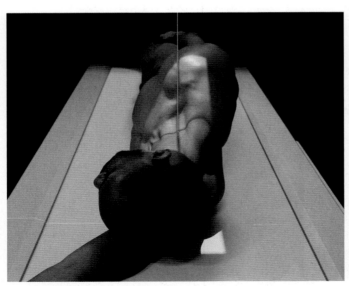

Fig. 9.64 Recumbent lateral cervicothoracic region: Pawlow method.

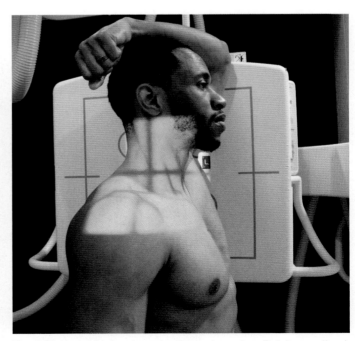

Fig. 9.65 Upright lateral cervicothoracic region: Twining method.

Collimation

- Adjust radiation field to 10 × 12 inches (24 × 30 cm) on the collimator. Place the side marker in the collimated exposure field.

▌ COMPENSATING FILTER

This projection may benefit from the use of a compensating filter because of the extreme difference between the thin lower neck and the very thick upper thoracic region. With the use of a specially designed filter, the C7–T1 area can be shown on one image.

Structures shown

The cervicothoracic vertebrae between the shoulders (Figs. 9.66 and 9.67).

EVALUATION CRITERIA

The following should be clearly seen:

- Evidence of proper collimation and presence of the side marker placed clear of anatomy of interest
- Adequate x-ray penetration through the shoulder region demonstrating the lower cervical and upper thoracic vertebra, not appreciably rotated from lateral position
- Humeral heads minimally superimposed on vertebral column
- Bony trabecular detail and surrounding soft tissues

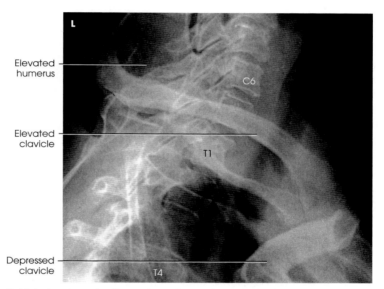

Fig. 9.66 Lateral cervicothoracic region: swimmer's technique with Ferlic filter.

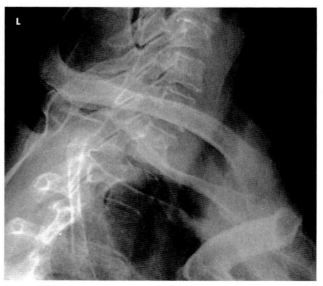

Fig. 9.67 Lateral cervicothoracic region: swimmer's technique with Ferlic filter showing bony structures.

457

⚹ AP PROJECTION

Image receptor + grid: Positioned by manufacturer or department protocol for proper anatomy display orientation; CR plate: 14 × 17 inches (35 × 43 cm) lengthwise.

Position of patient
- Place the patient in the supine or upright position.
- Place the patient's arms along the sides of the body, and adjust the shoulders to lie in the same horizontal plane.
- If the patient is supine, let the head rest directly on the table or on a thin pillow to avoid accentuating the thoracic kyphosis. If possible, orient the patient so the lower thorax is at the cathode end of the x-ray tube. This orientation takes advantage of the "anode heel effect" to ensure a more uniform exposure of the thoracic anatomy.
- If the upright position is used, ask the patient to sit or stand up as straight as possible.

Position of part
- Center the MSP of the body to the midline of the grid.
- For the *supine position,* to reduce kyphosis, flex the patient's hips and knees to place the thighs in vertical position. Immobilize the feet with sandbags (Fig. 9.68).
- If the patient's limbs cannot be flexed, support the knees to relieve strain.
- For the *upright position,* have the patient stand so that the patient's weight is equally distributed on the feet to prevent rotation of the vertebral column.
- If the patient's lower limbs are of unequal length, place a support of the correct height under the foot of the shorter side.
- Place the superior edge of the IR 1½ to 2 inches (3.8 to 5 cm) above the shoulders on an average patient. This positions the IR so that T7 appears near the center of the image and all thoracic vertebrae are shown.

- *Shield gonads.*
- *Respiration:* Suspended at the end of full expiration. This minimizes the air in the lungs, which results in less attenuation differences and more uniform exposure of the thoracic anatomy.

Central ray
- Perpendicular to the IR. The center of the central ray should be approximately halfway between the jugular notch and the xiphoid process (see Fig. 9.68).
- Collimate closely to the spine.

Collimation
- Adjust radiation field to 7 × 17 inches (18 × 43 cm) on the collimator. Place the side marker in the collimated exposure field.

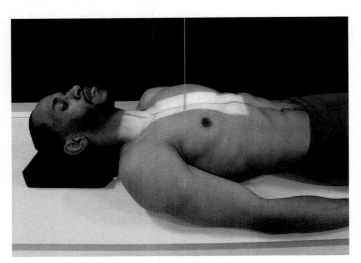

Fig. 9.68 AP thoracic vertebrae.

NOTE: As suggested by Fuchs,[16] a more uniform exposure of the thoracic vertebrae can be obtained if the "heel effect" of the tube is used (Figs. 9.69 and 9.70). With the tube positioned so that the cathode end is toward the feet, the greatest percentage of radiation goes through the thickest part of the thorax.

Structures shown

The thoracic bodies, intervertebral disk spaces, transverse processes, costovertebral articulations, and surrounding structures (see Fig. 9.69). The thoracic spine can be difficult to evaluate with radiography for extremely large patients and those with a fluid-filled chest. CT is often used to see the vertebrae in detail (Fig. 9.71).

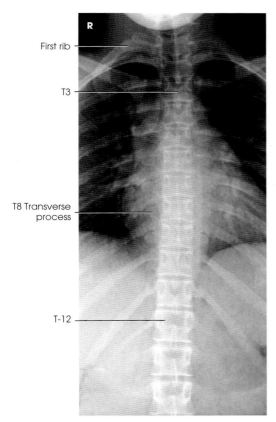

Fig. 9.69 Cathode end of x-ray tube over lower thorax (more uniform exposure).

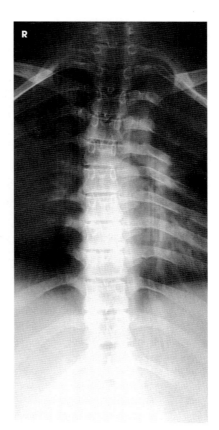

Fig. 9.70 Cathode end of x-ray tube over upper thorax (nonuniform exposure).

▼ COMPENSATING FILTER

This projection can be improved significantly with the use of a compensating filter. Various wedge filters are available to assist in providing an even exposure of the entire thoracic spine, without the need to window.

EVALUATION CRITERIA

The following should be clearly seen:
- Evidence of proper collimation and presence of the side marker placed clear of anatomy of interest
- All 12 thoracic vertebrae

- No rotation as demonstrated by spinous processes at the midline of the vertebral bodies
- Vertebral column aligned to the middle of the image
- Bony trabecular detail and surrounding soft tissues

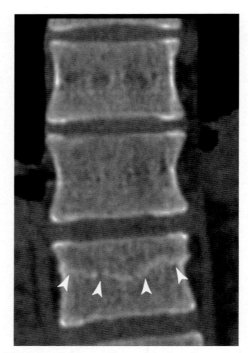

Fig. 9.71 CT thin-section scan thoracic spine shows unstable injury at T-5 after car accident. *Arrows* show various fractures.

✺ LATERAL PROJECTION

Right or left position

Image receptor + grid: Positioned by manufacturer or department protocol for proper anatomy display orientation; CR plate: 14 × 17 inches (35 × 43 cm) lengthwise.

Position of patient

- Place the patient in the lateral recumbent position. (*Note:* Oppenheimer[17] also suggests the use of the upright position.)
- If possible, use the left lateral position to place the heart closer to the IR, which minimizes superimposition of the vertebrae by the heart.
- Have the patient dressed in an open-backed gown so that the vertebral column can be exposed for adjustment of the position.

Position of part

- Place a firm pillow under the patient's head to keep the long axis of the vertebral column horizontal.
- Flex the patient's hips and knees to a comfortable position.
- Place the superior edge of the IR 1½ to 2 inches (3.8 to 5 cm) above the relaxed shoulders. Center the posterior half of the thorax to the midline of the grid and at the level of T7 (Fig. 9.72). T7 is at the inferior angle of the scapulae.
- With the patient's knees exactly superimposed to prevent rotation of the pelvis, a small sponge or cloth may be placed between the knees.
- Adjust the patient's arms at right angles to the long axis of the body to elevate the ribs enough to clear the intervertebral foramina.

- If the long axis of the vertebral column is not horizontal, elevate the lower or upper thoracic region with a radiolucent support (Fig. 9.73). This is the *preferred method*.
- *Shield gonads.*
- *Respiration:* The exposure can be made while the patient continues to breathe normally, the "breathing technique," to blur the pulmonary vascular markings and ribs or after breathing is suspended at the end of expiration.
- When the breathing technique is used, the patient should be instructed not to move during the exposure. An increased exposure time, preferably 2 to 3 seconds (with a corresponding decrease in mA), is needed to ensure the pulmonary vasculature and ribs will be blurred.

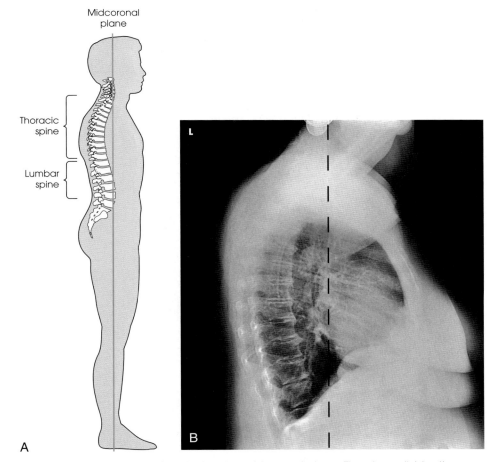

Fig. 9.72 (A) Lateral view of body showing midcoronal plane. The plane divides the thorax in half, and thoracic vertebrae lie in posterior half. Centering for lateral thoracic vertebrae is on posterior half of thorax. (B) Lateral chest showing entire thorax. Thoracic vertebrae are located in posterior half of thorax.

Central ray

- Perpendicular to the center of the IR at the level of T7 (inferior angles of the scapulae). The central ray enters the *posterior half* of the thorax.
- If the vertebral column is not elevated to a horizontal plane when the patient is in a recumbent position, angle the tube to direct the central ray perpendicular to the long axis of the thoracic column, and then center it at the level of T7. An average angle of 10 degrees cephalad is sufficient in most female patients; an average angle of 15 degrees is satisfactory in most male patients because of their greater shoulder width (Fig. 9.74). Fig. 9.75 shows positioning of the central ray for an upright lateral thoracic spine.

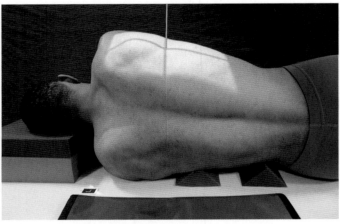

Fig. 9.73 Recumbent lateral thoracic spine. Support placed under lower thoracic region; perpendicular central ray. This is the preferred method of positioning.

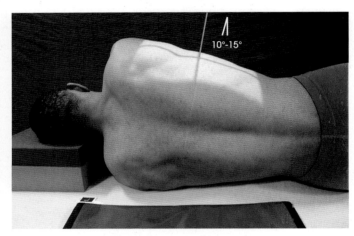

Fig. 9.74 No support under lower thoracic spine; central ray angled 10 to 15 degrees cephalad.

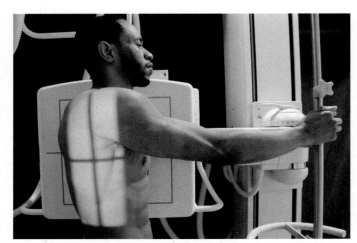

Fig. 9.75 Upright lateral thoracic spine.

Collimation

• Adjust the radiation field to 7 × 17 inches (18 × 43 cm) on the collimator. Place the side marker in the collimated exposure field.

Improving radiographic quality

In addition to close collimation, the quality of the radiographic image can be improved in several ways. A 48-inch (112-cm) or greater SID is recommended to reduce the magnification inherent in this image, because OID of the thoracic spine is significant in this projection. In addition, if a sheet of leaded rubber is placed on the table behind the patient (see Figs. 9.73 and 9.74), the lead absorbs the scatter radiation coming from the patient and prevents table scatter from affecting the image. Scatter radiation decreases the quality of the radiograph and darkens the

image of the spinous processes. More important, with automatic exposure control (AEC), the scatter radiation coming from the patient is often sufficient to terminate the exposure prematurely. The resulting image may be underexposed because of the effect of the scatter radiation on the AEC device.

Structures shown

The thoracic bodies, intervertebral disk spaces, intervertebral foramina, and lower spinous processes. Because of the overlapping shoulders, the upper vertebrae may not be shown in this position (Figs. 9.76 and 9.77). If the upper thoracic area is of interest, a *swimmer's lateral* may be included with the examination. The younger the patient, the easier it is to show the upper thoracic bodies.

The following should be clearly seen:

■ Evidence of proper collimation, posterior field shielding and presence of the side marker placed clear of anatomy of interest

■ Vertebrae clearly seen through rib and lung shadows

■ Twelve thoracic vertebrae centered on the IR. Superimposition of the shoulders on the upper vertebrae may cause underexposure in this area. The number of vertebrae visualized depends on the size and shape of the patient. T1 to T3 are not well seen.

■ Ribs superimposed posteriorly to indicate that the patient was not rotated

■ Open intervertebral disk spaces

■ Bony trabecular detail and surrounding soft tissues

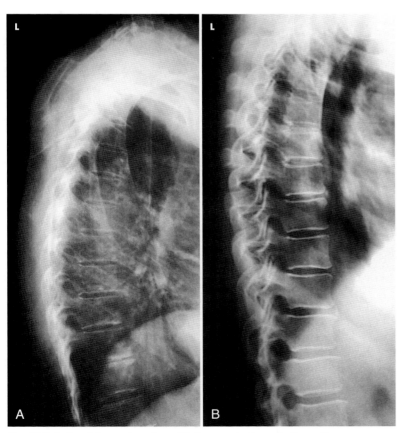

Fig. 9.76 Lateral thoracic spine. (A) Suspended respiration with exposure of ½ second. (B) Breathing technique with exposure of 1½ seconds. Note that lung's vascular markings are blurred.

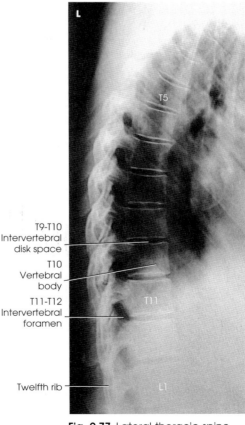

T9-T10 Intervertebral disk space
T10 Vertebral body
T11-T12 Intervertebral foramen
Twelfth rib

Fig. 9.77 Lateral thoracic spine with breathing technique.

AP OR PA OBLIQUE PROJECTION
RAO and LAO or RPO and LPO
Upright and recumbent positions

The thoracic zygapophyseal joints are examined using PA oblique projections, as recommended by Oppenheimer,[17] or using AP oblique projections, as recommended by Fuchs.[18] The joints are well shown with either projection. AP obliques show the joints *farthest* from the IR, and PA obliques show the joints *closest* to the IR. Although the difference in OID between the two projections is not great, the same rotation technique is used bilaterally.

Upright position

> **Image receptor + grid:** Positioned by manufacturer or department protocol for proper anatomy display orientation; CR plate: 14 × 17 inches (35 × 43 cm) lengthwise.

Position of patient
- Place the patient, standing or sitting upright, in a lateral position before a vertical grid.

Position of part
- Rotate the body 20 degrees anterior (PA oblique) or posterior (AP oblique) so that the coronal plane forms an angle of 70 degrees from the plane of the IR.
- Center the patient's vertebral column to the midline of the grid, and have the patient rest the adjacent shoulder firmly against it for support.
- Adjust the height of the IR 1½ to 2 inches (3.8 to 5 cm) above the shoulders to center the IR to T7.

- For the PA oblique, flex the elbow of the arm adjacent to the grid and rest the hand on the hip. For the AP oblique, the arm adjacent to the grid is brought forward to avoid superimposing the humerus on the upper thoracic vertebrae.
- For the PA oblique, have the patient grasp the side of the grid device with the outer hand (Fig. 9.78). For the AP oblique, have the patient place the outer hand on the hip.
- Adjust the patient's shoulders to lie in the same horizontal plane.
- Have the patient stand straight to place the long axis of the vertebral column parallel with the IR.
- The weight of the patient's body must be equally distributed on the feet, and the head must not be turned laterally.
- *Shield gonads.*
- *Respiration:* Suspend at the end of expiration.

NOTE: See p. 436 for the Summary of Oblique Projections.

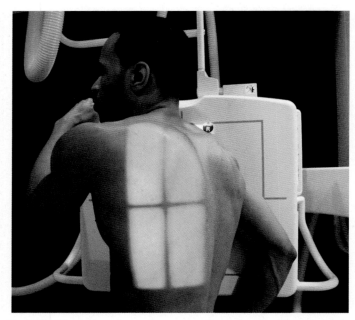

Fig. 9.78 PA oblique thoracic zygapophyseal joints: RAO for joints closest to the IR.

Recumbent position

> **Image receptor + grid:** Positioned by manufacturer or department protocol for proper anatomy display orientation; CR plate: 14 × 17 inches (35 × 43 cm) lengthwise.

Position of patient

- Place the patient in a lateral recumbent position.
- Elevate the head on a firm pillow so that its MSP is continuous with that of the vertebral column.
- Flex the patient's hips and knees to a comfortable position.

Position of part

- For the PA oblique, place the lower arm behind the back and the upper arm forward with the hand on the table for support (Fig. 9.79).
- For the AP oblique, adjust the lower arm at right angles to the long axis of the body, flex the elbow, and place the hand under or beside the head. Place the upper arm posteriorly and support it (Fig. 9.80).
- Rotate the body slightly, either anteriorly or posteriorly 20 degrees, so that the coronal plane forms an angle of 70 degrees with the horizontal.
- Center the vertebral column to the midline of the grid.

- Center the IR $1\frac{1}{2}$ to 2 inches (3.8 to 5 cm) above the shoulders to center it at the level of T7.
- If needed, apply a compression band across the hips, but be careful not to change the position.
- *Shield gonads.*
- *Respiration:* Suspend at the end of expiration.

Central ray

- Perpendicular to the IR exiting or entering the level of T7

Collimation

- Adjust radiation field to 7 × 17 inches (18 × 43 cm) on the collimator. Place the side marker in the collimated exposure field.

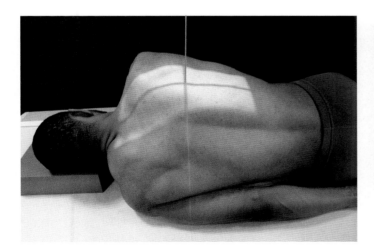

Fig. 9.79 PA oblique thoracic zygapophyseal joints: LAO for joints closest to the IR.

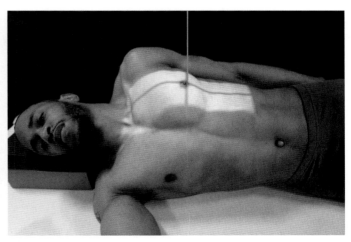

Fig. 9.80 AP oblique thoracic zygapophyseal joints: RPO for joints farthest from the IR.

Structures shown

The thoracic zygapophyseal joints (*arrows* on Figs. 9.81 and 9.82). The number of joints shown depends on the thoracic curve. A greater degree of rotation from the lateral position is required to show the joints at the proximal and distal ends of the region in patients with an accentuated dorsal kyphosis. The inferior articular processes of T12, having an inclination of about 45 degrees, are not shown in this projection. (See the Summary of Oblique Projections on p. 436.)

EVALUATION CRITERIA

The following should be clearly seen:
- Evidence of proper collimation and presence of the side marker placed clear of anatomy of interest
- All 12 thoracic vertebrae
- Zygapophyseal joints closest to the IR on PA obliques and the joints farthest from the IR on AP obliques
- Bony trabecular detail and surrounding soft tissues

NOTE: The AP oblique projection shows the cervicothoracic spinous processes well and is used for this purpose when the patient cannot be satisfactorily positioned for a direct lateral projection.

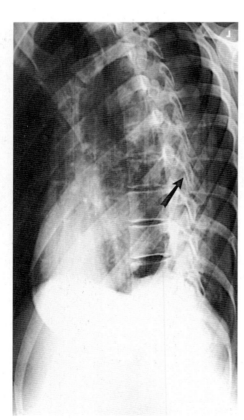

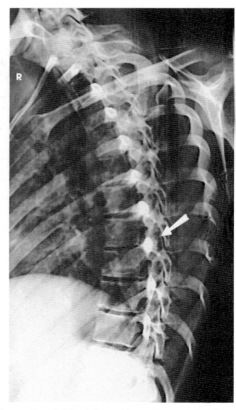

Fig. 9.81 Upright PA oblique thoracic zygapophyseal joints: LAO position. *Arrow* indicates articulation that is closest to the IR.

Fig. 9.82 Recumbent AP oblique thoracic zygapophyseal joints: RPO position. *Arrow* indicates articulation that is farthest from the IR.

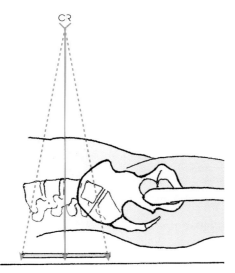

Fig. 9.83 Lumbar spine showing intervertebral disk spaces are not parallel; diverging CR.

⚜ AP PROJECTION
PA PROJECTION (OPTIONAL)

If possible, gas and fecal material should be cleared from the intestinal tract for examination of bones lying within the abdominal and pelvic regions. The urinary bladder should be emptied just before the examination to eliminate superimposition caused by the secondary radiation generated within a filled bladder.

An AP or PA projection may be used, but the AP projection is more commonly employed. The AP projection is generally used for recumbent examinations. The extended limb position accentuates the lordotic curve, resulting in distortion of the bodies and poor delineation of the intervertebral disk spaces (Figs. 9.83 and 9.84). This curve can be reduced by flexing the patient's hips and knees enough to place the back in firm contact with the radiographic table (Figs. 9.85 and 9.86).

The PA projection places the intervertebral disk spaces at an angle closely paralleling the divergence of the beam of radiation (Fig. 9.87; also see Fig. 9.84C). This projection also reduces the dose to the patient by decreasing the abdominal thickness when prone, which requires less mAs, and by placing the gonads farther from the beam entrance to the body. However, this position does result in a slight increase in bone marrow dose in the spine.[19]

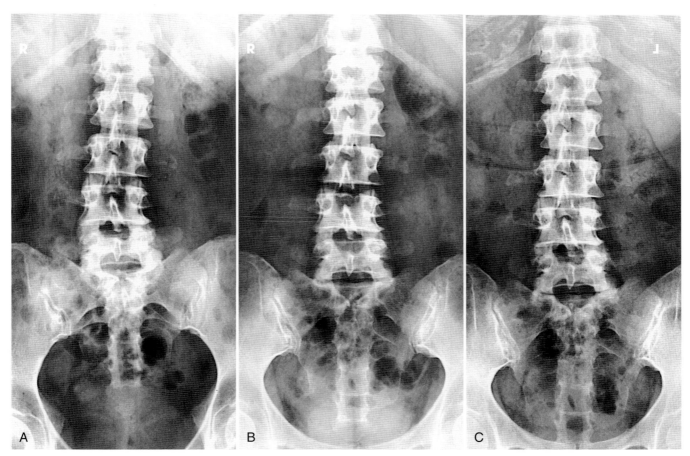

Fig. 9.84 Lumbar spine: AP and PA comparison on same patient. (A) AP with limbs extended. (B) AP with limbs flexed. (C) PA.

Special positioning

- If a patient is having *severe* back pain and a radiographic room with a tilting table is available, place a footboard on the radiographic table, and stand the table upright before beginning the examination.
- Have the patient stand on the footboard, and position the part for the projection.
- Turn the table to the horizontal position for the exposure, and return it to the upright position for the next projection.
- Although this procedure takes a few minutes, the patient appreciates the decrease in pain.

Image receptor + grid: Positioned by manufacturer or department protocol for proper anatomy display orientation; CR plate: 14 × 17 inches (35 × 43 cm) lengthwise.

SID: 48 inches (122 cm) is suggested to reduce distortion and open the intervertebral disk spaces more completely.

Position of patient

- Examine the lumbar or lumbosacral spine with the patient recumbent.

Position of part

- Center the MSP of the patient's body to the midline of the grid.
- Adjust the patient's shoulders and hips to lie in the same horizontal plane.
- Flex the patient's elbows, and place the hands on the upper chest so that the forearms do not lie within the exposure field.
- A radiolucent support under the lower pelvic side can be used to reduce rotation when necessary.

- Reduce lumbar lordosis by flexing the patient's hips and knees enough to place the back in firm contact with table (see Fig. 9.86).
- To show the lumbar spine and sacrum, center the 14 × 17 inches (35 × 43 cm) IR at the level of the iliac crests (L4).
- To show the lumbar spine only, center the IR 1.5 inches (3.8 cm) above the iliac crest (L3).
- *Shield gonads.*
- *Respiration:* Suspend at the end of expiration.

Central ray

- Perpendicular to the IR at the level of the iliac crests (L4) for a lumbosacral examination or 1.5 inches (3.8 cm) above the iliac crest for the lumbar spine only

Collimation

- Adjust to 8 × 17 inches (18 × 43 cm) on the collimator for the lumbosacral spine. Ensure that the sacroiliac joints are included. For lumbar spine only, collimation can be reduced to 8 × 14 inches (18 × 35 cm). Place the side marker in the collimated exposure field.

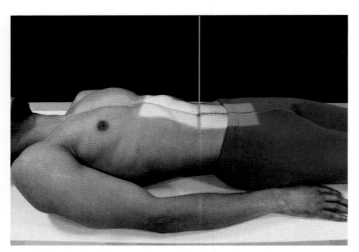

Fig. 9.85 AP lumbar spine with limbs extended, creating increased lordotic curve.

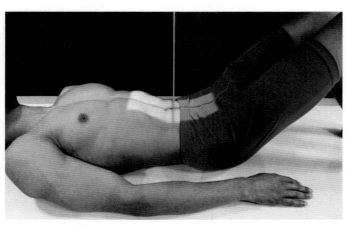

Fig. 9.86 AP lumbar spine with limbs flexed, decreasing lordotic curve.

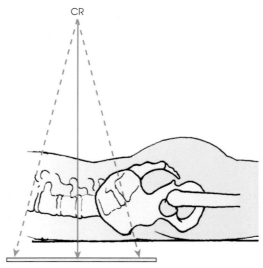

Fig. 9.87 Lumbar spine showing intervertebral disk spaces nearly parallel with divergent PA x-ray beam.

Structures shown, AP and PA

The lumbar bodies, intervertebral disk spaces, interpediculate spaces, laminae, and spinous and transverse processes (Fig. 9.88). The images may include one or two of the lower thoracic vertebrae, the sacrum, coccyx, and the pelvic bones. Because of the angle at which the last lumbar segment joins the sacrum, this lumbosacral disk space is not shown well in the AP projection. The projections used for this purpose are described later in this chapter.

CT (Fig. 9.89) and magnetic resonance imaging (MRI) are used often to identify pathology.

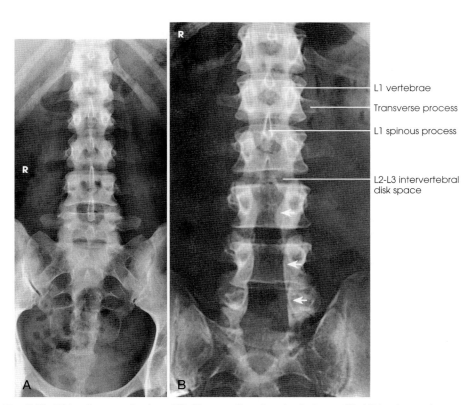

Fig. 9.88 AP lumbosacral spine. (A) Close collimation technique. (B) AP lumbar spine showing spina bifida (arrows).

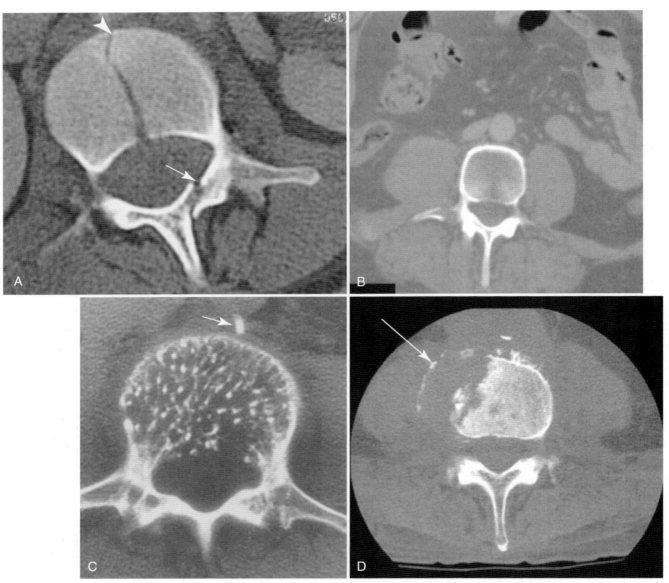

Fig. 9.89 Value of using CT for further evaluation of lumbar spine. Axial images. (A) Burst fracture of L2. Fracture of vertebral body *(arrowhead)* and fracture of left lamina *(arrow)*. (B) Fracture of transverse process of L4. (C) Hemangioma of L3 with no involvement of pedicles or laminae. *Arrow* points to catheter in common third artery for CT angiography. (D) Osteomyelitis seen in L3. *Arrow* points to tuberculous abscess with paravertebral calcification in wall.

⚜ LATERAL PROJECTION
Right or left position

Image receptor + grid: Positioned by manufacturer or department protocol for proper anatomy display orientation; CR plate: 14 × 17 inches (35 × 43 cm) lengthwise.

Position of patient
- For the lateral position, use the same body position (recumbent or upright) as for the AP or PA projection.
- Have the patient dressed in an open-backed gown so that the spine can be exposed for final adjustment of the position.

Position of part
- Ask the patient to turn onto the affected side and flex the hips and knees to a comfortable position.
- When examining a thin patient, adjust a suitable pad under the dependent hip to relieve pressure.

- Align the midcoronal plane of the body to the midline of the grid and ensure that it is vertical. On most patients, the long axis of the bodies of the lumbar spine is situated in the midcoronal plane (Fig. 9.90).
- With the patient's elbow flexed, adjust the dependent arm at right angles to the body.
- To prevent rotation, superimpose the knees exactly, and place a small sponge or cloth between them.
- Place a suitable radiolucent support under the lower thorax, and adjust it so that the long axis of the spine is *horizontal* (Fig. 9.91A). This is the *preferred method* of positioning the spine.
- Center the IR at the level of the iliac crest (L4) for the lumbosacral spine.
- To show the lumbar spine only, center the IR 1.5 inches (3.8 cm) above the iliac crest (L3).
- *Shield gonads.*
- *Respiration:* Suspend at the end of expiration.

Central ray
- Perpendicular; at the level of the iliac crest (L4) for the lumbosacral spine or 1.5 inches (3.8 cm) above the iliac crest (L3) for the lumbar spine only. The central ray enters the midcoronal plane (see Fig. 9.91A).

- When the spine cannot be adjusted so that it is horizontal, angle the central ray caudad so that it is perpendicular to the long axis (see Fig. 9.91B). The degree of central ray angulation depends on the angulation of the lumbar column and the breadth of the pelvis. In most instances, an average caudal angle of 5 degrees for men and 8 degrees for women with a wide pelvis is used. CR placement must be adjusted slightly based on the angle used.

Collimation
- Adjust radiation field to 8 × 17 inches (18 × 43 cm) on the collimator. For lumbar spine only, collimation can be reduced to 8 × 14 inches (18 × 35 cm). Place the side marker in the collimated exposure field.

Structures shown
The lumbar bodies and their intervertebral disk spaces, the spinous processes, and the lumbosacral junction (Fig. 9.92). This projection gives a profile image of the intervertebral foramina of L1–L4. The L5 intervertebral foramina (right and left) are not usually well seen in this projection because of their oblique direction. Consequently, oblique projections are used for these foramina.

EVALUATION CRITERIA
The following should be clearly seen:
- ▪ Evidence of proper collimation and presence of the side marker placed clear of anatomy of interest
- ▪ Area from the lower thoracic vertebrae to the coccyx for lumbosacral spine procedure
- ▪ Area from the lower thoracic vertebrae to proximal sacrum for lumbar only
- ▪ Vertebrae aligned down the middle of the image
- ▪ No rotation
  - ☐ Superimposed posterior margins of each vertebral body
  - ☐ Nearly superimposed crests of the ilia when the x-ray beam is not angled
  - ☐ Spinous processes in profile
- ▪ Open intervertebral disk spaces and intervertebral foramina (L1–L4)
- ▪ Bony trabecular detail and surrounding soft tissues

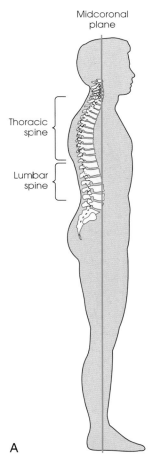
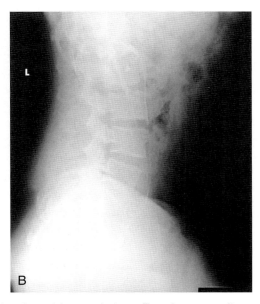

Midcoronal plane

Thoracic spine

Lumbar spine

A   B

Fig. 9.90 (A) Lateral view of body showing midcoronal plane. The plane goes through lumbar bodies. (B) Lateral abdomen showing lumbar bodies located near midcoronal plane.

Improving radiographic quality

In addition to close collimation, the quality of the radiographic image can be improved in several ways. A 48-inch (112-cm) or greater SID is recommended to reduce the magnification inherent in this image, because OID of the lumbar spine is significant in this projection. In addition, if a sheet of leaded rubber is placed on the table behind the patient (see Fig. 9.91), the lead absorbs scatter radiation coming from the patient and prevents table scatter. Scatter radiation decreases the quality of the radiograph and darkens the image of the spinous processes. More important, with AEC, scatter radiation coming from the patient is often sufficient to terminate the exposure prematurely. As a result, the image may be underexposed.

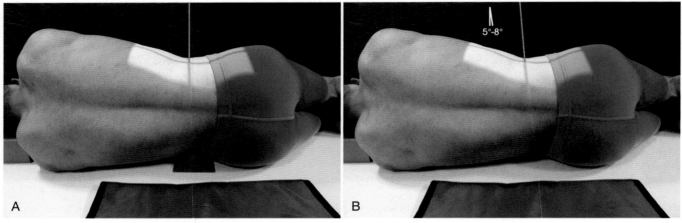

Fig. 9.91 Lateral lumbar spine. (A) Horizontal spine and perpendicular central ray. This is the preferred method of positioning. (B) Spine is angled and central ray is directed caudad to be perpendicular to long axis of spine.

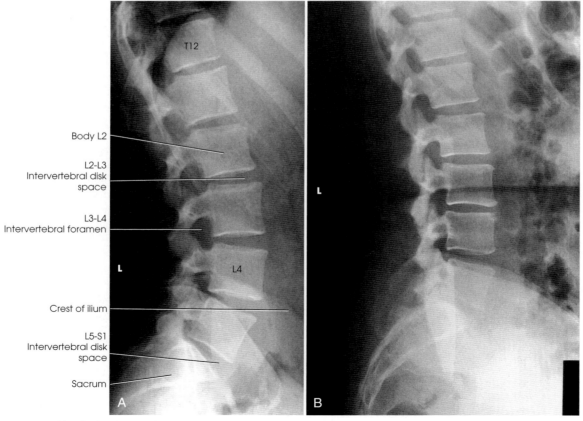

Fig. 9.92 (A) Lateral lumbar spine, 11 × 14 inches (28 × 35 cm) IR. (B) Lateral lumbosacral spine, 14 × 17 inches (35 × 43 cm) IR.

✿ LATERAL PROJECTION
Right or left position

Image receptor + grid: Positioned by manufacturer or department protocol for proper anatomy display orientation; CR plate: 10 × 12 inches (24 × 30 cm) lengthwise.

Position of patient

- Examine the L5–S1 lumbosacral region with the patient in the lateral recumbent position.

Position of part

- With the patient in the recumbent position, adjust the pillow to place the MSP of the head in the same plane with the spine.
- Adjust the midcoronal plane of the body (passing through the hips and shoulders) so that it is perpendicular to the IR.
- Flex the patient's elbow, and adjust the dependent arm in a position at right angles to the body (Fig. 9.93A).

- Flex the patient's hips and knees, superimpose the knees, and place a support between them.
- As described for the lateral projection, place a radiolucent support under the lower thorax and adjust it so that the long axis of the spine is *horizontal* (see Fig. 9.93A). This is the *preferred method*.
- *Shield gonads.*
- *Respiration:* Suspend.

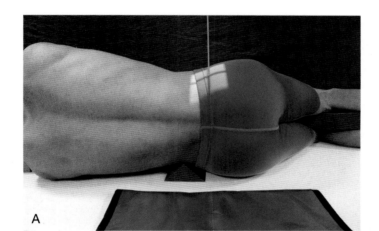

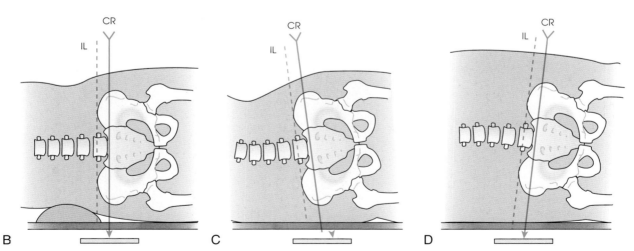

Fig. 9.93 (A) Lateral L5–S1. (B) Optimal L5–S1 joint position. Lower abdomen is blocked to place spine parallel with the IR. Interiliac *(IL)* line is perpendicular, and CR is perpendicular. (C) Typical lumbar spine curvature. If blocking cannot be used, angle CR caudad and parallel to IL. (D) Typical lumbar spine position in a patient with a large waist. IL shows that CR must be angled cephalad to open joint space.

(Modified from Francis C: Method improves consistency in L5–S1 joint space films. *Radiol Technol* 63:302, 1992.)

Central ray

- The elevated anterior superior iliac spine (ASIS) is easily palpated and found in all patients when lying on the side. The ASIS provides a standardized and accurate reference point from which to center the L5–S1 junction.
- Center on a coronal plane 2 inches (5 cm) posterior to the ASIS and 1.5 inches (3.8 cm) inferior to the iliac crest.
- Center the IR to the central ray.
- When the spine cannot be positioned horizontal, the central ray is angled 5 degrees caudally for male patients and 8 degrees caudally for female patients.

- Francis[20] identified an alternative technique to show the open L5–S1 intervertebral disk space when the spine is not horizontal:
  1. With the patient in the lateral position, locate both iliac crests.
  2. Draw an imaginary line between the two points (interiliac plane).
  3. Adjust central ray angulation to be parallel with the interiliac line (see Fig. 9.93B–D).

Collimation

- Adjust radiation field to 6 × 8 inches (15 × 20 cm) on the collimator. This is a high-scatter projection. Close collimation is essential. Place the side marker in the collimated exposure field.

Structures shown

The lumbosacral junction, the lower one or two lumbar vertebrae, and the upper sacrum (Fig. 9.94).

EVALUATION CRITERIA

The following should be clearly seen:
- Evidence of proper collimation and presence of the side marker placed clear of anatomy of interest
- Lumbosacral joint in the center of the image
- Open lumbosacral intervertebral disk space
- Crests of the ilia closely superimposing each other when the x-ray beam is not angled
- Bony trabecular detail and surrounding soft tissues

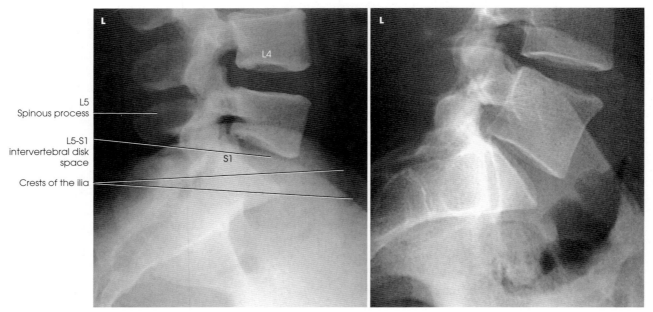

Fig. 9.94 Lateral L5–S1.

☀ AP OBLIQUE PROJECTION
RPO and LPO positions

The plane of the zygapophyseal joints of the lumbar vertebrae forms an angle of 30 to 60 degrees to the MSP in most patients. The angulation varies from patient to patient, however, and from cephalad to caudad in the same patient (see Table 9.3). For comparison, both oblique radiographs are obtained.

> **Image receptor + grid:** Positioned by manufacturer or department protocol for proper anatomy display orientation; CR plate: 10 × 12 inches (24 × 30 cm) or 14 × 17 inches (35 × 43 cm) lengthwise.

Position of patient

- When oblique projections are indicated, they are generally performed immediately after the AP projection and in the same body position (recumbent or upright).

Position of part

- Have the patient turn from the supine position toward the side of interest approximately 45 degrees to show the joints *closest* to the IR. An oblique body position 60 degrees from the plane of the IR may be needed to show the L5–S1 zygapophyseal joints.
- Adjust the patient's body so that the long axis of the patient is parallel with the long axis of the radiographic table.
- Center the patient's spine to the midline of the grid. In the oblique position, the lumbar spine lies in the longitudinal plane that passes 2 inches (5 cm) medial to the elevated ASIS.
- Ask the patient to place the arms in a comfortable position. A support may be placed under the elevated shoulder, hip, and knee to avoid patient motion (Figs. 9.95 and 9.96).
- *Shield gonads.*
- *Respiration:* Suspend at the end of expiration.

NOTE: Although the customary 45-degree oblique body position shows most L3–S1 zygapophyseal joint spaces, 25% of L1–L2 and L2–L3 joints are shown on an AP projection, and a small percentage of L4–L5 and L5–S1 joints are seen on a lateral projection.[21]

Central ray
Lumbar region

- Perpendicular to enter 2 inches (5 cm) medial to the elevated ASIS and 1 to 1.5 inches (2.5 to 3.8 cm) above the iliac crest (L3)

L5–S1 zygapophyseal joint

- Perpendicular to enter 2 inches (5 cm) medial to the elevated ASIS and to a point midway between the iliac crest and the ASIS
- Center the IR to the central ray.

Collimation

- Adjust radiation field to:
  - 9 × 12 inches (23 × 30 cm) on the collimator for 10 × 12 inches (24 × 30 cm) IR
  - 9 × 14 inches (23 × 35 cm) on the collimator for 14 × 17 inches (35 × 43 cm) IR
  - 8 × 10 inches (18 × 24 cm) on the collimator for L5–S1 zygapophyseal joint
- Place the side marker in the collimated exposure field.

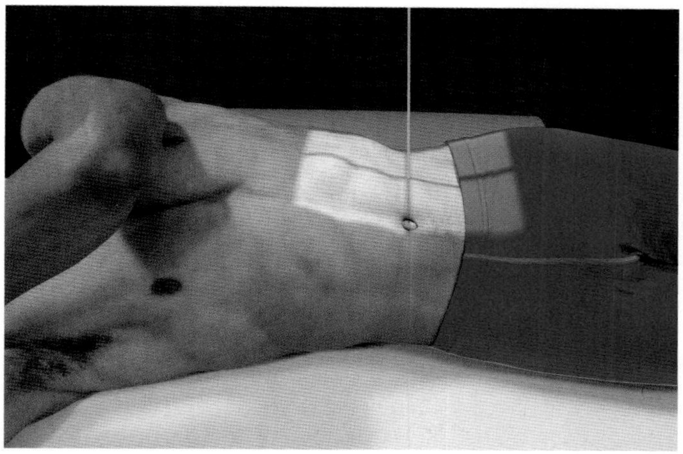

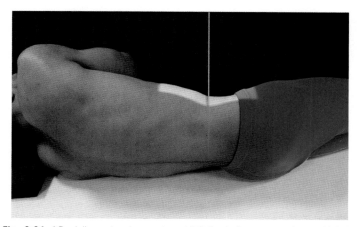

Fig. 9.95 AP oblique lumbar spine: RPO for right zygapophyseal joints.

Fig. 9.96 AP oblique lumbar spine: LPO for left zygapophyseal joints.

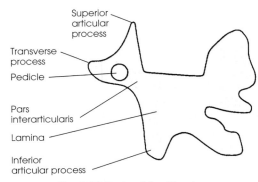

Fig. 9.97 Parts of Scottie dog.

Labels: Superior articular process, Transverse process, Pedicle, Pars interarticularis, Lamina, Inferior articular process

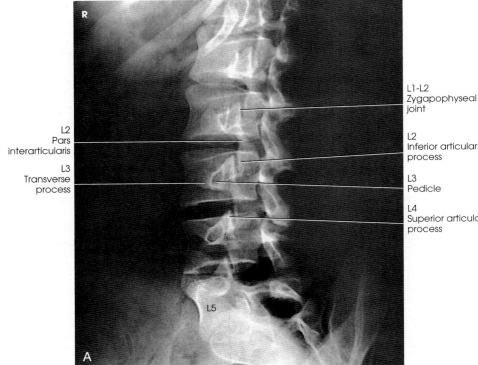

Labels: L1-L2 Zygapophyseal joint, L2 Pars interarticularis, L2 Inferior articular process, L3 Transverse process, L3 Pedicle, L4 Superior articular process, L5

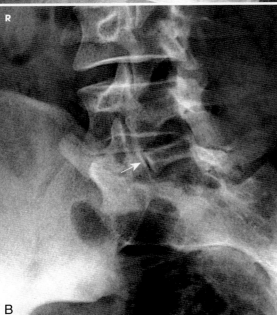

Fig. 9.98 (A) AP oblique lumbar spine: RPO for right zygapophyseal joints. (Note Scottie dogs.) (B) AP oblique lumbar spine: RPO showing L5–S1 zygapophyseal joint *(arrow)* using a 60-degree position.

Structures shown

The lumbar or lumbosacral spine or both, showing the articular processes of the side closest to the IR. Both sides are examined for comparison (Figs. 9.97 and 9.98).

When the body is placed in a 45-degree oblique position and the lumbar spine is radiographed, the articular processes and the zygapophyseal joints are shown. When the patient has been properly positioned, images of the lumbar vertebrae have the appearance of Scottie dogs. Fig. 9.97 shows the vertebral structures that compose the Scottie dog. (See the Summary of Oblique Projections, p. 436.)

EVALUATION CRITERIA

The following should be clearly seen:
- Evidence of proper collimation and presence of the side marker placed clear of anatomy of interest
- Area from the lower thoracic vertebrae to the sacrum
- Zygapophyseal joints closest to the IR—open and uniformly visible through the vertebral bodies
- When the joint is not well seen, and the pedicle is *anterior* on the vertebral body, the patient is not rotated enough (Fig. 9.99A).
- When the joint is not well seen, and the pedicle is *posterior* on the vertebral body, the patient is rotated too much (see Fig. 9.99B).
- Vertebral column parallel with the tabletop so that T12–L1 and L1–L2 intervertebral joint spaces remain open
- Bony trabecular detail and surrounding soft tissues

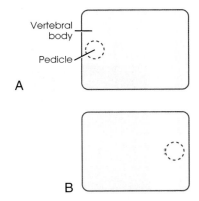

Fig. 9.99 *Box* represents vertebral body, and *circle* represents pedicle. (A) Pedicle is anterior on vertebral body, which means that the patient is not rotated enough. (B) Pedicle is posterior on vertebral body, which means that the patient is rotated too much.

Side text: Vertebral Column

♠ PA OBLIQUE PROJECTION
RAO and LAO positions

Image receptor + grid: 10 × 12 inches (24 × 30 cm) or 14 × 17 inches (35 × 43 cm) lengthwise.

Position of patient
- Examine the patient in the upright or recumbent prone position. The recumbent position is generally used because it facilitates immobilization.
- Greater ease in positioning the patient and a resultant higher percentage of success in duplicating results make the semiprone position preferable to the semisupine position. The OID is increased, however, which can affect resolution.

Position of part
- From the prone position, have the patient turn away from the side of interest approximately 45 degrees to show the zygapophyseal joints furthest farthest from the IR and support the body on the forearm and flexed knee. An oblique body position 60 degrees from the plane of the IR may be needed to show the L5–S1 zygapophyseal joints.

- Adjust the patient's body so that the long axis of the patient is parallel with the long axis of the radiographic table.
- Center the patient's spine to the midline of the grid. In the oblique position, the lumbar spine lies in the longitudinal plane that passes 2 inches (5 cm) lateral to the spinous processes (Fig. 9.100).
- *Shield gonads.*
- *Respiration:* Suspend at the end of expiration.

Central ray
Lumbar region
- Perpendicular to enter the elevated side approximately 2 inches (5 cm) lateral to the palpable spinous process and 1 to 1.5 inches (2.5 to 3.8 cm) above the iliac crest.
L5-S1 zygapophyseal joint
- Perpendicular to enter the elevated side 2 inches (5 cm) lateral to the spinous process and to a point midway between the iliac crest and the ASIS.
- Center the IR to the central ray.

Collimation
- Adjust radiation field to:
  - 9 × 12 inches (23 × 30 cm) on the collimator for 10 × 12 inches (24 × 30 cm) IR
  - 9 × 14 inches (23 × 35 cm) on the collimator for 14 × 17 inches (35 × 43 cm) IR
  - 8 × 10 inches (18 × 24 cm) on the collimator for L5–S1 zygapophyseal joint
- Place the side marker in the collimated exposure field.

Structures shown
The lumbar or lumbosacral vertebrae, showing the articular processes of the side farther from the IR (Figs. 9.101–9.103). The T12–L1 articulation between the twelfth thoracic and first lumbar vertebrae, having the same direction as those in the lumbar region, is shown on the larger IR. The fifth lumbosacral joint is usually well shown in oblique positions (see Fig. 9.103).

When the body is placed in a 45-degree oblique position, and the lumbar spine is radiographed, the articular processes and zygapophyseal joints are shown. When the patient has been properly positioned, images of the lumbar vertebrae have the appearance of Scottie dogs. Fig. 9.101 identifies the vertebral structures that compose the Scottie dog. (See the Summary of Oblique Projections, p. 436.)

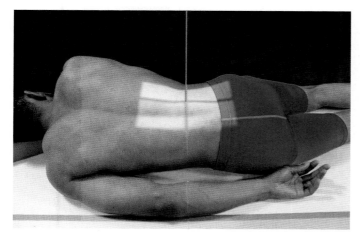

Fig. 9.100 PA oblique lumbar spine: LAO for right zygapophyseal joint.

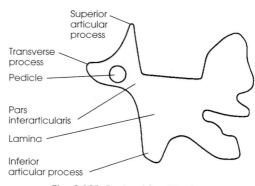

Fig. 9.101 Parts of Scottie dog.

Superior articular process
Transverse process
Pedicle
Pars interarticularis
Lamina
Inferior articular process

EVALUATION CRITERIA

The following should be clearly seen:
- Evidence of proper collimation and presence of the side marker placed clear of anatomy of interest
- Area from the lower thoracic vertebrae to the sacrum
- Zygapophyseal joints *farthest* from the IR
  - When the joint is not well seen and the pedicle is quite anterior on the vertebral body, the patient is not rotated enough.
  - When the joint is not well seen and the pedicle is quite posterior on the vertebral body, the patient is rotated too much.
- Vertebral column parallel with the tabletop so that the T12–L1 and L1–L2 intervertebral joint spaces remain open
- Bony trabecular detail and surrounding soft tissues

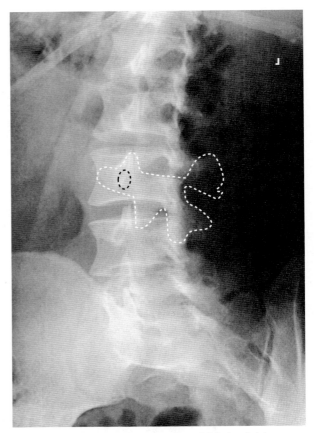

Fig. 9.102 PA oblique lumbar spine: LAO for right zygapophyseal joints. (Note Scottie dog.)

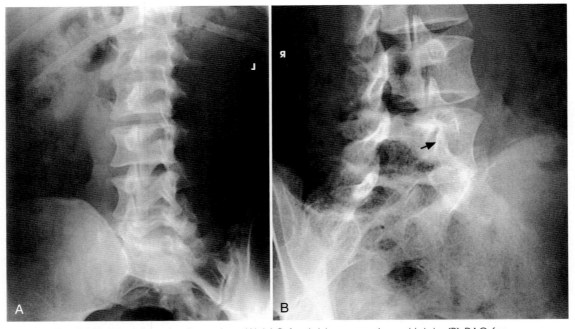

Fig. 9.103 PA oblique lumbar spine. (A) LAO for right zygapophyseal joints. (B) RAO for left L5 zygapophyseal joint *(arrow).*

AP OR PA AXIAL PROJECTION
FERGUSON METHOD[22]

Image receptor + grid: Positioned by manufacturer or department protocol for proper anatomy display orientation; CR plate: 10 × 12 inches (24 × 30 cm) lengthwise.

Position of patient
- For the AP axial projection of the lumbosacral and sacroiliac joints, position the patient in the supine position.

Position of part
- With the patient supine and the MSP centered to the grid, extend the patient's lower limbs or abduct the thighs and adjust in the vertical position (Fig. 9.104).
- Ensure that the pelvis is not rotated.
- *Shield gonads.*
- *Respiration:* Suspend.

Central ray
- Directed through the lumbosacral joint at an average angle of 30 to 35 degrees cephalad.[23]
- An angulation of 30 degrees in male patients and 35 degrees in female patients is usually satisfactory. By noting the contour of the lower back, unusual accentuation or diminution of the lumbosacral angle can be estimated, and the central ray angulation can be varied accordingly.
- The central ray enters the MSP at a point about 1.5 inches (3.8 cm) superior to the pubic symphysis or 2 to 2.5 inches (5 to 6.5 cm) inferior to the ASIS (Fig. 9.105).
- Ferguson originally recommended an angle of 45 degrees.
- Center the IR to the central ray.

Collimation
- Adjust radiation field to 8 × 10 inches (18 × 24 cm) on the collimator. Place the side marker in the collimated exposure field.

Structures shown
The lumbosacral joint and a symmetric image of both sacroiliac joints free of superimposition (Fig. 9.106).

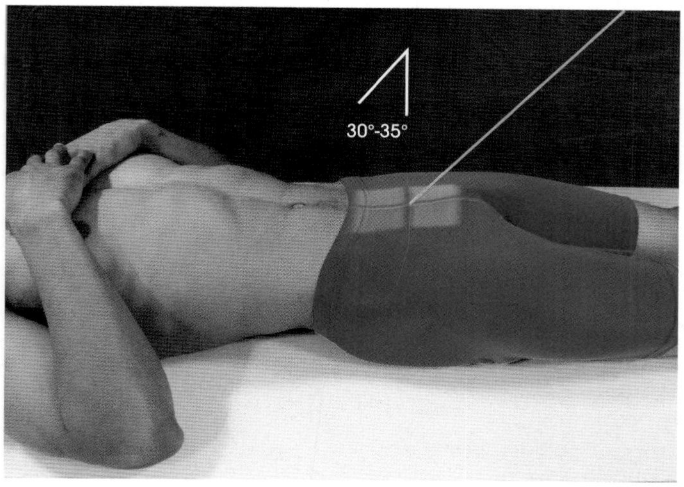

Fig. 9.104 AP axial lumbosacral junction and sacroiliac joints: Ferguson method.

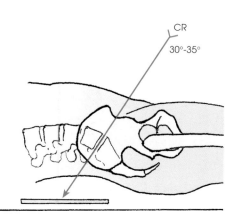

Fig. 9.105 AP axial sacroiliac joints: Ferguson method.

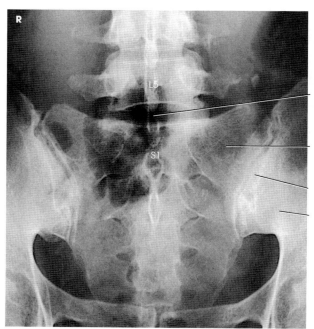

L5-S1 intervertebral disk space

Sacrum

Sacroiliac joint

Ilium

Fig. 9.106 AP axial lumbosacral junction and sacroiliac joints: Ferguson method.

EVALUATION CRITERIA

The following should be clearly seen:

■ Evidence of proper collimation and presence of the side marker placed clear of anatomy of interest
■ Lumbosacral junction and sacrum
■ Open intervertebral disk space between L5 and S1
■ Both sacroiliac joints
■ Bony trabecular detail and surrounding soft tissues

NOTE: The PA axial projection for the lumbosacral junction can be modified in accordance with the AP axial projection just described. With the patient in the prone position, the central ray is directed through the lumbosacral joint to the midpoint of the IR at an average angle of 35 degrees caudad. The central ray enters the spinous process of L4 (Figs. 9.107 and 9.108).

Meese[24] recommended the prone position for examinations of the sacroiliac joints because their obliquity places them in a position more nearly parallel with the divergence of the beam of radiation. The central ray is directed perpendicularly and is centered at the level of the ASIS. It enters the midline of the patient about 2 inches (5 cm) distal to the spinous process of L5 (Fig. 9.109).

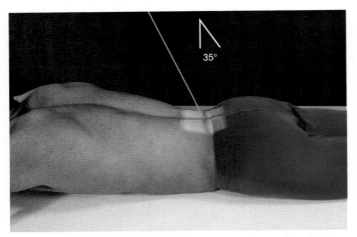

Fig. 9.107 PA axial lumbosacral junction and sacroiliac joints.

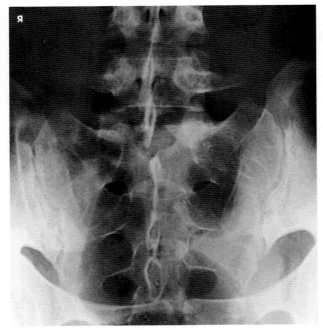

Fig. 9.108 PA axial lumbosacral junction and sacroiliac joints.

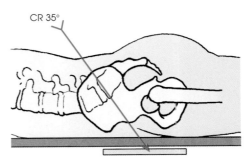

Fig. 9.109 PA axial lumbosacral junction and sacroiliac joints.

⚘ AP OBLIQUE PROJECTION
RPO and LPO positions

Image receptor + grid: Positioned by manufacturer or department protocol for proper anatomy display orientation; CR plate: 10 × 12 inches (24 × 30 cm) lengthwise. Both obliques are usually obtained for comparison.

Position of patient
- Place the patient in the supine position, and elevate the head on a firm pillow.

Position of part
- Elevate the side of interest approximately 25 to 30 degrees, and support the shoulder, lower thorax, and upper thigh (Figs. 9.110 and 9.111).
- The side being examined is farther from the IR. Use the LPO position to show the right joint and the RPO position to show the left joint.
- Adjust the patient's body so that its long axis is parallel with the long axis of the radiographic table.

- Align the body so that a sagittal plane passing 1 inch (2.5 cm) medial to the ASIS of the elevated side is centered to the midline of the grid.
- Check the rotation at several points along the back.
- Center the IR at the level of the ASIS.
- *Shield gonads.* Collimating close to the joint may shield the gonads in male patients. It may be difficult to use contact shielding in female patients.
- *Respiration:* Suspend.

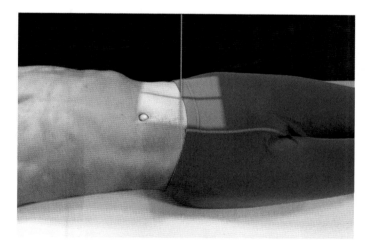

Fig. 9.110 AP oblique sacroiliac joint. RPO shows left joint.

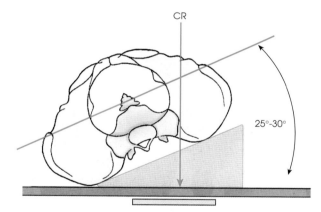

Fig. 9.111 Degree of obliquity required to show sacroiliac joint for AP oblique projection.

Central ray

- Perpendicular to the center of the IR, entering 1 inch (2.5 cm) medial to the elevated ASIS

Collimation

- Adjust radiation field to 6 × 10 inches (15 × 24 cm) on the collimator. Place the side marker in the collimated exposure field.

Structures shown

The sacroiliac joint *farthest* from the IR and an oblique projection of the adjacent structures. Both sides are examined for comparison (Fig. 9.112). (See the Summary of Oblique Projections, p. 436.)

EVALUATION CRITERIA

The following should be clearly seen:

- Evidence of proper collimation and presence of the side marker placed clear of anatomy of interest
- Open sacroiliac joint space with minimal overlapping of the ilium and sacrum
- Joint centered on the radiograph
- Bony trabecular detail and surrounding soft tissues

NOTE: An AP axial oblique can be obtained by positioning the patient as described. For the AP axial oblique, the central ray is directed at an angle of 20 to 25 degrees cephalad, entering 1 inch (2.5 cm) medial and 1½ inches (3.8 cm) distal to the elevated ASIS (Fig. 9.113).

NOTE: Brower and Kransdorf[25] summarized difficulties in imaging the sacroiliac joints because of patient positioning and variability.

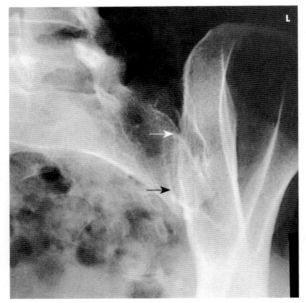

Fig. 9.112 AP oblique sacroiliac joint. RPO shows left joint *(arrows)*.

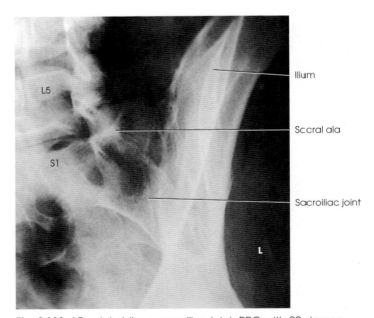

Fig. 9.113 AP axial oblique sacroiliac joint. RPO with 20-degree cephalad angulation shows left joint.

♠ PA OBLIQUE PROJECTION
RAO and LAO positions

Image receptor + grid: Positioned by manufacturer or department protocol for proper anatomy display orientation; CR plate: 10 × 12 inches (24 × 30 cm) lengthwise. Both obliques are usually obtained for comparison.

Position of patient
- Place the patient in a prone position.
- Place a small, firm pillow under the head.

Position of part
- Adjust the patient by rotating the side of interest toward the radiographic table until a body rotation of 25 to 30 degrees is achieved. Have the patient rest on the forearm and flexed knee of the elevated side.

- The side being examined is *closer* to the IR. Use the RAO position to show the right joint and the LAO position to show the left joint.
- Check the degree of rotation at several points along the anterior surface of the patient's body.
- Adjust the patient's body so that its long axis is parallel with the long axis of the table.

- Center the body so that a point 1 inch (2.5 cm) medial to the ASIS closest to the IR is centered to the grid (Figs. 9.114 and 9.115).
- Center the IR at the level of the ASIS.
- *Shield gonads.* Collimating close to the joint may shield the gonads in male patients. It may be difficult to use contact shielding in female patients.
- *Respiration:* Suspend.

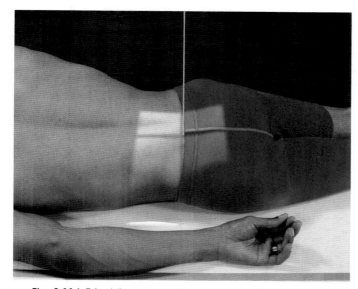

Fig. 9.114 PA oblique sacroiliac joint. LAO shows left joint.

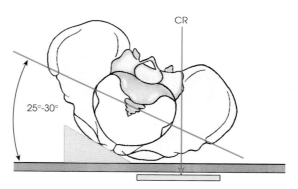

Fig. 9.115 Degree of obliquity required to show sacroiliac joint for PA oblique projection.

Central ray

- Perpendicular to the IR and centered 1 inch (2.5 cm) medial to the ASIS closest to the IR

Collimation

- Adjust radiation field to 6 × 10 inches (15 × 24 cm) on the collimator. Place the side marker in the collimated exposure field.

Structures shown

The sacroiliac joint closest to the IR (Fig. 9.116). (See the Summary of Oblique Projections, p. 436.)

EVALUATION CRITERIA

The following should be clearly seen:

- Evidence of proper collimation and presence of the side marker placed clear of anatomy of interest
- Open sacroiliac joint space closest to the IR or minimal overlapping of the ilium and sacrum
- Joint centered on the radiograph
- Bony trabecular detail and surrounding soft tissues

NOTE: A PA axial oblique can be obtained by positioning the patient as described previously. For the PA axial oblique, the central ray is directed 20 to 25 degrees caudad to enter the patient at the level of the transverse plane, pass 1½ inches (3.8 cm) distal to the L5 spinous process, and exit at the level of the ASIS (Fig. 9.117).

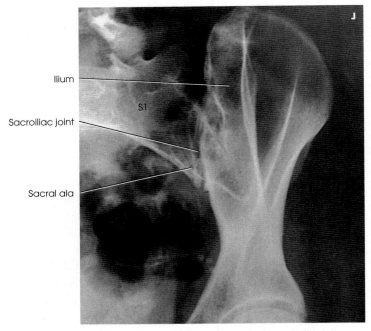

Fig. 9.116 PA oblique sacroiliac joint. LAO shows left joint.

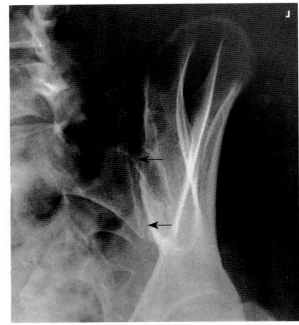

Fig. 9.117 PA axial oblique sacroiliac joint. LAO with 20-degree caudal central ray shows left joint (arrows).

AP AND PA AXIAL PROJECTIONS

Bowel content may interfere with radiography of the sacrum and coccyx. The urinary bladder should be emptied before the examination.

Image receptor + grid: Positioned by manufacturer or department protocol for proper anatomy display orientation; CR plate: 10 × 12 inches (24 × 30 cm) lengthwise.

Position of patient

- Place the patient in the supine position. The prone position can be used without appreciable loss of detail and is particularly appropriate for patients with a painful injury or destructive disease.

Position of part

- With the patient either supine or prone, center the MSP of the body to the midline of the table grid.
- Adjust the patient so that both ASIS are equidistant from the grid.
- Have the patient flex the elbows and place the arms in a comfortable, bilaterally symmetric position.
- When the supine position is used, place a support under the patient's knees.
- *Shield gonads* on men. Women cannot be shielded for this projection.
- *Respiration:* Suspend.

Central ray

Sacrum

- With the patient supine, direct the central ray 15 degrees cephalad and center it to a point 2 inches (5 cm) superior to the pubic symphysis (Figs. 9.118–9.120).
- With the patient prone, angle the central ray 15 degrees caudad and center it to the clearly visible sacral curve (Fig. 9.121).

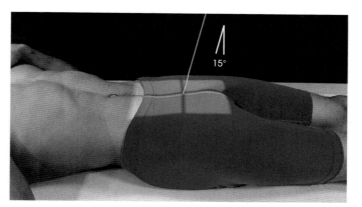

Fig. 9.118 AP axial sacrum.

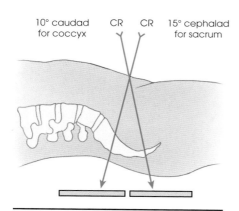

Fig. 9.119 CR angles for AP axial sacrum and coccyx.

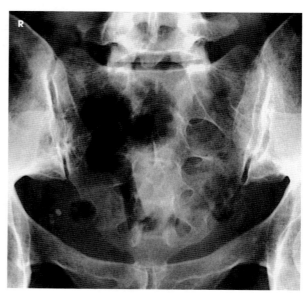

Fig. 9.120 AP axial sacrum.

Vertebral Column

Coccyx

- With the patient *supine,* direct the central ray 10 degrees caudad and center it to a point about 2 inches (5 cm) superior to the pubic symphysis (see Figs. 9.121 and 9.122).
- With the patient *prone,* angle the central ray 10 degrees cephalad and center it to the easily palpable coccyx.
- Center the IR to the central ray.

Collimation

- Adjust radiation field to:
  - *Sacrum:* 10 × 12 inches (24 × 30 cm) on the collimator
  - *Coccyx:* 8 × 10 inches (18 × 24 cm) on the collimator
- Place the side marker in the collimated exposure field.

Structures shown

The sacrum or coccyx free of superimposition (see Figs. 9.120 and 9.123; see also Fig. 9.121).

EVALUATION CRITERIA

The following should be clearly seen:
- Evidence of proper collimation and presence of the side marker placed clear of anatomy of interest
- Bony trabecular detail and surrounding soft tissues

Sacrum

- Sacrum centered and seen in its entirety
- Sacrum free of foreshortening, with the sacral curvature straightened
- Pubic bones not overlapping the sacrum
- No rotation of the sacrum, as demonstrated by symmetric alae

Coccyx

- Coccyx centered and seen in its entirety
- Coccygeal segments not superimposed by pubic bones
- No rotation of coccyx, as demonstrated by distal segment in line with pubic symphysis

Radiation protection

- Because the ovaries lie within the exposure area, use close collimation for female patients to limit the irradiated area and the amount of scatter radiation.
- For male patients, use gonad shielding in addition to close collimation.

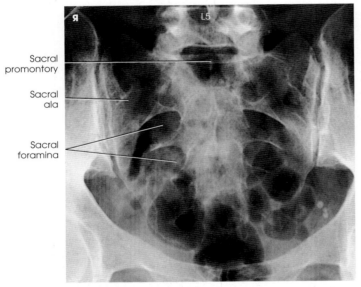

Sacral promontory

Sacral ala

Sacral foramina

Fig. 9.121 PA axial sacrum.

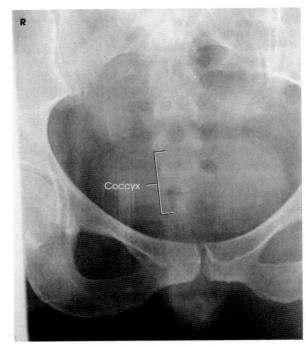

Coccyx

Fig. 9.123 AP axial coccyx.

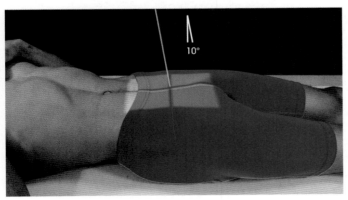

10°

Fig. 9.122 AP axial coccyx.

⚜ LATERAL PROJECTION
Right or left position

Image receptor + grid: Positioned by manufacturer or department protocol for proper anatomy display orientation; CR plate: 10 × 12 inches (24 × 30 cm) lengthwise.

Position of patient
- Ask the patient to turn onto the indicated side, and flex the hips and knees to a comfortable position.

Position of part
- Adjust the arms in a position at right angles to the body.
- Superimpose the knees, and, if needed, place positioning sponges under and between the ankles and between the knees.
- Adjust a support under the body to place the long axis of the spine horizontal. The interiliac plane should be perpendicular to the IR.
- Adjust the pelvis and shoulders so that the true lateral position is maintained (i.e., no rotation) (Figs. 9.124 and 9.125).
- To prepare for accurate positioning of the central ray, center the sacrum or coccyx to the midline of the grid.
- *Shield gonads.*
- *Respiration:* Suspend.

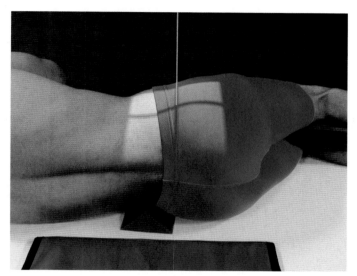

Fig. 9.124 Lateral sacrum.

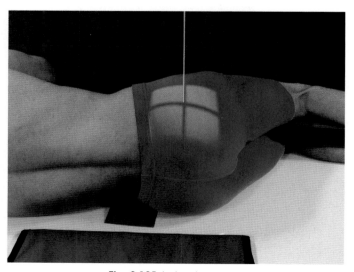

Fig. 9.125 Lateral coccyx.

Central ray

- The elevated ASIS is easily palpated and found on all patients when they are lying on their side and provides a standardized reference point from which to center the sacrum and coccyx (Fig. 9.126).

Sacrum

- Perpendicular and directed to the level of the ASIS and to a point 3.5 inches (9 cm) posterior. This centering should work with most patients. The exact position of the sacrum depends on the pelvic curve.

Coccyx

- Perpendicular and directed toward a point 3.5 inches (9 cm) posterior to the ASIS and 2 inches (5 cm) inferior. This centering should work for most patients. The exact position of the coccyx depends on the pelvic curve.
- Center the IR to the central ray.

Collimation

- Adjust radiation field to:
  - *Sacrum:* 10 × 12 inches (24 × 30 cm) on the collimator.
  - *Coccyx:* 6 × 8 inches (15 × 20 cm) on the collimator.
- Place the side marker in the collimated exposure field.

Structures shown

The sacrum or coccyx (Figs. 9.127 and 9.128).

EVALUATION CRITERIA

The following should be clearly seen:
- Evidence of proper collimation, presence of a lead rubber absorber behind the sacrum and presence of the side marker placed clear of anatomy of interest
- Sacrum and coccyx
- Closely superimposed posterior margins of the ischia and ilia, demonstrating no rotation
- Bony trabecular detail and surrounding soft tissues

Improving radiographic quality

The quality of the radiograph can be improved if a sheet of leaded rubber is placed on the table behind the patient (see Figs. 9.124 and 9.125). The lead absorbs the scatter radiation coming from the patient. Scatter radiation decreases the quality of the radiograph. More important, with AEC, the scatter radiation coming from the patient is often sufficient to terminate the exposure prematurely resulting in an underexposed radiograph. For the same reason, close collimation is necessary for lateral sacrum and coccyx images.

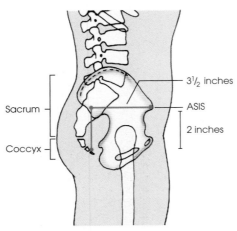

Fig. 9.126 Lateral sacrum, coccyx, and ilium *(dashed outline)* showing centering points. ASIS provides a standardized reference point for central ray positioning.

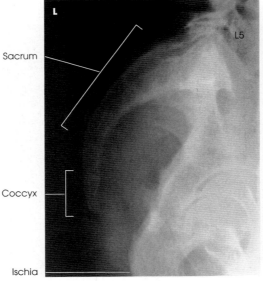

Fig. 9.127 Lateral sacrum.

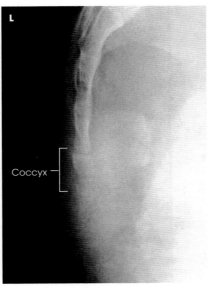

Fig. 9.128 Lateral coccyx.

Vertebral Column

PA PROJECTION
WEIGHT-BEARING METHOD
Right and left bending

> **Image receptor + grid:** Positioned by manufacturer or department protocol for proper anatomy display orientation; CR plate: 14 × 17 inches (35 × 43 cm) lengthwise.

Position of patient

- Perform this examination with the patient in the standing position. Duncan and Hoen[26] recommended that the PA projection be used because in this direction the divergent rays are more nearly parallel with the intervertebral disk spaces.

Position of part

- With the patient facing the vertical grid device, adjust the height of the IR to be centered at the level of L3.
- Adjust the patient's pelvis for rotation by ensuring that the ASIS are equidistant from the IR.
- Center the MSP of the patient's body to the midline of the vertical grid device (Fig. 9.129).
- Let the patient's arms hang unsupported by the sides.
- Make one radiograph with the patient bending to the right and one with the patient bending to the left (Fig. 9.130).

- Have the patient lean directly lateral as far as possible without rotation and without elevation of the foot. The degree of bending must not be forced, and the patient must not be supported in position.
- Ensure that the MSP of the lower lumbar spine and sacrum remains centered to the grid device as the upper portion moves laterally.
- *Shield gonads.*
- *Respiration:* Suspend.

Central ray

- Directed perpendicular to L3 or through the L4–L5 or L5–S1 intervertebral disk spaces, if these are the areas of interest

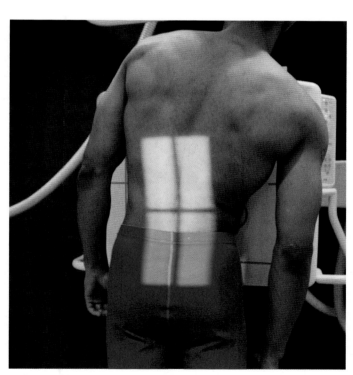

Fig. 9.129 PA lumbar intervertebral disks with right bending.

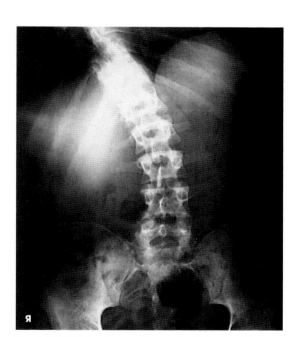

Fig. 9.130 PA lumbar radiograph. Note that the pelvis is straight and only the lumbar spine is bent.

Collimation

- Adjust radiation field to 8 × 17 inches (20 × 43 cm) on the collimator. Place the side marker in the collimated exposure field.

Structures shown

The lower thoracic region and the lumbar region for demonstration of the mobility of the cartilaginous intervertebral joints (see Fig. 9.130). In patients with disk protrusion, this type of examination is used to localize the involved joint, as shown by limitation of motion at the site of the lesion.

EVALUATION CRITERIA

The following should be clearly seen:
- Evidence of proper collimation and presence of the side marker placed clear of anatomy of interest
- Area from the lower thoracic intervertebral disk spaces to all of the sacrum
- No rotation of the patient in the bending position
- Bending direction correctly identified on the image with appropriate lead markers
- Bony trabecular detail and surrounding soft tissues

Radiation protection

The PA projection is recommended instead of the AP projection whenever the clinical information provided by the examination is not compromised. With the PA projection, the patient's gonad area and breast tissue receive significantly less radiation than when the AP projection is used. In addition, proper collimation reduces the radiation dose to the patient. Lead shielding material should be placed between the x-ray tube and a male patient's gonads to protect this area further from unnecessary radiation.

⚕ PA AND LATERAL PROJECTION

FRANK ET AL. METHOD[27-29]

The method described has been endorsed by the American College of Radiology, the Academy of Orthopedic Physicians, and the Center for Development and Radiation Health of the Department of Health and Human Services. Endorsement includes use of the PA projection, compensating filters, and lateral breast protection, and nonuse of graduated screens.

Scoliosis is an abnormal lateral curvature of the vertebral column with some associated rotation of the vertebral bodies at the curve. This condition may be caused by disease, surgery, or trauma, but it is frequently idiopathic. Scoliosis is commonly detected in the adolescent years. If not detected and treated, it may progress to the point of debilitation.

Radiographic diagnosis and monitoring of scoliosis usually consist of PA (or AP) and lateral images taken in the upright position with a special ruler placed adjacent to the spine to allow accurate measurements to be made. Some of the newer scoliosis radiography systems do not require use of a ruler because software allows accurate measurements to be made from the digital data sets. Supine and bending studies may be included when dictated by patient condition. The PA (or AP) and lateral upright projections show the amount or degree of curvature that occurs with the force of gravity acting on the body and allow precise measurements to be taken. Spinal fixation devices, such as Harrington rods, may also be evaluated. Bending studies may be included to differentiate between primary and compensatory curves. Primary curves do not change when the patient bends, whereas secondary curves do change with bending.

Radiation protection

In 1983, Frank et al.[27] described use of the PA projection for radiography of scoliosis. Also in 1983, Frank and Kuntz[30] described a simple method of protecting the breasts during radiography of scoliosis. By 1986, the federal government had endorsed the use of these techniques in an article by Butler et al.[31]

Radiation protection is crucial. Collimation must be closely limited to irradiate only the thoracic and lumbar spine. The gonads should be shielded by placing a lead apron at the level of the ASIS between the patient and the x-ray tube. The breasts should be shielded with leaded rubber or leaded acrylic, or the breast radiation exposure should be decreased by performing PA projections.

Image receptor + grid: Positioned by manufacturer or department protocol for proper anatomy display orientation. A variety of devices and IR holders have been developed for both CR and DR systems. All systems allow multiple images encompassing the entire spine to be captured without the need for repositioning of the patient. The acquired images are combined, or "stitched," by the computer system into a composite image that demonstrates the entire spine in one image.

Position of patient

- This procedure is usually performed with the patient in the upright position.

Position of part

PA (or AP)

- Patient faces the vertical grid device for the PA or rests the back against the device for the AP.
- Adjust the patient's pelvis for rotation by ensuring that the ASIS are equidistant from the IR.

- Center the MSP of the patient's body to the midline of the vertical grid device (Fig. 9.131A).
- Let the patient's arms hang by the sides.
- Position the special ruler adjacent to the spine, if needed.
- *Shield gonads and breasts as appropriate.*
- *Respiration:* Suspend.

Lateral

- Place the patient's side against the vertical grid device.
- Adjust the position of the patient so that the MSP of the body is parallel with the IR and the adjacent shoulder is touching the grid device.
- Center the thorax to the grid; the midcoronal plane should be perpendicular and centered to the midline of the grid (see Fig. 9.131B).
- Position the special ruler adjacent to the spine, if needed.
- Have the patient extend the arms upward to prevent superimposition over the spine.
- *Shield gonads and breasts as appropriate.*
- *Respiration:* Suspend.

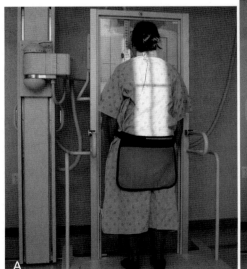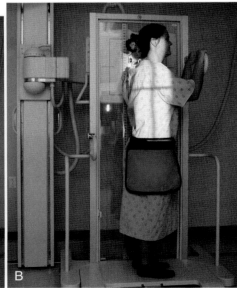

Fig. 9.131 Standing full-spine radiography for evaluation of scoliosis. (A) PA projection: Frank et al. method. (B) Lateral projection.

Central ray

- Perpendicular to the center of the IR. The centering points for each radiographic in the sequence will be dictated by the system used.
- A two- (or three-) image sequence is performed for both the PA and lateral projections (Figs. 9.132 and 9.133).

Collimation

- Extent of collimation depends on the type of imaging system used, as well as the extent of the patient's scoliosis. Care should be taken to include only the anatomy of interest. If possible, the width of the collimated field should be less than the width of the IR. Always check previous examination images to determine extent of curvature.

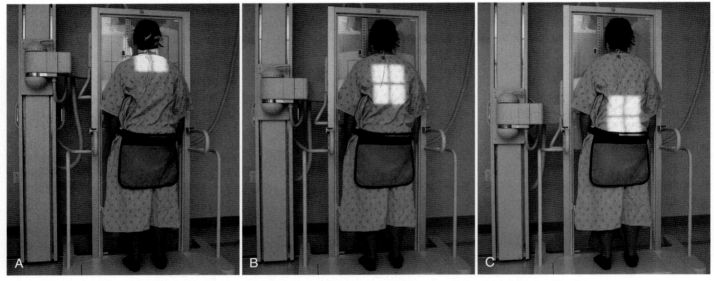

Fig. 9.132 Standing full-spine radiography for evaluation of scoliosis. (A) PA projection to include the cervical spine. (B) PA projection to include the thoracic spine. (C) PA projection to include the lumbar spine and sacroiliac joints.

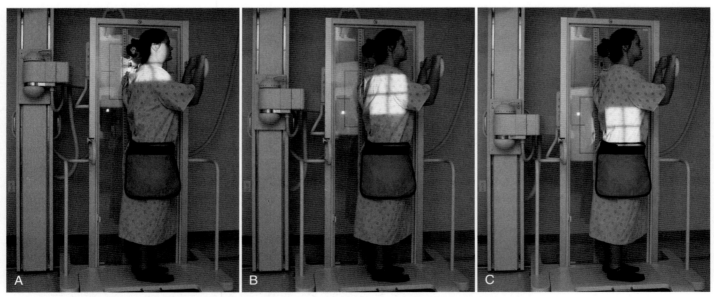

Fig. 9.133 Standing full-spine radiography for evaluation of scoliosis. (A) Lateral projection to include the cervical spine. (B) Lateral projection to include the thoracic spine. (C) Lateral projection to include the lumbar spine and sacroiliac joints.

Structures shown

The entire spine from base of skull to tip of coccyx (Fig. 9.134).

EVALUATION CRITERIA

The following should be clearly seen:

- Evidence of proper collimation, presence of special ruler if used, and presence of the side marker placed clear of anatomy of interest
- Entire cervical, thoracic, and lumbosacral spines
- Vertebral column aligned down the center of the image
- Bony trabecular detail and surrounding soft tissues

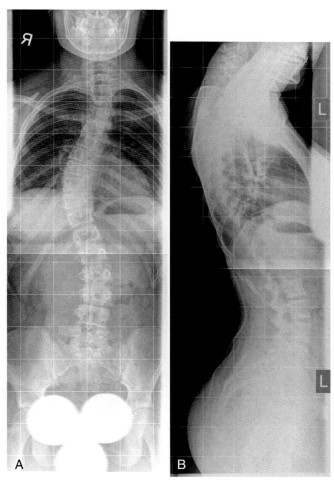

Fig. 9.134 Standing full-spine radiography. Multiple images were combined digitally to create these composite images. (A) PA projection. (B) Lateral projection.

Microdose procedure

Large children's hospitals may have a low-dose slit scanning system (Fig. 9.135) that allows upright PA and lateral images (Fig. 9.136) to be acquired simultaneously. These systems are capable of delivering microdose exposures for repeat procedures where less detail is needed.

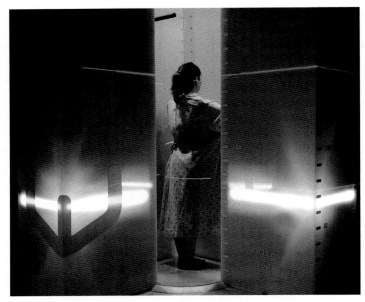

Fig. 9.135 Standing full-spine radiography using a microdose slit-scanning unit. Both PA and lateral projections can be acquired simultaneously.

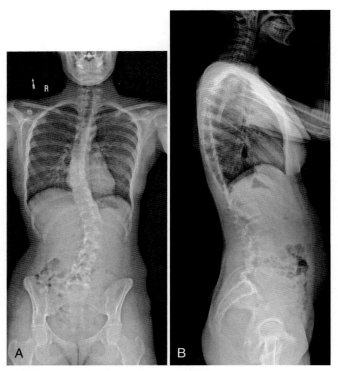

Fig. 9.136 Standing full-spine radiographs acquired by the microdose unit in Fig. 9.135. (A) PA projection. (B) Lateral projection.

PA PROJECTION
FERGUSON METHOD[32]

The patient should be positioned to obtain a PA projection (in lieu of the AP projection) to reduce radiation exposure[27] to selected radiosensitive organs. The decision whether to use a PA or AP projection is often determined by physician or institutional policy.

> **Image receptor + grid:** Positioned by manufacturer or department protocol for proper anatomy display orientation. A variety of devices and IR holders have been developed for both CR and DR systems. All systems allow multiple images encompassing the entire spine to be captured without the need for repositioning of the patient. The acquired images are combined, or "stitched," by the computer system into a composite image that demonstrates the entire spine in one image.

Position of patient
- For a PA projection, place the patient in a seated or standing position in front of a vertical grid device (Fig. 9.137).

Position of part
First radiograph
- Adjust the patient in a normally seated or standing position to check the spinal curvature.
- Center the MSP of the patient's body to the midline of the grid.
- Allow the patient's arms to hang relaxed at the sides. If the patient is seated, flex the elbows and rest the hands on the lap (Fig. 9.138).
- Do not support the patient.
- *Shield gonads.*
- *Respiration:* Suspend.

Second radiograph
- Elevate the patient's hip or foot on the convex side of the primary curve approximately 3 or 4 inches (7.6 to 10.2 cm) by placing a block, a book, or sandbags under the buttock or foot (Fig. 9.139). Ferguson[32] specified that the elevation must be sufficient to make the patient expend some effort in maintaining the position.
- Do not support the patient.
- *Shield gonads.*
- *Respiration:* Suspend.
- Obtain additional radiographs (if needed) with elevation of the hip on the side opposite the major or primary curve (Fig. 9.140), or with the patient in a recumbent position (Fig. 9.141).

Central ray
- Perpendicular to the midpoint of the IR. The centering points for each radiographic in the sequence will be dictate by the system used.

Collimation
- Extent of collimation depends on the type of imaging system used, as well as the severity of the patient's scoliosis. Care should be taken to include only the anatomy of interest. The width of the collimated field must be less than the width of the IR. Always check previous examination images to determine the extent of curvature.

Structures shown
The thoracic and lumbar vertebrae, for comparison to distinguish the deforming or primary curve from the compensatory curve in patients with scoliosis (see Figs. 9.138–9.141).

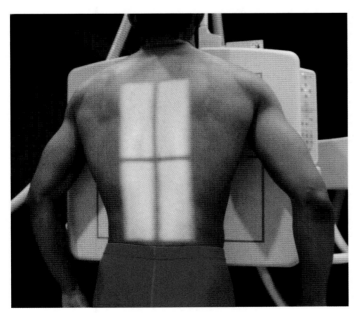

Fig. 9.137 PA thoracic and lumbar spine for scoliosis, upright.

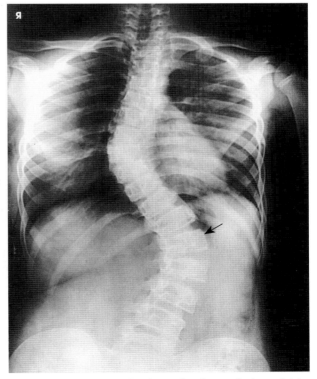

Fig. 9.138 PA thoracic and lumbar spine for scoliosis, upright, showing structural (major or primary) curve *(arrow)*.

EVALUATION CRITERIA

The following should be clearly seen:

- Evidence of proper collimation and presence of the side marker placed clear of anatomy of interest
- Thoracic and lumbar vertebrae to include about 1 inch (2.5 cm) of the iliac crests
- Vertebral column aligned down the center of the image
- Bony trabecular detail and surrounding soft tissues

NOTE: Another widely used scoliosis series consists of four images of the thoracic and lumbar spine: a direct PA projection with the patient standing, a direct PA projection with the patient prone, and PA projections with alternate right and left lateral flexion in the prone position. The right and left bending positions are described in the next section.

NOTE: Young et al.[33] described their application of this scoliosis procedure in detail. They recommended the addition of a lateral position, made with the patient standing upright, to show spondylolisthesis or to show exaggerated degrees of kyphosis or lordosis. Kittleson and Lim[34] described the Ferguson and Cobb methods of measurement of scoliosis.

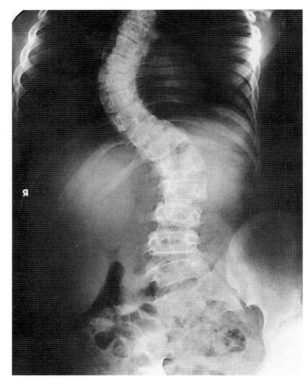

Fig. 9.139 PA thoracic and lumbar spine with left hip elevated.

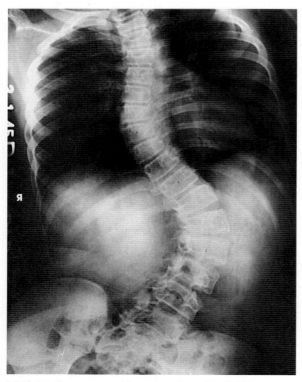

Fig. 9.140 PA thoracic and lumbar spine with right hip elevated.

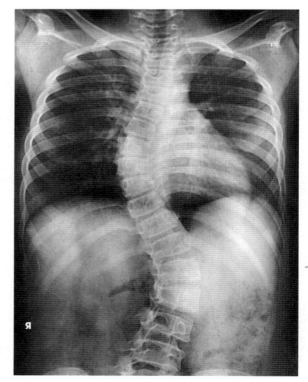

Fig. 9.141 PA thoracic and lumbar spine for scoliosis, prone.

AP PROJECTION
Right and left bending

Image receptor + grid: Positioned by manufacturer or department protocol for proper anatomy display orientation; CR plate: 10 × 12 inches (24 × 30 cm) or 14 × 17 inches (35 × 43 cm) lengthwise for each exposure. IR size is determined by number of vertebral segments to be imaged.

Position of patient
- Place the patient in the supine position, and center the MSP of the body to the midline of the grid. These bending positions can also be performed with the patient upright.

Position of part
- Make the first radiograph with maximum right bending, and make the second radiograph with maximum left bending.

- To obtain equal bending force throughout the spine when the patient is supine, cross the patient's leg on the opposite side to be flexed over the other leg. A right bending requires the left leg to be crossed over the right.
- Move both of the patient's heels toward the side that is flexed. Immobilize the heels with sandbags.
- Move the shoulders directly lateral as far as possible without rotating the pelvis (Fig. 9.142).
- *Shield gonads.*
- *Respiration:* Suspend.

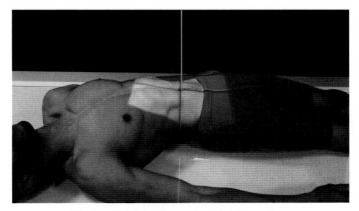

Fig. 9.142 AP lumbar spine, right bending.

Central ray

- Perpendicular to the level of the third lumbar vertebra, 1 to 1.5 inches (2.5 to 3.8 cm) above the iliac crest on the MSP
- Center the IR to the central ray.

Collimation

- Adjust radiation field to 10 × 12 inches (24 × 30 cm) or 14 × 17 inches (35 × 43 cm) on the collimator. Place the side marker in the collimated exposure field.

Structures shown

The lumbar vertebrae, in maximum right and left bending (lateral flexion) (Figs. 9.143 and 9.144). These studies are used to evaluate the integrity of a spinal fusion and are usually performed 6 months after the fusion procedure. This procedure may also be used in patients with early scoliosis to determine the presence of structural change when bending to the right and left. The studies may be used to localize a herniated disk, as shown by limitation of motion at the site of the lesion.

EVALUATION CRITERIA

The following should be clearly seen:

- Evidence of proper collimation and presence of the side marker placed clear of anatomy of interest
- Site of the spinal fusion centered and including the superior and inferior vertebrae
- No rotation of the pelvis (symmetric ilia)
- Bending directions correctly identified with appropriate lead markers
- Bony trabecular detail and surrounding soft tissues

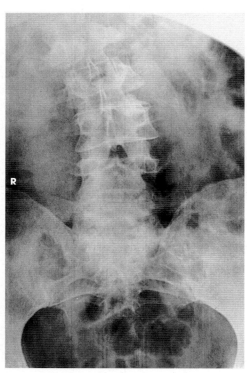

Fig. 9.143 AP lumbar spine, right bending spinal fusion series.

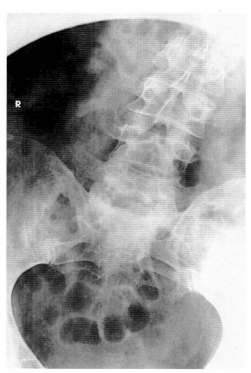

Fig. 9.144 AP lumbar spine, left bending spinal fusion series.

🦅 LATERAL PROJECTION
Right or left position
Flexion and extension

Image receptor + grid: Positioned by manufacturer or department protocol for proper anatomy display orientation; CR plate: 14 × 17 inches (35 × 43 cm) lengthwise for each exposure.

Position of patient
- Adjust the patient in the upright or lateral recumbent position.
- Center the midcoronal plane to the midline of the grid.

Position of part
Flexion
- Ask the patient to bend forward, to flex the spine as much as possible (Fig. 9.145).

Extension
- Ask the patient to bend backward, to extend the spine as much as possible (Fig. 9.146).
- Immobilize the patient to prevent movement, if needed.
- Center the IR at the level of the spinal fusion.
- *Shield gonads.*
- *Respiration:* Suspend.

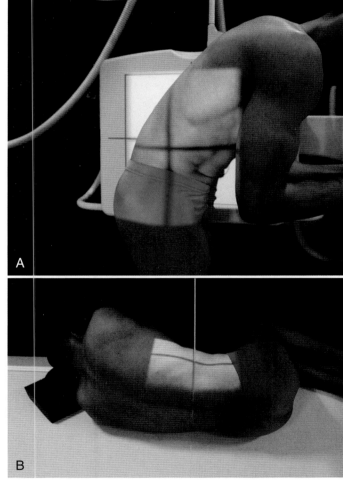

Fig. 9.145 Lateral lumbar spine in flexion. (A) Upright position. (B) Recumbent position.

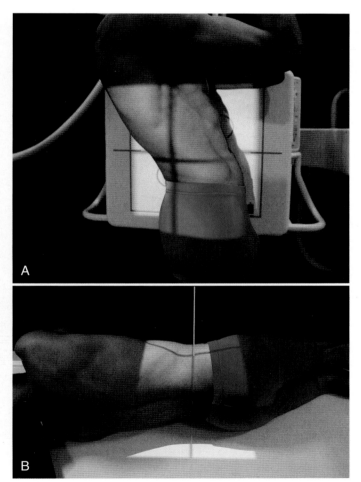

Fig. 9.146 Lateral lumbar spine in extension. (A) Upright position. (B) Recumbent position.

Lumbar Spine: Spinal Fusion

Central ray

• Perpendicular to the spinal fusion area or L3.

Collimation

• Adjust radiation field to 14 × 17 inches (35 × 43 cm) on the collimator. Place the side marker in the collimated exposure field.

Structures shown

Two lateral projections of the spine are taken in flexion (Fig. 9.147A) and extension (see Fig. 9.147B), to determine whether motion is present in the area of a spinal fusion, indicating a nonunion, or to localize a herniated disk as shown by limitation of motion at the site of the lesion.

EVALUATION CRITERIA

The following should be clearly seen:

■ Evidence of proper collimation and presence of the side marker placed clear of anatomy of interest
■ Site of the spinal fusion in the center of the radiograph
■ No rotation of the vertebral column (posterior margins of the vertebral bodies are superimposed)
■ Hyperflexion and hyperextension identification markers correctly used for each respective projection
■ Bony trabecular detail and surrounding soft tissues

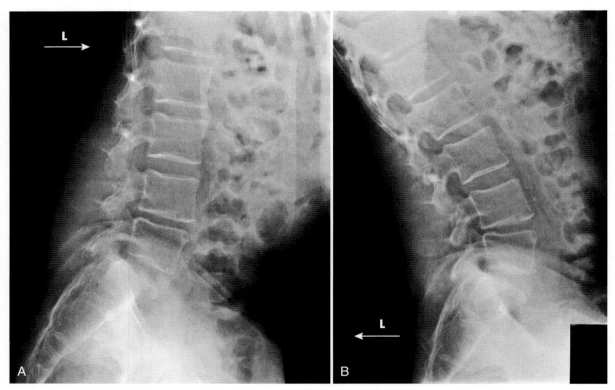

Fig. 9.147 (A) Lateral with hyperflexion. (B) Lateral with hyperextension. Note position of markers and accurate use of *arrows*.

References

1. Fuchs AW: Cervical vertebrae (part 1), *Radiogr Clin Photogr* 16:2, 1940.
2. Albers-Schönberg HE: *Die Röntgentechnik*, ed 3, Hamburg, 1910, Gräfe & Sillem.
3. George AW: Method for more accurate study of injuries to the atlas and axis, *Boston Med Surg J* 181:395, 1919.
4. Grandy CC: A new method for making radiographs of the cervical vertebrae in the lateral position, *Radiology* 4:128, 1925.
5. Barsóny T, Koppenstein E: Eine neue Method zur Röntgenuntersuchung der Halswirbelsäule, *Fortschr Roentgenstr* 35:593, 1926.
6. Barsóny T, Koppenstein E: Beitrag zur Aufnah-metechnik der Halswirbelsäule; Darstellung der Foramina intervertebralia, *Röntgenpraxis* 1:245, 1929.
7. Boylston BF: Oblique roentgenographic views of the cervical spine in flexion and extension: an aid in the diagnosis of cervical subluxations and obscure dislocations, *J Bone Joint Surg Am* 39:1302–1309, 1957.
8. Dorland P, Frémont J: Aspect radiologique normal du rachis postérieur cervicodorsal (vue postérieure ascendante), *Semaine Hop* 1457, 1957.
9. Abel MS: Moderately severe whiplash injuries of the cervical spine and their roentgenologic diagnosis, *Clin Orthop* 12:189–208, 1958.
10. Dorland P, Fremont J, Parer, et al: Techniques d'examen radiologique de l'arc postérieur des vertebres cervicodorsales, *J Radiol* 39:509–519, 1958.
11. Twining EW: Lateral view of the lung apices, *Br J Radiol* 10:123, 1937.
12. Pawlow MK: Zur Frage über die seitliche Strahlenrichtung bei den Aufnahmen der unteren Hals und oberen Brustwirbel, *Rüntgenpraxis* 1:285, 1929.
13. Bartsch GW: Radiography of the upper dorsal spine, *X-ray Tech* 10:135, 1938.
14. Fletcher JC: Radiography of the upper thoracic vertebrae: lateral projection, *Radiogr Clin Photogr* 14:10, 1938.
15. Monda LA: Modified Pawlow projection for the upper thoracic spine, *Radiol Technol* 68:117–121, 1996.
16. Fuchs AW: Thoracic vertebrae, *Radiogr Clin Photogr* 17:2, 1941.
17. Oppenheimer A: The apophyseal intervertebral articulations roentgenologically considered, *Radiology* 30:724, 1938.
18. Fuchs AW: Thoracic vertebrae (part 2), *Radiogr Clin Photogr* 17:42, 1941.
19. Heriard JB, Terry JA, Arnold AL: Achieving dose reduction in lumbar spine radiography, *Radiol Technol* 65:97–103, 1993.
20. Francis C: Method improves consistency in L5-S1 joint space films, *Radiol Technol* 63:302–305, 1992.
21. Bogduk N, Twomey L: *Clinical anatomy of the lumbar spine*, ed 3, London, 1997, Churchill Livingstone.
22. Ferguson AB: The clinical and roentgenographic interpretation of lumbosacral anomalies, *Radiology* 22:548, 1934.
23. Lisbon E, Bloom RA: Anteroposterior angulated view, *Radiology* 149:315–316, 1983.
24. Meese T: Die dorso-ventrale Aufnahme der Sacroiliacalgelenke, *Fortschr Roentgenstr* 85:601, 1956.
25. Brower AC, Kransdorf MJ: Evaluation of disorders of the sacroiliac joint, *Appl Radiol* 21:31, 1992.
26. Duncan W, Hoen T: A new approach to the diagnosis of herniation of the intervertebral disc, *Surg Gynecol Obstet* 75:257, 1942.
27. Frank ED, Stears JG, Gray JE, et al: Use of the posteroanterior projection: a method of reducing x-ray exposure to specific radiosensitive organs, *Radiol Technol* 54:343–347, 1983.
28. Frank ED, et al: A method of reducing x-ray exposure to specific radiosensitive organs, *Can J Radiol* 15(2):10, 1984.
29. Gray JE, Stears JG, Frank ED: Shaped, lead-loaded filters for use in diagnostic radiology, *Radiology* 146(3):825–828, 1983.
30. Frank ED, Kuntz JI: A simple method of protecting the breasts during upright lateral radiography for spine deformities, *Radiol Technol* 55:532, 1983.
31. Butler PF, Thomas AW, Thompson WE, et al: Simple methods to reduce patient exposure during scoliosis radiography, *Radiol Technol* 57:411–417, 1986.
32. Ferguson AB: *Roentgen diagnosis of the extremities and spine*, New York, 1939, Harper & Row.
33. Young LW, Oestreich AE, Goldstein LA: Roentgenology in scoliosis: contribution to evaluation and management, *Radiology* 97:778–795, 1970.
34. Kittleson AC, Lim LW: Measurement of scoliosis, *AJR Am J Roentgenol* 108:775–777, 1970.

10

BONY THORAX

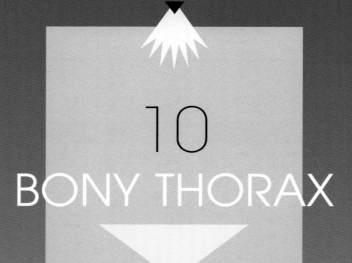

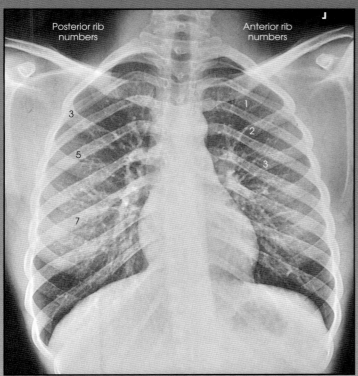

Posterior rib numbers

Anterior rib numbers

PROJECTIONS, POSITIONS, AND METHODS

Page	Essential	Anatomy	Projection	Position	Method
516	♠	Sternum	PA oblique	RAO	
518		Sternum	PA oblique	Modified prone	MOORE
520	♠	Sternum	Lateral	R or L	
522		Sternoclavicular articulations	PA		
523		Sternoclavicular articulations	PA oblique	RAO or LAO	BODY ROTATION
524		Sternoclavicular articulations	PA oblique	RAO or LAO	CENTRAL RAY ANGULATION
527	♠	Upper anterior ribs	PA		
529	♠	Posterior ribs	AP		
531	♠	Axillary ribs	AP oblique	RPO or LPO	
533	♠	Axillary ribs	PA oblique	RAO or LAO	

The icons in the Essential column indicate projections that are frequently performed in the United States and Canada. Students should be competent in these projections.
AP, Anteroposterior; *L*, left; *LAO*, left anterior oblique; *LPO*, left posterior oblique; *PA*, posteroanterior; *R*, right; *RAO*, right anterior oblique; *RPO*, right posterior oblique.

Bony Thorax

The *bony thorax* supports the walls of the pleural cavity and diaphragm used in respiration. The thorax is constructed so that the volume of the thoracic cavity can be varied during respiration. The thorax also protects the heart and lungs.

The bony thorax is formed by the sternum, 12 pairs of ribs, and 12 thoracic vertebrae. The bony thorax protects the heart and lungs. Conical in shape, the bony thorax is narrower above than below, more wide than deep, and longer posteriorly than anteriorly.

Sternum

The *sternum*, or breastbone, is directed anteriorly and inferiorly and is centered over the midline of the anterior thorax (Figs. 10.1–10.3). A narrow, flat bone about 6 inches (15 cm) in length, the sternum consists of three parts: manubrium, body, and xiphoid process. The sternum supports the clavicles at the superior manubrial angles and provides attachment to the costal cartilages of the first seven pairs of ribs at the lateral borders.

The *manubrium*, the superior portion of the sternum, is quadrilateral in shape and is the widest portion of the sternum. At its center, the superior border of the manubrium has an easily palpable concavity termed the *jugular notch*. In the upright position, the jugular notch of the average person lies anterior to the interspace between the second and third thoracic vertebrae. The manubrium slants laterally and posteriorly on each side of the jugular notch, and an oval articular facet called

T2,T3

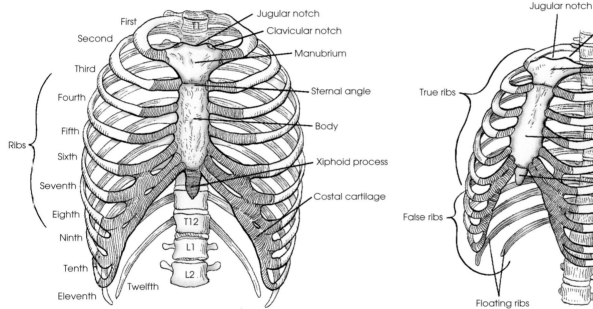

Fig. 10.1 Anterior aspect of bony thorax.

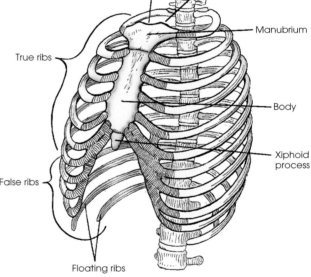

Fig. 10.2 Anterolateral oblique aspect of bony thorax.

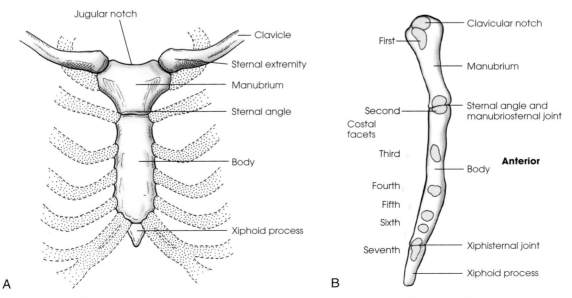

Fig. 10.3 (A) Anterior aspect of sternum and sternoclavicular joints. (B) Lateral sternum.

the *clavicular notch* articulates with the sternal extremity of the clavicle. On the lateral borders of the manubrium, immediately below the articular notches for the clavicles, are shallow depressions for attachment of the cartilages of the first pair of ribs.

The *body* is the longest part of the sternum (4 inches [10.2 cm]) and is joined to the manubrium at the *sternal angle*, an obtuse angle that lies at the level of the junction of the second costal cartilage. The manubrium and the body contribute to the attachment of the second costal cartilage. The succeeding five pairs of costal cartilages are attached to the lateral borders of the body. The sternal angle is palpable; in the normally formed thorax, it lies anterior to the interspace between the fourth and fifth thoracic vertebrae when the body is upright.

The *xiphoid process*, the distal and smallest part of the sternum, is cartilaginous in early life and partially or completely ossifies, particularly the superior portion, in later life. The xiphoid process is variable in shape and often deviates from the midline of the body. In the normal thorax, the xiphoid process lies over the tenth thoracic vertebra and serves as a useful bony landmark for locating the superior portion of the liver and the inferior border of the heart.

Ribs

The 12 pairs of ribs are numbered consecutively from superiorly to inferiorly (Fig. 10.4; also see Figs. 10.1 and 10.2). The rib number corresponds to the thoracic vertebra to which it attaches. Each rib is a long, narrow, curved bone with an anteriorly attached piece of hyaline cartilage, the *costal cartilage*. The costal cartilages of the first through seventh ribs attach directly to the sternum. The costal cartilages of the eighth through tenth ribs attach to the costal cartilage of the seventh rib. The ribs are situated in an oblique plane slanting anteriorly and inferiorly so that their anterior ends lie 3 to 5 inches (7.6 to 12.5 cm) below the level of their vertebral ends. The degree of obliquity gradually increases from the first to the ninth rib and then decreases to the twelfth rib. The first seven ribs are called *true ribs* because they attach directly to the sternum. Ribs 8 to 12 are called *false ribs* because they do not attach directly to the sternum. The last two ribs (eleventh and twelfth ribs) are often called *floating ribs* because they are attached only to the vertebrae. The spaces between the ribs are referred to as the *intercostal spaces*.

The number of ribs may be increased by the presence of cervical or lumbar ribs, or both. *Cervical ribs* articulate with the C7 vertebra but rarely attach to the sternum.

Cervical ribs may be free or may articulate or fuse with the first rib. Lumbar ribs are less common than cervical ribs. *Lumbar ribs* can lend confusion to images. They can confirm the identification of the vertebral level, or they can be erroneously interpreted as a fractured transverse process of the L1 vertebra.

Ribs vary in breadth and length. The first rib is the shortest and broadest; the breadth gradually decreases to the twelfth rib, the narrowest rib. The length increases from the first to the seventh rib and then gradually decreases to the twelfth rib.

A typical rib consists of a *head*, a flattened *neck*, a *tubercle*, and a *body* (Figs. 10.5 and 10.6). The ribs have *facets* on their heads for articulation with the vertebrae. The facet is divided on some ribs into superior and inferior portions for articulation with demifacets on the vertebral bodies. The tubercle also contains a facet for articulation with the transverse process of the vertebra. The eleventh and twelfth ribs do not have a neck or tubercular facets. The two ends of a rib are termed the *vertebral end* and the *sternal end*.

From the point of articulation with the vertebral body, the rib projects posteriorly at an oblique angle to the point of articulation with the transverse process. The rib turns laterally to the *angle* of the body, where the bone arches anteriorly, medially, and inferiorly in an oblique plane. Located along the inferior and internal border of each rib is the *costal groove*, which contains costal arteries, veins, and nerves. Trauma to the ribs can damage these neurovascular structures, causing pain and hemorrhage.

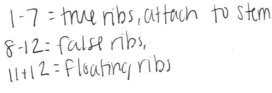

1-7 = true ribs, attach to stem.
8-12 = false ribs,
11+12 = Floating ribs

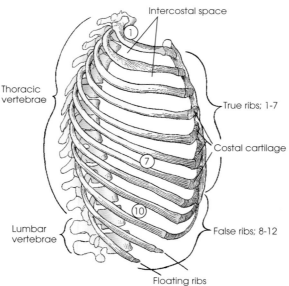

Fig. 10.4 Lateral aspect of bony thorax.

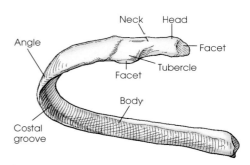

Fig. 10.5 Typical rib viewed from posterior.

Bony Thorax Articulations

The eight joints of the bony thorax are summarized in Table 10.1. A detailed description follows.

The *sternoclavicular* joints are the only points of articulation between the upper limbs and the trunk (Fig. 10.3). Formed by the articulation between the sternal extremity of the clavicles and the clavicular notches of the manubrium, these *synovial gliding* joints permit free movement (the gliding of one surface on the other). A circular disk of fibrocartilage is interposed between the articular ends of the bones in each joint, and the joints are enclosed in articular capsules.

TABLE 10.1
Joints of the bony thorax

| Joint | Structural classification | | |
	Tissue	Type	Movement
Sternoclavicular	Synovial	Gliding	Freely movable
Costovertebral:			
1st–12th ribs	Synovial	Gliding	Freely movable
Costotransverse			
1st–10th ribs	Synovial	Gliding	Freely movable
Costochondral			
1st–10th ribs	Cartilaginous	Synchondroses	Immovable
Sternocostal			
1st rib	Cartilaginous	Synchondroses	Immovable
2nd–7th ribs	Synovial	Gliding	Freely movable
Interchondral			
6th–9th ribs	Synovial	Gliding	Freely movable
9th–10th ribs	Fibrous	Syndesmoses	Slightly movable
Manubriosternal	Cartilaginous	Symphysis	Slightly movable
Xiphisternal	Cartilaginous	Synchondroses	Immovable

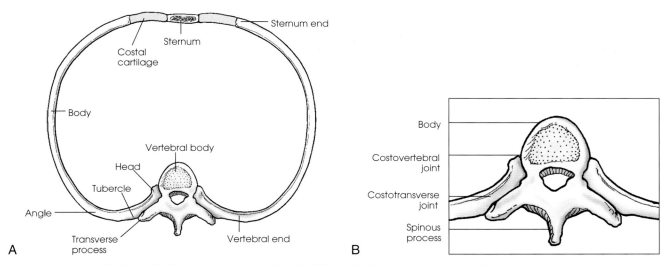

Fig. 10.6 (A) Superior aspect of rib articulating with thoracic vertebra and sternum. (B) Enlarged image of costovertebral and costotransverse articulations.

Posteriorly, the head of a rib is closely bound to the demifacets of two adjacent vertebral bodies to form a synovial gliding articulation called the *costovertebral joint* (Figs. 10.6 and 10.7A). The first, tenth, eleventh, and twelfth ribs all articulate with only one vertebral body.

The tubercle of a rib articulates with the anterior surface of the transverse process of the lower vertebra at the *costotransverse joint*, and the head of the rib articulates at the costovertebral joint. The head of the rib also articulates with the body of the same vertebra and articulates with the vertebra directly above. The costotransverse articulation is also a *synovial gliding* articulation. The articulations between the tubercles of the ribs and the transverse processes of the vertebrae permit only superior and inferior movements of the first six pairs. Greater freedom of movement is permitted in the succeeding four pairs.

Costochondral articulations are found between the anterior extremities of the ribs and the costal cartilages (see Fig. 10.7B). These articulations are *cartilaginous synchondroses* and allow no movement. The articulations between the costal cartilages of the true ribs and the sternum are called *sternocostal* joints. The first pair of ribs, rigidly attached to the sternum, forms the first sternocostal joint. This is a *cartilaginous synchondrosis* type of joint, which allows no movement. The second through seventh sternocostal joints are considered synovial gliding joints and are freely movable. *Interchondral* joints are found between the costal cartilages of the sixth and seventh, seventh and eighth, and eighth and ninth ribs (see Fig. 10.7C). These interchondral joints are *synovial gliding* articulations. The interchondral articulation between the ninth and tenth ribs is a *fibrous syndesmosis* and is only slightly movable.

The *manubriosternal* joint is a *cartilaginous symphysis* joint, and the *xiphisternal* joints are *cartilaginous synchondrosis* joints that allow little or no movement (Figs. 10.3B and 10.7B-C).

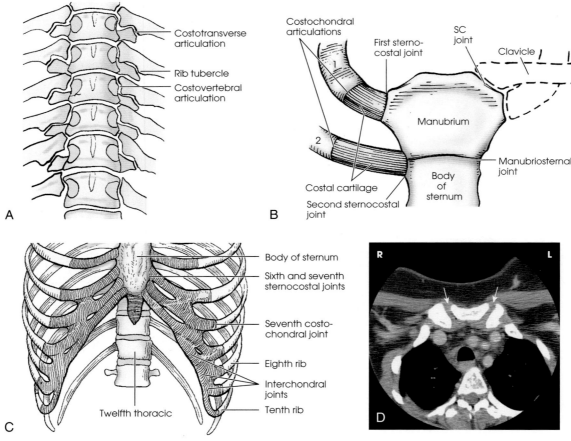

Fig. 10.7 Rib articulations. (A) Anterior aspect of thoracic spine, showing costovertebral articulations. (B) Anterior aspect of manubrium, sternum, and first two ribs, showing articulations. (C) Lower sternum and ribs, showing intercostal, costochondral, and sternocostal joints. (D) CT cross-section image of upper thorax showing manubrium and angulation of sternoclavicular joints *(arrows)*.

RESPIRATORY MOVEMENT

The normal oblique orientation of the ribs changes little during quiet respiratory movements; however, the degree of obliquity *decreases* with deep *inspiration* and *increases* with deep *expiration*. The first pair of ribs, which are rigidly attached to the manubrium, rotates at its vertebral end and moves with the sternum as one structure during respiratory movements.

On deep inspiration, the anterior ends of the ribs are carried anteriorly, superiorly, and laterally while the necks are rotated inferiorly (Fig. 10.8A). On deep expiration, the anterior ends are carried inferiorly, posteriorly, and medially, while the necks are rotated superiorly (see Fig. 10.8B). The last two pairs of ribs are depressed and are held in position by the action of the diaphragm when the anterior ends of the upper ribs are elevated during respiration.

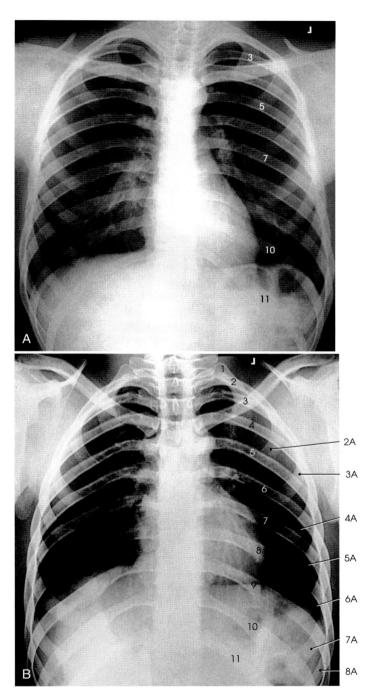

Fig. 10.8 Respiratory lung movement. (A) Full inspiration with posterior ribs numbered. (B) Full expiration with ribs numbered. Anterior ribs are labeled with *A*.

DIAPHRAGM

The ribs located above the diaphragm are best examined radiographically through the air-filled lungs, whereas the ribs situated below the diaphragm must be examined through the upper abdomen. Because of the difference in penetration required for the two regions, the position and respiratory excursion of the diaphragm play a large role in radiography of the ribs.

The position of the diaphragm varies with body habitus: it is at a higher level in hypersthenic patients and at a lower level in asthenic patients (Fig. 10.9). In sthenic patients of average size and shape, the right side of the diaphragm arches posteriorly from the level of about the sixth or seventh costal cartilage to the level of the ninth or tenth thoracic vertebra when the body is in the upright position. The left side of the diaphragm lies at a slightly lower level. Because of the oblique location of the ribs and the diaphragm, several pairs of ribs appear on radiographs to lie partly above and partly below the diaphragm.

The position of the diaphragm changes considerably with the body position, reaching its lowest level when the body is upright and its highest level when the body is supine. For this reason, it is desirable to place the patient in an upright position for examination of the ribs above the diaphragm and in a recumbent position for examination of the ribs below the diaphragm.

The respiratory movement of the diaphragm averages about 1½ inches (3.8 cm) between deep inspiration and deep expiration. The movement is less in hypersthenic patients and more in hyposthenic patients. Deeper inspiration or expiration and greater depression or elevation of the diaphragm are achieved on the second respiratory movement than on the first. This greater movement should be taken into consideration when the ribs that lie at the diaphragmatic level are examined.

When the body is placed in the supine position, the anterior ends of the ribs are displaced superiorly, laterally, and posteriorly. For this reason, the anterior ends of the ribs are less sharply visualized when the patient is radiographed in the supine position.

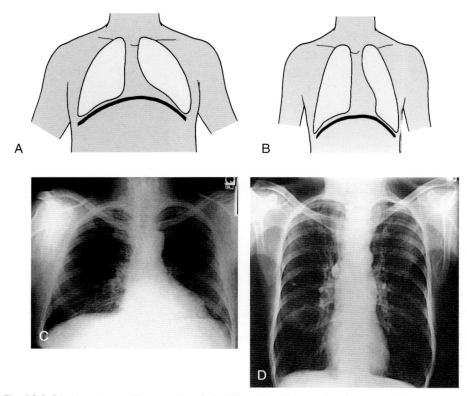

Fig. 10.9 Diaphragm position and body habitus. (A) A hypersthenic patient has a diaphragm positioned higher. (B) An asthenic patient has a diaphragm positioned lower. (C) Chest radiograph of a hypersthenic patient. (D) Chest radiograph of an asthenic patient. Note position of diaphragm on these extremely different body types.

BODY POSITION

Although in rib examinations it is desirable to take advantage of the effect that body position has on the position of the diaphragm, the effect is not of sufficient importance to justify subjecting a patient to a painful change from the upright position to the recumbent position or vice versa. Even minor rib injuries are painful, and slight movement frequently causes the patient considerable distress. Unless the change in position can be effected by a tilting radiographic table, patients with recent rib injury should be examined in the position in which they arrive in the radiology department. An ambulatory patient can be positioned for recumbent images with minimal discomfort by bringing the tilt table to the vertical position for each positioning change. The patient stands on the footboard, is comfortably adjusted, and is then lowered to the horizontal position.

TRAUMA PATIENTS

The first and usually the only requirement in the initial radiographic examination of a patient who has sustained severe trauma to the rib cage is the need to take AP and lateral projections of the chest. These projections are obtained not only to show the site and extent of rib injury, but also to investigate the possibility of injury to underlying structures by depressed rib fractures. Patients are examined in the position in which they arrive, usually recumbent on a stretcher. If it is deemed necessary to show the presence of air or fluid levels in the chest, the dorsal decubitus position is preferred.

SUMMARY OF ANATOMY

Bony thorax	Ribs	Bony thorax articulations
Sternum	Costal cartilage	Sternoclavicular
Ribs (12)	True ribs	Costovertebral
Thoracic vertebrae (12)	False ribs	Costotransverse
	Floating ribs	Costochondral
Sternum	Cervical ribs	Sternocostal
Manubrium	Lumbar ribs	Interchondral
Jugular notch	Intercostal spaces	Manubriosternal
Clavicular notch	Head	Xiphisternal
Body	Neck	
Sternal angle	Tubercle	
Xiphoid process	Body	
	Facets	
	Vertebral end	
	Sternal end	
	Angle	
	Costal groove	

SUMMARY OF PATHOLOGY

Condition	Definition
Fracture	Disruption of the continuity of bone
Metastasis	Transfer of a cancerous lesion from one area to another
Osteomyelitis	Inflammation of bone due to a pyogenic infection
Osteopetrosis	Increased density of atypically soft bone
Osteoporosis	Loss of bone density
Paget disease	Thick, soft bone marked by bowing and fractures
Tumor	New tissue growth where cell proliferation is uncontrolled
Chondrosarcoma	Malignant tumor arising from cartilage cells
Multiple myeloma	Malignant neoplasm of plasma cells involving the bone marrow and causing destruction of bone

Eponymous (named) pathologies are listed in nonpossessive form to conform to the *AMA manual of style: a guide for authors and editors*, ed 10, Oxford, 2009, Oxford University Press.

SAMPLE EXPOSURE TECHNIQUE CHART ESSENTIAL PROJECTIONS

These techniques were accurate for the equipment used to produce each exposure. However, use caution when applying them in your department because "there is considerable variability in image receptor response owing to varying scatter sensitivity, the use of grids with different grid ratios, collimation, beam filtration, the choice of kilovoltage, source-to-image distance, and IR size."[1]

This chart was created in collaboration with Dennis Bowman, AS, RT(R), Clinical Instructor, Community Hospital of the Monterey Peninsula, Monterey, CA. http://digitalradiographysolutions.com/.

BONY THORAX

Part	cm	kVp[a]	SID[b]	Collimation	CR[c] mAs	CR[c] Dose (mGy)[e]	DR[d] mAs	DR[d] Dose (mGy)[e]
Sternum—*PA oblique*[f]	20	81	30"	6" × 11" (15 × 28 cm)	6.3[g]	0.76.5	3.2[g]	0.383
Sternum—*lateral*[f]	29	81	40"	5" × 11" (13 × 28 cm)	20[g]	2.790	10[g]	1.395
Sternoclavicular articulations—*PA*[f]	17	81	40"	6" × 4" (15 × 10 cm)	7.1[g]	0.670	3.6[g]	0.337
Sternoclavicular articulations—*PA oblique*[f]	18	81	40"	6" × 4" (15 × 10 cm)	10[g]	0.963	5[g]	0.479
Upper anterior ribs—*PA*[f]	21	81	72"	9" × 17" (23 × 43 cm)	20[g]	0.625	10[g]	0.312
Posterior ribs—*AP upper*[f]	21	81	72"	9" × 17" (23 × 43 cm)	20[g]	0.625	10[g]	0.312
Posterior ribs—*AP lower*[f]	21	85	40"	9" × 12" (23 × 30 cm)	25[g]	3.540	12.5[g]	1.779
Ribs: axillary—*AP oblique*[f]	23	81	72"	11" × 17" (28 × 43 cm)	36[g]	1.180	16[g]	0.522
Ribs: axillary—*PA oblique*[f]	23	81	72"	11" × 17" (28 × 43 cm)	36[g]	1.181	16[g]	0.523

[1]ACR-AAPM-SIMM Practice Parameter for Digital Radiography, revised 2017.
[a]kVp values are for a high-frequency generator.
[b]40-inch minimum; 44–48 inches recommended to improve spatial resolution (mAs increase needed, but no increase in patient dose will result).
[c]AGFA CR MD 4.0 General IP, CR 75.0 reader, 400 speed class, with 6:1 (178LPI) grid when needed.
[d]GE Definium 8000, with 13:1 grid when needed.
[e]All doses are skin entrance for average adult (160 to 200 pounds male, 150 to 190 pounds female) at part thickness indicated.
[f]Bucky/Grid.
[g]Small focal spot.

The position of the sternum with respect to the denser bony and soft tissue thoracic structures makes it difficult to radiograph. Few problems are involved in obtaining a lateral projection. However, in a PA or AP projection, the sternum would be projected directly over the thoracic spine, so little useful diagnostic information could be obtained from these projections. To separate the thoracic vertebrae and sternum, it is necessary to rotate the body from the prone position or to angle the CR medially. The exact degree of required rotation or angulation depends on the depth of the chest; deep chests require less rotation or angulation than shallow chests (Fig. 10.10 and Table 10.2).

Rotation of the body or angulation of the CR to project the sternum to the right of the thoracic vertebrae clears the sternum of the vertebrae but superimposes it over the posterior ribs and the lung markings (Fig. 10.11). If the sternum is projected to the left of the thoracic vertebrae, it is projected over the heart and other mediastinal structures (Fig. 10.12). The superimposition of the homogeneous density of the heart can be used to advantage (compare Figs. 10.11 and 10.12). For this reason, the PA oblique projection in the right anterior oblique (RAO) position is recommended.

The pulmonary structures, particularly in elderly persons and heavy smokers, can cast confusing markings over the sternum, unless the motion of *shallow* breathing is used to eliminate them. If motion is desired, the exposure time should be long enough to cover several phases of shallow respiration (Figs. 10.13 and 10.14). The milliampere (mA) must be relatively low to achieve the desired milliampere-second (mAs).

When female patients with large, pendulous breasts are imaged, the inferior portion of the sternum may be obscured. They should be instructed to separate the breasts laterally, where they can be held in place with a wide bandage to prevent them from overlapping the sternum and to position the sternum closer to the IR. This positioning strategy for patients with pendulous breasts is also suggested for chest radiography. Pendulous breasts can also obscure the inferior portion of the sternum on the lateral projection and may need to be repositioned.

Radiation Protection

Protection of the patient from unnecessary radiation is a professional responsibility of the radiographer (see Chapter 1 for specific guidelines). In this chapter, the *Shield gonads* statement indicates that the patient is to be protected from unnecessary radiation by restricting the radiation beam using proper collimation. In addition, placement of lead shielding between the gonads and the radiation source is appropriate when the clinical objectives of the examination are not compromised.

TABLE 10.2

Sternum: thickness versus rotation/ CR angulation

Depth of thorax (cm)	Amount of rotation or CR angulation
15	22
16.5	21
18	20
19.5	19
21	18
22.5	17
24	16
25.5	15
27	14
28.5	13
30	12

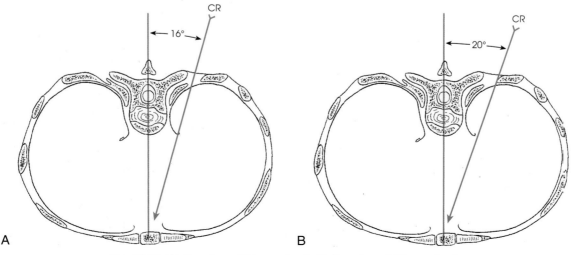

Fig. 10.10 (A) Drawing of 24-cm chest. (B) Drawing of 18-cm chest.

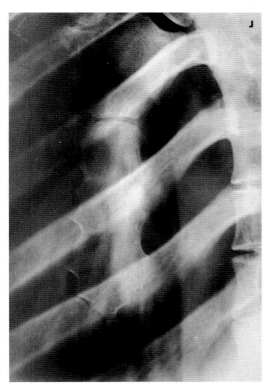

Fig. 10.11 PA oblique sternum, LAO position.

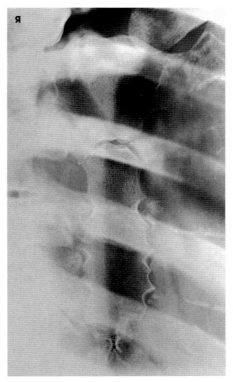

Fig. 10.12 PA oblique sternum, RAO position.

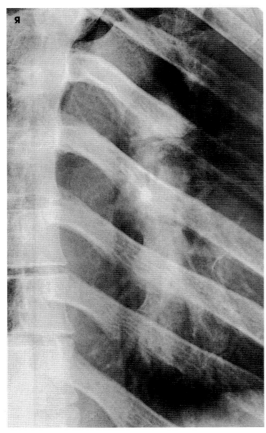

Fig. 10.13 Suspended respiration.

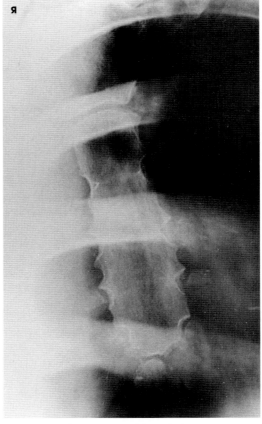

Fig. 10.14 Shallow breathing during exposure.

PA OBLIQUE PROJECTION
RAO position

Image receptor + grid: Positioned by manufacturer or department protocol for proper anatomy display orientation; CR plate: 10 × 12 inches (24 × 30 cm) lengthwise.

NOTE: This position may be difficult to perform on trauma patients. Use an upright position if possible.

SID: A 30-inch (76-cm) SID is recommended to blur the posterior ribs. See page 29, Chapter 1, for information on use of a 30-inch (76-cm) SID.

- 30" SID to magnify sternum

- increase SID, decrease magnification

Position of patient
- With the patient prone or upright facing the IR, adjust the body into RAO position to use the heart for contrast as previously described.
- Have the patient support the body on the forearm and flexed knee, if recumbent.

Position of part
- Adjust the elevation of the left shoulder and hip so that the thorax is rotated just enough to prevent superimposition of the vertebrae and sternum.
- Estimate the amount of rotation with sufficient accuracy by placing one hand on the patient's sternum and the other hand on the thoracic vertebrae to act as guides while adjusting the degree of obliquity. The average rotation is about 15 to 20 degrees (Fig. 10.15).
- Align the patient's body so that the long axis of the sternum is centered to the midline of the grid.
- Place the top of the IR about 1½ inches (3.8 cm) above the jugular notch.
- *Shield gonads.*
- *Respiration:* When a breathing technique is to be used, instruct the patient to take slow, shallow breaths during the exposure. When a short exposure time is to be used, instruct the patient to suspend breathing at the end of expiration to minimize the visibility of the pulmonary vasculature.

NOTE: For trauma patients who are recumbent and unable to lie prone, obtain this projection with the patient in the left posterior oblique (LPO) position, resulting in an AP oblique projection.

- ~~bony thorax~~ sternum
- PA oblique
- RAO 15°-20°
- CR 1" lateral to msp @ level T7
  - top of IR 1½" above jug. notch
- breathe normally during exposure
  OR
- hold on expiration for short exposure time

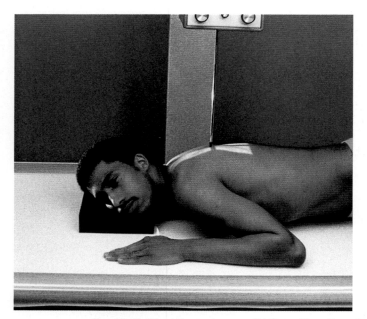

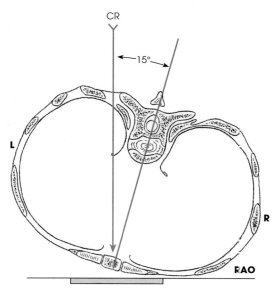

Fig. 10.15 PA oblique sternum, RAO position. Line drawing is an axial view (from feet upward).

Central ray

- Perpendicular to IR. The CR enters the *elevated side* of the posterior thorax at the level of T7 and approximately 1 inch (2.5 cm) lateral to the MSP.

Collimation

- Adjust radiation field to 10 × 12 inches (24 × 30 cm) on the collimator. Place side marker in the collimated exposure field.

Structures shown

A slightly oblique projection of the sternum (Fig. 10.16). The detail depends largely on the technical procedure employed. If a breathing technique is used, the pulmonary markings are obliterated.

The following should be clearly seen:

- Evidence of proper collimation and presence of side marker placed clear of anatomy of interest
- Entire sternum from jugular notch to tip of xiphoid process
- Sternum projected over the heart, but free of superimposition from the thoracic spine
- Minimally rotated sternum and thorax, as shown by the following:
  - □ Sternum projected just free of superimposition from vertebral column
  - □ Minimally obliqued vertebrae to prevent excessive rotation of the sternum
  - □ Lateral portion of manubrium and sternoclavicular joint free of superimposition by the vertebrae
- Blurred pulmonary markings, if a breathing technique was used
- Bony trabecular detail and surrounding soft tissues

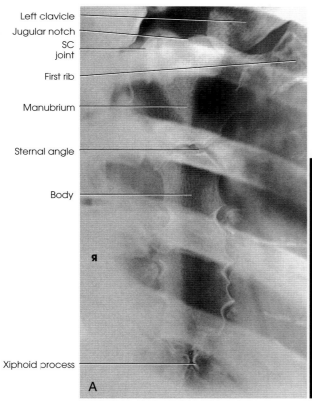

Left clavicle
Jugular notch
SC joint
First rib
Manubrium
Sternal angle
Body
Xiphoid process

A

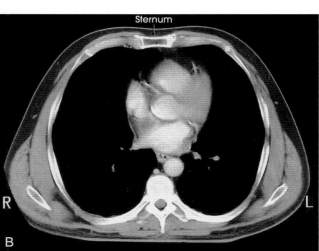

Sternum

R   L

B

Fig. 10.16 (A) PA oblique sternum, RAO position. (B) CT is often used today to image the sternum. Image shows sternum in axial plane.

(B, Modified from Kelley LL, Petersen CM: *Sectional anatomy for imaging professionals,* ed 2, St. Louis, 2007, Mosby.)

PA OBLIQUE PROJECTION
MOORE METHOD
Modified prone position

Image receptor + grid: Positioned by manufacturer or department protocol for proper anatomy display orientation; CR plate: 10 × 12 inches (24 × 30 cm) lengthwise.

SID: A 30-inch (76-cm) SID is recommended. This short distance assists in blurring the posterior ribs.

Radiography of the sternum can be difficult to perform on an ambulatory patient who is having acute pain. The alternative positioning method described by Moore[1] employs a modified prone position, which makes it possible to produce a high-quality sternum image in a more comfortable manner for the patient.

Position of patient

- Before positioning the patient, place the IR crosswise in the Bucky tray. Place the x-ray tube at a 30-inch (76-cm) SID, angle it 25 degrees, and direct the CR to the center of the IR. The x-ray tube is positioned over the patient's right side.
- Place a marker on the tabletop near the patient's head to indicate the exact center of the IR.
- Have the patient stand at the side of the radiographic table directly in front of the Bucky tray.
- Ask the patient to bend at the waist, and place the sternum in the center of the table directly over the previously positioned IR.

Position of part

- Place the patient's arms above the shoulders and the palms down on the table. The arms act as a support for the side of the head (Fig 10.17).
- Ensure that the patient is in a true prone position and that the midsternal area is at the center of the radiographic table.
- *Shield gonads.*
- *Respiration:* A shallow breathing technique produces the best results. Instruct the patient to take slow, shallow breaths during the exposure. A low mA setting and an exposure time of 1 to 3 seconds are recommended. When a low mA setting and long exposure time cannot be employed, instruct the patient to suspend respiration at the end of expiration to minimize the visibility of the pulmonary vasculature.

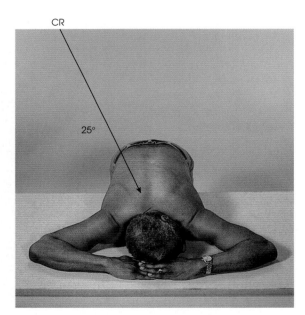

Fig. 10.17 PA oblique projection: Moore method.

Central ray

- The CR is already angled 25 degrees and centered to the IR. If patient positioning is accurate, the CR enters at the level of T7 and approximately 2 inches (5 cm) to the right of the spine. This angulation places the sternum over the lung to maintain maximum contrast of the sternum.
- The x-ray tube angulation can be adjusted for extremely large or small patients. Large patients require *less* angulation and thin patients require *more* angulation than the standard 25-degree angle.

Collimation

- Adjust radiation field to 10 × 12 inches (24 × 30 cm) on the collimator. Place side marker in the collimated exposure field.

Structures shown

A slightly oblique projection of the sternum (Fig. 10.18). The degree of detail shown depends largely on the technique used. If a breathing technique is used, the pulmonary markings are obliterated.

The following should be clearly seen:

- Evidence of proper collimation and presence of side marker placed clear of anatomy of interest
- Entire sternum from the jugular notch to the tip of the xiphoid process
- Sternum projected free of superimposition from the thoracic spine
- Blurred pulmonary markings if a breathing technique was used
- Blurred posterior ribs if a reduced SID was used
- Bony trabecular detail and surrounding soft tissues

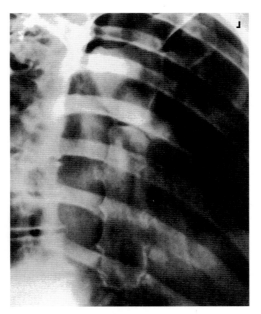

Fig. 10.18 PA oblique projection: Moore method.

♠ LATERAL PROJECTION
Right or left position

Image receptor + grid: Positioned by manufacturer or department protocol for proper anatomy display orientation; CR plate: 10 × 12 inches (24 × 30 cm) lengthwise.

SID: 72-inch (183-cm) SID to reduce magnification and distortion of the sternum.

Position of patient
- Place the patient in a lateral position, either upright (seated or standing) or recumbent. A dorsal decubitus position may be used if needed because of the patient's condition.

Position of part
- Center the sternum to the midline of the grid.
Upright
- Adjust the patient in a true lateral position so that the broad surface of the sternum is perpendicular to the plane of the IR (Fig. 10.19).

- Rotate the shoulders posteriorly, and have the patient lock the hands behind the back.
- Being careful to keep the MSP of the body vertical, place the patient close enough to the grid that the shoulder can be rested firmly against it.
- Large breasts on female patients should be drawn to the sides and held in position with a wide bandage so that their shadows do not obscure the lower portion of the sternum.
Recumbent
- Extend the patient's arms over the head to prevent them from overlapping the sternum (Fig. 10.20).
- Rest the patient's head on the arms or on a pillow.
- Place a support under the lower thoracic region to position the long axis of the sternum horizontally.
- *Shield gonads.*
- *Respiration:* Suspend deep inspiration. This provides sharper contrast between the posterior surface of the sternum and the adjacent structures.

Central ray
- Perpendicular to the center of the IR and entering the lateral border of the midsternum

Collimation
- Adjust radiation field to 10 × 12 inches (24 × 30 cm) on the collimator. Place side marker in the collimated exposure field.

Structures shown
A lateral image of the entire length of the sternum shows the superimposed sternoclavicular joints and medial ends of the clavicles (Fig. 10.21).

EVALUATION CRITERIA
The following should be clearly seen:
- ▪ Evidence of proper collimation and presence of side marker placed clear of anatomy of interest
- ▪ Sternum in its entirety
- ▪ Manubrium free of superimposition by the soft tissue of the shoulders
- ▪ Sternum free of superimposition by the ribs
- ▪ Lower portion of the sternum unobscured by the breasts of a female patient
- ▪ Bony trabecular detail and surrounding soft tissues

[Handwritten notes:]
Projection: lateral
position: right/left lateral
CR: centered to lateral
   border of midsternum
— upright (seated/standing)
   or recumbent

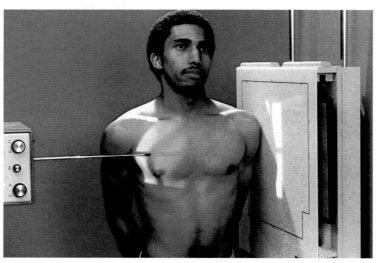

Fig. 10.19 Lateral sternum.

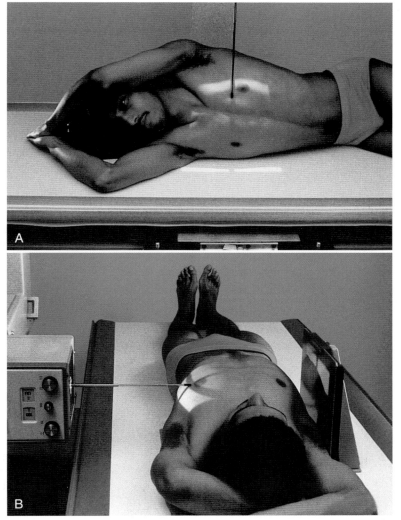

Fig. 10.20 (A) Lateral sternum. (B) Dorsal decubitus position for lateral sternum.

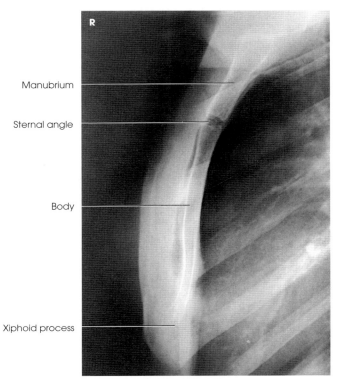

Manubrium

Sternal angle

Body

Xiphoid process

Fig. 10.21 Lateral sternum.

PA PROJECTION

NOTE: This position may be difficult to perform on trauma patients. Use the upright position if the patient is able.

Image receptor + grid: Positioned by manufacturer or department protocol for proper anatomy display orientation; CR plate: 10 × 12 inches (24 × 30 cm) lengthwise.

Position of patient

- Place the patient in the prone (or upright) position.
- Center the MSP of the patient's body to the midline of the grid.
- Adapt the same procedure for use with a patient who is standing or seated upright.

Position of part

- Center the IR at the level of the spinous process of the third thoracic vertebra, which lies posterior to the jugular notch.
- Place the patient's arms along the sides of the body with the palms facing upward.
- Adjust the shoulders to lie in the same transverse plane.
- For a bilateral examination, rest the patient's head on the chin and adjust it so that the MSP is vertical.
- For a unilateral projection, ask the patient to turn the head to face the affected side and rest the cheek on the table (Fig. 10.22). Turning the head rotates the spine slightly away from the side being examined and provides better visualization of the lateral portion of the manubrium.

- *Shield gonads.*
- *Respiration:* Suspend at the end of expiration.

Central ray

- Perpendicular to the center of the IR and entering T3

Collimation

- Adjust radiation field to 6 × 8 inches (15 × 20 cm) on the collimator. Place side marker in the collimated exposure field.

Structures shown

The sternoclavicular joints and the medial portions of the clavicles (Figs. 10.23 and 10.24).

EVALUATION CRITERIA

The following should be clearly seen:
- Evidence of proper collimation and presence of side marker placed clear of anatomy of interest
- Both sternoclavicular joints and the medial ends of the clavicles
- No rotation present on bilateral examination; slight rotation present on unilateral examination
- Bony trabecular detail and surrounding soft tissues

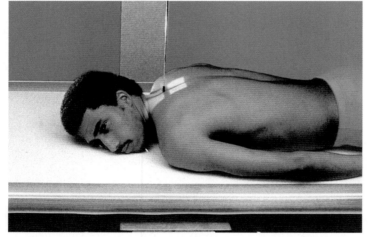

Fig. 10.22 Unilateral examination to show left sternoclavicular articulation.

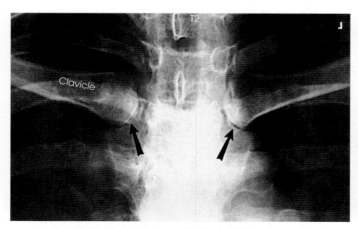

Fig. 10.23 Bilateral sternoclavicular joints *(arrows)*.

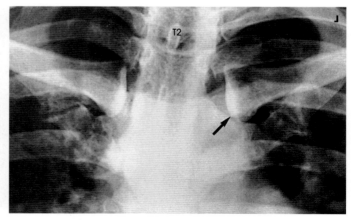

Fig. 10.24 Unilateral sternoclavicular joint *(arrow)*.

PA OBLIQUE PROJECTION
BODY ROTATION METHOD
RAO or LAO position

NOTE: This position may be difficult in trauma patients. Use the upright position if the patient is able.

Image receptor + grid: Positioned by manufacturer or department protocol for proper anatomy display orientation; CR plate: 10 × 12 inches (24 × 30 cm) lengthwise.

Position of patient
- Place the patient in a prone or seated-upright position.

Position of part
- Keeping the affected side adjacent to the IR, position the patient at enough of an oblique angle to project the vertebrae well behind the sternoclavicular joint closest to the IR. The angle is usually about 10 to 15 degrees.
- Adjust the patient's position to center the joint to the midline of the grid.
- Adjust the shoulders to lie in the same transverse plane (Fig. 10.25A and B).
- *Shield gonads.*
- *Respiration:* Suspend at the end of expiration.

Central ray
- Perpendicular to the sternoclavicular joint closest to the IR. The CR enters at the level of T2-3 (about 3 inches [7.6 cm] distal to the vertebral prominens) and 1 to 2 inches (2.5 to 5 cm) lateral from the MSP. If the CR enters the right side, the left sternoclavicular joint is shown, and vice versa (see Fig. 10.25B).
- Center the IR to the CR.

Collimation
- Adjust radiation field to 6 × 8 inches (15 × 20 cm) on the collimator. Place side marker in the collimated exposure field.

Structures shown
A slightly oblique sternoclavicular joint (see Fig. 10.25C).

EVALUATION CRITERIA
The following should be clearly seen:
- Evidence of proper collimation and presence of side marker placed clear of anatomy of interest
- Sternoclavicular joint of interest in the center of the radiograph, with the manubrium and the medial end of the clavicle included
- Open sternoclavicular joint space
- Sternoclavicular joint of interest immediately adjacent to the vertebral column with minimal obliquity
- Bony trabecular detail and surrounding soft tissues

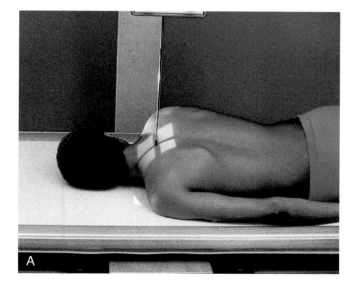

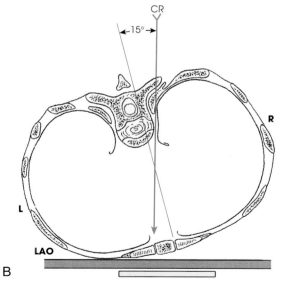

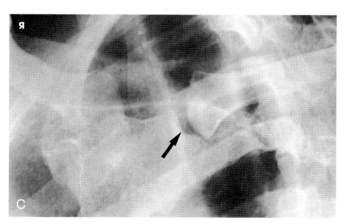

Fig. 10.25 (A) PA oblique sternoclavicular joint, LAO position: Body rotation method. (B) Axial view (from feet upward) of central ray position in relation to spine and sternoclavicular joint. (C) PA oblique sternoclavicular joint, LAO position. The joint closest to the IR is shown *(arrow)*.

PA OBLIQUE PROJECTION
CR ANGULATION METHOD

Image receptor: Positioned by manufacturer or department protocol for proper anatomy display orientation; CR plate:10 × 12 inches (24 × 30 cm) lengthwise.

NOTE: For this projection, the joint is closer to the IR, and less distortion is obtained than when the previously described body rotation method is used. A grid IR placed on the tabletop enables the joint to be projected with minimal distortion. This position may be difficult to perform on trauma patients. Use the upright position if the patient is able.

Position of patient
- Place the patient in the prone position on a grid IR positioned directly under the upper chest.
- Center the grid to the level of the sternoclavicular joints.
- To avoid grid cutoff, place the grid on the radiographic table with its long axis running *perpendicular* to the long axis of the table.

Position of part
- Extend the patient's arms along the sides of the body with the palms of the hands facing upward.
- Adjust the shoulders to lie in the same transverse plane.
- Ask the patient to rest the head on the chin or to rotate the chin toward the side of the joint being radiographed (Fig. 10.26).

Central ray
- From the side opposite the side being examined, direct to the midpoint of the IR at an angle of 15 degrees toward the MSP. A small angle is satisfactory in examinations of sternoclavicular articulations because only slight anteroposterior overlapping of the vertebrae and these joints occurs.
- The CR should enter at the level of T2-3 (about 3 inches [7.6 cm] distal to the vertebral prominens) and 1 to 2 inches (2.5 to 5 cm) lateral to the MSP. If the CR enters the left side, the right side is shown, and vice versa.

Collimation
- Adjust radiation field to 6 × 8 inches (15 × 20 cm) on the collimator. Place side marker in the collimated exposure field.

Structures shown
A slightly oblique sternoclavicular joint (Figs. 10.27 and 10.28).

EVALUATION CRITERIA
The following should be clearly seen:
- Evidence of proper collimation and presence of side marker placed clear of anatomy of interest
- Sternoclavicular joint of interest in the center of the radiograph, with the manubrium and the medial end of the clavicle included
- Open sternoclavicular joint space
- Sternoclavicular joint of interest immediately adjacent to the vertebral column with minimal obliquity
- Bony trabecular detail and surrounding soft tissues

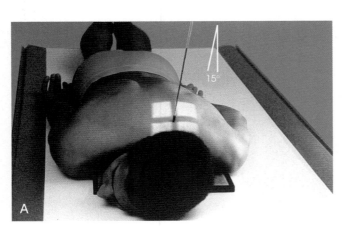

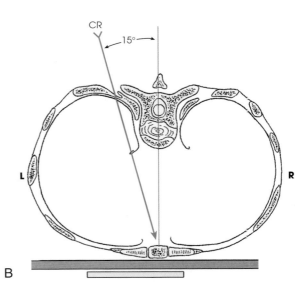

Fig. 10.26 PA oblique sternoclavicular joint: CR angulation method. CR enters left side to show right joint.

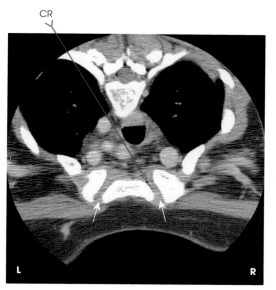

Fig. 10.27 CT axial image with patient prone, showing sternoclavicular joints *(white arrows)* and path of CR. View is from feet looking upward.

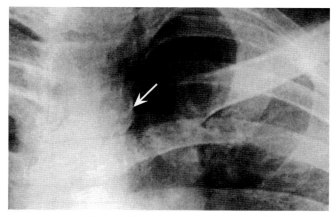

Fig. 10.28 Central ray angulation method for sternoclavicular joint farthest from x-ray tube *(arrow)*.

(From Kurzbauer R: The lateral projection in the roentgenography of the sternoclavicular articulation, *AJR Am J Roentgenol* 56:104, 1946.)

In radiography of the ribs, an IR 14 × 17 inches (35 × 43 cm) should be used to identify the ribs involved and to determine the extent of trauma or the pathologic condition. Projections can be made in recumbent and upright positions.

After the lesion is localized, the next step is to determine (1) the position required to place the affected rib region parallel with the plane of the IR, and (2) whether the radiograph should be made to include the ribs above or below the diaphragm.

The anterior portion of the ribs, usually referred to simply as the *anterior ribs*, is often examined with the patient facing the IR for a PA projection. The posterior portion of the ribs—the *posterior ribs*—is more commonly radiographed with the patient facing the x-ray tube in the same manner as for an AP projection.

The axillary portion of the ribs is best shown using an oblique projection.

Because the lateral projection results in superimposition of the two sides, it is generally used only when fluid or air levels are evaluated after rib fractures.

When the ribs superimposed over the heart are involved, the body must be rotated to obtain a projection of the ribs free of the heart, or the radiographic exposure must be increased to compensate for the density of the heart. Although the anterior and posterior ends are superimposed, the left ribs are cleared of the heart when the LAO position or the right posterior oblique (RPO) position is used. These two body positions place the right-sided ribs parallel with the plane of the IR and are reversed to obtain comparable projections of the left-sided ribs. Lower kVp, compared with that used for chest radiography, should be used to increase beam attenuation in the ribs. The kVp chosen will vary based on expected rib mineralization of the patient.

RESPIRATION

In radiography of the ribs, the patient is usually examined with respiration suspended in either full inspiration or full expiration. Occasionally, shallow breathing may be used to obliterate lung markings. If this technique is used, breathing must be shallow enough to ensure that the ribs are not elevated or depressed, as described in the anatomy portion of this chapter.

Rib fractures can cause a great deal of pain and hemorrhage because of the closely related neurovascular structures. This situation commonly makes it difficult for the patient to breathe deeply for the required radiograph. Deeper inspiration is attained if the patient fully understands the importance of expanding the lungs, and if the exposure is taken after the patient takes the second deep breath.

⚘ PA PROJECTION

Image receptor + grid: Positioned by manufacturer or department protocol for proper anatomy display orientation; CR plate: 14 × 17 inches (35 × 43 cm) lengthwise.

Position of patient

- Position the patient either upright or recumbent, facing the IR.
- Because the diaphragm descends to its lowest level in the upright position, use the standing or seated-upright position for projections of the upper ribs when the patient's condition permits (Fig. 10.29). The upright position is also valuable for showing fluid levels in the chest.

Position of part

- Center the MSP of the patient's body to the midline of the grid.
- Adjust the IR position to project approximately 1½ inches (3.8 cm) above the upper border of the shoulders. Less may be required for hypersthenic patients and for those with very muscular shoulders.
- Rest the patient's hands against the hips with the palms turned outward to rotate the scapulae away from the rib cage.
- Adjust the shoulders to lie in the same transverse plane.

- If the patient is prone, rest the head on the chin and adjust the MSP to be vertical (Fig. 10.30).
- For hypersthenic patients with wide rib cages, it may be necessary to move the patient laterally to include the entire lateral surface of the affected rib area on the radiograph.
- *Shield gonads.*
- *Respiration:* Suspend at full inspiration to depress the diaphragm as much as possible.

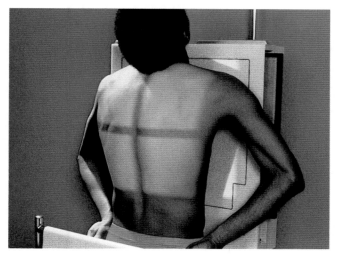

Fig. 10.29 PA ribs, upright position.

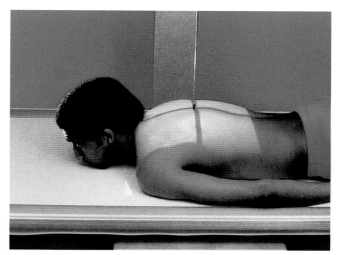

Fig. 10.30 PA ribs, recumbent position.

Central ray

- Perpendicular to the center of IR. If the IR is positioned correctly, the CR is at the level of T7.
- A useful option for showing the seventh, eighth, and ninth ribs is to angle the x-ray tube about 10 to 15 degrees caudad. This angulation aids in projecting the diaphragm below the affected ribs.

Collimation

- Adjust radiation field to 14×17 inches (35×43 cm) on the collimator. Place side marker in the collimated exposure field.

Structures shown

The anterior ribs above the diaphragm (Figs. 10.31 and 10.32). Although the posterior ribs are seen, the anterior ribs are shown with greater detail because they are closer to the IR.

The following should be clearly seen:

- Evidence of proper collimation and presence of side marker placed clear of anatomy of interest
- First through ninth ribs in their entirety, with posterior portions lying above the diaphragm
- First through seventh anterior ribs from both sides, in their entirety and above the diaphragm
- In a unilateral examination, ribs from the opposite side possibly not included in their entirety
- Bony trabecular detail and surrounding soft tissues

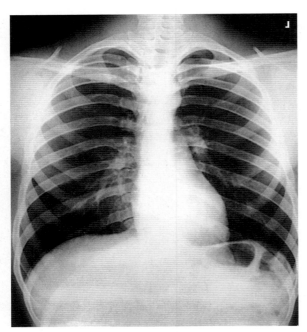

Fig. 10.31 PA ribs, normal centering.

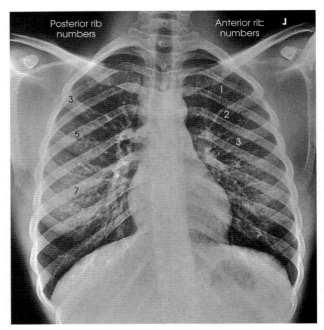

Fig. 10.32 PA ribs, with 10- to 15-degree caudal angulation.

⚛ AP PROJECTION

Image receptor + grid: Positioned by manufacturer or department protocol for proper anatomy display orientation; CR plate: 14 × 17 inches (35 × 43 cm) lengthwise.

Position of patient
- Have the patient face the x-ray tube in either an upright or a recumbent position.
- When the patient's condition permits, use the upright position to image ribs above the diaphragm and the supine position to image ribs below the diaphragm to permit gravity to assist in moving the patient's diaphragm.

Position of part
- Center the MSP of the patient's body to the midline of the grid.

Ribs above diaphragm
- Place the IR lengthwise 1½ inches (3.8 cm) above the upper border of the *relaxed* shoulders.
- Rest the patient's hands, palms outward, against the hips. This position moves the scapula off the ribs. Alternatively, extend the arms to the vertical position with the hands under the head (Fig. 10.33).
- Adjust the patient's shoulders to lie in the same transverse plane, and rotate them forward to draw the scapulae away from the rib cage.
- *Shield gonads.*
- *Respiration:* Suspend at *full inspiration* to *depress* the diaphragm.

Ribs below diaphragm
- Place the IR crosswise in the Bucky tray, centered to a point halfway between the xiphoid process and the lower rib margin. The lower edge of the IR will be near the level of the iliac crests. This positioning ensures inclusion of the lower ribs because of the divergent x-rays.
- Adjust the patient's shoulders to lie in the same transverse plane.
- Place the patient's arms in a comfortable position (Fig. 10.34).
- *Shield gonads.*
- *Respiration:* Suspend at *full expiration* to *elevate* the diaphragm.

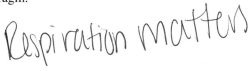

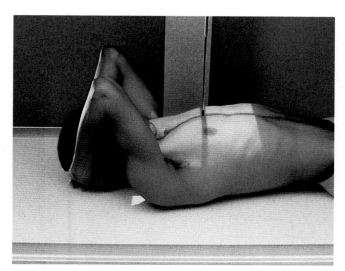

Fig. 10.33 AP ribs above diaphragm.

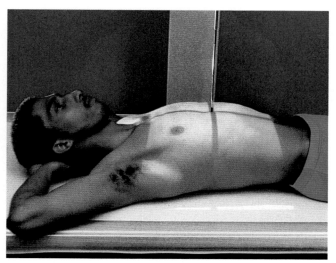

Fig. 10.34 AP ribs below diaphragm.

Bony Thorax

Central ray

- Perpendicular to the center of the IR

NOTE: Refer to the Exposure Technique Chart on p. 513 for the different exposure settings for the upper and lower rib projections.

Collimation

- Adjust radiation field to 14 × 17 inches (35 × 43 cm) on the collimator. Place side marker in the collimated exposure field.

Structures shown

The posterior ribs above or below the diaphragm, according to the region examined (Figs. 10.35 and 10.36). Although the anterior ribs are seen, the posterior ribs are shown in greater detail because they are closer to the IR.

EVALUATION CRITERIA

The following should be clearly seen:
- Evidence of proper collimation and presence of side marker placed clear of anatomy of interest
- For ribs above the diaphragm, first through tenth posterior ribs from both sides in their entirety
- For ribs below the diaphragm, eighth through twelfth posterior ribs on both sides in their entirety
- Ribs visible through the lungs or abdomen, according to the region examined
- In a unilateral examination, ribs from the opposite side possibly not included in their entirety
- Bony trabecular detail and surrounding soft tissues

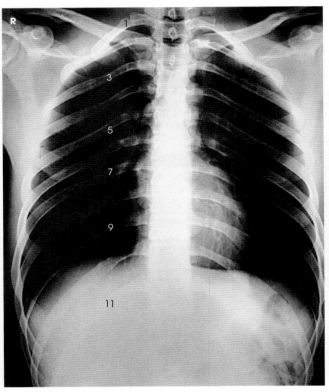

Fig. 10.35 AP ribs above diaphragm.

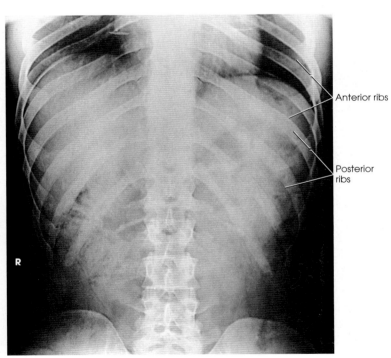

Fig. 10.36 AP lower ribs.

🌲 AP OBLIQUE PROJECTION
RPO or LPO position

Image receptor + grid: Positioned by manufacturer or department protocol for proper anatomy display orientation; CR plate: 14 × 17 inches (35 × 43 cm) lengthwise.

Position of patient
- Examine the patient in the upright or recumbent position.
- Unless contraindicated by the patient's condition, use the upright position to image ribs above the diaphragm, and use the recumbent position to image ribs below the diaphragm. Gravity assists by moving the diaphragm.

Position of part
- Position the patient's body for a 45-degree AP oblique projection using the RPO or LPO position. Place the *affected* side closest to the IR.
- Center the affected side on a longitudinal plane drawn midway between the MSP and the lateral surface of the body.
- Position this plane to the midline of the grid.
- If the patient is in the recumbent position, support the elevated hip.
- Abduct the arm of the affected side, and elevate it to carry the scapula away from the rib cage.

- Rest the patient's hand on the head if the upright position is used (Fig. 10.37), or place the hand under or above the head if the recumbent position is used (Fig. 10.38).
- Abduct the opposite limb with the hand on the hip.
- Center the IR with the top 1½ inches (3.8 cm) above the upper border of the relaxed shoulder to image ribs above the diaphragm or to a point halfway between the xiphoid process and the lower rib margin to image ribs below the diaphragm.
- *Shield gonads.*
- *Respiration:* Suspend at the end of *full inspiration* for ribs *above* the diaphragm and at the end of *deep expiration* for ribs *below* the diaphragm.

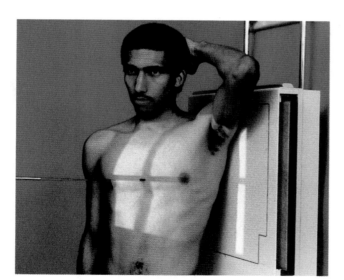

Fig. 10.37 Upright AP oblique ribs, LPO position.

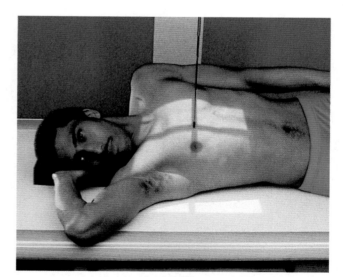

Fig. 10.38 Recumbent AP oblique ribs, RPO position.

Central ray
- Perpendicular to the center of IR
- Closest to IR

Collimation
- Adjust radiation field to 14 × 17 inches (35 × 43 cm) on the collimator. Place side marker in the collimated exposure field.

Structures shown
The axillary portion of the ribs *closest* to the IR is projected free of superimposition with the thoracic spine (Fig. 10.39). The posterior ribs closest to the IR are also well shown.

The following should be clearly seen:
- Evidence of proper collimation and presence of side marker placed clear of anatomy of interest
- Approximately twice as much distance between the vertebral column and the lateral border of the ribs on the affected side as is present on the unaffected side
- Axillary portion of the ribs free of superimposition with the thoracic spine
- First through tenth ribs visible above the diaphragm for upper ribs
- Eighth through twelfth ribs visible below the diaphragm for lower ribs
- Ribs visible through the lungs or abdomen according to the region examined
- Bony trabecular detail and surrounding soft tissues

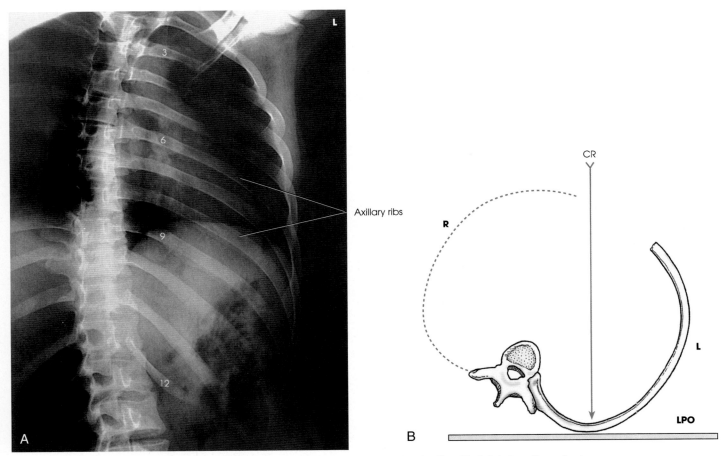

Fig. 10.39 (A) AP oblique ribs. LPO position shows left-side ribs. (B) Axial view (from feet upward) of ribs and CR, LPO position.

⚔ PA OBLIQUE PROJECTION
RAO or LAO position

Image receptor + grid: Positioned by manufacturer or department protocol for proper anatomy display orientation; CR plate: 14 × 17 inches (35 × 43 cm) lengthwise.

Position of patient
- Examine the patient in the upright or recumbent position.
- Unless contraindicated by the patient's condition, use the upright position to image ribs above the diaphragm and use the recumbent position to image ribs below the diaphragm. Gravity assists by moving the diaphragm.

Position of part
- Position the body for a 45-degree PA oblique projection using the RAO or LAO position. Place the affected side away from the IR (Fig. 10.40).
- If the recumbent position is used, have the patient rest on the forearm and flexed knee of the elevated side (Fig. 10.41).
- Align the body so that a longitudinal plane drawn midway between the midline and the lateral surface of the body side up is centered to the midline of the grid.

- Center IR with the top 1½ inches (3.8 cm) above the upper border of the shoulder to image ribs above the diaphragm or to a point halfway between the xiphoid process and the lower rib margin to image ribs below the diaphragm.
- *Shield gonads.*
- *Respiration:* Suspend at the end of *full expiration* for ribs *below* the diaphragm and at the end of *full inspiration* for ribs *above* the diaphragm.

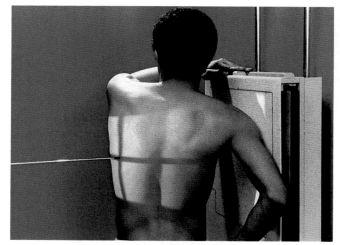

Fig. 10.40 Upright PA oblique ribs, RAO position.

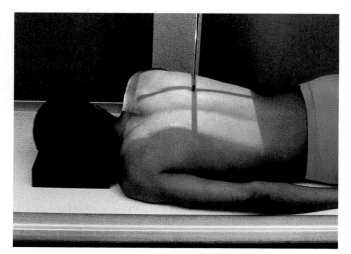

Fig. 10.41 Recumbent PA oblique ribs, LAO position.

Central ray

- Perpendicular to center of IR

Collimation

- Adjust radiation field to 14 × 17 inches (35 × 43 cm) on the collimator. Place side marker in the collimated exposure field.

Structures shown

The axillary portion of the ribs *farthest* from the IR is projected free of bony superimposition with the thoracic spine (Fig. 10.42). The anterior ribs farthest from the IR are also shown.

EVALUATION CRITERIA

The following should be clearly seen:
- Evidence of proper collimation and presence of side marker placed clear of anatomy of interest
- Approximately twice as much distance between the vertebral column and the lateral border of the ribs on the affected side as is present on the unaffected side
- Axillary portion of the ribs free of superimposition with the thoracic spine
- First through tenth ribs visible above the diaphragm for upper ribs
- Eighth through twelfth ribs visible below the diaphragm for lower ribs
- Ribs visible through the lungs or abdomen according to the region examined

Reference

1. Moore TF: An alternative to the standard radiographic position for the sternum, *Radiol Technol* 60:133, 1988.

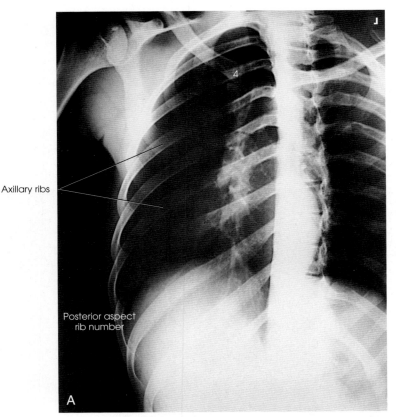

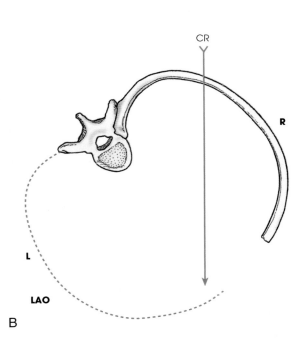

Axillary ribs

Posterior aspect rib number

Fig. 10.42 (A) PA oblique ribs. LAO position shows right-side ribs. PA projection radiograph is placed in the anatomic position for display. (B) Axial view (from feet upward) of ribs and CR with the patient in LAO position.

ADDENDUM A
SUMMARY OF ABBREVIATIONS, VOLUME ONE

AAA	Abdominal aortic aneurysm	IOML	infraorbitomeatal line	OR	operating room
AC	acromioclavicular	IP[b]	image plate	PA	posteroanterior
AEC	automatic exposure control	IP[b]	interphalangeal (hand and foot)	PIP	proximal interphalangeal (hand and foot)
AP	anteroposterior	IR	image receptor		
ARRT	American Registry of Radiologic Technologists	kVp	kilovolt peak	PTC	Percutaneous transhepatic cholangiography
		L	left		
ASIS	anterior superior iliac spine	LAO	left anterior oblique	R	right
ASRT	American Society of Radiologic Technologists	LLQ	left lower quadrant	RA	radiologist assistant
		LPO	left posterior oblique	RAO	right anterior oblique
CAMRT	Canadian Association of Medical Radiation Technologists	LUQ	left upper quadrant	RLQ	right lower quadrant
		mA	milliamperage	RPA	radiology practitioner assistant
CDC	Centers for Disease Control and Prevention	mAs	milliampere second	RPO	right posterior oblique
		MC	metacarpal	RUQ	right upper quadrant
cm	centimeter	MCP	metacarpophalangeal	SC	sternoclavicular
CMC	carpometacarpal	MMD	mean marrow dose	SI	sacroiliac
CR[a]	central ray	MRI	magnetic resonance imaging	SID	source–to–image receptor (IR) distance
CR[a]	computed radiography	MSP	Midsagittal plane		
CT	computed tomography	MTP	metatarsophalangeal	SMV	submentovertical
DIP	distal interphalangeal (hand and foot)	NCRP	National Council on Radiation Protection	SSD	source–to–skin distance
				TEA	top ear attachment
DR	direct digital radiography	NPO	Nil per os (nothing by mouth)	TMT	tarsometatarsal
EAM	external acoustic meatus	OD	optical density	US	ultrasound
ERCP	Endoscopic retrograde cholangiopancreatography	OID	object-to-image receptor (IR) distance	VSM	verticosubmental
HNP	herniated nucleus pulposus	OML	orbitomeatal line		

[a]Note: CR has two different meanings.
[b]Note: IP has two different meanings.

535

INDEX

Page numbers followed by "*f*" indicate figures, "*t*" indicate
tables, and "*b*" indicate boxes. Boldface numbers indicate
the volume.

Index

Index

Index

Greater sciatic notch, anatomy of, **1:**379*f*, **1:**380, **1:**382*f*
Greater trochanter
    anatomy of, **1:**278*f*, **1:**380*f*, **1:**381, **1:**382*f*, **1:**385*f*
    with obese patients, **1:**45
    sectional anatomy of, **3:**199–200, **3:**199*f*
Greater tubercle
    anatomy of, **1:**148*f*, **1:**149
    defined, **1:**62*f*
Greater wing of sphenoid
    anatomy of, **2:**4*f*, **2:**10*f*–11*f*, **2:**11
    sectional anatomy of, **3:**162–163, **3:**164*f*, **3:**166*f*
Greenstick fracture, **1:**70*f*, **3:**100
Grenz rays, **3:**458
Grids, **1:**17–18, **1:**17*f*
    for mammography, **2:**359
    in mobile radiography, **3:**3–4, **3:**4*f*
    for obese patients, **1:**48, **1:**48*f*
    in trauma radiography, **2:**113
Groove, **1:**70
Ground state, **3:**391, **3:**429
Growth plate fractures, **3:**101
Gruntzig, Andreas, **3:**274
Guidewires, for angiography, **3:**288, **3:**288*f*, **3:**354
"Gull wing" sign, **1:**392
Gynecography, **2:**344, **2:**348, **2:**348*f*
Gynecologic applications, of ultrasonography, **3:**374–376
    anatomic features and, **3:**374, **3:**374*f*
    endovaginal transducers for, **3:**363*f*, **3:**376, **3:**376*f*,
        3:385
    indications for, **3:**375–376
    of ovaries, **3:**361*f*, **3:**363*f*, **3:**376, **3:**377*f*
    transabdominal, **3:**375, **3:**375*f*
    of uterus, **3:**375*f*–377*f*, **3:**376
Gynecomastia, **2:**414
Gyri, **3:**160–161

H

Haas method, for PA axial projection of skull, **2:**50–51,
    2:50*f*
    central ray, **2:**50
    collimation of, **2:**51
    position of part, **2:**50, **2:**50*f*
    position of patient in, **2:**50
    structures shown in, **2:**51, **2:**51*b*, **2:**51*f*
Half-life (T1/2), **3:**391, **3:**429
Half-value layer, **3:**458
Hamartoma, **2:**374*f*, **2:**382*t*–383*t*
Hamate, **1:**145*f*, **1:**146
Hamulus, **1:**70
Hand
    anatomy of, **1:**145–146, **1:**145*f*–146*f*
    articulations of, **1:**149–151, **1:**149*f*–151*f*, **1:**149*t*
    digits of. *See* Digit(s)
    fan lateral projection of, **1:**172–173
        evaluation criteria for, **1:**173*b*
        position of part for, **1:**172, **1:**172*f*
        position of patient for, **1:**172, **1:**172*f*
        structures shown on, **1:**173, **1:**173*f*
    lateromedial projection in flexion of, **1:**174, **1:**174*b*,
        1:174*f*
    mediolateral or lateromedial projection in extension of,
        1:172–173
        evaluation criteria for, **1:**173*b*
        position of part for, **1:**172, **1:**172*f*
        position of patient for, **1:**172, **1:**172*f*
        structures shown on, **1:**173, **1:**173*f*
    Norgaard method, for AP oblique projection, in medial
        rotation of, **1:**174–175
        evaluation criteria for, **1:**175*b*
        position of part of, **1:**174–175, **1:**175*f*
        position of patient for, **1:**174
        structures shown on, **1:**175, **1:**175*f*
    PA oblique projection in, lateral rotation of, **1:**170–171
        evaluation criteria for, **1:**171*b*
        position of part for, **1:**170
            to show joint spaces, **1:**170, **1:**170*f*
            to show metacarpals, **1:**170, **1:**170*f*
        position of patient for, **1:**170
        structures shown on, **1:**171, **1:**171*f*
    PA projection of, **1:**168
        evaluation criteria for, **1:**168*b*
        position of part for, **1:**168, **1:**168*f*
        position of patient for, **1:**168
        special techniques for, **1:**168
        structures shown on, **1:**168, **1:**169*f*
    position, effects on proximal humerus, **1:**228*t*

Hand *(Continued)*
    reverse oblique projection of, **1:**171
    tangential oblique projection of, **1:**171
Handwashing, **1:**5
Hangman's fracture, **1:**434*t*
Hard palate, anatomy of, **2:**180, **2:**180*f*, **2:**182, **2:**183*f*
Harris-Beath method for axial projection of calcaneus,
    1:319, **1:**319*f*
Haustra, **2:**190, **2:**190*f*
Haustral folds, **3:**198
Head. *See also* Skull
    of bone, **1:**70
    CT of, **2:**149
    three-dimensional CT of, **3:**154*f*
    trauma, CT of, **2:**122, **2:**122*f*
Head circumference, fetal ultrasound for, **3:**378, **3:**378*f*
Health Insurance Portability and Accountability Act of
    1996 (HIPAA), **2:**500
Hearing impairment, in older adults, **3:**139
Heart, **3:**278
    AP oblique projection of, **1:**118
    CT angiography for, **3:**228–230, **3:**229*f*–230*f*
        gated, **3:**230*f*
    echocardiography of, **3:**381–384
        for congenital heart lesions, **3:**384
        indications for, **3:**381
        pathology in, **3:**381–384, **3:**384*f*
        procedure for, **3:**381, **3:**383*f*
    lateral projection with barium of, **1:**114
    PA chest radiographs with barium of, **1:**110
    PA oblique projection with barium of, **1:**117
    in radiography of sternum, **1:**514
    sectional anatomy of, **3:**174, **3:**179–181, **3:**182
Heart shadows, **1:**112*f*
Heat trauma, **2:**112
Heel, bone densitometry of, **2:**499*f*
Helical CT, **3:**243
    multislice, **3:**210, **3:**227–228, **3:**227*f*–228*f*
    single-slice, **3:**210
Helix, **2:**16*f*, **2:**17
Hematologic system disorders, in older adults, **3:**143
Hematoma, **2:**382*t*–383*t*, **3:**354
    during catheterization, **3:**292
Hematopoietic tissue, cancer arising from, **3:**435*t*
Hemodynamics, **3:**354
Hemostasis, **3:**354
Hepatic arteriogram, **3:**298, **3:**298*f*
Hepatic artery
    anatomy of, **2:**192
    ultrasonography of, **3:**365*f*
Hepatic ducts, anatomy of, **2:**193
Hepatic flexure
    anatomy of, **2:**190*f*, **2:**191
    sectional anatomy of, on coronal plane, **3:**194*f*, **3:**202,
        3:202*f*
Hepatic veins
    anatomy of, **2:**192, **2:**193*f*
    sectional anatomy of, **3:**189, **3:**189*f*
Hepatic venography, **3:**316, **3:**316*f*
Hepatitis B virus (HBV), cancer and, **3:**434
Hepatitis C virus, cancer and, **3:**434
Hepatopancreatic ampulla
    anatomy of, **2:**188, **2:**189*f*, **2:**193, **2:**193*f*
    sphincter of, **2:**193, **2:**193*f*
Hereditary nonpolyposis colorectal cancer syndrome,
    3:435
Hernia, hiatal
    AP projection of, **2:**232, **2:**233*f*
    PA oblique projection of (Wolf method), **2:**234–235,
        2:234*f*–235*f*, **2:**235*b*
    upright lateral projection of, **2:**233*f*
Herniated nucleus pulposus (HNP), **1:**422, **1:**434*t*, **3:**262*t*
Heterogeneous structure/mass, in ultrasonography, **3:**362,
    3:362*f*, **3:**385
Hiatal hernia, **2:**198*t*–199*t*
    AP projection of, **2:**232, **2:**233*f*
    PA oblique projection of (Wolf method), **2:**234–235,
        2:234*f*–235*f*, **2:**235*b*
    upright lateral projection of, **2:**233*f*
Hickey method, for mediolateral projection of hip, **1:**400,
    1:400*b*, **1:**400*f*–401*f*
Hickman catheter placement, **3:**44*f*
High-dose-rate (HDR) brachytherapy, **3:**437, **3:**458
Highlighting, in CT, **3:**208*f*
High-osmolality contrast agents (HOCAs), in children,
    3:86

High-resolution scans, in CT, **3:**223–224, **3:**225*f*, **3:**243
Hill-Sachs defect, **1:**226*t*
Hilum, **1:**89–90, **1:**89*f*, **1:**96*f*
Hindbrain, **2:**164, **2:**175
Hindfoot, **1:**274
Hinge (ginglymus) joint, **1:**68, **1:**69*f*
Hip(s), **1:**377–415
    abbreviations in, **1:**386*b*
    alternative positioning landmark for, **1:**386–387
    anatomy of, **1:**379–387, **1:**386*b*
        summary of, **1:**386*b*
    AP projection of, **1:**398–399, **1:**398*f*
        evaluation criteria for, **1:**399*b*
        structures shown in, **1:**399, **1:**399*f*
    axiolateral projection of, Danelius-Miller method for,
        1:402–403, **1:**402*f*–403*f*, **1:**403*b*
        Clements-Nakamaya modification of, **1:**404–405,
            1:404*f*–405*f*, **1:**405*b*
        compensating filter for, **1:**403
        for trauma, **2:**136, **2:**136*f*
    in children, **3:**95–96
        developmental dysplasia of, **2:**155*t*, **3:**112, **3:**112*f*
        general principles of, **3:**95–96, **3:**95*f*
        image evaluation for, **3:**93*t*
        initial images in, **3:**95
        positioning and immobilization for, **3:**96, **3:**96*f*
        preparation and communication for, **3:**96
    congenital dislocation of
        Andren-von Rosén approach for, **1:**397
        AP projection of, **1:**391, **1:**391*f*
        contrast arthrography of, **2:**154*f*
    developmental dysplasia of, **2:**155*t*
    fluoroscopic procedures for, **3:**48–50, **3:**48*f*–50*f*, **3:**50*b*
    in geriatric patients, **3:**149, **3:**149*f*
    lateral projection of, **1:**392–393, **1:**392*f*–393*f*
        evaluation criteria for, **1:**393*b*
    localizing anatomic structures in, **1:**385–387, **1:**385*f*
    mediolateral projection of, Lauenstein and Hickey
        methods for, **1:**400, **1:**400*b*, **1:**400*f*–401*f*
    modified axiolateral projection (Clements-Nakayama
        modification) of, for trauma, **2:**137, **2:**137*f*
    MRI of, **3:**266*f*
    radiation protection for, **1:**388, **1:**388*f*
    radiography of, **1:**388–413
    sample exposure technique chart essential projections
        for, **1:**387*t*
    summary of projections for, **1:**378
    trauma radiography of
        axiolateral projection (Danelius-Miller method) in,
            2:136, **2:**136*f*
        modified axiolateral projection (Clements-Nakayama
            modification) in, **2:**137, **2:**137*f*
Hip arthrography, **2:**160
    AP, **2:**160*f*–161*f*
    axiolateral "frog," **2:**160*f*
    with congenital dislocation, **2:**154*f*
    digital subtraction technique for, **2:**160, **2:**161*f*
Hip bone, anatomy of, **1:**379–380, **1:**379*f*
Hip fractures, in osteoporosis, **2:**473
Hip joint, **1:**383*f*
    replacement, mobile radiography procedures for, in
        operating room, **3:**64*f*
    sectional anatomy of, **3:**203*f*
Hip pads, **2:**473
Hip pinning, **3:**48–50, **3:**48*f*–50*f*, **3:**50*b*
Hip prosthesis, contrast arthrography of, **2:**160, **2:**161*f*
    digital subtraction technique for, **2:**160, **2:**161*f*
Hip screws, cannulated, **3:**48–50, **3:**48*f*–50*f*, **3:**50*b*
HIPAA. *See* Health Insurance Portability and
    Accountability Act of 1996
Hirschsprung disease, **2:**198*t*–199*t*
Histogram, in CT, **3:**208*f*
Histoplasmosis, **1:**97*t*
History, for trauma patient, **2:**119
Holly method, for tangential projection, of sesamoids,
    1:296, **1:**297*f*
Holmblad method, for PA axial projection, of
    intercondylar fossa, **1:**352–353, **1:**352*f*
    evaluation criteria for, **1:**353*b*
    position of part for, **1:**353, **1:**353*f*
    position of patient for, **1:**352, **1:**352*f*
    structures shown on, **1:**353, **1:**353*f*
Homeostasis, **3:**390, **3:**429
Homogeneous structure/mass, in ultrasonography, **3:**362,
    3:362*f*, **3:**385
Hook of hamate, **1:**146, **1:**146*f*

Index

Index

Weight-bearing method, for PA projection, of lumbar intervertebral joints, **1:**489–490, **1:**489*f*, **1:**490*b*

West Point method, for inferosuperior axial projection, of shoulder girdle, **1:**240*f*–241*f*, **1:**241, **1:**241*b*

White matter
anatomy of, **2:**164
sectional anatomy of, **3:**160–161

Whole-body imaging, in nuclear imaging, **3:**402, **3:**402*f*

Wilms tumor, **2:**288*t*

Window level, **3:**216, **3:**216*t*, **3:**244

Window width, in CT, **3:**216, **3:**216*t*, **3:**244

Wolf method, for PA oblique projection, of superior stomach and distal esophagus, **2:**234–235, **2:**234*f*–235*f*, **2:**235*b*

Wrist, **1:**176–189
anatomy of, **1:**146, **1:**146*f*
AP oblique projection in, medial rotation of, **1:**181, **1:**181*b*, **1:**181*f*
AP projection of, **1:**177, **1:**177*b*, **1:**177*f*
articulations of, **1:**149–151, **1:**150*f*
lateromedial projection of, **1:**178–179
with carpal boss, **1:**179, **1:**179*f*
central ray for, **1:**178
collimation for, **1:**178
evaluation criteria for, **1:**179*b*
position of part for, **1:**178, **1:**178*f*
position of patient for, **1:**178
structures shown on, **1:**178–179, **1:**178*f*–179*f*
PA oblique projection in, lateral rotation of, **1:**180, **1:**180*b*, **1:**180*f*
PA projection of, **1:**176, **1:**176*b*, **1:**176*f*
with radial deviation, **1:**183, **1:**183*b*, **1:**183*f*
with ulnar deviation, **1:**182, **1:**182*b*, **1:**182*f*
scaphoid of, **1:**184–185

Wrist *(Continued)*
anatomy of, **1:**145*f*, **1:**146
Rafert-Long method for scaphoid series (PA and PA axial projections with ulnar deviation), **1:**186, **1:**186*b*, **1:**186*f*–187*f*
Stecher method for, PA axial projection of, **1:**184–185, **1:**184*b*, **1:**184*f*–185*f*
surgical radiography of, **3:**67*f*–68*f*
tangential projection of
carpal bridge, **1:**189, **1:**189*b*, **1:**189*f*
Gaynor-Hart method for, **1:**190
evaluation criteria for, **1:**191*b*
inferosuperior, **1:**190, **1:**190*f*–191*f*
superoinferior, **1:**191, **1:**191*f*

Wrist arthrogram, **2:**162, **2:**162*f*

X

Xenon-133 (^{133}Xe), in nuclear medicine, **3:**394*t*
Xenon-133 (^{133}Xe) lung ventilation scan, **3:**409
Xerography, **2:**358, **2:**358*f*
Xeromammogram, **2:**358, **2:**358*f*
Xiphisternal joints, **1:**508
Xiphoid process
anatomy of, **1:**505*f*, **1:**506
as surface landmark, **1:**57*f*
X-ray modified barium swallow, **2:**205

Y

Yellow marrow, **1:**62
Yolk sac, ultrasonography of, **3:**376, **3:**377*f*–378*f*

Z

Zenker diverticulum, **2:**198*t*–199*t*
Z-score, in DXA, **2:**481, **2:**502

Zygapophyseal joints, **1:**422, **1:**432
cervical
anatomy of, **1:**425, **1:**425*f*
positioning rotations needed to show, **1:**425*t*
lumbar
anatomy of, **1:**428, **1:**428*f*–429*f*, **1:**429*t*
AP oblique projection of, **1:**475–476, **1:**475*f*–476*f*, **1:**476*b*
PA oblique projection of, **1:**477, **1:**477*f*–478*f*, **1:**478*b*
positioning rotations needed to show, **1:**425*t*, **1:**428*f*
sectional anatomy of, **3:**173*f*, **3:**182–183, **3:**183*f*
thoracic
anatomy of, **1:**426–427, **1:**427*f*
AP or PA oblique projection of, **1:**464–466, **1:**464*f*–466*f*, **1:**466*b*
positioning rotations needed to show, **1:**425*t*

Zygomatic arch, **2:**19
anatomy of, **2:**18*f*, **2:**19, **2:**21, **2:**21*f*, **2:**56*f*
AP axial projection of (modified Towne method), **2:**79, **2:**79*b*, **2:**79*f*–80*f*
modified parietoacanthial projection of, **2:**68*f*
parietoacanthial projection of, **2:**66*f*
sectional anatomy of, **3:**167*f*
submentovertical projection of, **2:**75–76, **2:**75*f*–76*f*, **2:**76*b*
tangential projection of, **2:**77–78, **2:**77*f*–78*f*, **2:**78*b*

Zygomatic bones
acanthioparietal projection of, **2:**70*f*
sectional anatomy of, **3:**157, **3:**166

Zygomatic process
anatomy of, **2:**14, **2:**14*f*
sectional anatomy of, **3:**156–157

Zygote, **2:**339

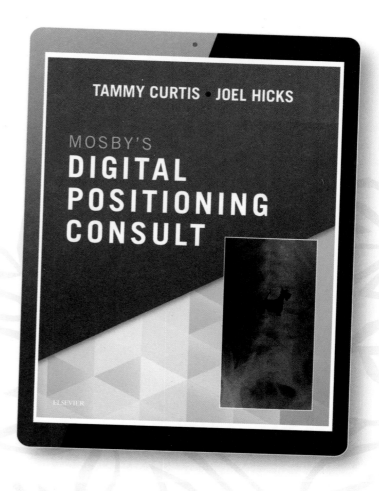
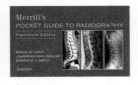
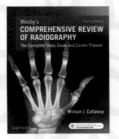
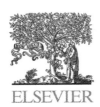

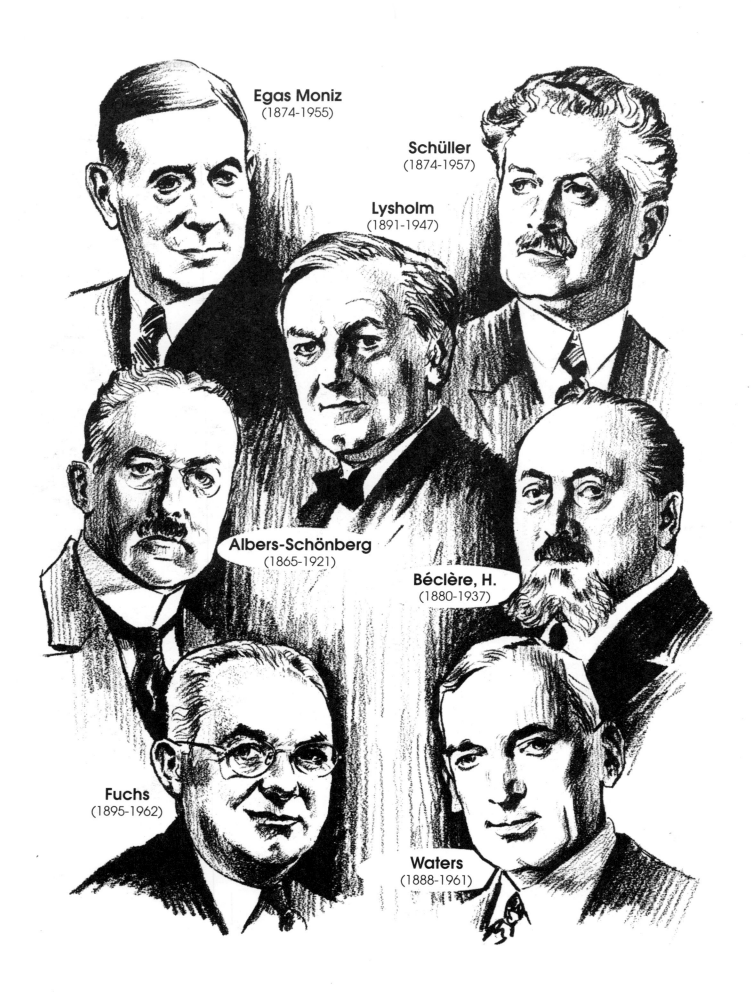

Egas Moniz
(1874-1955)

Schüller
(1874-1957)

Lysholm
(1891-1947)

Albers-Schönberg
(1865-1921)

Béclère, H.
(1880-1937)

Fuchs
(1895-1962)

Waters
(1888-1961)